TEACHING COMPREHENSIVE MEDICAL CARE

THE AUTHORS

This study was jointly conducted by members of the staffs of the Behavior Research Laboratory and the School of Medicine of the University of Colorado. Dr. Hammond was Research Director and Drs. Crow, Groesbeck, and Gyr were Research Associates of the Behavior Research Laboratory. Dr. Kern was Director and Dr. Githens Associate Director of the General Medical Clinic; Lyle Saunders, a sociologist, was Associate Professor in the School of Medicine.

Teaching Comprehensive Medical Care

A PSYCHOLOGICAL STUDY OF A CHANGE IN MEDICAL EDUCATION

Kenneth R. Hammond and Fred Kern, Jr., M.D.

WAYMAN J. CROW

JOHN H. GITHENS, M.D.

BYRON GROESBECK

JOHN W. GYR

LYLE H. SAUNDERS

PUBLISHED FOR THE COMMONWEALTH FUND
BY HARVARD UNIVERSITY PRESS
CAMBRIDGE, MASSACHUSETTS, 1959

Published for
The Commonwealth Fund
By Harvard University Press
Cambridge, Massachusetts

For approximately a quarter of a century THE COMMONWEALTH FUND, through its Division of Publications, sponsored, edited, produced, and distributed books and pamphlets germane to its purposes and operations as a philanthropic foundation. On July 1, 1951, the Fund entered into an arrangement by which HARVARD UNIVERSITY PRESS became the publisher of Commonwealth Fund books, assuming responsibility for their production and distribution. The Fund continues to sponsor and edit its books, and cooperates with the Press in all phases of manufacture and distribution.

Distributed in Great Britain
By Oxford University Press, London

LIBRARY OF CONGRESS CATALOG CARD NO. 59-11518

MANUFACTURED IN THE UNITED STATES OF AMERICA

To

Ward Darley, M.D.

Foreword

If medicine is to reach its full potential as a function of society, there must be a proper balance between the discovery of knowledge, the application of knowledge, and the education necessary to foster both.

Since World War II the amount of research in the physical and biological sciences basic to medicine has been increasing prodigiously; but the contribution of this to the ultimate effectiveness of medicine will depend upon the degree to which the resultant knowledge can be put to use through the more adequate education of medical personnel and the discovery of improved ways of rendering medical service. And if we are to achieve a satisfactory balance, it is essential that medical education and medical service be subjected to the same study and experimentation that has been accorded the scientific aspects of medicine. In other words, the time has come when we must realize that if medicine is to be of maximum effectiveness, we must accept research in medical care and medical education as being just as basic to medicine as are such things as the investigation of electrolyte and fluid balance or the elucidation of the mechanisms of heredity.

The General Medical Clinic of the University of Colorado has been an experiment in both medical care and medical education.

The incentive for the project was a feeling on the part of the medical school administration and faculty that medicine and, a priori, medical education, while they should not neglect the diagnosis and treatment of illness, should show more concern for the individual in whom illness occurs. The objectives of the project were to create an environment that would not only foster thorough and deliberate teaching and learning, but also involve students, faculty, and patients in a clinic committed to the continuing, comprehensive care of the individual and the cultivation of a patient-student-teacher relationship in which environmental, psychological, and cultural, as well as pathological, factors would play a very deliberate role in the formation of medical judgments. It was decided to see if a clinic that would satisfy these objectives could be successfully designed and established and, if it could, to determine whether experience in such a clinic was of educational benefit to students.

Attempts to realize this combination of objectives encountered many complications.

As an experiment in medical care, the new clinic injected a philosophy foreign to long-standing trends and practices into two situations: first, a medical school organized around departments and divisions which reflected the advanced stage of present day specialism and the corresponding fragmentation of teaching and of service to patients; and second, a clinic located in a city hospital, staffed but not controlled by the medical school, in which the organization of clinics and services reflected this same fragmentation. Besides this, the hospital's large patient load and small budget necessitated a service program sharply limited to emergency and episodic care.

As an experiment in medical education, the new clinic had to deal with a multitude of complexities, none of which easily lent themselves to controlled study. The criteria to be measured had to be defined; many of the tools and methods to be used in criteria measurement had to be devised and evaluated; and it was necessary to insure the comparable application of these criteria and study methods to both the control and experimental groups. In addition to all this, there was the problem of rotating into and out of the clinic hundreds of individuals, each playing his part, some more, some less, in contributing to program harmony and study continuity. Because the individuals concerned—students, residents, teachers, researchers, administrators, and patients—came from so many groups and represented such a variety of motivations, objectives, and fears, such different intellectual, social, and personality resources, this was not the easiest of situations. The willingness of those in authority to launch this project against a stream of contrary philosophy and practice, and of the students, teachers, and researchers to participate, deserves high praise. It should be gratifying to all that after five years the clinic has seemed to justify continued operation.

Now if I may swing to the use of the first person, singular, I am personally proud that this venture developed and progressed to fruition while I was associated with the University of Colorado, first as dean of the school of medicine and later as president. While I am no longer with the university, I know I speak the truth when I express the university's appreciation to the many agencies and individuals that made the project possible: the Commonwealth Fund;

the City of Denver; the school of medicine; the department of psychology; those who were close to the administration of the service, research, and teaching aspects of the clinic; and last but not least the hundreds of students in both the control and experimental groups, whose patience, interest, and active cooperation were so essential.

I believe that the most important medical development during the years immediately ahead can be in the field of preventive medicine; but if this is to happen, continuing, comprehensive care must be effectively practiced. And if, in its turn, this is to happen, all physicians, irrespective of their specialties, should have first-hand appreciation of the importance of this concept as a result of their educational experience in medical school.

I believe also that the medical school should take the lead in developing advanced programs so that the family physicians of tomorrow can be well prepared to take the major responsibility for translating the implications of the concept of continuing, comprehensive care into service. This kind of medicine can easily qualify for specialty status, and complete preparation for its practice will require a carefully integrated experience beyond the M.D. degree that is as long and as arduous as that for any of the other specialties. If physicians are to become interested and competent in this kind of service, students at both medical school and advanced levels must be placed in a setting that will provide the necessary education. And if this setting is to subscribe to continuing, comprehensive care, it must also provide for continuing, comprehensive education. Neither patient care nor physician education should be subjected to layering or segmentation.

For these reasons I think teaching units such as the General Medical Clinic represent a giant step forward. But as I read this report, it seemed to me that, aside from the many frustrating and time-consuming operational difficulties, certain very significant obstacles stood in the way of a thoroughly satisfactory experience. As I analyze the implications of these obstacles, it seems to me that they point to many of the flaws, other than those reflected in the primary objectives of the clinic itself, that presently exist throughout the fabric of medical education and also to the direction in which the correction of these flaws might move.

Before I go into this, it is important to remember that the students in the General Medical Clinic were given an opportunity to conduct an unhurried study of their patients and of all the exogenous and endogenous factors that might be involved in the promotion of their health as well as in the cause and aggravation of their illness. The degree of student responsibility was very considerable, and the opportunities for study and supervision which this kind of responsibility requires were provided. Unfortunately, it was not possible to select patients of both sexes representing a wide range of ages and clinical conditions, but an effort was made to hold the clinical load for each student to a reasonable size. Since extreme indigency was a requirement for admission to the hospital and its clinics, the students had no opportunity to study individuals other than those whose socio-economic situations were well-nigh hopeless.

By contrast, students in the control group were working in the classical medical school set-up. These students were regularly and frequently moved from clinic to clinic, and the time they spent with each patient was correspondingly short. Clinical assignments were upon a rotation, next-student-up basis, irrespective of the patient's age, sex, or clinical entity. The students' clinical load was light or heavy, depending upon the number of patients presenting themselves for care. While far from ideal, the socio-economic situation of these patients was somewhat better than in the General Medical Clinic. Of course, student responsibility was considerable, but rarely if ever did this go far enough to permit the significant student-patient relationship that was possible in the General Medical Clinic.

What are the flaws in medical education suggested by the experience of the General Medical Clinic? And also what are the remedies implied? I will discuss these two questions in each of four sections.

In the first place, I believe that the General Medical Clinic experience reflects the unfortunate custom of using only persons in poor socio-economic circumstances for teaching purposes. This was particularly true as regards realization of the satisfactions inherent in the concept of continuing, comprehensive care. I say this because the unfavorable living conditions and the lack of financial resources, both usually associated with educational and social inadequacy, so interfered with the management of patients and with their cooperation that the students' interest and effort were too frequently nullified. This is not good education. Socio-economic factors, those both of want and of plenty, have an important selective influence upon the etiology, course, and prognosis of illness and also upon the evaluation and management of health. And as a consequence, there is every reason for placing all students of medicine in a responsible relationship with individuals, both sick and well, from all walks of life.

In the second place, the contrasting experiences of the control and experimental groups of students suggested the important part that "free" or "unstructured" study can play in education for the practice of medicine. In the control clinic the range and depth of study were considerably limited by the size of the patient load in relation to the amount of student time available. Such was not the case in the General

Medical Clinic. Early in their clinic service the students seemed to enjoy and profit from this "freedom," but as they approached the end of the clinic experience (the end of their senior year) they became apprehensive, first because they knew their classmates in the control clinic were seeing many more cases of illness than they and hence might be learning more facts, and second because they feared that as a result their capacity to pass state and national board examinations and to compete for internships and residencies might be impaired. And yet in spite of this, the tests administered in connection with the experiment revealed that in the accumulation and regurgitation of factual information General Medical Clinic students compared favorably with the others. So, from the standpoint of the assimilation of factual information, the students in the General Medical Clinic lost nothing.

This suggests that we would be justified in freeing medical education from the rigid and over-stuffed curriculum that is presently emphasizing what to learn instead of how to learn, and thus constricting and distorting the potential of its product. To continue in this vein means that facts learned today may no longer apply tomorrow, and progress is accordingly hindered. The rapidity with which medical knowledge is cutting more and more deeply across more and more scientific disciplines, and also the rapidity with which change is taking place in the milieu in which medical service must be rendered, are reaching the point where the inflexibility of our old concepts of education must be replaced with something better. This "something better" might well come out of carefully studied ventures specifically aimed at finding more satisfactory ways and means of freeing students' time and energy so that both teaching and learning can be geared to the differing intellectual and personality strengths and weaknesses which individual students must carry through their medical careers. We should do more to create conditions where responsibility for self and patients will stimulate habits of learning and reasoning and the capacity for judgment that will encourage effective life-long medical scholarship. As our medical schools may develop such projects (and some of them are), perhaps some of the criteria and methods of criteria measurement reported in this volume will help with their evaluation.

The third flaw, together with its remedy, to which the General Medical Clinic experience seems to point concerns the place that the patient-physician relationship and the art of medicine should and can occupy in the practice of medicine in general and in the practice of continuing, comprehensive care in particular. Careful evaluation revealed that the General Medical Clinic fostered favorable attitudes toward comprehensive care: the interest the General Medical Clinic students had developed in this kind of care before they came to the clinic was not lost. Such was not the case with the control students, for most of them not only lost interest in the concept of comprehensive care but developed hostility toward it.

In my opinion, the problem this points to is both involved and serious. I strongly feel that it is time a determined effort was made to give real substance to the patient-physician relationship and the art of medicine. Unless this is done, I do not see how we can bring the concept of continuing, comprehensive care to fruition. The solution to this problem is a function of the time per patient and how this time is used. Our present preoccupation with the growing body of physical and biological medical knowledge and with ways and means of increasing efficiency in the translation of such knowledge into medical service is cutting in on this time. But there must be a limit beyond which increased efficiency, at the expense of time per patient, will impair effectiveness. A certain amount of time per patient is essential, if for no other reason than to permit the physician to apply his scientific and technical knowledge properly. This certain amount of time does not necessarily mean an adequate amount of time. I say this because in spite of our scientific and administrative progress, the actual therapeutic value of the interpersonal relationship between the physician and his patient should stand as an indispensable tool in effective medical care. The effective use of this tool does not readily lend itself to time limitation. But even if there were no factors limiting the time per patient, I think we would still be up against the question of the lack of substance in the patient-physician relationship and the art of medicine. I say this because we do not have commonly accepted working definitions of these two terms and because we do not have a body of knowledge sufficient or sufficiently collated and recorded to make working definitions meaningful. I believe this report makes it abundantly clear that the faculty responsible for the General Medical Clinic, and also the students, were repeatedly frustrated by this lack of definition and knowledge.

While scientific facts and technical procedures play an important role in medicine's effectiveness, it still takes a human being to apply the fact and use the procedure to solve another human being's problem. No two human beings are alike or respond alike to the same situation. Scientific information and technical procedures represent the only fixed quantities in an equation in which both the human patient and the human physician are variable considerations. In the last analysis, the ultimate situation in medical care is one in which two human beings are working together on the basis of a close interpersonal relationship —the physician-patient relationship. And it seems to me that the deliberate development, control, and constructive use of this relationship, in proper combination with the application of scientific and technical knowledge and procedures, might be called the art of medicine.

Chapter 12 of this book presents a thoughtful discussion of the difference between humanitarianism and knowledge about human behavior. The authors conclude that the two are not necessarily related and that the one is neither cause nor substitute for the other. Therefore, even though humanitarianism may be a desirable characteristic of the physician, it alone cannot take the place of knowledge and techniques that can be applied in the area of human behavior.

A great deal of knowledge about human behavior is scattered through the disciplines of sociology, psychology, and psychiatry. It is time that this was pulled together in one place so that with this as a point of reference the research that is needed to increase our ability to manipulate the doctor-patient relationship and apply the art of medicine in the patient's favor can be started. And as this project is developed, the dangers of both misuse and abuse of the patient-physician relationship as well as its use for good must be kept in mind. I think we must concede the possibility that humanitarianism without a knowledge of human behavior can do harm; also that the intelligent application of knowledge of human behavior, without great capacity for humanitarianism, can result in good. The physician's knowledge and understanding of human behavior must encompass his own behavior as well as that of his patient. I believe that the time has come when illness as it may be caused or aggravated, and health as it may be potentiated, by iatrogenic factors, should be subjected to careful and intensive study. As I write in this vein, I realize that I am touching upon a most complex situation—perhaps the most complex of all the situations facing either behavioral or medical science. Our tools for the study and measurement of human behavior, particularly behavior that is distorted by threat to life and health, are still crude and hence far from satisfactory. Here is an opportunity not only for those who are qualified to conduct the needed investigation, but also for those who might provide the necessary financial support.

The fourth situation which the General Medical Clinic experience emphasizes is one that medical educators are constantly aware of every time they consider any of the problems of medical teaching and learning. It has to do with the selection of the kinds of students who, from the standpoint of both intellect and personality, can cope with the non-spoon-feeding type of education, the intellectual and emotional discipline, and the human sensitivity, which professional competence of the future will demand. Fortunately, this area is presently commanding a great deal of research attention, both individually on the part of many schools and collectively by all the schools through the basic, behavioral research program of the Association of American Medical Colleges. It is to be hoped that this research will progress so that by 1962 or 1963, the number of applicants who can satisfy improved selection methods will probably have increased so that we can develop stronger student bodies, and because of this, stronger educational programs.

In concluding this foreword, I should acknowledge the premise that medical education should be geared to meet both demands and needs as they are reflected in medical practice. I am afraid that the demand for continuing, comprehensive care does not approach my estimate for its need. As a consequence, I believe that as we look to the goals of medical education, we find ourselves cast upon the horns of a dilemma. Should these goals be geared to the demands of the moment or to the satisfaction of needs which will or should be the demands of the future? With the total field of medicine in a state of flux, I should like to hope that, at least for the moment, we can skip all the present tensions and compromises and look to the future, asking and seeking the answer to one question: What are the components that should constitute adequate medical care? A secure answer to this question would be of inestimable help to medical educators planning for the future. Much has been written about this subject, particularly about the need for enough health facilities and personnel and for economical and efficient means of bringing medical service to the people. But little consideration has been given to the place among these components of the concept of continuing, comprehensive care and the things that must go with it. As this nation stands upon the threshold of increasing its medical manpower, the role which this concept is to play as a component of adequate medical care must be decided, for if this concept is important, our programs in medical education will need to be adjusted accordingly.

WARD DARLEY, M.D., Executive Director
Association of American Medical Colleges

Preface

During the twentieth century there has been an extremely rapid growth of the many sciences that compose the foundation of modern medicine. One necessary consequence has been the inclusion of a progressively larger body of facts in the formal education of a physician. The medical student must acquire knowledge of anatomy, physiology, biochemistry, pharmacology, genetics, immunology, biophysics, and pathology, to name only some of the basic scientific disciplines. In addition he must learn fundamentals of the clinical sciences which are accumulating at an incredibly fast rate. As these sciences have grown, large quantities of new knowledge and even whole new courses have been crowded into the medical school curriculum, which in most schools has not changed in length in fifty years.

In the past decade some medical educators have been concerned lest the emphasis on scientific advances lead to underemphasis or indifference to other equally important aspects of medicine. Specifically, some have come to believe that the central objective of medicine, the care of the patient, may not be sufficiently emphasized in the teaching of medical students. Concerned over this underemphasis on the teaching of patient care, the University of Colorado School of Medicine introduced into the curriculum a new program, the General Medical Clinic, designed to encourage the medical student to learn comprehensive medical care. Comprehensive medical care involves an approach to the care of patients in which the patient is regarded not only as a complex biological entity with a disease, but also as a living person who is part of a family and of a larger society. It implies the conviction that psychological and social factors are important influences on the well-being of the patient and that they may be the immediate and most important concern of the attending physician.

As plans for this teaching program were discussed, questions arose.

Would the program really teach what it was supposed to? Would the experience induce change in students' attitudes? Would the emphasis on total patient care interfere with learning the necessary medical knowledge? Since these and many other questions were regarded as vitally important, the program was organized so that they could be answered. A research project designed to answer such questions was established.

The research project was in itself a major undertaking. It required considerable developmental work, which involved extensive theoretical and methodological explorations, as well as the collection and analysis of large amounts of data over a three-year period.

This book describes the whole undertaking—the experimental teaching program, the control program with which it was compared, and the research project developed to study these programs.

The first part of the book discusses the educational issues involved and describes in detail the clinic in which comprehensive care was taught—the educational philosophy, the curriculum, the staff, the patients—and compares it with the control clinic. The remainder of the book describes the findings which emerged from the research. It also describes the theoretical and methodological work undertaken in the effort to evaluate the relative effectiveness of the two approaches including a study of the day-to-day operation of the teaching programs, as well as a study of the students who participated in them.

The book is a large one. It is large because we have presented the full details of both the teaching program and the effort to develop a research project for the evaluation of the effectiveness of the teaching program. Thus, the substance of the book is mainly factual, rather than persuasive. It is our aim to let the facts speak for themselves as much as possibile.

As soon as we began organizing our materials for publication, a dilemma presented itself. We found ourselves addressing two quite different groups of readers—medical educators and psychologists. Thus, we were faced with a choice. We could write two books, each addressed to a special reader, or write one book addressed to both. Writing two books would eliminate the disadvantages inherent in attempting to speak to two different and highly specialized groups, but would create the disadvantage of separating what was in fact a joint undertaking—the teaching program and the research project. More important, the separation of the material into two books would make it difficult to achieve our aim of a full factual presentation. The medical educator who was curious about the factual bases for evaluations would have to discover them in another book, and the psychologist or sociologist who was curious about the implications of comprehensive care would have to find these in a separate book. Because we felt that such curiosity should be encouraged rather than discouraged, the decision was made in favor of a single volume, despite the difficulties of addressing two quite different groups of readers.

This work was carried out jointly by members of the staffs of the Behavior Research Laboratory and the School of Medicine of the University of Colorado. The Behavior Research Laboratory was represented by Kenneth R. Hammond, professor of psychology, who was director of research. Wayman J. Crow, Byron L. Groesbeck, and John W. Gyr were research associates in the Behavior Research Laboratory, and each was in charge of a section of the research project. The school of medicine was represented by Dr. Fred Kern, Jr., associate professor of medicine, who was director of the General Medical Clinic. Dr. John H. Githens, associate professor of pediatrics, was associate director of the clinic, and Mr. Lyle H. Saunders, associate professor of preventive medicine and public health, was a consultant to the General Medical Clinic with regard to the sociological aspects of medical care. Drs. Kern and Githens, as well as Mr. Saunders, were also involved in the research project.

Although there was definite separation of responsibility, the work was truly collaborative.

THE AUTHORS

Boulder and Denver, Colorado
June 1959

Acknowledgments

The educational program and research project described in this volume were made possible only by the cooperation and support of many members of the administration and faculty of the University of Colorado School of Medicine and the administration of Denver General Hospital. It is not feasible to acknowledge our gratitude to each individual who contributed to the project, but to some we are particularly indebted.

Our dedication of this book indicates our warm regard for Dr. Ward Darley, who initiated the General Medical Clinic at the time he was director of the medical center and vice-president of the University of Colorado. Later, as president of the university, he was a never-failing source of advice and encouragement. Dr. Robert Lewis, then dean of the medical school, provided crucial assistance in several phases of the work. The Research Advisory Committee, consisting of Dr. John Benjamin, Dr. Alfred Washburn, Dr. Gordon Meiklejohn, Dr. Herbert Gaskill, Dr. Francis Manlove, Professor David Hawkins, Dean Robert Glaser, and Dr. Robert Alway, not only provided considerable research assistance during the five years the project was under way, but was a constant source of support within the medical school. Special thanks are due Dr. Alfred Washburn and Dr. John Benjamin, who were consulted frequently and who read early drafts of the manuscript.

Several psychologists, Lee J. Cronbach, Allen L. Edwards, John R. P. French, Jr., E. Lowell Kelly, David Krech, Jane Loevinger, Lawrence I. O'Kelly, Nevitt Sanford, and James W. Taylor, were consulted at various stages of the research project and provided valuable suggestions. Jeremiah Allen, Jr., assisted in the preparation of the manuscript. Without his unstinting efforts, the early organization and preparation of the manuscript would not have been accomplished.

All members of the teaching staff of the clinic gave steady and faithful service, but Dr. Eugene S. Turrell, Dr. Murray S. Hoffman, Dr. Stanley M. White, and Mrs. Genevieve B. Short deserve special thanks.

Two physicians, Dr. Gerald J. Conlin, and Dr. E. Michael Flaherty, were members of the research staff. They analyzed and rated over two hundred recorded student-teacher conferences. Perhaps no part of the project was more crucial—certainly none was carried out with greater care and painstaking attention to detail.

Graduate students in psychology who participated in the project were: Harriette S. Atkinson, Stuart E. Atkinson, Marian Roco Binner, Paul R. Binner, William O. Brown, Garth Buchanan, Patrick J. Capretta, Josephine Cohen, Donald Conrad, Eleanor G. Crow, Vernon J. Damm, John R. Davis, Robert C. Fadeley, Jack W. Fleming, Willie Mae Gillis, Jack H. Goldfarb, Theodore D. Graves, Irene Hunt, George J. Ivans, J. L. Khanna, Prabha Khanna, Thomas K. Landauer, Joel Levy, Albert J. Lott, Anne Mathews, Richard T. Putney, Alan H. Roberts, James Selkin, Stanley E. Shively, John R. Thompson, Frederick J. Todd, Benjamin B. Weybrew, Virgil Willis, JoAnn Zaynor, and Wesley Zaynor. Special thanks are due Ernest G. Jackson, Jr., Dorothy R. Neal, and Elene R. Maginnis for their efforts.

The processing of the data was handled with skill and ingenuity by Frank L. Garland. Valmai Gruber analyzed hundreds of interviews with medical students with thoroughness and perceptiveness.

We gratefully acknowledge the kindness of the following authors and publishers in giving permission to reproduce material: Dr. Reed Boswell, Dr. Harrison G. Gough, Dr. Gerard Neuman, Dr. R. B. Zajonc, the University of California Institute of Personality Assessment and Research, the University of California Press, the Consulting Psychologists Press, the Hafner Publishing Company, the Journal of Medical Education, the University of Michigan Research Center for Group Dynamics, the University of Minnesota Press, the Psychological Corporation, and John Wiley and Sons. We particularly wish to thank Professor Robert K. Merton for permission to use part of a questionnaire developed at the Bureau of Applied Social Research, Columbia University.

It is impossible to record our debt to our secretaries, Mrs. Dolores Chrysler and Mrs. Carolyn Householder, who stayed with the project from beginning to end.

The Commonwealth Fund of New York provided generous grants to the university for support of the educational and research programs. It was a pleasure to work with the editorial staff of The Commonwealth Fund in the preparation of this volume.

THE AUTHORS

Contents

FOREWORD, *by Ward Darley, M.D.* vii
PREFACE xv
ACKNOWLEDGMENTS xix

Part I. The Educational Program

CHAPTER 1. The Program to Teach Comprehensive Medical Care 3
CHAPTER 2. The Curriculum 8
CHAPTER 3. The Staff 15
CHAPTER 4. Social Characteristics of the Patients 24
CHAPTER 5. The Patients as Teaching Material 44
CHAPTER 6. The Family and Home Care Program 60
CHAPTER 7. Other Teaching Techniques (Conferences and Special Programs) 80
CHAPTER 8. Changes in the GMC Program 87
CHAPTER 9. General Problems 92

Part II. The Research Program

INTRODUCTION TO PART II 101
CHAPTER 10. Description of the Research Program 102
CHAPTER 11. Summary of Findings and Conclusions 129
CHAPTER 12. Implications of the GMC Program 153

Part III. Methodology

INTRODUCTION TO PART III 165
CHAPTER 13. Dependent Variables 166
CHAPTER 14. Independent Variables 210
CHAPTER 15. Individual Differences 278

Part IV. Findings and Conclusions

INTRODUCTION TO PART IV 309
CHAPTER 16. Medical Knowledge 312
CHAPTER 17. Medical Skill 329
CHAPTER 18. Medical Attitudes 341
CHAPTER 19. Psychological Knowledge 370
CHAPTER 20. Psychological Skill 389
CHAPTER 21. Psychological Attitudes 409
CHAPTER 22. Sociological Knowledge and Skill 447
CHAPTER 23. Sociological Attitudes 459

Part V. Special Studies

INTRODUCTION TO PART V 479
CHAPTER 24. Students' Performance in the GMC 480
CHAPTER 25. The Scheduling Effect 550
CHAPTER 26. Relations between Individual Attributes and Performance in Medical School 563

Appendices

APPENDIX 1. Sound-Film Interview Test 577
APPENDIX 2. Medical Attitudes Test 587
APPENDIX 3. Staff Description Checklists 597
APPENDIX 4. Questionnaire Used in Connection with Dependent Variables Measures 598
APPENDIX 5. Measures of Individual Attributes 615
APPENDIX 6. Students' Response to the GMC Program 624
INDEX 637

Part I

THE EDUCATIONAL PROGRAM

Chapter I

The Program to Teach Comprehensive Medical Care

During the last half century the body of knowledge necessary for the intelligent practice of medicine has expanded greatly. The rapid accumulation of scientific facts has made it possible for the physician equipped with these facts and associated skills to bring to his patients far better medical care than did his predecessors. The better understanding of disease, the more fully developed diagnostic procedures, and the more rational therapy of today, however, have not been applied to the maintenance of health without some sacrifice of the qualities that distinguished the practice of medicine in the past. The physician who attempts to acquire a thorough understanding of any field of medicine soon learns that he must restrict his interests and concentrate his energy in that one area if he is to become truly competent. Such restriction has naturally led to specialization in medicine. Because of the increasing specialization by teachers and practitioners, medical educators and others became concerned that the physician's interest in the patient as the central figure in medical care was being replaced by his interest in his specialty. Thus there was recognized a need to return to a broader concept of medicine and medical care. An interest in teaching such a concept, commonly called comprehensive medical care, has developed in a number of American medical schools during the past seven to eight years. In 1953 the University of Colorado School of Medicine initiated a General Medical Clinic for teaching comprehensive medical care. This program was undertaken in the spirit of scientific inquiry. It was regarded not as a favored and protected project or a crusade to save medicine, but rather as an experiment in medical education. As such, from the outset plans were made to study and evaluate the program. The major questions asked were: To what extent did the clinic teaching program achieve its goals, and did the clinic represent an improvement in the teaching of medicine?

Definition of Comprehensive Medical Care

Like many similar terms, "comprehensive medical care" has been subject to much confusion. It is therefore necessary to define it before proceeding further. As used in this book, the term "comprehensive medical care" is essentially synonymous with sound, or perhaps ideal, medical practice. It means simply that the physician (together with his associates) assumes responsibility for his patient's total health. All the implications of the foregoing definition cannot be enumerated here, but the principal ones can be indicated. First, it is obvious that the scientific knowledge, intellectual curiosity, conscientious attention to detail, and constant stimulation of research that have long been responsible for the high quality of all medicine are necessary components of comprehensive medicine. In addition to these, there is needed an awareness of the psychological and social factors affecting the patient's total health, and the ability and willingness to bring to bear on the patient's problems all the available resources of modern medicine. The physician practicing comprehensive care, in addition to utilizing his own knowledge and skills, must become a channel through which other specialized knowledge and advice can, when necessary, be directed for the benefit of the patient. He must recognize the importance of social and psychological factors to the patient's total health and must be aware of the value of preventive techniques in comprehensive medical care. Finally, it is essential that the practitioner of comprehensive medicine assume and maintain a central role in all consultations, so that responsibility for the patient is not divided among several individuals.

From the foregoing definition it is apparent that the practice of comprehensive medical care is primarily a matter of the attending physician's attitude: the assumption by him of a broadened responsibility for his patient's health. To be sure, special knowledge and skill, particularly concerning social and psychological factors, are involved, but in these areas, as in others, it is not possible for the physician to attain the proficiency of an expert; he simply has to be able to recognize the necessity or desirability of calling in specialized assistance when it is appropriate.

Goals and Philosophy of the Program

The over-all goal of the General Medical Clinic Program was to teach the techniques and philosophy of comprehensive medical care. The approach and organization of the clinic were shaped by that goal and by the underlying philosophy that comprehensive medical care is primarily a set of attitudes toward the practice of medicine.

More specifically, the goals of the GMC[1] were threefold: (1) to provide an opportunity for the medical student to learn at least as much about fundamental medical concepts, facts, and skills as in the classically organized medical clinics; (2) to provide the student with that additional knowledge and those additional skills, particularly in the areas of psychology and sociology, essential to the practice of comprehensive medical care; and (3) to provide a setting in which the attitudes leading to the practice of comprehensive medical care would be developed and maintained.

With respect to the first specific goal, it was postulated from the outset that the new program must entail no sacrifice of the large body of scientific and empirical knowledge necessary in modern medical education and practice. The quality of instruction would have to be as good as that in other sections of the medical school. Patients with the same types of diseases would have to be seen. The stimulation to learn would have to be as great as or greater than that found in other, comparable programs.

The second and third specific goals dictated the unique features of the over-all approach and methods of the clinic. These are described below.

Approach and Methods of the Program

In order to achieve the specific goals of the General Medical Clinic Program six general policies were worked out and followed as much as possible: (1) the student was given the maximum possible responsibility for his patients; (2) the time available for uninterrupted contact between student and patient was increased; (3) the importance of interpersonal relations within the family as a factor in medical care was stressed; (4) preventive medical techniques were incorporated in clinical teaching; (5) the importance of social and psychological problems in medicine was stressed; and (6) the student was given ample time to investigate and manage the problems presented by the patient. Most important of all, the above policies were incorporated into an active clinical program; they were not merely taught didactically, but learned in meaningful situations.

Regarding the first policy, it was believed most important that the student be given the fullest possible responsibility for the patient's total care. It is well known that the greatest stimulus to learning medicine is having responsibility for patients; broadening this responsibility

[1] This abbreviation of General Medical Clinic will be used throughout this book.

to include total medical care would help to make the student conscious of the scope of comprehensive medical care. Furthermore, it is essential to the successful practice of comprehensive medical care that the physician develop an appropriate relation with his patients, and such a relation can be achieved only when the student is made to feel responsible for his patient. At first glance, giving such responsibility to a student might seem to conflict with the need for close supervision of the student. However, if both the student and the staff physician clearly understand their specific functions, student responsibility and adequate supervision can, as experience has shown, exist simultaneously.

Closely related to the above was the second policy, that of lengthening the time of continued student-patient contact. This, it was thought, would promote the student's feeling of responsibility for his patient and enable him to develop a satisfactory physician-patient relation. It would contribute to the acquisition of a useful knowledge of the patient as an individual, as well as to an understanding of the course of his disease, and would thus bring home to the student the importance of psycho-social factors in medical care.

The third policy, that of stressing the importance of interpersonal relations within the family as a factor in medical care, was the basis of the Family and Home Care Program discussed in a later chapter. The purpose of this program was to give each student an opportunity to provide closely supervised home care for a carefully selected family. In this way, it was hoped, the student would gain insight, essential to the practice of complete medical care, into the social structure of his patients' families.

The techniques of preventive medicine were not treated as a separate discipline. Rather, it was the aim of the program to include as an integral part of the clinical practice all preventive measures of proved importance.

The social and psychological aspects of medical care were treated not as separate entities, but as component parts of the philosophy and practice of comprehensive medical care. Social and psychological problems were considered in the same manner as organic complaints, and their relative importance was determined individually for each patient. The evaluation and treatment of psycho-social problems were an important part of the GMC teaching program.

Finally, one of the most important policies of the GMC was to give the student ample time to investigate and manage all of the many problems his patients presented. It was felt that if the student was overburdened with patients and other duties, he would not have time to reflect on these problems and to do the necessary reading, and in that case, most of the goals of the program would not be achieved.

The achievement of the three major specific goals and the implementation of the policies discussed above required a specially qualified staff, a suitable hospital environment, and an appropriate patient population to work with. Each of these requirements (and the degree to which each was met) will be discussed in detail in a separate chapter. It should be repeated here, by way of summary, that the specific methods, policies, and programs of the GMC all evolved from the basic concepts of comprehensive medicine, and that the primary consideration at all times was to provide a setting favorable to the development of the appropriate attitudes on the part of the student. Fundamentally, the practice of comprehensive medical care is an attitude of the physician toward his patients.

Chapter 2

The Curriculum

Before the introduction of the General Medical Clinic, the third- and fourth-year curricula at the University of Colorado School of Medicine resembled the classic design of the curricula of many other medical schools. The academic year was divided into four twelve-week quarters. Of the three quarters they spent in school, the junior students devoted one quarter to medicine, including psychiatry; one quarter to surgery; and one quarter to a combination of pediatrics and obstetrics and gynecology. These clerkships, except surgery, were ward clerkships; the time assigned to surgery was divided among the various surgical specialty clinics.

During the senior year the schedule differed from that of the other years in that each student had as free time one quarter of the year. Accordingly, each quarter of the year, one fourth of the class was out of school and three fourths were in school. The senior students devoted one quarter to medicine, one quarter to surgery, one half of a quarter to pediatrics, and one half of a quarter to obstetrics and gynecology. In surgery the senior-year experience was a ward clerkship; in obstetrics and gynecology it was a combination of inpatient and outpatient experience; in pediatrics it was entirely outpatient; and in medicine it was two thirds outpatient and one third inpatient. The senior medical clerkship will be described in more detail later.

Curriculum of the GMC

In planning the curriculum of the General Medical Clinic, which was to be an experimental means of introducing the philosophy of comprehensive medical care into the education of medical students, three objectives were regarded as fundamental: (1) the advantages of existing educational philosophies and programs could not be sacrificed; (2) the new program should be designed so as to fit into the existing framework with a minimum of disruption; (3) an objective and controlled study of the new program as an educational experiment should be provided for.

On the basis of these objectives, three tentative plans were considered: (1) limited participation in the new program extending over both the third and fourth years; (2) slightly more intensive participation over the entire senior year; (3) the assignment of students for a block of time during the senior year.

The plan of having both third- and fourth-year students attend the GMC one half-day session per week was the first considered. This would make possible an almost continuous relation between students and patients for two years. It had the further advantage of being readily acceptable to all clinical departments because it could be put into effect without disturbing the already existing clerkships. Each department would merely allow one fifth of its assigned students to attend the GMC each day. Because of these advantages, much attention was given to this scheme. It soon became clear, however, that this plan involved many disadvantages for both the students and the clinic. For the students, the one-day-a-week attendance at a clinic with a special and difficult philosophy of medical care would not have much positive value. They would probably look upon the clinic simply as a nuisance that detracted from the time devoted to their more interesting clerkships. From the point of view of the clinic, it appeared impossible to achieve the complex organization necessary for presenting the concept of comprehensive medical care to ten different groups of students a week. Moreover, much of the idea of total care would probably be lost upon junior students, who were still working diligently and slowly to master the fundamental techniques of history-taking and physical examination. For these reasons, and for the additional important reason that such a system made impossible any sort of evaluation or objective study of the new program, this curricular design was abandoned.

After it was decided that junior students should not be included in the program, attention was directed toward a similar plan which involved assigning all senior students to the GMC for a small part of each week during the entire year. This second plan was attended by many of the advantages and disadvantages mentioned above, since it differed from the first plan simply by reducing the number of students at each clinic session and by eliminating the more inexperienced juniors. Although with these two changes the plan was feasible, it still did not provide for a controlled study. Furthermore, this plan was administratively impracticable because of the interruption in the senior year resulting from the off-quarter arrangement described above and because the department of surgery felt it necessary to maintain intact the ward clerkship in surgery.

Table 2.1. Sample schedule

	Student groups scheduled for:				
Quarter	General Medical Clinic	Surgery	Medicine	Pediatrics, obstetrics and gynecology	Free quarter
Summer	5, 7	3, 4	6	8	1, 2
Fall	5, 7	1, 2	8	6	3, 4
Winter	1, 3	7, 8	2	4	5, 6
Spring	1, 3	5, 6	4	2	7, 8

The third plan, assigning senior students to the GMC for a block of time, was then considered and adopted. This made possible the continuous and intensive participation of senior students in the clinic for two consecutive academic quarters (approximately six months). To permit evaluation of the new program, it was decided to divide the class so that one half would participate in the GMC and the other half would participate in the old program and serve as a control group. A second teaching hospital with already established medical clinics was used for the control clinic.

To put this plan into effect the senior class was divided equally: one half was assigned to the GMC for two of the three academic quarters and to surgery for the other quarter; the other half continued with the pre-existing senior program. Students were roughly matched for class standing and allocated to the two groups at random. The division of the class was carried out by the dean of the medical school, who made certain that each third of the class was equally represented in each section. The decision as to which half would be assigned to which program was made by lot in the presence of the entire class in the spring of the junior year. The same procedures for dividing the class and assigning the sections were followed for each of the three years.

Each class was further subdivided into eight groups of ten students each, and the groups were numbered 1 through 8, as shown in the sample schedule (Table 2.1). The odd-numbered groups represent the GMC half of the class, and the even-numbered groups represent the other half.

Distribution of Time of the GMC Students

During the two quarters (twenty-four weeks) devoted to the General Medical Clinic the student's time was apportioned as illustrated in Figure 2.1 and as outlined below. For the first twelve weeks he spent five half-days in the GMC and four half-days on the medical service. For the next six weeks he spent five half-days in the GMC and four half-days on the pediatric service. For the last six weeks he spent two

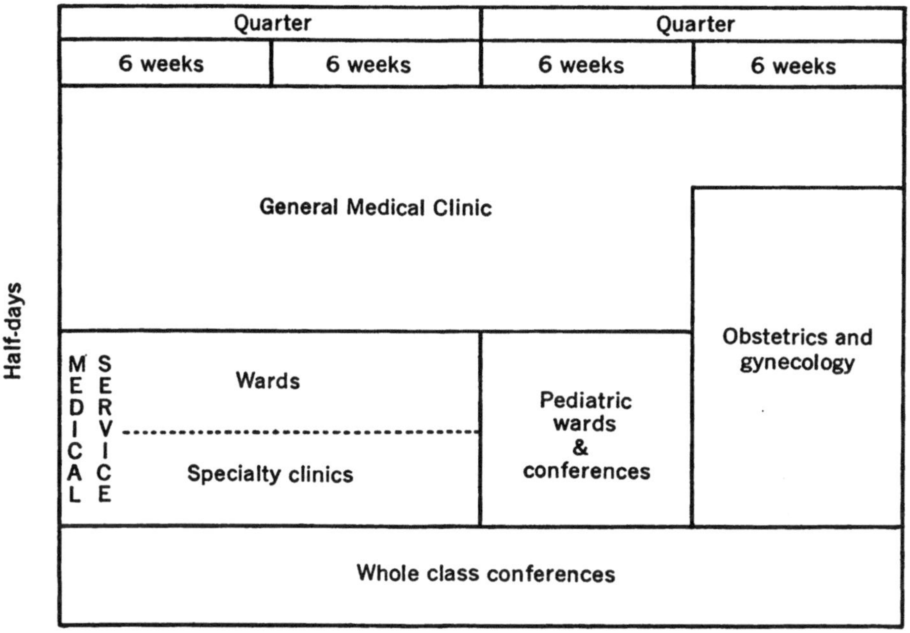

Figure 2.1. Distribution of time of the General Medical Clinic student

half-days in the GMC and seven half-days on the obstetrics and gynecology service. For the whole twenty-four weeks, the other two half-days per week were devoted to conferences attended by the entire senior class (grand rounds, clinical pathological conference, therapy conference, etc.).

Thus, the student was in the GMC five half-days per week for eighteen weeks and two half-days per week for six weeks; the remainder of his time was spent outside the GMC and was divided among the medical, pediatric, and obstetrics-gynecology services.

The four half-days per week for twelve weeks that the GMC student spent on the medical service were divided between the wards at Denver General Hospital and certain medical specialty clinics at Colorado General Hospital. Since it was believed that the patients at Denver General Hospital would not provide an adequate educational experience in neurology, dermatology, hematology, and endocrinology, the GMC student was assigned to specialty clinics in each of those fields for a number of sessions. These specialty clinics accounted for two half-days per week. The other two half-days per week, supplemented by two nights per week—one in the emergency room and one on the ward—were devoted to a modified clinical clerkship on the medical wards at Denver General Hospital. During this ward experience, the student was assigned to his clinic patients who had been hospitalized, and in addition acquired new ward patients admitted through the emergency room or elsewhere. All the student's ward patients were discharged to him in the clinic so that the student had experience with the same patients both in and out of the hospital. Because of the twelve week duration of this clerkship, each student was able to follow patients through protracted illnesses. Although the duration of this ward clerkship was limited, it seemed to serve a useful purpose in the education of students.

The four half-days per week for six weeks that the GMC student was assigned to pediatrics were devoted to attendance at several types of pediatric ward rounds and conferences.

It will be noted that the student was assigned to the regular obstetrics and gynecology clerkship as well as to the GMC.

The important features of the educational program of the GMC in which these students spent most of their time are listed below. They will be described in detail in later chapters.

1. Continuity of student-patient relation for as long as six months
2. Emphasis on thorough understanding of a few patients, rather than superficial contact with a large number of patients
3. Concern with all the patient's problems
4. Development of the student's sense of responsibility for patients
5. Development of patient-physician relation by student, instead of staff
6. Frequent opportunity for the student to deal with family groups as patients
7. Some experience with home care
8. Obstetrical program including long-term prenatal care, delivery of the baby, and postpartum care of the mother and newborn
9. Long-term well-child care
10. Supervision by a medical team: internist, pediatrician, psychiatrist, obstetrician, social service worker, public health nurse

Distribution of Time of the Control Students

The experience of the student in the other half of the class, the control group, differed considerably from that of the student in the General Medical Clinic (Figure 2.2). The control student was assigned for short periods of time to medical and pediatric clinics at Colorado General Hospital. The medical clinic assignment consisted of several half-days per week for three to eight weeks in a non-specialized medical clinic and one to two half-days per week for three to four weeks in each of a number of medical specialty clinics, including cardiac, pulmonary, gastrointestinal, hematology, endocrinology, arthritis, neurology, and

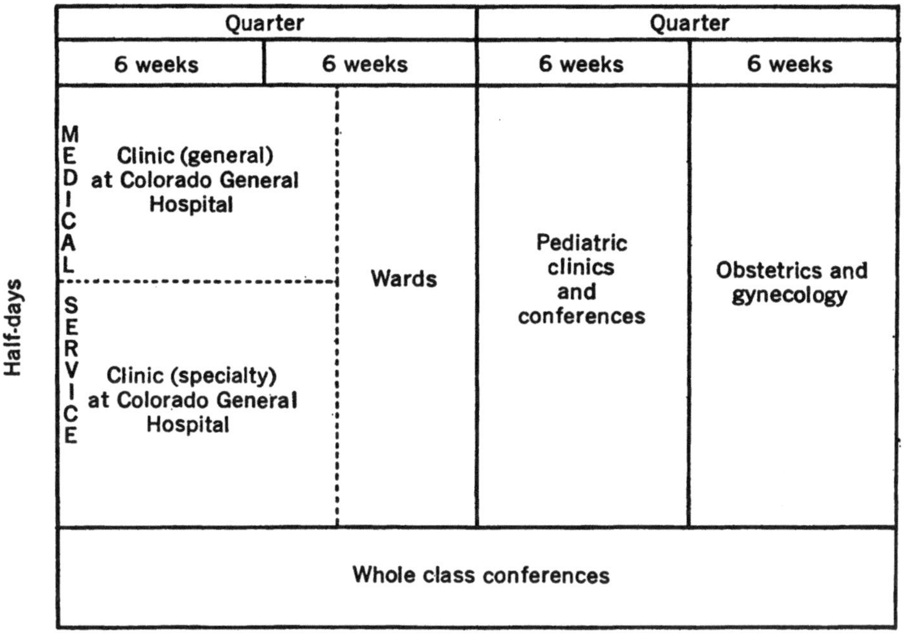

Figure 2.2. Distribution of time of the control student

dermatology. In addition, the student spent one month in a ward clerkship at Denver General Hospital.

The pediatric experience of the control student was six weeks long. It included three half-days per week in a general pediatric clinic, two half-days per week in a well-baby clinic, one half-day per week in a pediatric cardiac clinic, one half-day per week making home visits with a visiting nurse, and two half-days in conferences.

It is apparent that the student in the control half of the class did not have the opportunity to maintain continued contact with the same patients or to see more than one member of the same family; nor did he have immediately available to him the skill of consultants in other specialties.

The role of the control student differed considerably from that of the GMC student. In the GMC the student was made to feel responsible for his patients. Although the student was closely supervised, every effort was made to have the patient dependent upon the student (not the staff) and to encourage a student-patient relation that would make this possible. This was not a goal of the control program. Because of the short time the student spent in each clinic, effective medical care was frequently possible only by making it clear to the patient that the instructor was his physician.

The most important difference, however, was the difference in philosophy of patient care. This difference was most apparent in the medical specialty clinics, where the principal interest of the clinician was apt to center about the disease rather than the patient. In a specialty clinic expert knowledge is brought to bear on the patient's illness, but often there is neither time nor opportunity for concern with the patient's other medical problems, or his social and psychological problems. In fact, these problems, when they are not ignored altogether, are frequently considered to be a nuisance, to make the patient less desirable. Of course, the physician instructor in such a clinic generally believes in the principles of total medical care; however, he realizes that since the student is not likely to see the patient again, attempts to teach such a concept may be meaningless. Moreover, he frequently does not have time for this more complicated and lengthy approach, and may feel that his teaching effort should not be diverted from his field of expert knowledge. Therefore, he may be unable or unwilling to spend time teaching the principles of comprehensive care.

Chapter 3

The Staff

The success or failure of any program in medical education obviously depends in large measure on the staff that does the teaching. This is particularly true in the present case, where the educational program aimed at developing attitudes and beliefs in addition to knowledge and skills. These special requirements of the General Medical Clinic Program modified both the composition of the staff and the criteria used in selecting individual staff members.

Composition of the Staff

The interest of the General Medical Clinic Program in teaching comprehensive medical care made necessary a larger staff than is usual in a medical clinic. Teaching the student the correct approach to all his patients' problems could be done most effectively only by a staff of teachers skilled in general medicine or pediatrics and their specialties. Although there are exceptions, in most teaching clinics consultation is obtained by referring the patient from the general medical clinic to consultants elsewhere. This procedure appeared to be inconsistent with the goals of the GMC, and accordingly arrangements were made for having the consultants present in the clinic. The specific advantages of this system were: (1) it allowed the student to be completely the physician for his patient—as the patient's doctor he gave the patient the advice and recommendations of the specialist; (2) it reduced greatly the possibility of losing the patient by his being referred to a specialty clinic; (3) it provided a valuable learning experience for the student; (4) the availability of consultants made their utilization easy and simple so that advice was readily sought for minor problems.

During most of the period of operation of the GMC the following staff members were in attendance at each clinic session: four or five internists, one or two pediatricians, one psychiatrist, two or three social workers, and one public health nurse. In addition, a number of special consultants were in the clinic two to four sessions per week. These were: an obstetrician-gynecologist, a surgeon, and internists with special interests (cardiologists, hematologists, endocrinologists, etc.).

Need for a Separate Staff

As has been shown, the GMC's needs for staff varied somewhat from those of a conventional medical clinic. Still, there was considerable overlap, and the need for a separate, special staff might be questioned: Why not use the regular full-time and volunteer faculty who were responsible for the remainder of the clinical teaching program, adding only the relatively few special personnel required by the new program? There were good reasons for doing so, and to some extent the GMC was staffed in this way; but there were also some excellent reasons for using a special faculty group to teach in this type of program.

It cannot be emphasized too strongly that an outpatient clinic designed to teach continuing total patient care to medical students must be organized around the needs of the student and the patient—not the staff. This student-focused orientation of the clinic is in contrast to that of most teaching clinics and is an important reason for having a separate staff. In many teaching clinics the customary practice is for the attending physician to come to clinic late and to check rapidly the several students who, having completed the examinations of their patients, have waited for his arrival. In this way the physician utilizes his time efficiently; he does not have to wait for the student. Such a procedure was incompatible, however, with the goals of the GMC. At every clinic session some students were seeing new patients and others were seeing patients on return visits. This meant that students became ready to be checked by the instructor at an irregular and to some extent unpredictable pace. Each student had a schedule of appointments to fill his time, and if he had to wait for an instructor, he would be unable to adhere to that schedule. In that event not only would the patients be kept waiting unnecessarily long, but the student, as yet an inexperienced physician, was likely to react badly to the pressure imposed upon him to finish his work before the end of the day. He might lose his poise and attempt to hurry with his remaining patients without regard for the desired patient-care objectives. Thus, if total patient care was to be encouraged, it would be necessary for the staff to be present in the clinic for almost the entire clinic session. There were many days when they were constantly busy working with students, but on other days the smooth flow of students and patients was disrupted by the broken appointments, unscheduled patient visits, and other unforeseen events of any medical practice. Frequently, this resulted in periods of time when one or more members of the staff were unoccupied. Instructors whose primary interest was elsewhere, either in other academic duties or in private practice, were annoyed and inclined to feel that such a "waste of time" was intolerable. On the other hand, instructors whose academic interest was in this particular teaching program understood and tolerated such unavoidable delays. Therefore, it was regarded as highly desirable to maintain a special, separate staff for the GMC, and as far as was feasible this was done.

Criteria for Selection of Staff Members

The selection of teachers for the clinic presented a particularly difficult problem. The difficulties involved in choosing the best teachers of a concrete body of knowledge are generally recognized. It was clear that no rigid criteria could or should be established for the selection of a faculty for an educational program as broad as that of the GMC. The guiding criteria, therefore, were chosen and weighed on a somewhat subjective basis, and the actual selection of staff was modified to an appreciable extent by practical considerations. The general characteristics sought in the medical staff of the GMC were: professional competence as demonstrated by customary standards, a zest for at least some of the intellectual problems of medicine, an interest in and understanding of the comprehensive medicine concept, a broad social philosophy, interest and proven ability in teaching medical students, and such personal qualities as make for harmonious relations during prolonged close contact with students and with other members of the staff. Thus, although the traditional dominant criterion was not dispensed with, others were introduced and possibly given more weight than in the usual medical school situation. With experience, more was learned about the special problems and requirements of teaching in a general medical clinic program, and these criteria were modified somewhat; but in general they served very well.

Problems of Teaching Comprehensive Medical Care

The criteria enumerated above derived to a considerable extent from the special conditions and problems encountered in attempting to teach comprehensive medical care. One of these has been mentioned above: the student-focused orientation of the clinic, which necessitated that the staff members be willing to devote long periods of time to working with students in the clinic and that they possess the personal qualities conducive to working harmoniously with other members of the group. Aside from this consideration, however, the teaching of comprehensive medical care is difficult in itself. It makes many demands upon the staff in addition to the expenditure of time. Although it is often satisfying to the instructor, it may frequently be frustrating and unsatisfying.

One of the important difficulties is inherent in comprehensive medicine, which requires the physician to deal with complex, intangible problems that he does not fully understand. Not only must he cope with them, but he must also teach the student to recognize and manage them. Teaching students about diseases of unknown etiology and about clinical phenomena that are poorly understood are everyday activities of the medical instructor. This does not present any particular difficulty; indeed, it is somewhat stimulating to recognize that one has extended one's own knowledge to the boundary, that one has a fairly complete grasp of a subject and knows exactly what the problems are. One is cognizant of available knowledge and knows that beyond a certain point, ignorance is universal. Admitting such ignorance to a student is not traumatic. It is quite a different situation, however, to be confronted with a patient whose complaints are multiple and whose history, physical examination, and laboratory tests provide data that cannot be formulated into a fairly concrete problem or set of problems. The pain may be vague and ill defined; its relation to activity, eating, and other events in the patient's life may not be consistent or clear-cut. The combination of complaints may be unorthodox. The patient's personality may be poorly understood. His needs, his conflicts, his reactions to his environment, and his culturally determined behavior patterns may somehow be related to his complaints; but establishing these relations as facts is extremely difficult and often impossible. And this is the type of situation that was faced time and again in the GMC.

Other types of difficult clinical situations tended to arise in the GMC. For example, there were many patients with clear-cut organic disease for which specific curative or effective palliative therapy exists, but whose complaints were largely unrelated to that disease. If, as in conventional teaching clinics, such patients are seen once or even twice by the student and instructor, it is generally assumed that the complaints are related to the specific disease and that the patient will respond to appropriate therapy. However, in the GMC the protracted student-patient relation brought the student and the instructor face to face with the disconcerting fact that the patients' complaints often were *not* the result of the diagnosed disease and hence did not respond to therapy. Similarly, many patients at the GMC presented, at first visit, a pattern of findings that suggested a probable diagnosis, and the student assumed such a diagnosis to be correct. However, after diagnostic studies had been completed, it often became apparent that the assumed disease was not present. Thus, the prolonged contact with patients, which was an essential element of the GMC, led to the accumulation of more and more patients with complex, poorly understood problems. Yet it was fundamental to the clinic's philosophy of comprehensive medicine that every effort should be made to understand these patients, and that all the facets of their lives bearing on their health should be of concern to the physician.

Such patients are common in any type of medical practice. They were numerous in the GMC, and many of them were more than usually difficult to understand and manage because of the failure of communication that resulted from the social class differences between the patients on one hand and the students and staff on the other (see Chapter 4).

The GMC full-time and half-time staff believed heartily and sincerely in the validity and worth of the comprehensive approach to patients. They generally performed excellently in teaching this doctrine. Nevertheless, repeated confrontation with difficult patient problems resulted in the intermittent appearance of two types of undesirable reactions on the part of the staff:

1. Inappropriate persistence in trying to establish an organic diagnosis. Fear of overlooking some subtle or obscure organic disease is a response common to all conscientious physicians at one time or another. Fundamental to the practice and teaching of good medicine is an extremely careful and meticulous examination of all clinical facts and their relations. Equally important is a thorough familiarity with uncommon and exotic diseases so that the clues to their presence are not overlooked. Notwithstanding the importance of these principles, unwise and inappropriate persistence in attempting to establish a diagnosis of organic disease tends to direct the student's attention away from the more important and more pertinent social and psychological features of a patient's illness. In some instances the instructor's reaction to the constant repetition of difficult clinical problems described above was a dogged determination to establish a definite diagnosis of organic disease, even when one did not exist.

2. Frustration and hostility toward patients. From time to time the clinic staff became so frustrated by failures in dealing with patients that hostility toward the patients became evident. The failure to make a specific diagnosis, the failure to explain symptoms adequately, the failure to treat the illness effectively, and the failure to return the patient to useful employment contributed to this frustration.

Frustration and hostility on the part of the staff also resulted from the patient's apparent lack of motivation to get well and his general apathy about his health. These attitudes were not universal but, as pointed out in Chapter 4, they were frequently present among GMC patients. Although the development of a satisfying relation with a patient depends upon many things, a necessary condition for such a relation is a cooperative patient, strongly motivated to recover and to maintain his health. Since a satisfactory physician-patient relation is necessary for the practice of comprehensive medical care, efforts to teach and practice this approach to patient care were frequently frustrated, causing staff and students to feel hostile toward patients. The hostility became somewhat less as understanding of the reasons for the patient's behavior increased.

This hostility was not conducive to teaching comprehensive medical care, but fortunately it was almost always temporary. The over-all attitude of the clinic staff toward patients created an atmosphere in which hostile behavior was immediately conspicuous. The reasons for it were easily recognized, and although it recurred, it did not represent a serious or sustained handicap to effective teaching.

Training Requirements for the Staff

Another vital aspect of the problem of staff selection was the question of training. What formal training should the teachers of comprehensive medicine have? Ideally, the internists and pediatricians should be prepared by a broader-than-usual education. In addition to the customary residency and fellowship experience in internal medicine or pediatrics, they should have further training to familiarize them with the available knowledge of psychosomatic medicine and give them an understanding of the basic concepts underlying patient-physician relations. Moreover, the internists and pediatricians could profit considerably from supervised experience with psychoneurotic patients.

Similarly, the psychiatrist who teaches comprehensive medicine in a general medical clinic should have training in internal medicine or pediatrics. His understanding of physiological and clinical processes would thus enable him to integrate his teaching of emotional and psychiatric aspects of medicine into the total clinical picture.

All three, the internist, pediatrician, and psychiatrist, should also have a more-than-superficial knowledge of sociology. This knowledge can be acquired through either undergraduate college courses, special seminars, or independent reading. The need for such sociological knowledge was demonstrated by experience in the GMC, where it was most valuable for staff members to have available a sociologist who contributed to their understanding of the particular cultural and subcultural groups from which the patients were derived.

Since comprehensive medical care is focused on the total health of the individual, it naturally includes prevention as well as treatment of disease. This fact has implications for the training of staff members in a general medical clinic. Specifically what, if any, advanced training in the discipline of preventive medicine and public health is necessary for teachers in a setting such as the GMC, and what should be the role in such a program of a department of preventive medicine and public health?

In a number of American medical schools this department has taken the lead in similar educational programs.[1] Indeed, in some schools departments of preventive medicine and public health have independently organized and operated courses in comprehensive medical care or family medical care. At the University of Colorado the department of preventive medicine and public health was active and influential in the early planning of the GMC. Despite the important stimulation furnished by the department, however, it was decided at the outset that the teachers in the clinic should be physicians whose experience and training were primarily in clinical medicine rather than in preventive medicine and public health. An active interest in preventive medicine is essential to the teaching of comprehensive medicine, but this is simply an integral part of ordinary good clinical medicine. A knowledge of community health resources and a willingness to call upon them for appropriate help is also essential to the successful teaching of comprehensive medicine. The experience with the GMC, however, did not lead to a belief that formal advanced training in preventive medicine and public health is needed as background for teaching comprehensive medicine.

Recruiting and Maintaining an Adequate Staff

In addition to the difficulty of recognizing good teachers of comprehensive medicine and the weaknesses inherent in depending upon arbitrary qualitative standards for their selection, there was yet another problem to be faced: the staff had to be selected within a limited amount of time, and the choices had to be made from among those who were available and interested in teaching comprehensive medicine. It was clear that the qualities desired in a teacher of comprehensive medicine were among those that also characterize the successful physician in other roles. Such individuals are apt to be successful in the private practice of medicine as well as in the more usual type

[1] See Robert E. Shank, "Three Years' Experience in the Coordinated Outpatient Program at Washington University," *Journal of Medical Education* 31:283, May 1956; also John Perry Hubbard, "Integrating Preventive and Social Medicine in the Medical Curriculum," *New England Journal of Medicine* 251:513–519, September 1954.

of academic career, and the vast majority are attracted to these pursuits rather than to teaching and research in an experimental educational program. Thus, recruiting and maintaining an adequate staff for the GMC was a very difficult practical problem.

This is most clearly illustrated in connection with staffing the clinic with internists. Although not a unique problem, it is of great importance in this type of program. Teaching comprehensive medicine is a time-consuming process. The instructor must become familiar with all the patient's problems; he must help the student apply his knowledge of basic sciences to the individual patient; and he must guide the student in planning the diagnostic work-up and treatment. All these functions can be performed satisfactorily only when adequate time is available to permit work without interruption and without hurry. Sufficient time is available only when there is a proper ratio of staff to students. The most desirable ratio is one to one; since this was impossible to attain, however, it was necessary to operate with the minimum acceptable ratio of one internist to two students.[2]

The internists with special interests in various fields of internal medicine such as cardiology or hematology initially came to the GMC once or twice a week to serve as consultants for the students and for the general internists. A patient with a particularly interesting or perplexing problem would be told to return the day the appropriate specialist would be in the clinic. At that time the student to whom the patient was assigned would present him to the specialist, who served as the student's consultant. This system served several very useful purposes, as outlined earlier.

In spite of the value of this part of the program, it had to be abandoned toward the end of the second year because it could not be made as attractive for the specialists as it was for the students and for the regular members of the GMC staff. The chief reason for the specialists' dissatisfaction was that to them such teaching seemed an inefficient use of their time. Often they spent an entire half-day in the clinic to see only two or three patients. As pointed out above, the clinic was organized around the needs of the student, not those of the staff. It was usually impossible to have a large number of patients lined up waiting for the specialist so that he and the student could see them quickly and he could feel that his time had been efficiently utilized. The specialist believed, and correctly from his point of view, that he

[2] Only those students seeing adult patients were considered in calculating this ratio. Since about one third of the patients at any clinic session were pediatric cases, about two thirds of student time was devoted to adult patients. For example, if twelve students were present in the clinic, only eight were regarded as spending their time with adults, and accordingly four internists were scheduled to be present.

could see these patients more conveniently in his own specialty clinic at Colorado General Hospital. (During these years each specialty section of the department of medicine was expanding its research, service, and teaching functions and thereby creating additional demands on the time of the faculty.) These reasons in combination led the specialists to omit the GMC from their weekly schedules.

Effectiveness of the Staff

The GMC full-time and half-time internists and pediatricians did not have the broad program of formal training outlined above as desirable for teachers of comprehensive medical care. (There are relatively few physicians in the United States with such training, but it is hoped that there will be more of them in the future.) The GMC was fortunate, however, in that the teaching staff possessed most of the other characteristics desired in teachers of comprehensive medicine.

The staff was composed of capable internists and pediatricians with a sincere interest in and dedication to the concepts of comprehensive medicine and to the educational goals of the clinic. All invested a considerable amount of time and thought in the effort to achieve these goals and generally performed excellently as teachers of comprehensive medical care. It was only the excellence of the staff that prevented the many practical problems associated with the General Medical Clinic from having a greater detrimental effect.

Chapter 4

Social Characteristics of the Patients

In the process of learning their profession medical students have occasion to interact with and learn from several kinds of people. The knowledge, skill, and attitudes that form part of the professional equipment of the physician are acquired not only from students' associations with their faculty mentors in planned learning activities, but also from association and interaction—both planned and unplanned—with the many kinds of people that are to be found in medical school, hospital, and clinic. As Robert Merton has pointed out, medical students learn "not only from precept, or even from deliberate example; they also learn—and it may often be, most enduringly learn—from sustained involvement in that society of medical staff, fellow-students, and patients which makes up the medical school as a social organization."[1]

Not the least important of the categories of persons from whom the student learns are the patients. From them he learns not only how the human organism reacts to disease and how it responds to efforts to set it right again, but also how people variously behave in sickness and health in accordance with their orientations, expectations, and learned needs.

Any patient will serve for teaching purposes if communication with him is possible, if he is motivated to get well, and if the problems he presents are comprehensible. That is to say—since ability to communicate, motivation, and problem complexity are functions of social as well as psychological and physical factors—any patient is an appropriate and effective teaching instrument provided he is suitable from a social as well as from a physical point of view. If, as is generally believed, the most effective learning requires that the student have

[1] Robert K. Merton, George G. Reader, and Patricia L. Kendall (eds.), *The Student-Physician: Introductory Studies in the Sociology of Medical Education* (Cambridge: Harvard University Press, 1957), p. 42.

experience with a variety of diseases and with a broad spectrum of both normal and pathological physical conditions, it may be equally important for his learning that he have opportunity to interact with a variety of social and cultural types representing the entire range of characteristics he is likely to encounter among patients in his subsequent practice.[2]

If it were possible to view patients solely as objects of technical significance—to exclude from attention everything about them except their diseases—it would perhaps make little difference what patients were used for teaching purposes so long as they collectively presented the student with the variety of clinical material necessary to the furtherance of his education. But it is not possible or, it has come to be believed, desirable to view patients in this way only. Students, and mature physicians as well, do not deal only with disease. They work with people, and they must take into account and cope with much more than disease processes. Even in the most disease-centered situations in medical education and practice, the cultural and personal characteristics of patients intrude themselves. *Who* patients are and *what* they are must be reckoned with. And who and what patients are assume added importance in a situation where a goal is the teaching of comprehensive medical care.

Over the years that the General Medical Clinic has operated, the staff, in the words of one of them, "have become increasingly aware that the success or failure of an outpatient program in medical education may be extremely dependent upon the type of patient that is available as teaching material and have come to believe that the socioeconomic background of the patient may be of almost equal importance with his medical problem in choosing patients for the teaching of comprehensive medicine." Almost from the beginning, the teaching staff of the GMC found themselves dissatisfied with the teaching potential of the patient group they had to work with. It was felt and frequently expressed that these patients were difficult to communicate with; that they tended to be too little concerned about their own health and that of members of their families; that they were frequently indifferent to attempts that were being made to help them; that they tended to rely heavily on the medical advice of family and friends; that they had little insight into their own personalities and problems; that many were not "really sick" and only wanted someone to tell their troubles to; that their lives were so complicated and the problems they

[2] In most medical schools considerable attention is given to the problem of assuring that students see patients with a wide range of diseases. The possible advantage to students of seeing patients from a variety of social backgrounds is not so well recognized, and relatively little effort is given to controlling this aspect of the educational experience.

presented so intricate and complex that little could be done to help them; and that their medical complaints were monotonously similar, limited in range, and only infrequently of such a nature as to arouse in students a keen interest in problems of diagnosis or therapy.[3]

Comments made in interviews at the end of their GMC experience indicate that students shared the staff's unfavorable opinions about the patients with whom they both worked. The expectations of most students were probably fairly well summed up in the comment of a member of the 1954 class: "I'm interested in patients that have a good therapeutic problem or a good diagnostic problem that is interesting." That the GMC patients did not entirely satisfy this expectation is indicated in the comments of other students about the patients they treated: "You just have to take them as they come, and a lot of them are just a lot of old crocks. Actually there is nothing wrong; just a multitude of complaints." "The patients I had during the summer were very monotonous. . . . They seemed to be all the same kind—old men, broke, retired." "They are all old crocks over there. You see them, and you are going to see them in practice too, but you kind of lose your interest. The same thing comes in time after time."

Since the patient group with whom the students interacted during their GMC experience was felt to influence the amount and kinds of knowledge, skill, and attitudes that students developed during this phase of their medical education, some general description of that group and some specification of characteristics that may have influenced the GMC effort either favorably or adversely is helpful in understanding the effect of the clinic on its students. And, since the control students worked with a different group of patients in another hospital, it is also of interest to review some of the ways in which the two patient groups were alike and different.

Demographic Characteristics of GMC and Control Patients

No special study of the patient group as a variable influencing the differential development of GMC and control students was undertaken. However, information about selected demographic characteristics of the GMC patients was routinely gathered, and comparable information about clinic patients at Colorado General Hospital was obtained for four brief sample periods. These data provided the basis for the following comparisons.[4]

[3] For a series of comments illustrating how GMC students viewed their patients, see Chapter 5.

[4] Information was available for 2,731 (75.7%) of the 3,607 patients new to the GMC during the calendar years 1954 and 1955. The remaining 24.3%, for whom no data were available, represented patients whose records could not be obtained for tabulation. A good proportion of these were obstetrical cases or others

The GMC patients are drawn from persons who are admitted to Denver General Hospital. Denver General is the facility of the City and County of Denver charged with the responsibility of providing emergency medical care to anyone requiring it and additional medical services to citizens of Denver who require such services but cannot pay for them elsewhere. During a good part of its operation—from its inception in 1953 until 1956—the GMC was assigned all adult ambulatory patients requiring medical (as opposed to surgical, psychiatric, or pediatric) service, plus a sufficiently large group of pediatric and obstetrical cases to give students the desired experience in these areas. During this period the obligation to provide service was so heavy that it was not possible to select patients carefully on the basis of their presumed suitability for teaching purposes.

Colorado General Hospital is the main teaching facility of the University of Colorado School of Medicine. As such it serves the entire

---

who, subsequent to being seen in the GMC, were admitted as bed patients to Denver General Hospital wards. Others were patients whose charts could not be obtained because of confusion resulting from a change in the medical record numbering system that took place during the 1954–1955 period. The direction and magnitude of any bias introduced by the failure to obtain information on nearly a quarter of the GMC patients are not known. No systematic factor, other than the transfer of patients requiring hospitalization to inpatient status, was observed to operate in the processes by which the records of some patients became available while those of others did not, so that it is unlikely that any considerable bias occurred.

The 367 Colorado General Hospital patients whose characteristics are described here were part of a larger group of 1,473 ambulatory and bed patients admitted to Colorado General Hospital during four two-week periods in October and November of 1955, and January and February of 1956. It was hoped that information might be obtained about all patients admitted to Colorado General Hospital during these four sample periods. This, however, was not possible. Among the 1,473 persons admitted were 193 (13.1%) newborns, who obviously could not be interviewed; their mothers, who represented separate admissions, were interviewed. Twenty-three patients were too sick to be interviewed on admission and subsequently died; 39 persons, although their names appear in the records, were found to be ineligible for service and were not admitted. A substantial group, 339 (23.0%), was missed either because they continued too sick to be interviewed during the time the interviewer was available or because they were too sick to talk when admitted and were subsequently discharged before the interviewer could get back to them. Of the 879 persons for whom information could be obtained, 367 were found to have been given service in clinics corresponding to the GMC. These 367, who were in clinics in which control students were working, were selected for comparison with the GMC patients.

The requirements of strictly random sampling could not be met in the selection of either the GMC or Colorado General Hospital clinic patient groups compared here. In view of the many uncontrolled factors in the sampling process, neither group can be demonstrated to be truly representative of the population from which it was obtained. However, since for many characteristics, the distributions here obtained closely parallel those obtained in other samples drawn from the Denver General Hospital and Colorado General Hospital clinic patient populations, it is not likely that any considerable systematic bias has been introduced.

state, admitting some patients whose care is partly paid for by local welfare departments, but, more importantly, receiving patients of any socio-economic circumstance who present diagnostic or treatment problems beyond the capabilities of the personnel or facilities available in their local areas.

Denver contributed heavily to the population of both the GMC (95.0%) and Colorado General Hospital clinic (45.2%). More than half (52.6%) the GMC patients came from eleven of Denver's forty-six census tracts. These tracts form a rough S-curve around the central part of the city, bounded on the north and west by the railroad yards, industrial areas, and the Platte River (Figure 4.1). They include a good part of the least desirable residential area of the city and a number of localities that have been slated for slum clearance and urban renewal activity. In an early study of the sections from which the GMC patients come,[5] it was found that the five tracts contributing the largest number of patients to the GMC had, as compared with the city as a whole, a lower median income, more persons per household, more broken homes, more single adult males, a lower level of education, a disproportionately high excess of males, a higher fertility ratio, a higher dependency ratio,[6] a higher concentration of Spanish-speaking and Negro people, fewer males in the labor force, and fewer employed persons among those in the labor force.

More than half the Colorado General Hospital clinic patients who lived in Denver came from twelve tracts, seven of which are among the eleven heavily supplying the GMC. These seven tracts (24, 17, 45, 12, 23, 36, 10) provided 36.6% of the GMC patients from Denver and 30.0% of the Colorado General Hospital clinic patients from Denver. Thus, there was some overlap in the areas from which patients were drawn, although the majority of Colorado General Hospital clinic patients came from outside Denver.

A comparison of the two groups of patients, by sex, is shown in Table 4.1. The GMC patient group, it will be noted, included a somewhat higher proportion of females than did the Colorado General Hospital clinic group.[7] This may have been due partly to the GMC practice of accepting some obstetrical cases; it may also be a reflection of the heavy concentration of GMC patients in upper age groups.

[5] Sam Schulman, "An Analysis of Selected Census Tracts in the City of Denver" (unpublished manuscript, 1955).

[6] The proportion of persons under fifteen and over sixty-five to those aged fifteen to sixty-five.

[7] The sex distribution of GMC patients was not greatly different from that of inpatients at Denver General. In 1955, 43.4% of all inpatients admitted to Denver General Hospital were males, and 56.6% were females; on the medical wards, however, the proportions were reversed (55.9% males and 44.1% females).

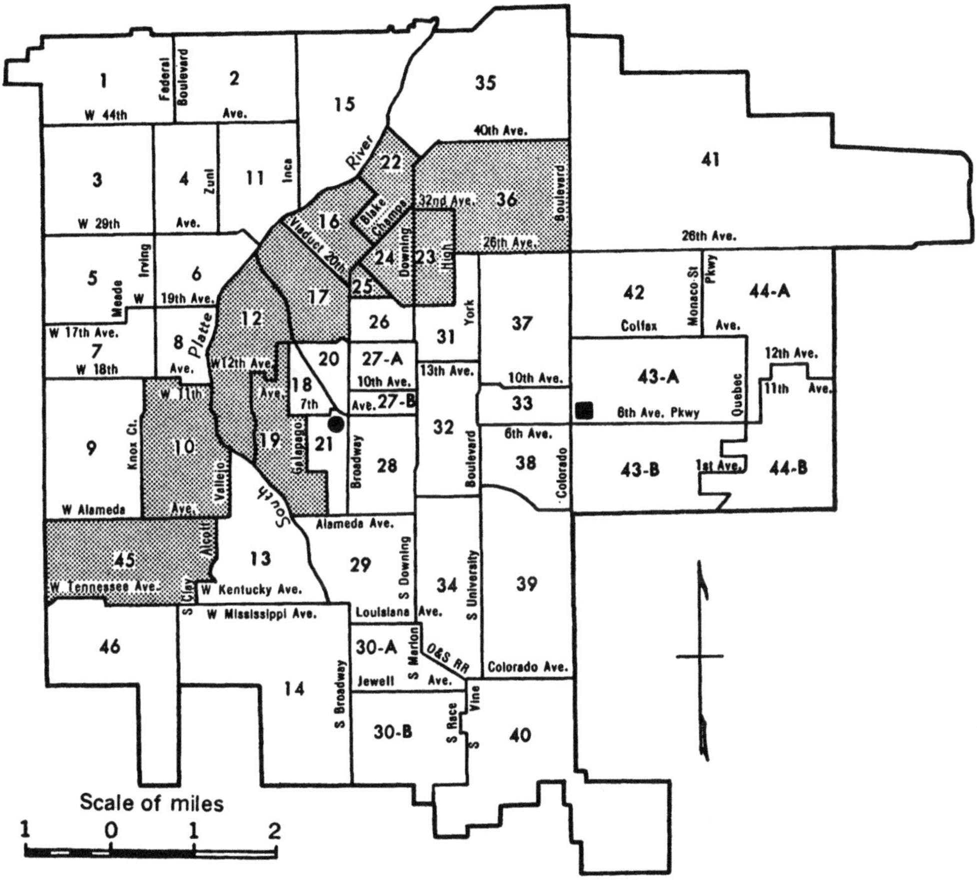

● Denver General Hospital

■ Colorado General Hospital

Shaded areas represent those eleven census tracts that together provide more than half the patients of the General Medical Clinic.

Figure 4.1. Denver, Colorado, by census tracts

Persons nineteen years of age and over made up 74.0% of the GMC patient group and 61.7% of the Colorado General Hospital clinic group. Within these proportions, however, the age distributions were quite dissimilar, as is shown in Table 4.2. The GMC had considerably fewer young adults, about the same proportion in the middle years, but nearly twice as high a proportion in the older age group. Even more striking is the comparison of the proportions of patients seventy-five years of age and older in the two clinics: 16.3% of the GMC patients aged nineteen or above were seventy-five or older, compared with 5.1% in the Colorado General Hospital clinic. Thus, one out of every six adult patients seen by GMC students was likely to be seventy-five or older; two out of five were likely to be sixty-five or older. By contrast, the control students, to the extent that these figures represent an accurate picture of the Colorado General Hospital clinic situation, were likely to see only one person seventy-five or older among each twenty adult patients, or one person sixty-five or older among each five adult patients.

As shown in Table 4.3, GMC students were more likely than control students to encounter among their patients members of minority ethnic groups. Both Spanish-speaking persons and Negroes were represented in the GMC patient group in a proportion several times greater than their concentration in the population of Denver.[8] At Colorado General Hospital clinics these ethnic groups were represented in a proportion which, while still somewhat above that in the population of either Denver or the entire state of Colorado, was considerably smaller than at the GMC. Thus, to the extent that differences in ethnic group membership hinders communication and interaction, GMC students may have found their patients somewhat harder to work with effectively than did the control students.

A comparison of marital status patterns among GMC and Colorado General Hospital clinic patients (Table 4.4) shows some notable differences. About the same proportion of adults were single, but the GMC had a much lower proportion of married patients and a correspondingly higher proportion of widowed, separated, and divorced patients. The high proportion of widowed among the GMC group was undoubtedly a reflection of the age distribution; the differences between the GMC and Colorado General Hospital clinic patients in the proportions married, divorced, and separated would seem to indicate more stability, less family disorganization, and probably fewer personality and emotional problems among Colorado General Hospital clinic patients.

Employment status is another indicator of family and personal stability. Table 4.5 presents data on the employment status of household heads in the homes of GMC and Colorado General Hospital clinic patients. Here again the differences are striking. The GMC patients were much less likely than the Colorado General Hospital clinic patients to come from households whose head (whether the patient or some other person) was regularly employed; they were much more likely to come from households where the principal bases of economic support

[8] The Spanish-speaking patients at both the GMC and the Colorado General Hospital clinic were largely Spanish-Americans. In 1950 Spanish-Americans made up 6.0% and Negroes 3.6% of the population of Denver.

Table 4.1. Comparison of GMC and Colorado General Hospital clinic patients, by sex

	GMC		CGH	
Sex	No.	%	No.	%
Male	1,124	41.2	169	46.0
Female	1,594	58.4	198	54.0
Sex not recorded	13	0.4	0	0.0
Total	2,731	100.0	367	100.0

$\chi^2 = 2.857$ (with "not recorded" omitted from calculation); $.10 > p > .05$.

Table 4.2. Comparison of GMC and Colorado General Hospital clinic adult patients, by age

	GMC		CGH	
Age	No.	%	No.	%
19–44	627	30.7	105	44.7
45–64	638	31.3	81	34.5
65 and over	775	38.0	49	20.8
Total	2,040	100.0	235	100.0

$\chi^2 = 30.087$; $.001 > p$.

Table 4.3. Comparison of GMC and Colorado General Hospital clinic patients, by ethnic group

	GMC		CGH	
Ethnic group	No.	%	No.	%
Spanish-speaking	807	29.5	64	17.4
Other white	1,493	54.7	269	73.3
Negro	398	14.6	30	8.2
Other	20	0.7	4	1.1
Not recorded	13	0.5	0	0.0
Total	2,731	100.0	367	100.0

$\chi^2 = 45.383$ (with "Negro, other, not recorded" combined); $.001 > p$.

Table 4.4. Comparison of GMC and Colorado General Hospital clinic adult patients, by marital status

	GMC*		CGH	
Marital status	No.	%	No.	%
Single	107	10.9	26	11.1
Married	348	35.4	147	62.6
Widowed	295	30.0	33	14.0
Divorced	110	11.2	18	7.7
Separated	124	12.6	11	4.7
Total	984	100.1	235	100.0

$\chi^2 = 66.057$; $.001 > p$.

* Patients new to the GMC during 1954. Comparable data are not available for the 1955 patient group.

Table 4.5. Comparison of GMC and Colorado General Hospital clinic patients, by employment status of household head

	GMC*		CGH	
Employment status	No.	%	No.	%
Regularly employed	229	19.1	186	52.1
Other employment status†	967	80.9	171	47.9
Subtotal	1,196	100.0	357	100.0
Employment status not recorded	206		10	
Total	1,402		367	

$\chi^2 = 154.105$ (with "not recorded" omitted from calculation; $.001 > p$.

* 1955 patients only. Comparable data not available for 1954 patients.
† Includes irregularly employed, unemployed, and retired persons, and housewives.

were intermittent employment (intermittent because of illness of the breadwinner, lack of occupational skills that would lead to job stability, or unstable personality organization), welfare payments, or retirement income.

The figures on employment status suggest the direction of the differences that may be expected in the family income distribution of GMC and Colorado General Hospital clinic patients. A high proportion of GMC patients, as might be expected from the age and employment distributions and from a knowledge of the eligibility policies of Denver General Hospital, had very low family incomes (nearly 30% were under $1,000 a year). The annual family incomes of Colorado General Hospital clinic patients, while not high, were substantially above those of GMC patients, four out of five of whom lived (in 1954 and 1955) in households with incomes of less than $2,000 per year.

Community support of one type or another was common for GMC patients. More than a quarter of them (26.5%) received either old age

Table 4.6. Comparison of GMC and Colorado General Hospital clinic patients, by annual family income

	GMC		CGH	
Annual income	No.	%	No.	%
Under $2,000	1,730	81.7	94	27.5
$2,000–$3,999	374	17.7	202	59.1
$4,000 and over	13	0.6	46	13.4
Subtotal	2,117	100.0	342	100.0
Income not recorded	614		25	
Total	2,731		367	

$\chi^2 = 541.515$ (with "not recorded" omitted from calculation); $.001 > p$.

Table 4.7. Comparison of GMC and Colorado General Hospital clinic patients, by public support status

	GMC		CGH	
Public support	No.	%	No.	%
Public assistance, including old age pension	1,652	65.7	88	24.2
Social Security	76	3.0	15	4.1
No public support	785	31.2	261	71.7
Subtotal	2,513	99.9	364	100
No information recorded	218		3	
Total	2,731		367	

$\chi^2 = 235.802$ (with "no information" omitted from calculation); $.001 > p$.

pensions or Social Security payments; nearly half (42.4%) received benefits from Aid to Dependent Children, Aid to Needy Disabled, General Assistance, or other categorical aid programs. By contrast, only 11.5% of the Colorado General Hospital clinic patients were living on old age pensions or Social Security, and only 16.7% were receiving any form of categorical welfare assistance.

In an effort to obtain a generalizing measure of socio-economic status, scores on the Hollingshead Two-Factor Index of Social Position[9] were computed for those patients for whom the necessary information on occupation and education of the household head could be obtained. The distributions are presented in Table 4.8. In terms of this measure, more than two thirds of the GMC patients, and half of the Colorado General Hospital clinic patients were in the lowest socio-economic category, the upper limits of which are nine years of schooling and a semi-skilled occupation. An additional quarter of the

[9] A. B. Hollingshead and F. C. Redlich, "Social Stratification and Psychiatric Disorders," *American Sociological Review* 18:163–169, April 1953. This article describes the use of a *three*-factor index of social position, using place of residence, occupation, and education as indicators. It was subsequently found by Hollingshead that relatively little efficiency was sacrificed by omitting place of residence from the formula. The two-factor index uses a 7-point scale for ranking each of the two indicators, education and occupation. Scale scores are weighted by factors of 4 and 7, respectively, and the results combined into a single index score. The possible range of scores is 11 to 77, with scores varying inversely with socio-economic status. The divisions used in Table 4.8 correspond to those used by Hollingshead and his colleagues in establishing boundaries of five social classes in New Haven. No position is taken here, however, with respect to social class boundaries in Denver. The categories used in Table 4.8 are simply those formed by breaking the data at convenient, though arbitrary, points on a socio-economic continuum. For a detailed discussion of the philosophy and method of validation of indices such as this, see A. B. Hollingshead, *Elmtown's Youth* (New York: Wiley, 1949); W. Lloyd Warner, Marchia Meeker, and Kenneth Eells, *Social Class in America* (Chicago: Science Research Associates, 1949); and A. B. Hollingshead and F. C. Redlich, *Social Class and Mental Illness* (New York: Wiley, 1958).

Table 4.8. Comparison of GMC and Colorado General Hospital clinic patients, by socio-economic status as measured by scores on two-factor index of social position

	GMC		CGH	
Scores	No.	%	No.	%
11–17	8	0.6	5	1.4
18–31	33	2.6	5	1.4
32–47	60	4.8	44	12.2
48–63	298	23.9	124	34.3
64–77	848	68.0	183	50.7
Subtotal	1,247	100.0	361	100.0
Information not available	1,484		6	
Total	2,731		367	

$\chi^2 = 37.601$ (categories 11–17 and 18–31 combined in calculations); $.001 > p$.

GMC patients and a third of the Colorado General Hospital clinic patients were in a category made up of those with partial or complete high school education and occupations ranging up to clerical and skilled work.

The GMC patient group, then, was made up largely of older persons living in some of the least desirable residential sections of Denver. Nearly half (44.1%) were either Spanish-speaking or Negro; more than half (53.8%) the adults were persons whose homes had been broken by death, divorce, or separation. Four fifths lived in households with yearly incomes under $2,000; two thirds received some form of public assistance; and nearly all were at or near the bottom of the socio-economic ladder.

The differences between the GMC and Colorado General Hospital clinic patient groups were numerous enough and of such magnitude as to justify the conclusion that, in statistical terms, these populations probably came from somewhat different universes. The attributes and qualities that each group brought to the respective clinic situations were factors in the judgments and opinions about patients formed by students and staff in the two institutions. There is evidence in the evaluation materials that the control students tended to view their patients more favorably than did the GMC students. If a difference in attitudes and feelings about patients did, in fact, exist between the two student groups, it may have been due, in part at least, to the circumstance that control students and their patients were more nearly alike—in age, in socio-economic background, in ethnic group membership, in education, in knowledge, values, and expectations—than were the GMC students and their patients.

The knowledge, skills, and attitudes that students develop through their association with patients and, conversely, the extent to which patients benefit or think they benefit from the association is, in part, a function of the quality of the interaction between them, i.e., the extent to which mutual expectations are met, communication is felt to be satisfactory to both, and the ends or objectives of both are thought to be approached. Relatively little, beyond a common-sense level, is known about the images medical students have of patients, their preferences with respect to patients, or the characteristics of patients that enhance or hinder student-patient interaction.[10] However, it may be not unreasonable to assume that, *everything else being equal*, students in general prefer to work with and accomplish most from association with patients who are under sixty-five years of age, rather than older than sixty-five; are of the same ethnic background as themselves; are of middle or higher social class status; are self supporting, rather than community supported; are reasonably well educated; come from a situation of good intra-family relations, rather than from broken homes or families with poor relations; have "interesting" rather than "ordinary" or "common" illnesses; have diseases for which there can be a favorable prognosis, rather than those for which the prognosis must be unfavorable; have illnesses of physical rather than emotional etiology; have relatively few rather than relatively many emotional complications; have and express confidence in the interest and competence of the practitioner; are motivated toward recovery, rather than not caring whether they get well or not; are "cooperative" rather than "uncooperative."

If characteristics such as these are essential to the development in students of a sense of accomplishment and satisfaction in their relations with patients, the GMC situation was far from ideally conducive to such development. Relatively few of the patients possessed all these characteristics; most were lacking in several.

The age and ethnic distributions, welfare and marital conditions of the GMC patients have already been mentioned. Details of their

[10] One exception to this statement is a study by William Martin, "Preferences for Types of Patients," in Robert K. Merton, George G. Reader, and Patricia L. Kendall, *op. cit.*, pp. 189–205. Martin is more concerned with the question of what types of students express preferences about patients than of what characteristics of patients are favorably or unfavorably regarded by medical students. One finding, however, is of interest here: ". . . the choice between patients with physical or with emotional illnesses is so heavily weighted that almost no student prefers the latter . . ." (p. 192). See also G. Saslow and I. N. Mensh, "Medical Student Attitudes toward Behavior Disorders," *Journal of Medical Education* 28:37–42, 1953; and Robert J. Stoller and Robert H. Geertsma, "Measurement of Medical Students' Acceptance of Emotionally Ill Patients," *Journal of Medical Education* 33:585–590, 1958.

illnesses and their behavior in the clinic will be presented in the immediately following chapters. Here, perhaps, some further description of the social characteristics of the GMC patients is indicated.

Social Characteristics of the GMC Patients

The GMC students came from families of middle or higher socio-economic status[11] or were persons who were well along in the process of achieving upward social mobility. They were moving into an occupation that is consistently ranked high in social prestige[12] and that commands the highest income of any professional group. They had or were acquiring many of the major value orientations of our society.[13] They were literate, verbally facile, problem-oriented, positively motivated, and optimistic in outlook. Most of them had had, prior to their medical school experience, relatively little intimate contact with persons from the social levels represented by the GMC patients.[14]

These patients, on the other hand, came largely from families of middle or lower socio-economic status or were persons who had dropped in the socio-economic scale. They pursued occupations that are consistently ranked low in social prestige and that provided them with only meager annual incomes. Relatively few of the adults had

[11] The fathers of 60.5% of the 1954 medical school seniors were either in the professions or in business. Seventeen per cent of the class had fathers who were M.D.'s; 77.8% had one or more relatives in a profession. For information on some aspects of the family backgrounds of students in fifteen medical schools, see Association of American Medical Colleges, *Questionnaire Analyses: Preparatory Materials for the 1957 Institute on Evaluation of the Student* (Evanston, Illinois: Association of American Medical Colleges, 1957).

[12] See Maryon K. Welch, "The Ranking of Occupations on the Basis of Social Status," *Occupations* 27:237–241, January 1949; and National Opinion Research Center, "Jobs and Occupations: A Popular Evaluation," *Opinion News* 9:3–13, September 1, 1947.

[13] For an extended discussion of these, see "Value Orientations in American Society," in Robin M. Williams, Jr., *American Society* (New York: Knopf, 1951), pp. 372–442. Among the values discussed by Williams are achievement and success, activity and work, efficiency and practicality, progress, material comfort, equality, freedom, external conformity, science and secular rationality.

[14] There is a large and growing literature on the social, cultural, and psychological characteristics of persons in the various socio-economic levels in the United States. Illustrative of the differences in attitudes, values, life styles, and goals between GMC students and patients are the descriptions in "Cultural Characteristics of the Five Classes," in A. B. Hollingshead, *Elmtown's Youth* (New York: Wiley, 1949), pp. 83–120. See also, W. Lloyd Warner and Paul S. Lunt, *The Social Life of a Modern Community* (New Haven: Yale University Press, 1941); W. Lloyd Warner, *American Life: Dream and Reality* (Chicago: University of Chicago Press, 1953); Richard Centers, *The Psychology of Social Classes* (Princeton: Princeton University Press, 1949); "Social Stratification in the United States," in Robin M. Williams, Jr., *op. cit.*, pp. 78–135; A. B. Hollingshead and F. C. Redlich, *op. cit.;* and for a recent bibliography, Harold W. Pfautz, "The Current Literature on Social Stratification: Critique and Bibliography," *American Journal of Sociology* 58:391–418, January 1953.

gone beyond high school; the formal education of most stopped with elementary or junior high school. Their attitudes, values, norms, motivations, orientations, and life styles, in the aggregate, differed considerably from those of the medical students and staff. They were not highly literate in any meaningful sense of that term, they communicated more easily about concrete than about abstract matters,[15] and they were likely to be concerned more about immediate than future circumstances.

Most of the GMC patients (about 90%) could be classified into two large subgroups, roughly corresponding in their characteristics to the lowest two of the five social classes described by Hollingshead in his Elmtown study.[16] One group was made up of persons who, in Hollingshead's words are "poor but honest, hard workers who pay their taxes, raise their children properly, but never seem to get ahead financially."[17] These were largely persons from families in which the household heads were semi-skilled or skilled manual workers or lower rank white-collar workers. They were often home owners or home buyers, tended to be regularly or frequently employed, had fairly stable family relations, and had rarely if ever been on welfare. They were persons who for everything but expensive illness could generally pay their own way and were proud that they could. They were concerned for respectability and for the maintenance and improvement of their position, but their economic situation was generally precarious, and they were vulnerable to even small reverses or misfortunes. The interests of wives tended to center in home and children; those of husbands in job and family. Television watching, informal visiting, puttering around, movie-going, "riding around" occupied their leisure time. Included in this subgroup were a few old age pensioners whose education and former occupation reflected a somewhat higher socioeconomic background, but who had become eligible for GMC care because of a combination of reduced income following retirement and a chronic illness that required long-term care. Within the limits of their resources and understanding of what was expected of them, those in this subgroup generally behaved in such a way as to earn approval as "cooperative" or "deserving" or "appreciative" patients.

The other subgroup was made up of persons at or near the bottom of the social class structure, persons who collectively represented nearly the whole gamut of social and emotional pathology. Here were included the chronically unemployed, the second—and in rare instances

[15] See Leonard Schatzman and Anselm Strauss, "Social Class and Modes of Communication," *American Journal of Sociology* 60:329–338, January 1955.
[16] *Op. cit.*, pp. 102–120.
[17] *Ibid.*, p. 103.

the third–generation of welfare recipients, the socially inadequate, the fatherless families, the heavy drinkers from Larimer Street, the chronic social agency clients, the unstable personalities—the whole range of types that Charles Booth, many years ago, lumped together in his designation "the submerged tenth." In this subgroup were those who, when employed, could obtain only the hard, monotonous, unrewarding jobs open to persons with little or no skill; many of those whose formal education had stopped at six or fewer grades; those who were, again in Hollingshead's words, "on the bottom . . . believe that they can do nothing to improve their position . . . [and] give the impression of being resigned to a life of frustration and defeat in a community that despises them for their disregard of morals, lack of 'success' goals, and dire poverty."[18] In this subgroup, too, were the neurotics, the anomic, the lonely aged needing someone or something to relate to, and a small number of what can only be described as "empty people," lacking in knowledge, skills, money, goals, prospects, and unable to form satisfying and enduring relations with other people. People from this subgroup, people whose medical conditions were complicated by social and psychological problems too great to be handled comprehensively with the resources of a single outpatient clinic, were those most frequently labelled "uncooperative," "unappreciative," or simply "crocks."

Nearly half (45%) the GMC patients were members of distinguishable minority groups. A tiny proportion was of Japanese-American or American Indian descent; one in seven was Negro; one in three was Spanish-American or Mexican-American.[19] In the absence of specific studies, it is difficult to assess accurately the effect on students of working with patients of ethnic backgrounds different from their own. But undoubtedly there was some effect. It would be somewhat surprising if, in their attitudes, opinions, and behavior, students and patients both did not reflect local, regional, and national evaluations of ethnic group statuses. In a clinic devoted to teaching and practicing comprehensive medical care, the minority status of nearly half the patient population must have exerted a strong influence on what students learned and how they evaluated their learning experiences.

It should be noted that, apart from the possible effects of their minority status and cultural difference, Negro and Spanish-American patients in the GMC may have come closer to being considered "good"

[18] *Ibid.*, p. 111.

[19] For an extended discussion of the cultural characteristics of Spanish-Americans and their implications for the giving or receiving of medical care, see Lyle Saunders, *Cultural Difference and Medical Care* (New York: Russell Sage Foundation, 1954).

teaching material than did the "other white" patients. For one thing they were younger. The median age of Spanish-American persons fifteen years of age or older was 40.8 years, and that of Negroes was 49.0 years, whereas 62.7 years was the median age of the "other white" group.[20] Nearly half (47.1%) the "other white" patients who were fifteen or older had reached or passed the age of sixty-five, as compared with only 13.2% of the Spanish-Americans and 26.6% of the Negroes. Household heads in Negro (25.4%) and Spanish-American (22.2%) families were more likely to be regularly employed than those in "other white" families (15.6%). Stable family relations were more common among the Spanish-Americans than among either Negroes or "other whites." Fifty-three per cent of the Spanish-American adults were married, as compared with 35.2% of the "other whites" and 32.4% of the Negroes. On the other hand, 56.6% of the Negro adults and 51.2% of "other whites" were either widowed, divorced, or separated, whereas only 39.2% of the Spanish-Americans were so classified.[21] The relatively stable family relations of Spanish-Americans was a factor in their being represented more than either of the other ethnic groups in families selected for the Family and Home Care Program (see Chapter 6). Somewhat fewer Spanish-Americans (69.1%) reported incomes under $2,000 per year than either "other whites" (86.3%) or Negroes (79.0%); their median income ($1,468) was higher than that of "other whites" ($1,233) and Negroes ($1,215). Relatively more "other whites" (71.0%) received some form of public support (including Social Security) than either Negroes (56.9%) or Spanish-Americans (57.3%). But although they were somewhat "better" patients in terms of age, marital stability, employment stability, and income than were the "other whites," Spanish-Americans tended to have lower socio-economic status as measured by the Hollingshead Two-Factor Index of Social Position. More Spanish-Americans (85.4%) and Negroes (70.2%) reported occupations and educational attainments for household heads that ranked them in the lowest socio-economic category than did "other whites" (54.3%). Taking all known factors into account, it is probable that the minority group status and associated characteristics of a substantial proportion of GMC patients served to complicate and make more difficult the students' task of relating to and working effectively with the patients assigned to them.

One important area in which the social characteristics of the pa-

[20] These comparisons are based on new patients seen in the GMC in 1955.

[21] In any of the ethnic groups the proportion of widowed, divorced, or separated was in part a reflection of differing age distributions in each of the ethnic groups among the GMC patients. It may also reflect some underreporting of the Spanish-Americans, among whom separation may be more casual and less final than among either of the other groups.

tients adversely affected the work of the students was communication. The doctor-patient relation is one that calls for the clear, precise, and complete transmission and reception of information. In arriving at a diagnosis and formulating a plan of treatment, the physician must elicit and use reliable information about the medical (and social) history of the patient. The patient, for his part, must understand what is asked of him and what is told to him if he is to cooperate fully with the physician in their common undertaking. When physician and patient come from the same socio-economic background and share membership in the same ethnic group, communication is likely to be easier and more effective than when they are separated by differences in cultural and subcultural background and identification, as were students and patients in the GMC. Hindrances to communication arising out of different social class and ethnic group identification include more than lack of a common language, although that too may be involved. They include differences in vocabulary within a common language; differences in ways of conceptualizing and organizing experience and information; differences in amount of knowledge about a given subject; reservations, tensions, anxieties, inhibitions arising from perceived status differences; differences in value orientations, motives, and objectives; and differences in ways of expressing and interpreting nonverbal cues. All these, to some extent, were present in the General Medical Clinic situation.

A very small number of Spanish-Americans were hindered in the GMC by their inability to speak or understand any English. A somewhat larger number were hampered by a limited knowledge of and proficiency in English which resulted in either inability or unwillingness to express themselves fully, or in imperfect comprehension of what was said to them. Still others, who knew English well, were limited in their attempts to communicate by their having, to some degree, the orientations, values, and points of view of another culture.[22] Both Spanish-American and Negro patients must have experienced communication difficulty as a result of their confusion about whether, in relation to "Anglo" or white clinic personnel, they should behave as patients or as minority group members.

The vocabulary levels of GMC patients are not known. However, some related information is available in the results of a study of other Denver General Hospital patients who came from the same population universe and were selected by the same means as patients

[22] In interviews with Denver General Hospital patients of Spanish-American background it was found that many such patients would express themselves much more fully in Spanish than in English, even when they knew English well, and that some would freely discuss in Spanish matters that they denied knowledge of when questioned in English.

in the GMC. A group of 125 patients was presented with a series of fifty simple statements each containing a word known to be used in doctor-patient conversations at Denver General Hospital. The statements were read to the patients to minimize lack of understanding that might arise from inability to read well. Patients were asked to explain for each statement what the selected word meant in the context of that statement.[23] Of the 6,250 responses (50 from each of 125 patients), only 57.7% indicated that the word was well enough understood by that patient for clear communication in the clinic situation. To the extent that the GMC patients' vocabulary levels were similar to those of this group of Denver General Hospital patients, the potential for imperfect communication due to simple lack of comprehension was constantly present in the clinic.

Differences in knowledge of the body and its workings and in ways of conceptualizing that knowledge was another factor hindering communication between GMC students and patients. Senior medical students, as compared with almost any lay group, are likely to be highly sophisticated and knowledgeable in the fields of anatomy, physiology, biochemistry, and the other biological sciences. The GMC patients, understandably, had little accurate knowledge in these matters.

Again there is little information about these particular patients, but there are data pertaining to other Denver General Hospital patients. A sample of 101 of Denver General Hospital inpatients was shown a "Trans-Vision"[24] representation taken from a junior high school text and asked to identify some of the principal organs. Only two thirds

[23] Illustrative of the statements are these: Take this medicine *orally*. This is a *routine* examination. Be sure that the bandage is *sterile*. I am going to *dilate* your eyes. Was the pain *persistent*? When did you first notice these *symptoms*? How is your *digestion*? In each instance the italicized word was the one selected for explanation by the patient. Responses were rated in one of four categories: (1) patient cannot give any indication of the meaning of the word; (2) patient recognizes the word but gives an incorrect meaning; (3) patient recognizes the word and attempts an explanation but his understanding is not good enough for clear communication in the clinic situation; (4) patient knows the word well enough for adequate communication in the clinic situation. The proportion of category 4 ratings for the words listed above was: *orally*, 34.4%; *routine*, 60.0%; *sterile*, 72.0%; *dilate*, 32.0%; *persistent*, 80.8%; *symptoms*, 71.2%; *digestion*, 43.2%. Illustrative of how far wrong some patients could be even on such ordinary words as these were such responses as: *Digestion* is appetite; normal elimination; going to the toilet regularly; sick feeling; your bowels; belching. *Routine* means one after another; rupture; special; full; continued; not thorough; fundamental; preliminary. *Orally* means in time; ordinary; at certain times; often; in order; regularly; as needed; on the hour (hearing confusion with hourly); quickly; steadily; correctly. *Dilate* means wash with medicine; check; test; straighten; take out; move; darken; cure; operate; treat.

[24] This is a pictorial representation in which the various organs are shown in a series of transparent overlays. The "Trans-Vision" reproductions used in this study were donated by Henry Holt and Company, publisher of the text-book in which they originally appeared: James H. Otto, Cloyd J. Julian, and J. Edward Tether, M.D., *Modern Health* (New York: Holt, 1955), pp. 406–407.

were able to identify the heart (66%) and the lungs (65%); slightly more than half (58%) could locate the kidneys and liver; and fewer than half (45%) were able to pick out the stomach. None of the respondents was able to identify all ten of the organs asked for; only a quarter of the group (26.7%) could identify six or more. When asked further to explain the functions of each of these organs, most respondents could give only the vaguest of replies. Nearly two thirds (61.4%) knew that the heart pumps blood—which means that more than a third apparently did not know or did not state that they knew even this elementary fact! Only one in nine (11.9%) could give a reasonably clear explanation of what goes on in the stomach, and only one in seven (14.9%) mentioned anything about the gas exchange that takes place in the lungs. The general level of knowledge about what goes on in the body can be estimated from some illustrative comments. About the stomach: "There's two, ain't they?" "That's your bowels." "You can't live without it because all your insides are there." "It holds your food and digests it by forcing it through the intestines." About the heart: "The blood is purified in the heart." "That's where your blood is stored." "It beats and works your body." "Sends electricity to the rest of the body." And about the lungs: "Lungs are helping to pump the blood." "They keep you breathing." "They support your back." "They're in your throat; they make you cough."

Most of the patients interviewed were equally vague about causal factors associated with various diseases, and they expressed little knowledge of or faith in preventive activities.[25] They tended to think that good health can be promoted or regained by "taking care of yourself," "eating right," "living right," but they were far from certain about just what specifically is involved in living up to any of these general precepts.

In knowledge and understanding of the processes of health and disease, GMC students and patients were worlds apart, and the communication difficulties resulting from this difference must have been numerous and complex.

In many ways besides these that have been mentioned, the GMC patients were a difficult group for students to work with. Some were not highly motivated to get well and tended to become impatient with the sometimes prolonged efforts of students to do the thorough work-up necessary for establishing a definitive diagnosis. Some wanted only relief from immediately troubling symptoms and were not sympathetic to either the objectives or activities involved in giving comprehensive care. Patients' expectations of the clinic process were not always in

[25] Fewer than 10% of 112 patients questioned thought that smallpox vaccination would surely prevent their getting that disease.

accord with what had to go on in order that the students might have opportunity to learn how to provide comprehensive care. Some patients misunderstood the meaning of and the need for diagnostic procedures and withheld their full cooperation. The moral and ethical standards of many patients were sharply at variance with those of students, some of whom—as is discussed in the following chapter—tended to become disturbed about such matters as the easy acceptance of welfare aid, excessive drinking, illegitimacy, desertion, quarreling, and neglect of children. Unawareness of or indifference to the emotional components of some illnesses made it difficult for some patients to understand or accept what they were being told or were being asked to do. Added to all this were the special problems of handling elderly, homeless, anomic men; of attempting to work with patients who were personally or socially inadequate; of having to reconcile the desire and the need to be helpful and hopeful with the realities of working with a substantial proportion of patients who were old, chronically ill, and largely lacking in both resources and prospects.

To summarize briefly, the GMC students and the control students worked with patient groups that differed in sex, age, and ethnic group distributions, marital status patterns, and socio-economic background. The direction of difference was such that the GMC students were more likely than the controls to encounter patients who were old in years, members of ethnic minority groups, welfare recipients, from unstable or broken families, persons with no family ties, from low-income families, or incumbents of low-valued socio-economic statuses. It is believed that these characteristics of the patient group resulted in complex communication barriers between the GMC students and their patients—barriers that, given the further factors of prolonged contact between student and patient and the requirement that the student take account of and deal with psychological and social factors in providing comprehensive medical care, could have made the educational experience of the GMC students more difficult and less satisfying than that of the control students.

In the following chapter the medical characteristics of patients—which were to an extent related to and derived from their social and cultural characteristics—will be described, and some of the specific problems arising out of the nature of the patient group will be discussed.

Chapter 5

The Patients as Teaching Material

Medical Characteristics of the Patients

The patients seen by the General Medical Clinic students differed medically as well as socially from those seen by the control students (Tables 5.1 and 5.2), thus contributing to the difference in the experience of the two groups. The medical differences are partly, at least, the result of the social differences described in Chapter 4. In this regard, the fact that a larger proportion of GMC patients than Colorado General Hospital clinic patients were over sixty-five years of age is important. (For one group of GMC students 44% of all visits by adults were made by patients over sixty-five.) The medical differences are also the result of differences in the sources from which the two groups of patients were referred to their respective clinics. During the three-year period of this study all the adult patients in Denver General Hospital who needed care in a medical clinic were referred to the GMC; there were no other medical or medical specialty clinics. These patients had come to Denver General either because it was the only medical facility available to them or because they had been referred by welfare agencies. Only rarely were patients from outside the hospital referred to the GMC for their teaching value or because their physicians believed they posed unusual diagnostic or therapeutic problems. In contrast, the patients seen at the Colorado General Hospital clinic had been referred from various sources. Some came from the same sort of social background as the GMC patients, but others had been referred to the medical school hospital by physicians from throughout the state who believed these patients posed diagnostic problems.

Because of these differences in social background, age, and source of referral, the adults seen by the GMC students presented fewer specific disease entities and more ill-defined complaints than did those seen by the control students.

Table 5.1. Comparison of common diagnoses among adult patients in the GMC and Colorado General Hospital clinic

Diagnosis	GMC (1,077) No.	GMC (1,077) %	CGH (203) No.	CGH (203) %
A. More common in GMC				
Obesity	117	10.8	14	6.8
Osteoarthritis	112	10.3	12	5.9
Generalized arteriosclerosis	82	7.6	9	4.4
Cerebral vascular accident	55	5.1	4	2.0
Diabetes mellitus	48	4.4	3	1.5
Alcoholism	34	3.1	2	1.0
Syphilis	26	2.4	1	0.5
B. More common in CGH				
Neuroses, psychoneuroses, personality disorders, psychoses	121	11.2	44	21.6
Chronic pulmonary disease	90	8.3	29	14.2
Gynecological disorders	69	6.4	22	10.8
Neurological diseases (excluding cerebral vascular accident)	55	5.1	37	18.2
Cardiovascular diseases (excluding arteriosclerotic heart disease and rheumatic heart disease)	45	4.1	17	8.3
Skin diseases	44	4.0	20	9.8
Functional gastrointestinal disorders	31	2.8	17	8.3
C. Occurring about equally				
Essential benign hypertension	125	11.6	26	12.8
Arteriosclerotic heart disease	87	8.0	18	8.8
Musculo-skeletal diseases	82	7.6	19	9.4
Diseases of veins	67	6.2	13	6.4
Peptic ulcer	55	5.1	14	6.8
Gall bladder disease	54	5.0	8	3.9
Hernias	46	4.2	9	4.4
Benign prostatic hypertrophy	45	4.1	9	4.4
Tuberculosis	37	3.4	5	2.4
Rheumatic heart disease	36	3.3	11	5.4
Asthma	33	3.0	7	3.4

Table 5.1, part A, lists the diagnoses that occurred considerably more commonly among the GMC adult patients than among the Colorado General Hospital clinic adult patients.[1] These diagnoses (obesity, osteoarthritis, generalized arteriosclerosis, cerebral vascular

[1] The data presented in Tables 5.1 and 5.2 were obtained as follows. The diagnoses of all new patients admitted to the GMC during a six-month period in 1955 were reviewed. These 1,077 patients represented all the new adult patients admitted to the GMC during the course of one student group's stay in the clinic. The patients were shared with the general practice residents, who took care of about half. The 203 Colorado General Hospital patients represent all new adult patients admitted to medical and medical specialty clinics of the outpatient department during an eight-week period. This does not include all new patients available to a particular control group, but is a sample of the adult patients seen in the clinic by these students. Since the tables include all diagnoses made on each patient, the total number of diagnoses is much greater than the total number of patients.

accident, diabetes mellitus, alcoholism, and syphilis) reflect the age distribution of the adult patients seen in the GMC, in that at least four of the seven are primarily diseases of the aged. The higher incidence of syphilis and alcoholism among GMC than among Colorado General Hospital clinic patients can probably be accounted for by the difference in social background of the two patient groups, although the percentage of patients with alcoholism and syphilis was small in both groups. Thirty-four GMC patients were diagnosed as alcoholics; although this number was only about 3% of all GMC patients, analysis of diagnoses by age and sex showed that alcoholism was the most common diagnosis among male GMC patients nineteen to sixty-four years of age. With the exception of diabetes and syphilis, the diagnoses that predominated in the GMC group represented somewhat ill-defined and relatively incurable complaints.

Table 5.1, part B, lists the diagnoses that occurred more commonly among the Colorado General Hospital clinic adult patients than among the GMC adult patients. The fact that 21% of the Colorado General Hospital clinic patients were diagnosed as having neuroses, psychoneuroses, personality disorders, or psychoses was probably a result of the hospital's referral-center function. All medical centers to which diagnostic problems are referred are apt to concentrate such patients. The other diagnoses found more often in the patients at the Colorado General Hospital clinic were chronic pulmonary disease, gynecological disorders, neurological diseases (excluding cerebral vascular accident), cardiovascular diseases, skin diseases, and functional gastrointestinal disorders. The majority of patients with these conditions were eventually referred from the Colorado General Hospital medical clinic to the appropriate specialty clinic.

Table 5.1, part C, lists other common diagnoses that occurred with approximately equal frequency among patients in both clinics. With the exception of peptic ulcer, gall bladder disease, rheumatic heart disease, and asthma, it is likely that these diagnoses represented associated findings rather than primary diseases. It is particularly interesting that the diagnosis of peptic ulcer was made almost as frequently in the GMC as in the Colorado General Hospital clinic, although referred cases might have been expected to increase the incidence in the latter clinic.

Analysis of the less common diagnoses of GMC patients reveals that some disease categories were very sparsely represented. For instance, although there were many patients with diabetes mellitus and some with thyroid disorders, there were practically no patients with any other endocrine diseases. During the sample period only twelve patients were diagnosed as having a hematologic disease. The paucity

Table 5.2. Comparison of common diagnoses among pediatric patients in the GMC and Colorado General Hospital clinic

Diagnosis	GMC (318) No.	GMC (318) %	CGH (142) No.	CGH (142) %
A. More common in GMC				
Cardiovascular diseases (including rheumatic fever)	16	5.0	3	2.1
B. More common in CGH				
Gastrointestinal disorders	25	7.9	19	13.3
Neurological diseases	14	4.4	14	9.9
Musculo-skeletal diseases	5	1.6	9	6.3
Allergies	3	0.9	9	6.3
Lower respiratory disease	11	3.5	9	6.3
Congenital disease (other than cardiac)	11	3.5	8	5.6
C. Occurring about equally				
Acute upper respiratory diseases	144	45.3	60	42.2
Well baby or child	75	23.6	40	28.2
Skin diseases	48	15.0	16	11.3
Genitourinary diseases	18	5.7	6	4.2
Behavior disorders	16	5.0	6	4.2
Chronic upper respiratory diseases	14	4.4	9	6.3

of patients with these diseases was of varying importance to the students. The first five GMC groups attended specialty clinics in neurology, hematology, endocrinology, and dermatology at Colorado General Hospital and thus were able to see patients with these problems. The 1956 II group, however, did not have this experience. The control students also had experience (more than half their time) with patients in medical specialty clinics, which over a period of years had collected large groups of patients with specific diseases. Since these patients were not new during the sample period, their diagnoses are not included in Table 5.1. All six control groups attended clinics in neurology, hematology, endocrinology, dermatology, gastroenterology, cardiology, arthritis, and chest diseases.

Table 5.2 compares the occurrence of the more common diagnoses found in pediatric patients in the GMC and the Colorado General Hospital clinic.[2] Only one disease was more common among the pediatric patients of the GMC than among those of Colorado General Hospital clinic: heart disease, including rheumatic fever, was diagnosed in 5% of GMC patients compared with 2% of Colorado General Hospital clinic patients. The GMC diagnoses were almost entirely rheumatic fever and rheumatic heart disease. This was probably owing to the deliberate selection of a large number of family units containing children with rheumatic fever for the Family and Home Care Pro-

[2] The data presented in Table 5.2 were obtained in the same way and at the same time as those presented in Table 5.1.

gram and may also reflect the social background of the GMC patients.

Six diseases were more common in the children admitted to the Colorado General Hospital pediatric clinic (Table 5.2, part B). Like the conditions found among the adult patients at Colorado General, these diagnoses represent fairly specific disease entities (gastrointestinal disorders, neurological diseases, musculo-skeletal diseases, allergies, lower respiratory diseases, and congenital anomalies). Many children were probably referred to the hospital for evaluation and treatment because they were believed to present difficult or uncommon problems.

Table 5.2, part C, lists the common diagnoses that occurred about as frequently in the GMC as in the Colorado General Hospital clinic. These diagnoses represent the usual problems of any group of pediatric patients: acute upper respiratory diseases and well babies account for the majority; the remainder were skin diseases, genitourinary diseases, behavior problems, and chronic upper respiratory diseases.

The pediatric patients, one third of all patients seen in the GMC, represented only a small proportion of the total number of children receiving care at Denver General Hospital. Those not seen in the GMC were cared for in the emergency room or in the pediatric outpatient department by the pediatric residents and staff. There was an adequate number of sick children to serve the training needs of both groups. A large number of GMC children were infants who had been referred from the hospital's nursery for well-child care. Many were members of the families of adult patients or other pediatric patients previously assigned to GMC students and brought in at the students' request for complete work-up. The control students, besides their regular work in the pediatric clinic, were assigned to the Rheumatic Fever Diagnostic Clinic for special experience in cardiology; however, they did not participate in other pediatric specialty clinics. Each control student followed two patients with behavior problems under the supervision of a member of the department of psychiatry, but the period of follow-up was limited to six weeks. Night duty in the hospital pediatric emergency rooms provided both groups with additional experience with acute illness and contagious diseases.

To summarize, the medical problems seen by the two groups of students differed. The GMC students' adult patients were older than the control students' patients. They presented more chronic illness, more ill-defined complaints, fewer disease entities, fewer diagnostic problems, and more serious problems of social and emotional adjustment. The pediatric patients of the two student groups differed little except that the GMC children presented fewer diagnostic problems.

The Student's Patient Load

The student's experience in the GMC was influenced by the number of patients he saw and the number of visits made by the same patient as well as by the medical characteristics of the patients. Since the clinic was designed to promote continuity of care, the student spent more of his time with patients making revisits than with new patients. Therefore, he saw fewer patients and fewer disease entities than did the control student. However, the opportunity to follow his patients over an extended period of time may have compensated for this.

Table 5.3 shows that in the GMC for four student groups (1954 II, 1955 I and II, 1956 I) the average number of new patients per student was 47, whereas the average number of patient visits per student was 137. An effort was made to apportion the student's time so that one third of his experience was with pediatric and two thirds with adult patients. As Table 5.3 shows, 31% of the GMC student's experience was with pediatric and 69% with adult patients. In order to maintain this 1:2 ratio, more than one third of all new patients had to be children, since pediatric patients made fewer revisits.

In spite of the fact that the average number of patient visits, the average number of patients per student, and the over-all ratio of pediatric to adult patients were fairly constant from one group of students to another, there was marked variation among individual students. Table 5.4 shows that in one group the total number of patients per student varied from 34 to 58, even though the average of 47 was comparable with that of the other groups. The total number of patient contacts varied from 107 to 159, but the average of 137 was again similar to that of the other groups. A large patient load for a GMC student was undesirable. When a student had to rush from one patient to another the amount of time for consultation with the staff was curtailed, resulting in poor teaching. This happened frequently with certain GMC groups, because of the recurring heavy service obligations of the clinic. The ratio of pediatric to adult patient contacts varied widely from one student to another. In the 1955 II group the proportion of patients in the pediatric age range varied from 16%

Table 5.3. Average patient load for GMC students, based on experience of four GMC groups (1954 II, 1955 I and II, 1956 I)

	New patients per student		Patient contacts per student	
	Av. no.	%	Av. no.	%
Adults	27.7	58.6	94.6	69.0
Children	19.6	41.4	42.4	31.0
Total	47.3	100.0	137.0	100.0

Table 5.4. Number of patients seen and number of patient contacts for each GMC student (1955 II)

Student	Total no. of patients (adult and pediatric)	Pediatric patients		Adult patients		Total no. of contacts (adult and pediatric)	Pediatric contacts		Adult contacts	
		No.	% of total	No.	% of total		No.	% of total	No.	% of total
A	51	26	50.9	25	49.1	159	73	45.9	86	54.1
B	43	18	41.9	25	58.1	122	47	38.5	75	61.5
C	34	15	44.1	19	55.9	107	33	30.8	74	69.2
D	40	18	45.0	22	55.0	134	46	34.3	88	65.7
E	49	20	40.9	29	59.1	133	54	40.6	79	59.4
F	47	21	44.7	26	55.3	135	44	32.6	91	67.4
G	42	16	38.1	26	61.9	107	29	27.1	78	72.9
H	42	17	40.5	25	59.5	157	59	37.6	98	62.4
I	57	21	36.8	36	63.2	141	36	25.5	105	74.5
J	58	23	39.7	35	60.3	143	44	30.8	99	69.2
K	48	23	47.9	25	52.1	148	56	37.8	92	62.2
L	56	28	50.0	28	50.0	159	67	42.1	92	57.9
M	52	26	50.0	26	50.0	158	63	39.9	95	60.1
N	54	23	42.6	31	57.4	139	54	38.9	85	61.1
O	43	15	34.9	28	65.1	131	25	19.1	106	80.9
P	44	14	31.8	30	68.2	122	20	16.4	102	83.6
Total	760	324		436		2,195	750		1,445	
Average per student	47.5	20.2	42.6	27.3	57.4	137.2	46.9	34.2	90.3	65.8

to 45%; the average for the group was 34%, almost exactly the 33.3% which was the goal.

Exact figures are not available concerning the control student's patient load. It is estimated, however, that the average control student had a greater number of patient contacts (both adult and pediatric) than did the average GMC student. He saw more individual patients, but fewer patients making revisits. In the medical and pediatric specialty clinics the student did not usually see the same patient twice, and in the pediatric clinic, where his total experience was limited to six weeks, there were but few revisits for each student. The total number of patients seen varied less from one student to another in the control clinic than in the GMC, and the proportion of pediatric to adult patients varied hardly at all.

Although the total number of patient contacts in the GMC was slightly less than at the Colorado General Hospital clinic, it should be remembered that the GMC student had experience outside the clinic in the Family and Home Care Program. The first five GMC groups also spent four half-days per week on the medical and pediatric wards and in four different medical specialty clinics. Thus, the total number of their patient contacts was probably as large as that of the control students. For the 1956 II group, however, the ward and specialty clinic experience was replaced by three half-days per week spent in electives. The total clinical experience for this group was certainly less than that of the control students in their class.

GMC Patients' Missed Appointments

Missed appointments were frequent enough to have a significant effect on the functioning of the GMC and on the utilization of the student's time. Even more important, the failure of the patient to keep his appointment meant the interruption of continuity of care and an incomplete case for the student.

Table 5.5 shows that during 1955 (January 1 through December 31), out of a total of 19,059 appointments made in the GMC, 3,748 or

Table 5.5. Missed appointments in the GMC during 1955, by type of patient contact

	No. of appointments made	No. of appointments missed	Percentage of appointments missed
First visit (new patient)	2,472	613	24.8
Revisit	16,587	3,135	18.9
Total	19,059	3,748	19.7

20%, were missed.[3] The proportion of missed appointments was higher for new patients (25%) than for patients making revisits (19%). As one might expect, the missed appointment rate was highest in winter. The proportion of appointments missed by adult patients (19%) was almost the same as the proportion missed by pediatric patients (22%).

Although missed appointments were a serious problem in the GMC, the rate in that clinic was far lower than in the other clinics of the Denver General Hospital outpatient department. Table 5.6 shows the missed appointment rate for a sample period (January 1 through May 31, 1955) in the various outpatient clinics at Denver General. The rate for all other adult clinics was 38% and for the pediatric clinic 59%. During the same period the missed appointment rate at the GMC was 22%.[4] This large discrepancy suggests that the GMC patients were better satisfied with their experiences in that clinic than were patients in the other Denver General clinics, and that there were significant differences between the patients' experiences in these clinics. The GMC differed from the other clinics in three ways that may have accounted for the lower missed appointment rate: (1) the patients were repeatedly seen by the same physicians, who were interested in them; (2) it was the only clinic which adhered as closely as possible to a strict appointment system on an hourly basis (although patients in the GMC sometimes had to wait, this problem was not so great as in other clinics); and (3) more time was spent with the patients in GMC than in other clinics.

A study of the factors influencing the GMC patients to keep or to break appointments revealed interesting findings.[5] Eighty-eight patients were interviewed: 44 who had consistently kept appointments over a period of six months and 44 who had missed at least three consecutive appointments over a period of six months. They were all questioned in an effort to determine the primary reasons for either keeping or missing their appointments.

In the delinquent group some patients reported that they could not afford transportation to the clinic or purchase of medication; others

[3] Missed appointments include only appointments broken without notification of the clinic. Cancelled appointments are not included. Figures regarding missed appointments in 1954 and 1956 are similar to those for 1955.

[4] Some of this difference can perhaps be explained by the fact that a few of the GMC patients were screened for their reliability before being referred. About 16% of the children seen in the GMC had been carefully chosen for well-child care, and the obstetrical patients seen in the GMC had also been selected for their reliability.

[5] Violet Zawalski, "A Study of the Motivation Factors which Led Patients Either to Keep or Not to Keep Appointments in a Selected Outpatient Department" (thesis submitted in partial fulfillment of requirements for a master's degree in nursing, 1956).

Table 5.6. Missed appointments in all Denver General Hospital clinics during sample period, January–May, 1955

Clinic	No. of appointments made	No. of appointments missed	Percentage of appointments missed
General Medical Clinic	8,242	1,831	22.2
Other adult clinics*	10,566	3,942	38.3
Pediatric clinic	2,826	1,677	59.3

* Includes gynecology, obstetrics, orthopedics, and surgery.

found it difficult to keep appointments because they had to work. Many of the patients came from families with small children and said they broke their appointments because they were unable to pay for or to find baby sitters.

The ethnic background of the patients was related to the rate of missed appointments. Spanish-American patients made up 30% of the delinquent group and only 12% of the group that kept appointments well. Twenty-seven delinquent patients listed assorted problems relating to unsatisfactory interpersonal relations with various hospital staff members or occasionally with their own physicians. Most of these problems appeared to be inherent in the clinic setting, as indicated by the following typical complaints: "Too many doctors examined me . . . "; "The clerk in the admission office was inconsiderate . . . "; "I felt I could get better medical care elsewhere." The remainder of the responses were more directly related to the communication difficulty between physician and patient: "The doctor never tells you what he is doing . . . "; "The doctor said nothing was wrong . . . "; "I couldn't understand the doctor . . . "; "The doctor said that he couldn't help me."

It is of particular interest that the 44 patients who kept appointments well listed good interpersonal relations as a primary reason for doing so. These patients almost unanimously expressed confidence in their physicians and were particularly pleased to see the same doctor on each visit. It seems likely that this reaction was the principal reason that a higher percentage of GMC patients kept appointments than did patients in the other clinics at the same hospital.

In spite of the fact that fewer appointments were missed in the GMC, the rate was high enough to interfere with the smooth functioning of the clinic. It was necessary to schedule approximately 25% more new patients for each clinic session than were actually desired in order to compensate for the 25% missed appointment rate among new patients. This often resulted in having too many new patients on some days and too few on other days. It was also necessary to have a fairly extensive and careful system of follow-up for patients who missed appointments.

The most unfortunate result of the missed appointments was the time wasted by the student when his patients failed to keep their revisit appointments or to cancel them in advance. Since approximately 20% of the patients making revisits did break appointments, about 20% of the student's time was wasted in this way. Often several members of one family would have consecutive appointments with a student at a single clinic session, and their combined missed appointments might well result in the loss of the entire clinic session to that student.

Importance of the Patients

Many members of the GMC staff felt that the patients played an extremely important role in determining whether the General Medical Clinic Program achieved its objectives. Some of the areas in which the influence of the patients seemed to be important to the student's learning process are described below. This discussion is based primarily on observations of the medical staff, the sociologist, the social service workers, and the students. The students' comments were obtained in conversations with the staff, particularly in the preceptorial meetings, and from the students' summaries of their experiences in the Family and Home Care Program.

It appears that the patients seen in the GMC were less desirable for teaching purposes than those seen in the Colorado General Hospital clinic. The GMC students were concerned because their patients presented fewer disease entities than patients in the control clinic. This dissatisfaction was expressed most strongly by the 1956 II group, for whom the GMC provided the only senior-year clinical experience in medicine and pediatrics. The students' Family and Home Care summaries indicate their discouragement. One student wrote: "There seems to be no hope for Mrs. H. She is like so many of the General Medical Clinic patients . . . lots of complaints, but nothing is really wrong with her." Another reported: "The chronic medical problem in this family is primarily the father's desire to remain ill. This seems to be motivated by his intense dislike of work. Any suggestion on the part of the doctor that he has recovered brings on a marked increase in his symptoms, even though we can no longer demonstrate evidence of organic disease."

Some students were so dissatisfied with their patients that they expressed the belief that all good medical material was referred elsewhere. This opinion was reported frequently to the staff, even though the GMC was the only medical clinic at Denver General Hospital. Much of this dissatisfaction seemed to relate to the importance the student attached to being able to make a clear-cut diagnosis and to carry out a successful therapeutic regime with a patient who was motivated to get well.

Students were frequently thwarted in completing diagnostic study because patients missed appointments or refused to cooperate. The repeated failure of a patient to keep clinic appointments prevented adequate diagnostic work-up. In many instances, a student reported that he had good clinical evidence of a diagnosis such as peptic ulcer, which might readily have been confirmed by x-ray, but because the patient repeatedly broke his clinic appointments, the x-ray was never obtained, and the patient was never seen again. The data on missed appointments suggest that students were able to complete the medical work-up and carry out a therapeutic regime in almost 80% of the cases, despite frequent frustrating delays attributed to the patients.

The Family and Home Care summaries indicate that patients' refusal to cooperate was one of the greatest disappointments encountered by the GMC students. This frustration is illustrated by the case of a six-year-old girl with severe congenital heart disease. Her mother refused to allow electrocardiographic or radiologic evaluation because she feared that the work-up might lead ultimately to surgery. The mother continued to bring the child to the clinic for symptomatic treatment, but the student expressed extreme frustration over being unable to confirm his clinical impressions and refer the child for corrective surgery. Several students reported unsatisfactory experiences in trying to manage inactive rheumatic fever patients because the patients did not appreciate the importance of continuing to take pills when they were completely free of symptoms. (In a few of these cases the parents showed even less understanding than the children themselves.) Particularly troublesome were patients with cirrhosis of the liver. Since most of them were homeless, unemployed, hopeless alcoholics, attempts to provide good medical care, which always requires the patient's cooperation, almost always were unsuccessful.

Although the staff, especially in pediatrics, tried to stress the importance of preventive measures in medical care, practical application was often unsuccessful because patients would not cooperate, particularly if they felt entirely well at the time. This attitude completely defeated the original program for well-child care in the GMC. Although the mothers of babies in the Denver General newborn nursery were carefully screened by the public health nurse to determine their willingness to bring their babies to the GMC for well-child care, the missed appointment rate was so high that another source of infants had to be found for this program.

The S family, as described in a student's summary, exemplified this problem. Although they had lived in Denver for eight years prior to coming to the GMC, the mother had failed to take any of the children regularly to the readily available city well-baby clinics or to a private physician for routine care. At the urging of the visiting nurse, she had taken Susan for one visit, but had not returned. Questioning revealed she had failed to return because Susan had had a slight febrile reaction to her first immunizing injection with DPT.[6] Even though the mother had been warned that this might happen, she could see no reason why she should take a well child to a clinic where she was made ill. This attitude existed in spite of the fact that the three older children had had severe pertussis. In this case, because of the good rapport that developed with the student physician, the mother finally accepted the need for preventive care and brought the younger children to the GMC.

Most of the mothers seemed receptive to the idea of immunization and would listen to advice about well-child care. Many of them, however, did not really comprehend the need for this type of clinic visit and therefore were not willing to put forth the effort to continue. It must also be remembered that for a large number of them the effort required would have been considerable.

The students' discouragement over frustration of their efforts to carry out preventive measures was expressed in their summaries: "This family has been quite unsatisfactory in providing experience in comprehensive care as a family unit. The mother's consistent failure to keep return appointments and both parents' lack of interest in attempting to bring their children in for well-child visits made them a difficult family." Another student said of his experience: "This family had not taken advantage of the facilities available to them. They like me as a physician, but I strongly suspect that the factors of apathy, underlying emotional problems, and ignorance may have come between them and their desire for medical attention." The staff and students both noted, however, that the cooperation of many families and the rate of kept appointments greatly improved as the physician-patient relation became better. This was often aided by a home visit, as noted in the following comment from a student's summary: "All members of this family are very independent people who do not readily follow medical directions. In the past they have cancelled numerous appointments and were quite unable to achieve the necessary insight into their problems. However, since a home visit, they have come to appreciate the medical care program as practiced in the General Medical Clinic and appear to be quite happy and satisfied with it."

Problems of communication, described in Chapter 4, made it particularly difficult and in some instances impossible for the student to

[6] Diphtheria, pertussis, and tetanus.

take an adequate history and frequently seemed to interfere with the development of a satisfactory physician-patient relation. Many patients, especially those of the Spanish-speaking group, were reluctant to discuss problems not directly related to the immediate illness. Some could give only a very vague account of their previous medical problems and symptoms. Discussion of the social and emotional aspects of their lives was often considered "out of bounds" by the patient, even though the student and staff felt that such information was frequently an essential part of the patient's illness. One student summed up his experiences as follows: "This family has always been quite friendly and appeared anxious to have me see them. But there was some barrier, partly language, which kept me from being able to establish rapport to the extent necessary to carry out effective therapeutic measures."

A frequent deterrent to the development of a good physician-patient relation was the great difference between the moral and ethical standards of the student and those of the patient. The patient was often expected to meet moral standards appropriate for the student and his society. The staff was concerned that some students were extremely judgmental, particularly in regard to alcoholism, the presence of illegitimate children in the family, and the acceptance of welfare assistance. Many of the Family and Home Care summaries reflected this critical attitude. One student wrote of his family: "I see no immediate solution to their problems, and feel certain that any appeal to their intellect, social consciousness, or consideration for others is destined to fail, because they simply do not possess the faculties to appreciate the simple virtues of society. The GMC has failed dismally to fulfill its functions in the case of this family, in spite of all of our efforts." Another student said: "I wish to impress the reader of this report that like most other people enjoying any benefit which welfare agencies have to offer, the H family received the clinic, their doctor, the social worker, the nurses, and all others with an attitude that discouraged the most ardent worker from continuing with an active interest in the maze of entanglements into which they interposed themselves." Another commented: "Mr. K's recreation consists of watching the family television set with an occasional interlude of general mistreatment of wife and family."

The problem of illegitimacy disturbed many students. Often they were critical of the clinic families in which illegitimacy was fairly commonplace: "The father of Josie was a serviceman who squired Jane for only a few months before his departure. He had moved away from Denver by the time she gave birth to Josie. Their relationship was admittedly not close, and Jane apparently felt ashamed concerning the episode, though not repentant."

The reluctance of many patients to discuss their emotional problems often interfered with the efforts of the student to carry out psychotherapy. Some patients did not perceive that minor emotional problems in themselves or in their children were a cause for concern. This was particularly true, for instance, of enuresis, which many mothers seemed to consider a part of normal childhood. It was rarely recognized as a symptom calling for medical assistance; thus, it was almost impossible for the student to work with the parents.

Students also reported that efforts in psychotherapy or medical management were sometimes handicapped by their inability to solve the serious socio-economic problems which many times were directly related to the psychological or medical problems. Often it was found that a GMC family had been known to many welfare agencies for a number of years, with the result that most of their social problems already had been considered and all available assistance had been given. A few students reported that they became involved with petty financial problems which were quite unrelated to the patients' medical problem. One mother asked her student-physician to write the welfare department on her behalf to suggest that more funds be allotted so that the family might purchase a new washing machine. However, there was in this family no specific medical problem relating directly to the breakdown of the old washing machine.

One of the most unfortunate effects of using this group of patients for teaching was that many students, because of repeated frustration of their efforts to deal with the social aspects of medical care, developed a defeatist attitude toward these matters. Some of the more rigid and censorial students seemed to become even less tolerant in their attitudes toward major social problems.

Since nearly all the patients came from the same low social group and had similar medical, social, and emotional difficulties, the student had little chance to work with patients who presented certain problems more common to other social groups. Even so, nearly every student had the opportunity to work with some patients on whom he could successfully practice comprehensive medical care.

The patients illustrated the need for preventive medicine more frequently than would patients of another social group. Some students, for instance, had the opportunity to observe the seriousness of pertussis in the small child who had not been immunized, or the effects of spreading shigella dysentery in a tenement house.

A number of summaries revealed a fairly active approach to the social situation on the part of the student. In one case, a young mother of a large family could be treated for her acute attack of rheumatic fever only at home because she refused to remain in the hospital.

The student solved this problem by making frequent home visits and arranging through the hospital's social service for the welfare department to place a housekeeper in the home to care for the children. Many families failed to understand either their medical problem or its treatment, and in these cases the students had to call upon the public health nurse to insure that the appropriate measures were carried out.

Most of the GMC students had an opportunity to work with patients, both adults and children, who had emotional problems. Despite the various communication difficulties discussed above, students reported gaining valuable educational experience from their attempts to help these patients through superficial, supportive psychotherapy. Certain students who impressed the staff as rigid and hostile were able to develop fairly good relations with a few of their GMC patients. Most patients expressed a great deal of confidence in their student physicians. Several tried to compensate the student with money or gifts in appreciation of the time he had spent with them. It was only the rare patient who requested a different student physician.

It can be seen that both the students and the staff felt that the GMC patients were unsuitable teaching material for a comprehensive care program. They presented a limited variety of disease entities and overwhelming social problems; they did not appear anxious to regain health and employment; and they broke appointments so frequently that clinic function was significantly affected. There was often a serious communication barrier between patient and student.

In the light of this experience it seems that a program devoted to teaching comprehensive care would be most effective if patients from a wide variety of social backgrounds were made available to the student.

The control students, whose experience was at Colorado General Hospital, shared many of these problems, since 85% of their patients came from the two lower socio-economic groups (compared with 92% of the patients in the GMC) and a fairly large proportion were Spanish-speaking (17% compared with 30% of the patients in the GMC). However, since the control students usually did not care for their patients over as long a period as did the GMC students, and since the specific educational goals of the control clerkship were different from those of the GMC, the social background of the patients was less important.

Chapter 6

The Family and Home Care Program

Comprehensive medical care frequently requires the physician to understand the interpersonal relations within the patient's family and to have more than superficial knowledge of the patient's social environment. The Family and Home Care Program was designed to provide the General Medical Clinic student with appropriate experience in these important areas of comprehensive medical care. Originally it was thought of as two programs—the Family Care Program and the Home Care Program—but in practice it amounted to a single program.

Experience in the care of an entire family was provided in the following manner. When a patient was assigned to a student, that student became responsible for the care not only of the patient but also of other members of the patient's family. Whenever the medical history showed that other members of the family required medical attention, either for current complaints or for preventive care, appointments were made for them with the student physician at the clinic. The other children in the families of many pediatric patients, for example, were brought into the clinic for a review of each child's need for routine immunization, tuberculin testing, and physical examination. Each patient was told, and reminded with a written note, that he would have the same physician at each clinic visit and that if he or members of his family should need medical care, they should request an appointment with that physician. A filing system was set up so that whenever a new patient visited the GMC a check could be made to determine whether any other member of his family had been treated there, in which case the new patient was assigned to the same student physician.

Thus, with few exceptions, all patients who were members of a single family were seen by the same student physician; moreover, unless the patient lived alone, each patient seen by a student represented a potential for family care.[1]

The second objective of this program was to provide the student with a better understanding of the relation between a patient's social and psychological environment and his medical problems. In the hope of achieving this, a single family was assigned to each student (or selected by him) for intensive medical care, including home care. Then, throughout the entire six-month period, the student served as family physician for that family. He not only saw the members of this one family each time they visited the clinic, but was also on call for medical service and advice at all times.

Selection of the Families

The method of selecting families for the Family and Home Care Program changed somewhat during the course of the period under study. Students in both 1954 groups were assigned families previously chosen by the staff. In spite of careful screening by the social service department and the medical staff, however, a significant number of the families chosen was, for various reasons, unsuitable.

It was therefore decided not to assign families to the next group of students (the 1955 I group) but rather to allow each student to choose his own family from among his regular patients. Under this arrangement many excellent families were obtained, but unfortunately some students either had no appropriate family in their patient load or acquired one so late in the clerkship that it was of little value in terms of a continued experience.

For the remaining students (the 1955 II, 1956 I, and 1956 II groups) a combination of the two previous methods was employed. At the beginning of his clerkship, each student was assigned a family chosen by the staff, but the student was permitted to choose a different family if, during the first six weeks of his clerkship, a more suitable one came to his attention. This method proved to be the most satisfactory.

Operation of the Program

The Family and Home Care Program operated in the following manner. As early in his clerkship as possible, the student saw and worked up the primary patient in his family. Appointments were then made for

[1] It should be pointed out here that this type of integrated care for entire family groups was possible only in a setting like the GMC, where adults and children were seen in a single clinic, under the combined supervision of the departments of medicine, pediatrics, psychiatry, and obstetrics; and where students could discuss the problems of several members of a family at conferences that often included at least two staff members representing different medical disciplines and a public health nurse or social worker.

the other members of the family whose needs for medical care required evaluation, and the student gave the family his name and telephone number, explaining that whenever any medical problem arose they were to call him. Each student was on call at all times; he was required to sign out to one of his colleagues for any period when he could not be available.

Whenever a student received a telephone call from the family, he discussed the problem with an appropriate consultant. (During the day the consultant was the appropriate member of the clinic staff; at night it was the house physician who was on call to the students for this service.) After this consultation the student took appropriate action: that is, he might give telephone advice only; he might make an appointment for the patient in the clinic; he might arrange to meet the patient at the Denver General Hospital emergency room; or he might make a home visit if one seemed indicated.

Each student was expected to make at least one home visit during his stay in the GMC. Since it was necessary from both the educational and legal standpoints to supervise these home visits very carefully, the following procedure was evolved. When a home visit appeared desirable, the student went to the home first and did the appropriate work-up of the patient. The resident physician on call for home visiting met the student at the home approximately one-half hour after the student's arrival. The case was reviewed by the resident, and the appropriate management carried out by the student.

The educational supervision of the family and home care work of the student was accomplished principally in the preceptorial meetings and the weekly comprehensive care conferences. The details and importance of these parts of the program are discussed in Chapter 7. At the end of his stay in the clinic, each student was asked to submit a written summary of his experience with his family.

Family and Home Care Patients

The Family and Home Care patients in the GMC Program differed, as one might expect, from the total clinic population, since this group had been carefully screened to include families that had at least one member with a chronic organic illness, had small children, and were composed of fairly reliable people interested in receiving medical care. The data presented below were compiled from 110 family units who participated in this program during 1954, 1955, and 1956. (Of these, 13 especially suitable families were used by more than one student group; thus the 110 family units represented 84 different families.)

Age of patients and structure of families. As shown in Table 6.1, a larger proportion of adult Family and Home Care patients than of the

Table 6.1. Comparison of Family and Home Care adult patients and total GMC adult population, by age

Age	Family and Home Care		Total GMC	
	No.	%	No.	%
19–44	130	89.1	627	30.7
45–64	16	10.9	638	31.3
65 and over	0	0.0	775	38.0
Total	146	100.0	2,040	100.0

total adult GMC population[2] was under forty-five years of age (89% compared with 31%).

The average size of the family units was six persons. Although every effort was made to have complete family units, only 72% were headed by a married couple; 28% of the "families" lacked a husband, primarily through separation or divorce. The high incidence of broken homes in the total GMC population made it difficult to find complete family units for this program.

Economic status and ethnic background. The annual income of 72% of the families in this program, was, as shown in Figure 6.1, between $1,500 and $2,999. Table 6.2 shows that the proportion of regularly employed household heads was considerably greater among the 110 Family and Home Care families (49%) than among the 1,402 sample families in the total clinic population (19%).[3] However, the income of families that were receiving welfare aid was much the same as of those whose heads were employed.

Figure 6.2 shows that the majority of the families paid between $20 and $60 rent per month. Since there was an average of six persons in a family, this suggests generally substandard housing conditions. Some of the families, however, lived in housing projects where adequate apartments were obtained for this rent.

The ethnic background of the Family and Home Care patients differed from that of the total GMC population: 49% of the former compared with 30% of the latter group were Spanish-American.

Medical characteristics. Since the presence of significant chronic illness was a criterion for a family's inclusion in the program, the incidence of organic disease was high. Table 6.3 lists the fifteen diagnoses most commonly found among these patients during the three-year period of this study. Forty-two of the 69 patients with diseases of the circulatory system had inactive rheumatic fever or rheumatic heart

[2] Data for the 2,040 GMC patients are derived from the sample discussed in Chapter 4, Table 4.2.

[3] Data for the 1,402 families in the total GMC population are derived from the 1954 and 1955 sample discussed in Chapter 4, Table 4.5.

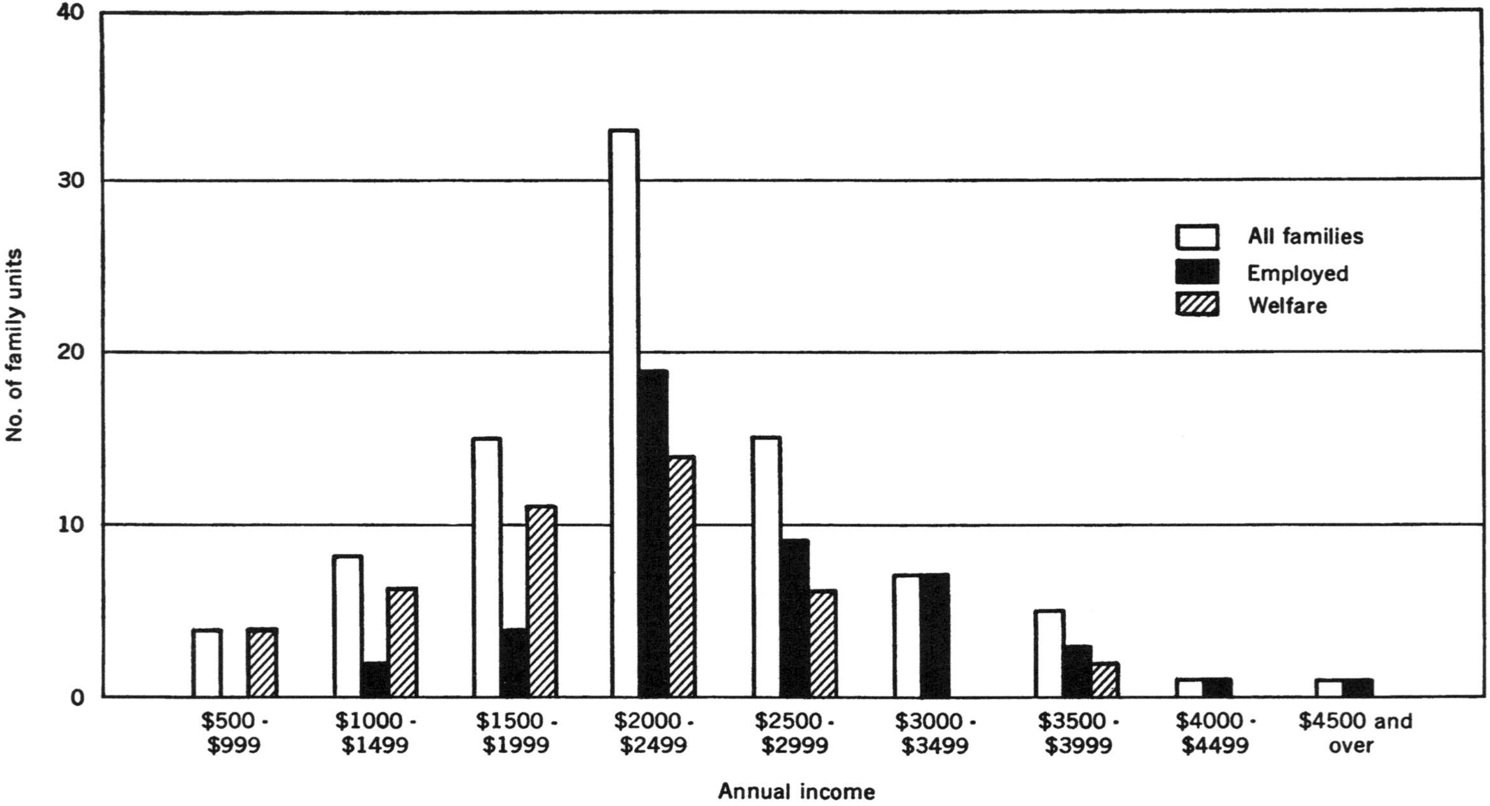

Figure 6.1. Annual income of families in Family and Home Care Program

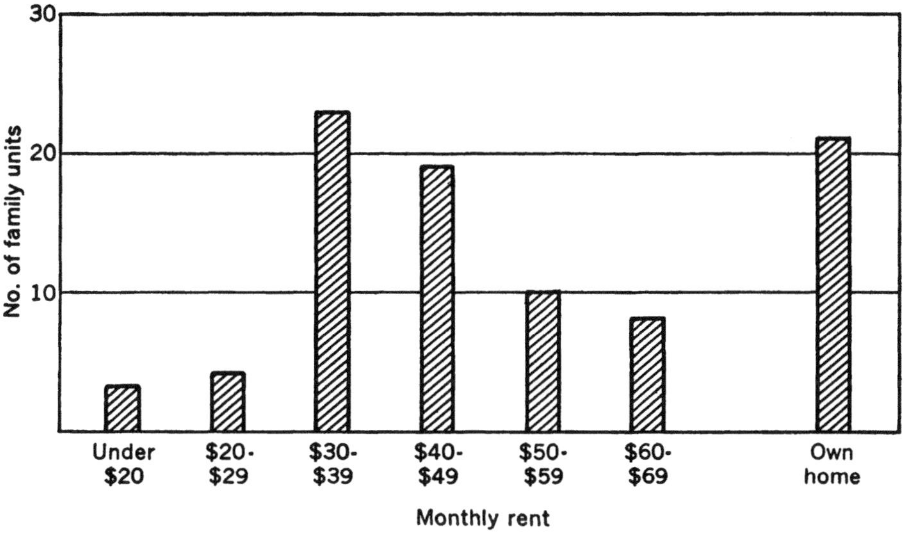

Figure 6.2. Monthly rent paid by families in Family and Home Care Program

disease; they were members of 29 families. Diseases of the respiratory system constituted the second most common diagnostic category, but most of these cases were acute respiratory infections that developed during the time the families were being followed by the students. Tuberculosis, included under "infectious and parasitic diseases," was present in 11 patients.

In spite of efforts to exclude families that presented major emotional or mental problems, psychoneuroses and personality disorders were fairly common; there were 2 patients with schizophrenia.

Patients with diseases of the digestive system included 9 patients with peptic ulcer, which was usually the primary chronic illness in the family. There were 10 patients with diabetes mellitus and 4 with myxedema. Among the patients with hematologic disorders were 2

Table 6.2. Comparison of Family and Home Care families and sample of total GMC families, by employment status of household head

	Family and Home Care		Total GMC	
Employment status	No.	%	No.	%
Regularly employed	52	49.1	229	19.1
Other*	54	50.9	967	80.9
Subtotal	106	100.0	1,196	100.0
Employment status not known	4		206	
Total	110		1,402	

* Includes irregularly employed, unemployed, and retired persons, and housewives.

Table 6.3. Fifteen diagnoses most commonly found in Family and Home Care patients (1954 to 1956)

Diagnosis	No. of patients
1. Diseases of the circulatory system	69
2. Diseases of the respiratory system	58
3. Well child	49
4. Infective and parasitic diseases	37
5. Allergic, endocrine, metabolic, and nutritional disorders	37
6. Diseases of nervous system and sense organs	36
7. Diseases of the genitourinary system	33
8. Mental, psychoneurotic, and personality disorders	27
9. Diseases of the digestive system	27
10. Deliveries and complications of pregnancy	20
11. Symptoms and ill-defined conditions	18
12. Diseases of blood and blood-forming organs	15
13. Well baby (under 1 year)	12
14. Diseases of skin and cellular tissue	11
15. Well adult	11

with hemophilia, 3 with chronic thrombocytopenic purpura, and 1 with Hodgkin's disease.

To summarize, a higher percentage of Family and Home Care patients had specific organic disease than did the total GMC population. Indeed, almost all available patients with certain diagnoses, such as tuberculosis, hemophilia, and rheumatic heart disease, were placed in the Family and Home Care Program.

Suitability of the Families to the Program

Considerable thought went into the selection of families for participation in the Family and Home Care Program. They were chosen on the basis of three criteria: (1) they should include at least one member with a chronic illness so that frequent clinic and/or home visits would be indicated; (2) they should include small children so that frequent acute problems would be likely to arise, as well as the chronic ones related to the basic illness; and (3) so far as possible families whose social or psychological problems were especially severe should be excluded. In an effort to ascertain how successful the staff had been in selecting suitable families, these families were evaluated on the basis of the students' summaries. A total of 87 such evaluations were made, the families being classified into three categories: satisfactory, partially satisfactory, and unsatisfactory. The judgment was based primarily on whether or not the student had been able to perform the role of family physician; successful performance of this role necessitated adequate illness in the family and their acceptance of the student as their doctor.

Of the 87 families evaluated, 48 appeared to have been satisfactory,

23 partially satisfactory, and 16 wholly unsatisfactory. Analysis of the families judged to be unsatisfactory or only partially satisfactory indicated that the difficulties were usually inherent in the family's shortcomings rather than in the student's inadequacy. As one might anticipate from the previous description of the GMC patients, the primary difficulty was related to their socio-economic and ethnic backgrounds.

Representative of the families that were wholly unsatisfactory is the G family, which illustrates several of the problems involved. This family consisted primarily of the mother and seven small children. Mr. G had been sentenced to jail in June 1953, for burglary, and the family was currently on relief. The primary medical problem was tuberculous adenitis in a three-year-old child. An effort was being made to treat this child at home with drugs. The children also contracted shigella dysentery while the family was connected with the program.

The G family, then, presented an adequate amount of disease. However, partly because of economic problems and partly as a result of their own attitudes, this family failed to provide the student with a satisfactory experience. For one thing, owing to the large size of her family and her inability to obtain a baby-sitter, Mrs. G was unable to keep appointments at the clinic. Thus, the student was obliged to make practically all contacts in the home. This in itself would not have been so serious a drawback if the family had taken a more intelligent and cooperative attitude toward their medical problems. However, they did not do so. For example, Mrs. G was quite indifferent to the problem of tuberculosis. In order to insure that the child would receive medication, the student found it necessary to count the number of pills left in the bottle at the time of his weekly visits to the home. Also, although he discussed general sanitary measures during the visit at which shigella dysentery was diagnosed and treated, no improvement resulted in this situation. The grandfather appeared to be the tuberculosis contact, but the student was unable to persuade this man to go to the hospital for an x-ray. At the time of the student's first visit, this family of eight was living in a two-room "outbuilding" behind Mr. G's parents' home. There was no running water, no toilet facilities, and no electricity in this building. With the student's aid, the family was moved to a housing project, but they kept their new apartment in the same state of disorder and uncleanliness, and used their meager welfare income to purchase a large floor-model television set. The student was greatly disappointed by this experience; he felt that this family had accepted him as merely another welfare agency, and he was frustrated and disturbed by his failure to achieve adequate medical management and to develop a good physician-patient relation. In the case of the G family, it would appear that social factors were largely responsible for their being unsatisfactory. Similar factors of a less severe nature resulted in other families' being only partially satisfactory.

The missed appointment problem, along with poor cooperation from the patient, accounted for the unsatisfactoriness of certain families. This is well exemplified by the R's, a moderately good family, but far from truly satisfactory. They presented a sufficiency of serious illness, including diabetes in both mother and father, active rheumatic fever in a twelve-year-old daughter, and severe congenital heart disease in a younger child. However, they were not wholly satisfactory in other respects, as the student's summary of his experience with this family indicated: "The General Medical Clinic has helped some to correct the medical problems and social problems of this family. Poor cooperation and missed appointments on the mother's part, however, made optimal care impossible. Nevertheless, the family members did seem to enjoy visits to the General Medical Clinic and to see me. Barbara, at least, stated that she wished I could continue to be her doctor and was concerned that I could not. This was gratifying, even in view of the rather incomplete medical care that could be given other members of the family because of poor cooperation."

In a few instances the difference between the students' and patients' social backgrounds proved a serious obstacle to a satisfactory experience in this program. In these cases, however, the primary difficulty seemed to be the students' inability to develop a satisfactory physician-patient relation with Spanish-American families. The linguistic and cultural barriers were important here.

A less frequent cause of a family's being unsuitable was that the medical problems were not sufficient to warrant an adequate number of clinic visits, telephone calls, or house calls during the six-month period. This problem occurred particularly when the students were allowed to choose their own families. For example, the H's only real medical problem was a convulsive disorder in one of the children, which was readily controlled and required only infrequent clinic visits. The student who worked with them reported: "The family has accepted my services and those of the General Medical Clinic very cooperatively and cheerfully. This was somewhat surprising to me, as they had been accustomed to the courtesies of private practice until two years ago. While my association with this family has been an enjoyable one, it has not been a very challenging or interesting medical experience because of the good health enjoyed by this family. For this reason I do not recommend their being used in the Family Care Program in the future." Another student summarized his experience with a similar family: "The reaction of the family to my activities as the family doctor has been more than cordial, but their need for care has been minimal. The fact that they were unable to persuade the mother to come to General Medical Clinic has made this family of limited value under the Family Care Plan." Since the mother in this situation was the one member with a chronic illness, this family's unsuitability was the result of lack of illness combined with lack of cooperation.

With many of the families it was a problem to find an adequate justification for a home visit. In most instances, however, some medical explanation could be given to justify at least one visit. In some families the opportunity made itself readily available as a result of acute illnesses in the children. However, many families had been accustomed to coming to the emergency room or the clinic with their acute problems, and it did not occur to them to call on their student physician for a home visit. Before the program was started, there was concern that some families might take advantage of home care and thus create an unnecessary burden for the student. The students' summaries, however, suggest that in almost no case did this occur; instead, many of the home calls were initiated by the student rather than requested by the patient.

A few families were unsatisfactory because the primary illness turned out to be entirely emotional in nature and of such a severe degree as to be more than the student could handle even under supervision. The reaction to such a family was expressed well by one of the students: "From the medical student's standpoint it has been a very frustrating experience to work with this family, realizing their potentialities and not being able to assist them." Another student put in a great deal of time with members of a very dependent, emotionally unstable family. He wrote: "In 1943 the J family moved to Denver from Kansas, where as rumrunners they had been financially successful. Their history in Denver has been one of rapid decline financially, rapid increase in family size, and worsening of social conditions. Mr. J has reacted by drunkenness, a poor employment record, irresponsibility, and anxiety; Mrs. J by outright psychosis." The student worked intensively with all members of the family, in particular with Mrs. J, and reported the following results: "Psychotherapy has been attempted under the guidance of the staff psychiatrist. Mrs. J has divulged a tremendous store of material regarding her mixed feelings: wanting the children and wishing to destroy them. However, any insight into the relationship of this to her symptoms has been very slow. Even more difficult is the task of getting any satisfactory adjustment to her very difficult situation. Having followed her through very trying times this summer, I am, however, convinced that supportive psychotherapy has a possibility of preventing another outright psychotic episode and that such prevention, if possible, is very probably of value to the family. I believe the probability of accomplishing more than this is very unlikely."

In a few cases the family appeared to be unsatisfactory or only moderately satisfactory because of problems relating to the student rather than the family itself. This was usually the result of lack of initiative on the part of the student, which resulted in an insufficient number of patient contacts. Sometimes, even though the number of contacts was adequate, the personalities of the student and the patient apparently made it difficult for them to develop an adequate relation. This situation was demonstrated particularly well by reports from two different students who had the same family for consecutive six-month periods. The first student commented: "Mrs. H is very pleased with the fact that she and her family are being carried as a unit in General Medical Clinic. She likes the idea of seeing one doctor for a six-month period rather than meeting a new doctor at each clinic visit. She seems to rely solely on that one person and can confide in him. This is an important aspect in the care of this family. She is very appreciative of the care given to her family by her doctor and speaks often of how wonderful both Doctors C and S were to her previously. I have enjoyed following this family very much and I believe that I benefited greatly both [in] increasing my medical knowledge and in bettering my relationship to patients." The student then went so far as to recommend a specific student in the next group that he felt would do a good job with this family. The second student summarized his experience as follows: "The role of the General Medical Clinic in the management of this family is merely one of a clearing-house in getting the members admitted to the hospital or as a follow-up after their admissions. There was some well-child supervision of the healthier members, some gynecological experience with the mother, and much sympathetic listening to the mother's problems. The family did not react strongly either toward or against the physician. I felt that I had gained less confidence from this family than from any other group I had seen in the General Medical Clinic. They are chronically public-supported and public-hospital-cared-for, and they give the impression of not becoming very reactive emotionally to any particular person. The mother was as willing to discuss all of her problems with the social worker, nurse, orderly, etc., as she was with the doctor, and I always had the feeling that she was seeing a new doctor every time she came to see me. I was not often contacted about the children, and the disease in this family is such that home care is usually not feasible, so that home visits were circumvented. For these reasons I do not believe this family is a good one for the Family Care Program."

It is interesting to note that the first student found occasion to have a total of 38 contacts and made 9 house calls as compared with 13 contacts and no house calls for the second student. It is probable that the second student's critical and judgmental attitude toward the family's way of life made it impossible for him to develop a satisfactory relation. This attitude appeared frequently in the summaries.

Another student expressed very clearly his own feeling of incompetence in establishing the physician-patient relation: "I should say that the family-physician relationship has not been satisfactory. This I attribute to my own shortcomings and partly to the family's independence or rather to their difficulty in trying to accept help. Another person might have had more success than I. I'm sure that this family has not felt that I was their physician, and I know that I have not played this role in the situation."

The majority of the families were moderately satisfactory in giving the student an opportunity to practice a comprehensive approach to medical care. These were the families who had an adequate medical problem that allowed frequent patient contacts, who kept their appointments, and who were generally cooperative in following the physician's recommendations for work-up and management. As a rule it was possible for the student to develop at least a moderately satisfactory patient-physician relation, so that the experience was gratifying to both him and members of the family. In most of the satisfactory families the psychological and social difficulties were not so overwhelming as to present insurmountable problems to the students. In general, families were considered satisfactory when it was possible to achieve some degree of success in improving either their physical health, their emotional status, or their social situation.

Patients' Reactions to the Program

Although no systematic study of the patients' reactions was made, it seems clear from the observations of both students and staff that the patients who participated in this program reacted very favorably. The medical staff was strongly of the opinion that the program provided the patients with better medical care than they would otherwise have received. The students' comments indicated that the patients shared this opinion. One student wrote: "Mrs. P has told me that it was a great relief to her and to her husband to know that all members of the family can be taken care of by one doctor. Both of them appreciate the value of the clinic for comprehensive care. They both know they are getting better medical care now than they have ever had in the past. This is primarily due to the fact that one doctor who is interested in the family is taking care of them." Another student reported: "Ruth has greatly enjoyed having a family physician in whom to confide and from whom to gain reassurance in regard to the medical problems which have occurred in this family. She also shows pride in having a personal physician in that she frequently has referred friends to me or to this clinic." Another said: "The family appeared very happy to have one doctor instead of many; the entire family has expressed this thought to me. All of them, and especially Mrs. A, appeared much more relaxed after two or three clinic visits and began to tell me about the problems with Mercy and Theresa. She also expressed her fears concerning pregnancy, which I do not believe she would have told if she had seen a different person at each visit." According to a fourth student: "Mrs. S expressed relief and gratitude that one doctor would see the family regularly. When first seen under the Family Plan, they registered absolute amazement when told that the same doctor would be available for night and emergency calls. She expressed continuing satisfaction with this system, probably partially because of the unhurried quality of the first two visits to the clinic and continuing attention of a certain individual. The advantages to the patient of a family physician are many. The consequent closer patient-doctor relationship in the General Medical Clinic as compared with other public clinics and the subsequent satisfaction with the medical care given should not be underestimated. Other patients have expressed even greater appreciation of the plan, even though changing doctors every six months is much oftener than they would like."

Students' Experiences in the Program

There was considerable difference in the total amount of time and effort expended by various student groups in this program. Figure 6.3 indicates the extent of participation in the Family and Home Care Program by each of the six student groups studied. This participation reflects the variations in the enthusiasm of the staff and students for the Family and Home Care Program during the three-year period of the study. There was a decrease in participation after the 1954 I group; then, except for the 1955 I group,[4] the others maintained a fairly uniform level of participation until the sharp decrease in the 1956 II group. The much greater participation by the first group of students probably reflected the initial enthusiasm of the staff for a new program. The explanation for the decreased interest of the 1956 II

[4] The decrease in participation by the 1955 I group is probably the result of hostility toward the principles and philosophy of the clinic overtly displayed by four of the students; among these four were the group leaders. Eight students in this group had very little family care experience, reporting four or fewer contacts with their families.

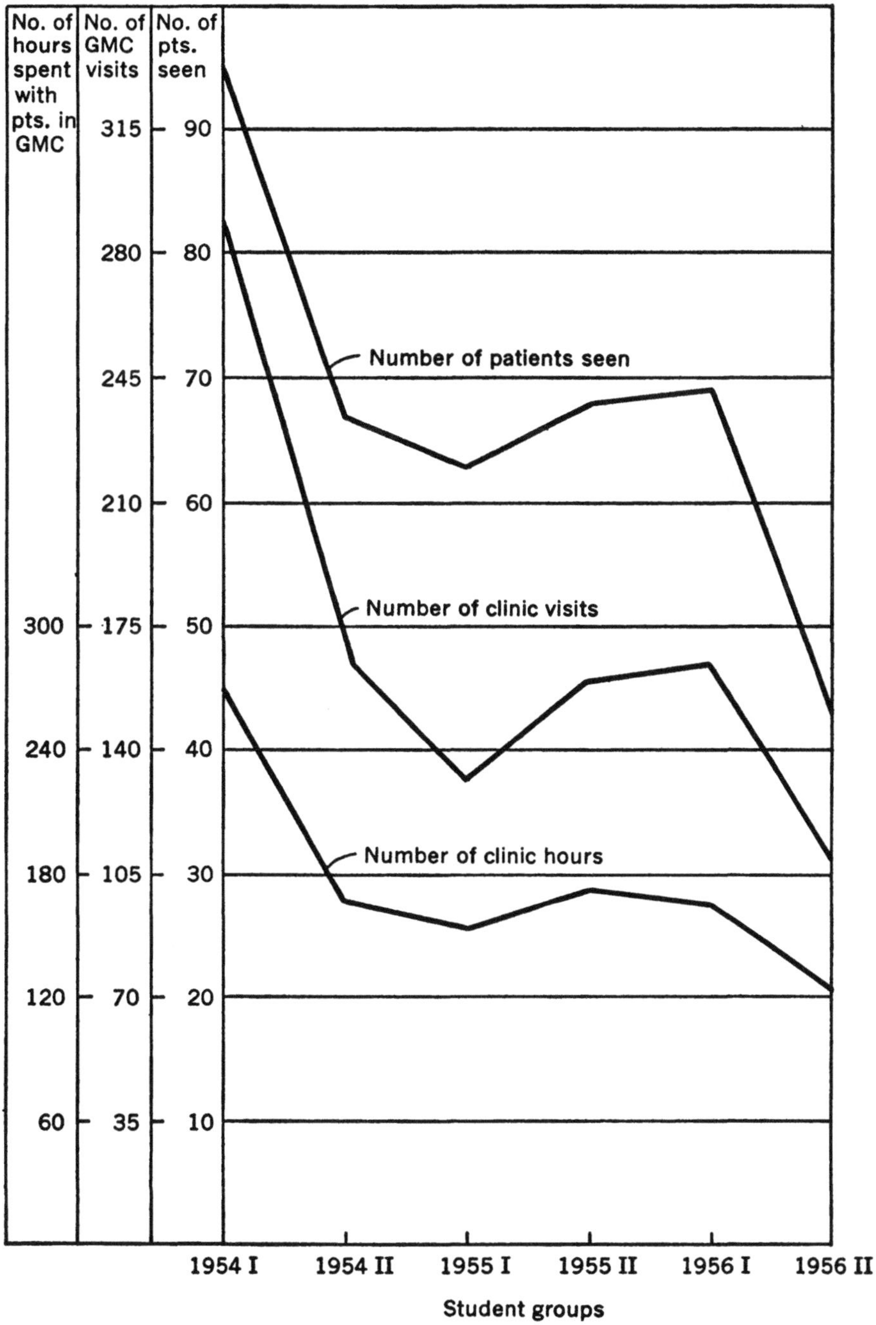

Figure 6.3. Total clinic contacts by students with Family and Home Care patients

Table 6.4. Average clinic contacts per student with Family and Home Care patients

Student group	No. of students	No. of students with families	Average no. of family visits per student*	Average clinic time per student on family care patients (hours)*
1954 I	21	21	13.7	13.7
1954 II	19	19	8.6	8.3
1955 I	20	19	6.6	7.7
1955 II	17	16	10.0	10.8
1956 I	18	18	9.3	9.3
1956 II	17	12	9.1	10.2

* Averages based on number of students who had families.

group is probably to be found in the changes that occurred in the GMC staff and curriculum at that time. The most important change (described in detail in a later section) was the abandonment of the comprehensive care conferences and the preceptorial meetings, which greatly diminished the opportunity for faculty and organizational stimulation of the students. The result was that 5 students out of the 1956 II group of 17 did not carry a family.

Tables 6.4 and 6.5 summarize student participation in the Family and Home Care Program. It will be noted that the average amount of clinic time per student spent on Family and Home Care patients varied from 13.7 hours for the 1954 I group to 7.7 for the 1955 I group. The average number of visits by each student making home visits varied from 1.6 for the 1955 I group to 4.0 for those students in the 1956 II group who had the initiative to undertake this program. The average amount of travel time varied roughly from one to two hours. The average amount of time spent on the home visit varied from 1.6 to 3.4 hours per visit.

Table 6.5. Average home contacts per student with Family and Home Care patients

Student group	No. of students	No. of students with families	No. of students making home visits	Average per student*: No. of home visits	Average per student*: Travel time (hours)	Average per student*: Time spent on home visits (hours)
1954 I	21	21	19	3.0	1.4	2.2
1954 II	19	19	15	2.3	2.1	3.3
1955 I	20	19	15	1.6	1.0	1.9
1955 II	17	16	12	3.5	1.4	2.3
1956 I	18	18	8	1.7	1.0	1.7
1956 II	17	12	7	4.0	2.0	3.4

* Averages based on number of students who had families.

Although the average amount of time for the students in each group did not show much variation, there was, over this three-year period, a tremendous amount of variation in the effort put into the Family and Home Care Program by individual students. Table 6.6 gives some idea of this variation. For those 6 students who had over 30 contacts with their families, this program probably took considerably more of their total time in the GMC than would have been ideal. For the 23 students with less than 5 contacts (including the 7 students who carried no family) the total experience was probably quite inadequate. However, for the large majority of the students the experience seemed to have involved about the right proportion of their total time.

Importance of the Program

The Family and Home Care Program was designed specifically to achieve several of the goals of the General Medical Clinic Program. There was no counterpart in the control clerkship, except for a day of home visits on which the student accompanied one of the Denver public health nurses on her regular rounds. Much of the data in the students' summaries suggested that the Family and Home Care Program provided at least some of the GMC students with an experience that was quite different from anything provided by the control clerkship.

In the first place, the summaries indicated that most of the students who had good families viewed this experience with feelings of satisfaction and accomplishment. Their most prevalent comment was that this program gave them a feeling of being real doctors. One student wrote: "In working with this family I have felt as though they regarded me as their own private physician, and I was often called upon as a consultant in many problems other than strictly medical. I'm sure that they appreciated my home visits, and it was gratifying and rewarding to see the children rush to the door and shout back to their mother, 'Here comes the doctor!'" Another student commented: "I was welcomed into their home on my visits. I was made to feel that I was liked and accepted by them as a competent physician."

The reader should not infer that the student's satisfaction was one

Table 6.6. Total number of contacts by all students with Family and Home Care patients

Total no. of family contacts	No. of students
31–41	6
21–30	8
11–20	50
5–10	25
0–5	23

of the goals of the clinic; it was merely a by-product of a concerted effort to give him as much responsibility as possible. However, it was the impression of the staff that in many instances this reaction had the advantage of stimulating greater initiative in the student and greater awareness of the comprehensive aspects of medical care. On the other hand, it may also have had the disadvantage of producing overconfidence in the student.

The summaries showed that most students were aware of the importance of social factors to the medical and psychological problems of the patient in at least their own families. The home environment and the social factors affecting the family were usually described, and the majority of students went on to correlate these factors with the medical problems. For example, the interaction between social factors, psychological factors, and organic illness was described in a report on a family in which the father had a duodenal ulcer and the mother had neurodermatitis. Because of the father's illness and the large size of the family, rather serious economic problems had arisen. The student recognized the cycle which began when the mother's worry regarding the economic problems aggravated her previously quiescent neurodermatitis into an active process. The husband's emotional problems were then amplified by the presence of the wife's dermatitis and his own inability to solve their economic difficulties. This in turn led to a severe exacerbation of his ulcer symptoms. The neurodermatitis and the ulcer so incapacitated the parents that the eldest child had to drop out of school to care for the younger children. The student, with the assistance of the social service department, was able to help the family solve some of their economic and housing problems. This reduced the emotional strain on the family and considerable improvement resulted in the neurodermatitis and the duodenal ulcer. The student stated: "There is no question but that the social agencies have played a tremendous role in aiding this family to get back on its feet. The economic aid provided by welfare has reduced many of the anxieties and perhaps prevented further medical and emotional problems which could have cost society even greater sums."

On occasion students became too preoccupied with social problems, and some of the summaries indicated that as a result of their experiences in this program, some of the more rigid students became even more judgmental in their attitudes toward indigent patients. The following comments regarding the social situation in two of the families are fairly typical. One student wrote: "The main problem confronting this family is social. Neither the mother nor the children have any pressing medical problems which are of major importance, and the minor problems are being solved. Social service has been of help in obtaining financial aid when this family was desperate, without making them a permanent relief family like so many others which have been created by over-zealous social workers and over-charitable city governments. The father is apparently able to work and will have to fulfill his social obligation in this respect." Another reported: "This family's major problem is obviously financial. The General Medical Clinic has fulfilled the family's medical needs very adequately, and the children are now provided for by Aid to Dependent Children. I feel that the family can expect no further improvement unless the father either leaves completely so that the family can obtain total welfare aid or else returns to the family and goes to work."

A few students were impressed with certain psychological factors related to both the physician-patient relation and the illness itself. The frequent contacts with a single family should have given the student considerable experience in developing physician-patient relations. On some occasions difficulty in this area was occasioned by the personality of the student himself, but more frequently the difference between student's and patient's social background was primarily responsible.

Case histories demonstrated that many of the patients in the GMC were extremely immature people with marked dependency needs. In some such situations the student became too involved with the patient. An extreme example of this was described by one of the female medical students: "I liked Joyce from the start and she seemed to like me. However, as time went by, she became extremely dependent upon me, so much so that it began to be embarrassing. For instance, the doctors on the GYN ward could not do anything unless she consulted me about it. On one occasion she made them revise their surgery schedule because I had told her I would be leaving town in September for a short vacation and she wanted me there for the surgery. On several occasions when she was taken to the operating room she created quite a fuss until I arrived. In fact, on the morning of her big operation I was upstairs in the delivery room. I rushed down to the operating room as soon as I could because I had said I would be there, and I found the surgical team, headed by the chief of the service, waiting for me—a senior student!"

The student himself often expressed concern about having to discontinue the relation with his family; he often felt that he was really just beginning to know them at the end of six months and was just getting to the point where he could perhaps help them with their emotional problems. One of the summaries stated: "All members of the family conveyed to me a feeling of appreciation for my immediate efforts, and it has been a pleasure dealing with these folks. I regret that I must leave them, for I am just beginning to understand them enough so that I can begin to help them." Another expressed almost the same thoughts: "I have enjoyed working with this family and especially wish I could continue in an effort to solve Joseph's problems, which I have only recently begun to understand more fully."

Insight into the family relations associated with psychosomatic problems was clearly expressed by many students. This was brought out with particular clarity in a family where the husband had very severe rheumatic heart disease with mitral stenosis and aortic insufficiency, and the wife had an active duodenal ulcer. The student described the mother's problem as follows: "Mrs. M is the thirty-four-year-old wife of Sam and the mother of his five children. Her medical problem, I feel, is very closely related to Sam's heart disease. About one year ago she had a duodenal ulcer demonstrated by x-ray. It seems that exacerbations of her symptoms are related in time with Sam's disposition and periods of increased symptomatology in his heart disease."

It is of interest that the student frequently did not become aware of the existence of serious emotional problems in his family until nearly the end of his time in the GMC. Many of the summaries suggested that, although almost no psychotherapy had been made available to the families, such treatment would be advisable in the future. Students also came to recognize that in many cases relatively little would be gained even from rather intensive work with their families: "I feel that more psychiatric aid should be offered the family, especially the mother to resolve some of her deep-seated conflicts. This would require an intensive effort, however, and I am not sure that the results would be commensurate with the effort." Two students carried families whose primary problem was a rather severe psychological one. Thus, as a result of the Family and Home Care Program, a few students had fairly impressive experiences in psychiatry under the supervision of one of the clinic psychiatrists.

The staff gained the impression from observations of the students, from comprehensive care conferences, and from the students' summaries, that the Family and Home Care Program had given at least some of the students an increased opportunity to develop physician-patient relations. They also noted that some students had clearly recognized and described the way in which family relations might produce psychosomatic or emotional symptoms. Most of the psychotherapy performed in the Family and Home Care Program consisted of sympathetic listening combined with the giving of assurance when needed. A survey of the students' summaries leaves the impression that many of the students felt that this type of activity had been extremely worth while to both the patients and themselves.

It seemed to the staff that much of the popularity of this program resulted from the fact that most students succeeded in developing more confidence in their ability to fill the role of physician. Although few of the students expressed this opinion, one wrote: "This was an excellent experience for me insofar as my medical education is concerned, in that much confidence in myself and my decisions was gained. Consequently, I am now of the opinion that I can better cope with similar situations as they will confront me in my future career."

The data from the students' summaries and the staff's observations suggest that for at least some of the students this program provided a good setting for achieving some of the goals of the GMC. These students clearly showed that they had become aware of the importance of social and psychological factors in the optimum care of a family of patients.

It was the impression of the staff that this type of Family and Home Care Program could be a valuable asset in stimulating the student to develop attitudes necessary for comprehensive medical care. The intensive relation with a single family afforded an adequate home care experience for the student, if at least one member of the family had a sufficient need for home care. Adequate stimulation of the students by the staff through frequent preceptorial meetings appeared to be necessary. The stimulus provided by the comprehensive care conferences also seemed essential to insure effective participation in this program by all the students. The students' summaries clearly indicated that the optimum success of such a program depends to a great extent upon the selection of appropriate families. In view of the many disadvantages of the GMC population for teaching comprehensive care (discussed in Chapters 4 and 5), it was encouraging to find that satisfactory patients could be found by careful screening. It was also the impression of the staff that the amount of contact between the student and the patient had an effect on the degree of satisfaction found by the student in dealing with patients of a different social background. In general, a limited relation, such as occurred in specialty clinics, produced very little reaction on the part of the student. Somewhat more extensive contact (of the type experienced with many of the GMC patients) led in some cases to dissatisfaction on the part of the student and a poor physician-patient relation. However, still further contact, such as some students had in the Family and Home Care Program, frequently led to a satisfactory physician-patient relation because the student developed better and more sympathetic understanding of the social and psychological factors involved.

Chapter 7

Other Teaching Techniques (Conferences and Special Programs)

Several special teaching techniques besides the Family and Home Care Program were employed in the General Medical Clinic. Since no parallel techniques existed in the control clerkship, these distinguishing characteristics of the GMC will be described in some detail. Two of these activities, the comprehensive care conferences and the preceptorial program were very closely related to the Family and Home Care Program. The other teaching techniques were the psychosomatic conferences, the medical and pediatric seminars, and the well-baby and obstetrical programs. These programs and conferences were conducted essentially as described below until marked changes were made in some of them for the 1956 II group. The changes are reviewed in detail in Chapter 8, since the over-all experience of the 1956 II students was considerably different from that of the previous groups.

Comprehensive Care Conferences

The primary aim of the comprehensive care conferences was to encourage the student to consider, discuss, and coordinate the social, psychological, and medical aspects of his patients' illnesses. The GMC staff believed that one such conference per week was necessary to teach successfully the philosophy of comprehensive medical care. All the conferences were informal; the students and staff sat around a large table rather than in a classroom. Since maximum participation by the students was encouraged, staff participation was kept to a minimum.

The method of achieving the aims of the comprehensive care conferences varied considerably during the three years of the study. Originally, the conferences dealt only with the patients in the Family and Home Care Program. A different family was discussed each week, and every student was given the opportunity to present his family at least once. An attempt was made to consider all the family's problems during the one-and-a-half-hour period. Details of the medical problem were emphasized as well as the social and psychological factors that were important in the total care of the family. The student and his preceptor usually planned the conference at least one week in advance so that the other students might know the subject and prepare themselves through appropriate reading. Whenever indicated, the student also consulted with the social worker, the psychiatrist, the public health nurse, or the sociologist, and most of these staff members usually participated in each conference.

The exact pattern of the conferences and the degree of student participation varied. Sometimes prepared discussions of the important aspects of the problem were presented by other members of the same preceptorial group as the student whose family was under consideration. In other conferences, particularly those led by an unusually capable student, there was more spontaneous discussion by all the students.

This type of conference, in which an attempt was made to discuss all aspects of the family's problems, was tried for the 1954 I group. It rapidly became apparent that the scope and complexity of the problems in each family were too great to be dealt with in the space of an hour and a half. This was, of course, related to the fact that the medical problems of many of the GMC patients were complicated by unusually serious social and psychological difficulties.

Thus, the form of the conferences was changed after the first group of students. A comprehensive care conference was held every other week and was alternated with a clinical medical conference. In both types of conferences student participation was emphasized. At the comprehensive care conferences the social and psychological aspects of a family's medical problems were stressed, and the purely medical aspects were discussed only in relation to these factors. At the medical conferences discussion was limited to the illnesses of patients who were not necessarily connected with the Family and Home Care Program.

The staff found that certain family problems provoked more stimulating comprehensive care conferences than others. A family in which there was a patient with a chronic illness (such as tuberculosis or rheumatic fever) in which social factors were important in the cause or management invariably made good conferences, provided the discussion was led by a student or staff member who could direct the thinking of the group along appropriate lines. A family in which the primary disease was one (such as peptic ulcer, asthma, or hypertension) that is generally considered to be influenced by psychological factors provided exceptionally good conferences. Chronic illnesses (such as diabetes and obesity) in which psychological factors were particularly important to the management of the patient provoked stimulating discussion of the illness. Although family problems that were entirely emotional occasionally produced stimulating conferences, the students often seemed opposed to purely psychiatric discussions.

The practice of alternating a comprehensive care conference with a medical conference was continued for the 1954 II, 1955 I, 1955 II, and 1956 I groups. The form of the comprehensive care conferences was changed drastically for the 1956 II group.

Seminars

Weekly teaching sessions of one hour were held for small groups of students. The aim of these seminars was to review with the students certain concepts and principles of the management of ambulatory patients. The more common medical and pediatric problems of the GMC patients were discussed. Before the seminars, the students were given a bibliography compiled by the staff and were encouraged to come prepared to participate actively in the discussion. The seminars were well attended by the students and were believed by the staff to be useful.

Psychosomatic Conferences

Psychosomatic conferences were conducted for the students in the GMC during part of the period covered by the study. Groups of four or five students participated in these conferences, with each student having the opportunity to attend approximately six. At these conferences one student presented a carefully prepared case from his GMC experience. The conferences were led by a staff psychiatrist and an internist (or pediatrician), but again maximum participation by the students was encouraged. These conferences were generally well liked by the students.

Preceptorial Program

Each General Medical Clinic student was assigned to a preceptorial group of approximately four or five students. Two staff physicians were assigned to each group as preceptors. As a rule one of these was an internist and the other a pediatrician.

The aims of the preceptorial system were: to make available to each student at least one member of the teaching staff with whom he could discuss freely any problems related to clinic function or to the care of his patients; to encourage and guide the student in his role as family physician in the Family and Home Care Program; to give the preceptors an opportunity to discuss in an entirely informal way the staff's concepts of the philosophy of comprehensive care. The groups met informally at least once a week for approximately one hour, immediately after the comprehensive care conference. A member of the social service department often joined the preceptorial groups.

In these meetings the status of each student's family was reviewed briefly, and an effort was made to stimulate the student's continuing active interest in the family. There was also considerable discussion of the comprehensive care conference that had just been completed. This gave the staff an excellent opportunity to discuss comprehensive care in general. Some time was usually spent planning a future comprehensive care conference that would be presented by members of the preceptorial group. Both the staff and the students participated actively and regularly in the preceptorial meetings during all of 1954 and 1955, and the first half of 1956. During the second half of 1956, these meetings, for reasons that will be discussed in Chapter 8, were for the most part discontinued.

Importance of the Conferences

The comprehensive care conferences had no counterparts in the control clerkship, and it was the impression of some of the medical staff that these conferences represented one important difference between the experience of the GMC students and that of the control students.

The reaction of the GMC students to these conferences was in general extremely unfavorable. This was expressed frequently in preceptorial meetings and in the course of the conferences. Students often commented that the social and psychological aspects of the problem did not need further emphasis and generally tried to plan their conferences to stress the purely medical factors. Considerable guidance by the preceptor was often needed to obtain a conference that did emphasize the broader aspects of the family's illnesses.

The comprehensive care conferences represented the only time in the student's GMC experience that the fundamental philosophy of the clinic was discussed in an organized manner by the entire student and staff group. The effect of these conferences was difficult to assess. It appeared that the open discussion of psychological and social problems, and the hopelessness of their solution, increased the antagonism of some students toward the idea of comprehensive medical care. Other students complained that only common-sense knowledge was being discussed, which was a waste of time. Nevertheless, the students did actively participate in the discussions and frequently became quite involved in debates about the role of the physician in society, the responsibility of the physician for his patients, and similar subjects. Almost every student actively studied the possible causes and solutions of the problems of the family he presented to the conference. For this reason the staff believed that students benefited from the conferences even though the only attitude acceptable to most student groups was one of dissatisfaction and tension.

The students appeared to be somewhat more satisfied with the comprehensive care conferences when these were alternated with medical conferences. This arrangement also allowed more adequate time for discussion of the social and psychological factors in one conference and the medical factors in the other.

An important by-product of the conferences was the stimulus they gave the student to get to know his family well. Frequently, when there had not previously been a good medical reason for making a home visit, the student would make one for the first time to prepare for his conference. In many instances a considerably more detailed history was obtained from various members of the family in order to have information that would be needed for the conference. The staff felt that the Family and Home Care Program was aided by using these families as the case material for the comprehensive care conferences.

Preceptorial meetings were regarded as important for a number of reasons. They gave the members of the medical staff a chance to know at least five students extremely well and gave the students a chance to know at least two of the staff members. Perhaps one of the most important contributions of these meetings was the opportunity they offered the students and staff to discuss informally the philosophy of comprehensive care. Some students were enthusiastic supporters of this approach, and others demonstrated increasing hostility toward it. The preceptorial meetings stimulated the students to think about comprehensive medicine and frequently provoked vigorous arguments. Most of the GMC students in the 1956 II group were denied this opportunity, as were all control students.

Although guiding the student in the care of his family was not a primary goal of the preceptorial meetings, the staff soon became aware that the success of the Family and Home Care Program depended to a very great extent on these meetings. It was often apparent to the preceptor, in the course of a discussion about the student's family, that the student still had insufficient information with which to assess the total needs of the family and carry out comprehensive care. The student often needed his preceptor's guidance and stimulus to serve effectively as family physician.

Importance of the Seminars

The importance of the seminars and the psychosomatic conferences was rather difficult to determine. Both students and staff seemed to react favorably to these activities, and the attendance and participation of the students was good. The psychosomatic conferences in particular provided a considerable period of time during which GMC students were exposed to a discussion of the available knowledge concerning the relations between emotion, body functions, and disease. No similar experience was offered to the control students.

Obstetrical Program

Each student was assigned responsibility for the care of two normal obstetrical patients during his stay in the General Medical Clinic. One patient was in early pregnancy and the other in the last trimester. Under the close supervision of the obstetrical consultant present at each clinic session, the student assumed full responsibility for the prenatal care and instruction of these patients. They were given the student's telephone number, and he was on call to them twenty-four hours a day as he was for his Family and Home Care patients.

If a student was called in regard to important obstetrical or gynecological problems when the GMC was not in session, he usually saw the patient in the Denver General Hospital emergency room under the supervision of the house staff. When his patient was admitted to the hospital in labor, the student was given the opportunity to follow her through the course of labor and to deliver her under the supervision of the obstetrical resident. In general, this system worked quite well.

The student was responsible for the postpartum care of the patients delivered by him as well as for that of the mothers of other newborn infants whom he was following as part of the well-baby program.

Well-Baby Program

As early in his GMC career as possible, each student was assigned two newborn infants (in addition to those described above) with the hope that he would be responsible for their care over a six-month period. These babies were chosen from the Denver General Hospital nursery. In addition, each student had as patients babies in other clinic families. All these infants were seen at approximately monthly intervals, and, under careful supervision, the student took full responsibility for their well-child care. He was also responsible for detailed observations regarding their physical, psychological, and motor development.

Despite careful screening by the social worker or public health nurse in an effort to appoint to the clinic only those babies whose mothers expressed interest in becoming GMC clients, an unusually high percentage failed to keep the first clinic appointment. As noted in Chapter 5, this was probably owing to lack of understanding of the need for preventive measures in an apparently well child. The majority of the students, however, did eventually have the opportunity to follow at least three or four well babies, but because of missed appointments the duration of follow-up was often limited to two or three months. Because of the extremely high missed appointment rate in this group, this source of patients was eventually abandoned.

Importance of the Obstetrical and Well-Baby Programs

The GMC provided the student with the long-term experience which seemed to be of particular value in prenatal and well-baby care. The obstetrical program was quite successful in meeting this objective, since the missed appointment rate was low, and the majority of the students followed at least two obstetrical patients for six months and delivered at least one of them. This experience seemed to contribute to the development of the student's sense of responsibility for his patients.

The well-baby program was a good facility for learning the principles of growth and development and of well-child care. The students expressed their confidence in being able to give adequate preventive care to infants and children. As noted above, however, this program was handicapped by the high rate of broken appointments. In spite of this difficulty, it was the general conclusion of the staff that prolonged follow-up of a few babies was a more satisfactory way of teaching well-child care, growth, and development than was the single-visit evaluation of many different babies.

Chapter 8

Changes in the GMC Program

During 1956 several important changes were made in the General Medical Clinic Program, primarily in the special teaching programs and conferences. Most of these changes affected only the 1956 II students. There were two reasons for making changes at that time. First, it was felt that a somewhat less rigid program was desirable for GMC students, and some of the changes aimed at achieving this effect. Second, many of the students in the first five groups had expressed dissatisfaction at spending conference time in discussions of the nonmedical aspects of patients' problems, and some of the changes were designed to make the emphasis on comprehensive care a little less formal and more spontaneous.

Since it seems likely that the resulting program was noticeably different from the experience of previous GMC groups, the important changes in the curriculum, the staff, the comprehensive care conferences, the preceptorial meetings, and the Family and Home Care Program are reported below. No comparable changes were made in the program of the control students.

Curriculum Changes

The curriculum changes in the General Medical Clinic Program affected only the 1956 II group. It will be remembered (see Chapter 2) that the original GMC curriculum consisted of five half-days per week spent in the General Medical Clinic itself (one of these being a conference period), two half-days spent in conferences attended by the entire class, and four half-days spent in medical specialty clinics and on the medical and pediatric wards. For the 1956 II group, however, the four half-days spent in the medical specialty clinics and on the medical and pediatric wards were eliminated. One of these half-days was added to the time spent in the GMC, to make a total of six half-days in that clinic, one of which was used for a conference. The other three half-days were made available for an elective course in some special area of medicine or pediatrics. These elective courses were under the supervision of faculty members in the departments of medicine and pediatrics and involved clinical work, research, or a combination of both. That is, a student taking his elective in diseases of the respiratory system might spend one half-day in the chest clinic, another half-day on the chest wards, and the third half-day working on a related research project. Alternatively, he might spend all three half-days in the clinic and on the ward, or he might devote two, or even all three, half-days to his research work. In general, the students tended to favor the clinical activity; only one elected to spend all three half-days in research work.

The above curriculum changes meant, among other things, that whereas previous GMC groups had received only about one half of their actual medical and pediatric experience in the GMC itself, the 1956 II group received its entire senior-year medical and pediatric experience in that clinic. This apparently led to some uneasiness among members of this group. Although a survey of student opinion indicated that in general the students enjoyed their electives and thought them worth while (an opinion shared by most of the staff), many students commented that the scheduling of the elective entailed the sacrifice of some of the more important aspects of their medical education. This student group also frequently expressed dissatisfaction with the GMC patients and seemed much more concerned about this problem than previous groups—probably because they realized that their GMC medical and pediatric experience would not be supplemented by contacts with other patients in the specialty clinics and on the hospital wards.

Staff Changes

There were a number of changes in the medical and pediatric staffs of both the General Medical Clinic and the control clerkship during all three years of the study, but most of these changes were routine personnel turnover and probably did not lead to any important differences in the teaching received by successive groups. A possible exception occurred during the third year of the study (1955–56); the principal member of the pediatric staff of the GMC became acting head of the department of pediatrics at the school of medicine. This meant that his services were in large measure lost to the GMC for that period, and as a consequence the instruction in pediatrics in the GMC was less systematically oriented toward the goals of comprehensive medical care. This was more obvious during the second half of 1956.

A reduction in the number of social workers available to the GMC also made a significant difference in the students' experience. During 1954 and 1955 three highly competent social workers were available at all times for consultation, help, and teaching. However, during the first half of 1956 only two of these workers were available and, more seriously, during the second half only one was available. This undesirable situation was caused by the shortage of qualified social workers; as first one, then two, of the social workers left, the vacant positions remained unfilled. The service load for the single worker during the end of 1956 was so great that her opportunities for teaching and consultation with the students were very severely limited. As a result, the role of the social worker and the importance of social factors in the total care of the patient was probably emphasized less effectively for the 1956 II students than for the students in the other five groups.

Changes in the Comprehensive Care Conferences

The comprehensive care conferences were rather profoundly changed during the second half of 1956 primarily because of the students' continued dissatisfaction with conferences based on a carefully planned discussion of a family's total problems. The staff hoped that the students would respond more readily to discussion of this type if it was allowed to come up spontaneously during the conference, rather than being planned in advance. Accordingly, the conferences were redesigned. Instead of families in the Family and Home Care Program, patients who had been hospitalized from the GMC were used as subjects for discussion; and instead of centering each conference around the presentation of a single family, as many patients were presented during each conference as time permitted.

The result of these changes was that although both the staff and the students enjoyed these conferences, relatively little time was devoted to the more comprehensive aspects of medical care; in most cases the discussion dealt almost exclusively with the medical problems. One reason for this tendency was that the students frequently knew so little about the patients' social and psychological history that discussion of these aspects was impossible, except on a purely speculative basis. Thus, for the 1956 II group the comprehensive care conferences involved considerably less discussion of comprehensive medical care than was the case with the first five groups.

Changes in the Preceptorial Meetings

The principal change in the preceptorial meetings was an indirect result of the changes in the curriculum. Although it had been planned to continue these meetings for the 1956 II group essentially as they had been conducted with the other five groups, various changes in the curriculum made it impossible to schedule a regular time for these meetings. Therefore, although the preceptorial groups were designated and weekly meetings were encouraged, there was such great difficulty in arranging a time convenient for all members of each group that the meetings were held much less frequently than with previous groups.

As a result, the staff and the students in this group did not come to know each other so well as in the other five groups, and the excellent opportunities for informal discussion of comprehensive care which the preceptorial meetings had provided in the past were for the most part lost. The students lost the guidance of one or two staff physicians in the management of their Family and Home Care patients, and the staff physicians lost the opportunity to encourage the students to make the most of their experience in this program.

Family and Home Care Program

No changes (in the sense of planned modifications) were made in the Family and Home Care Program during the second half of 1956. However, the effect on this program of the changes described above was so important that some discussion of it seems appropriate here.

There was a very marked decrease of interest and participation in the Family and Home Care Program among the 1956 II students (see Chapter 6). Many students did not participate at all in this program, and most of those who did became much less well acquainted with their families than had students in previous groups. In fact, the majority of the 1956 II students who carried families asked to be excused from preparing and submitting summaries of their experience in the program on the grounds that they had not come to know the families well enough to make such a project worth while. Only 6 members of this group of 17 students completed these summaries, whereas nearly every student in each of the previous groups did so.

This decrease of interest and participation in the Family and Home Care Program was caused almost entirely by the changes in the comprehensive care conferences and the virtual discontinuance of the preceptorial meetings. As noted in Chapter 7 the comprehensive care conferences stimulated the student to become more familiar with his family's problems. In order to present his family effectively at a conference, the student had to become acquainted with the members and their problems. As he became more involved with them and tried to work with them he gained valuable experience in this phase of comprehensive medical care. Similarly, the first five student groups devoted a considerable portion of their weekly preceptorial meetings to reviewing the status of each student's family. This impelled the student to see members of the family who had not been examined previously, to obtain more information about social and psychological factors, to make additional home visits, etc. The deterioration of the Family and Home Care Program in the second half of 1956, when these two sources of stimulation were removed, suggests that most students needed this kind of continuing stimulation and guidance to derive maximum benefit from such a program. In fact, many students obviously required this sort of prodding even to participate in the program. A considerable part of the 1956 II group missed all or some of the experience in comprehensive care that might have been gained through knowing and following one family very closely both in the clinic and in the home.

The changes in the General Medical Clinic Program, nearly all of which affected only the 1956 II group, occurred for a variety of reasons, but their over-all cumulative effect was to reduce the emphasis on comprehensive medical care. In particular, the changes in the comprehensive care conferences, together with the virtual discontinuance of the preceptorial meetings, by eliminating opportunities for formal and informal discussions of comprehensive care between students and staff, greatly reduced the effectiveness of the Family and Home Care Program. Because their entire senior-year education (in medicine and pediatrics) was confined to the GMC, the 1956 II students saw a slightly less varied group of medical entities than other GMC students. On the other hand, because of the elective offered them, they had somewhat more freedom to pursue their special interests and gain experience in research.

Chapter 9

General Problems

It was, of course, to be expected that the establishing of the General Medical Clinic would be accompanied by a number of problems. In this chapter the more important difficulties are discussed under the following headings: problems of communication, problems related to the medical school, and problems related to the hospital.

Problems of Communication

At the very outset an important problem of communication arose; indeed, this was the source of many of the more specific, practical difficulties that later arose in relation to the medical school and the hospital. The trouble was simply that the term *comprehensive medical care* (the goal of the General Medical Clinic) had different meanings to the various groups with which the GMC, as a complex, multidisciplinary program for total medical care, had to interact.

During a three-year period the proposal for the creation of a general medical clinic was drawn and redrawn repeatedly, and the idea of such an outpatient program was given much local publicity. During the next one and a half years, while the physical structure was being prepared and the staff being organized, the actual plans for operation were worked out. In these four and a half years the broad view of the GMC became known to the entire medical school and associated hospitals, and many groups became actually involved in planning the clinic. These included (at the medical school) the administration and the departments of internal medicine, pediatrics, psychiatry, surgery, obstetrics and gynecology, preventive medicine and public health, human growth, and graduate and postgraduate education; and (at the city department of health and hospitals) the administration, the nursing service, the visiting nurse service, the social service, the admissions office, the record room, the central laboratory, the x-ray department, the board of health and hospitals, the city budget and personnel office, the hospital personnel office, the mayor and the city council, the division of disease control, and the pharmacy. These groups were all striving for improvement; comprehensive medical care seemed obviously better than non-comprehensive medical care; so in the beginning they all enthusiastically acclaimed the establishment of the clinic. However, as plans became less general and more definite, it soon became apparent that each of these groups had its own concept of comprehensive care and its own views about what the purpose of the clinic should be, and that the actual objectives of the clinic were identical with none of these views.

For example, to some the notion of comprehensive medicine implied nothing more than a complete examination of all patients admitted to the Denver General Hospital emergency room and clinics. Others held that medical care would be comprehensive only if it included all the eligible people in the community. In some instances misunderstanding led not only to disappointment but to frustration and hostility.

Other types of communication problems arose as a by-product of the complexity of the GMC and its relation with many other groups. Frequently, those responsible for the clinic made plans to solve problems or devised better ways of doing things, only to be disconcerted at some later time by the failure of their plans. Investigation frequently revealed that someone had neglected to make the plan clear to one or more of the groups upon whom it depended—such as students or other members of the clinic staff.

Problems Related to the Medical School

The second group of problems that accompanied the establishment of the General Medical Clinic concerned relations between the GMC and other sections of the medical school. The establishment of a new educational program within the institutional structure of a medical school is likely to conflict with pre-existing values and goals. This, of course, is more apt to happen when the new program is introduced into a rigid, well-established, tradition-bound organization, and is less likely to occur in a young medical school not bound by tradition. The flexibility and tolerance of a young faculty in a young institution make the introduction of new ideas comparatively easy, but do not guarantee their support. Indeed, certain characteristics of a new institution contribute toward lack of support for any departure from the traditional.

For example, an institution that is rapidly expanding (as the University of Colorado School of Medicine was at the time of the GMC's development) is beset by many struggles and problems. These valuable and necessary struggles require vast expenditures of energy and thus drain away some of the potential strength that an older institution might call upon in support of a new educational program. The effort to establish the organization and procedures necessary to achieve high standards of medical education, medical research, and medical care concerns every member of every department and demands most of the mobilizable energy. The officials responsible for the administration and policy of the institution are frequently involved in these struggles. Departments and subdepartments strive to obtain the best possible staff, to establish themselves as functioning and identifiable entities, and to organize and support their programs of service, teaching, and research. The young full-time member of the clinical faculty tends to settle himself into his specialty, develop his clinical skills, expand his research staff, and publish research papers.

In such a setting it is clear that any general medical or pediatric outpatient department, particularly one organized primarily to teach a broad concept of medical care, is likely to have at best a secondary position. The goals and demands of such a clinic are sometimes at cross purposes with the goals and demands of the more usual research and clinical activities. When such conflict occurs, decisions are almost always made in favor of the established and time-honored activities—the clinical specialties and the inpatient service.

The GMC, an experimental outpatient program, was generously supported by outside funds and was widely publicized before it began, two facts which necessarily exerted pressure upon the university to facilitate its success. The university enthusiastically supported the clinic, and many members of the faculty gave their time freely to advise and to help solve its problems. There were many times, however, when GMC's needs for medical staff conflicted with the needs of the inpatient and specialty services. In almost every instance the decision was made in favor of the inpatient or specialty service. Moreover, most of the faculty were heavily committed to teaching assignments so that their assistance in the new program was necessarily limited.

Problems Related to the Hospital

The third group of problems stemmed from the fact that the General Medical Clinic, as mentioned in Chapter 2, was established, not in the medical school hospital (Colorado General) but in Denver General Hospital, an institution only secondarily devoted to medical education.

Denver General Hospital is a public hospital supported by the

City and County of Denver as an agency for providing medical care to the indigent and medically indigent of the city and county, and emergency medical care to anyone who applies. It had long been associated with the University of Colorado as a teaching hospital, but this affiliation had little meaning until 1947. At that time the newly elected mayor of Denver, Quigg Newton, and the progressive dean of the medical school, Dr. Ward Darley, with the able assistance of Doctors Florence Sabin, James Dixon, Lloyd Florio, and Solomon Kauvar, succeeded in establishing an intimate relation between Denver General Hospital and the University of Colorado School of Medicine. The major points of the resulting agreement were that all the patients of the hospital became available for medical school teaching; all the hospital staff were required to hold faculty appointments; the chiefs of the clinical services were appointed jointly by the hospital and the medical school; and the medical school provided the professional staff for the care of all Denver General Hospital patients.

During the next several years the ties between the two institutions became progressively stronger. Patient care at Denver General Hospital improved, and the laboratory and x-ray departments were expanded and improved. Full-time faculty representatives were employed by the medical school to organize the clinical services, and the scope and quality of graduate and undergraduate teaching at Denver General increased. By the time the GMC was begun in 1953, almost 50% of the medical school's undergraduate clinical teaching was done at Denver General Hospital.

However, nearly all the time, effort, and money devoted to improving Denver General Hospital were initially directed toward improving the inpatient service, including the x-ray department, the clinical laboratory, and the pathology department. The outpatient department was allowed to lag far behind. For the most part, it was a loosely organized collection of clinics, usually run by house officers alone. There was no place an adult patient could receive a complete medical work-up, and no organization for providing care for chronically ill patients. Recognition of the unsatisfactory state of the outpatient department and of the urgent need to improve it was the primary factor motivating Denver General Hospital to join the University of Colorado in proposing the GMC.

Discussion and planning of the actual operation of the clinic and the physical remodeling necessary to house the clinic began in early 1952. It very soon became clear that the objectives of a program designed to teach and practice total medical care often conflicted with the other primary objectives of Denver General Hospital. Despite the close association between the hospital and the medical school, and despite the evolution of Denver General Hospital into a teaching hospital, its major purpose continued to be the provision of medical care to the indigent and medically indigent.

The medical practice visualized by those who planned the clinic and who felt responsible for the education of the medical students could be realized only if certain conditions were fulfilled. The relation of some of these conditions to the customs of Denver General Hospital illustrates the basic conflict between education and service in this type of environment.

Any educational program in an outpatient clinic, and particularly one whose guiding philosophy is the idea of comprehensive medical care, must regulate the *type* and *number* of patients admitted. If these all-important variables are determined by any criteria except educational ones, the educational goals of the program are immediately compromised. The characteristics of the patients admitted to the GMC have been described in detail in Chapter 4. These patients represented the lowest socio-economic group, 90% being unemployed and 75% receiving community support. Lack of education, lack of occupational skills, lack of motivation to recover from illness, and unstable family structure were common. All efforts to modify the patient sample and make available to the student a more varied population of patients failed or at best received lukewarm support. The experience of the student was limited by the fact that his comprehensive care patients were nearly all restricted to a single social group. Certain characteristics of many patients and family groups made the practice of comprehensive care difficult, frustrating, and sometimes impossible.

Another example of this basic conflict, and probably a more important one, concerns the number of patients. It is clear that in any type of clinical teaching experience the number of patients must not be excessive. The pace of patient care must be regulated by the student's ability to participate fully and profitably in a program designed for him. This holds true for both undergraduate medical students and graduate physicians, but naturally is of greater importance for the medically less mature undergraduate. Good medical care and teaching are extremely difficult, if not impossible, when the student and the staff are burdened by a heavy caseload. The more time-consuming comprehensive approach in which the student is encouraged to spend as much time as is useful with his patients, and to discuss all his patients' problems with the appropriate consultant, is obviously impossible if the caseload is too heavy.

The GMC was usually burdened by too many patients. This was unavoidable because the primary reason for the existence and support of the hospital was service. All residents of Denver financially eligible for admission to Denver General Hospital, who needed medical care, had to be accepted; from June 1953 until June 1956 the only adult medical clinic at Denver General Hospital was the GMC; thus all patients who needed medical care were seen in the clinic. Various means of handling this growing load of chronically ill patients were improvised, each one being useful for a short time only. As each device became saturated, the pressure to see patients was apt to be transmitted to the students until a new method of coping with the problem could be put into effect. Thus, from time to time during these three years the teaching of comprehensive care was embarrassed by heavy patient-care demands.

In July 1956 the department of medicine of the medical school was able to inaugurate seven medical specialty clinics at Denver General Hospital, as well as a short-term medical care clinic for patients not suitable for the GMC or for the specialty clinics. These specialty clinics were undertaken with misgivings and doubts because the department already had a full set of specialty clinics at Colorado General Hospital. These additional clinics would solve the caseload problem of the GMC for the foreseeable future, but in the event of an economic depression that caused even a small increase in the number of patients eligible for admission to the city hospital, the facilities would be quickly swamped again. It would thus appear that good outpatient care and good teaching clinics can be maintained only if some means are provided of caring for the Denver General Hospital patients who overflow the teaching clinics. One obvious method of accomplishing this would be to secure the funds necessary to employ an adequate medical staff for this purpose. This should be a responsibility of the hospital rather than of the university. As pointed out by Deitrick and Berson in 1953,[1] and as is clearly obvious at the University of Colorado, university funds appropriated for the education and training of young physicians should not be syphoned off for this purpose, and faculty personnel should not be required to stretch their efforts any thinner than they are already doing.

[1] John E. Deitrick and Robert C. Berson, *Medical Schools in the United States* (New York: McGraw-Hill, 1953), pp. 139–156.

Part II

THE RESEARCH PROGRAM

Introduction to Part II

Chapter 10 includes a description of the purposes of the research project, the approach to the problem, the plan for evaluating the General Medical Clinic, and a discussion of certain limitations and problems encountered during the course of the research (1952–1957). Chapter 11 describes briefly the methods and procedures used in the research and summarizes the findings and conclusions. Detailed descriptions of methodology and findings are presented in Parts III and IV, respectively. Chapter 12, written jointly by the director and associate director of the General Medical Clinic, presents a general discussion of the clinic and of the research project, based on their five years' experience with both.

Chapter 10

Description of the Research Program

PURPOSES AND PLAN OF THE RESEARCH PROJECT

From the outset the research project was intended to serve two principal purposes: to evaluate the General Medical Clinic Program and to provide information relevant to medical education in general. In accomplishing these purposes, however, at least two other important though somewhat secondary aims would be achieved: as a pioneer study,[1] the project would explore the problems inherent in this type of research and it would answer questions about the value and feasibility of this type of psychological research.

The first purpose, to evaluate the GMC Program, did not, of course, extend to an evaluation of the *ends* of the program. It was concerned with answering two questions: Did the GMC Program enhance, impair, or have no effect on, the students' acquisition of traditional medical knowledge, and did the GMC Program result in the acquisition of knowledge, skill, and attitudes in addition to and different from those acquired through the traditional program?

The second purpose, to provide data relevant to medical education in general, concerned such questions as: What personality characteristics are associated with success in the GMC Program? What personality characteristics are associated with success in a traditional program of medical education? Can success or failure in such programs be predicted on the basis of personality measurement? The relevance of such information to the selection of medical students is obvious. It was assumed that data pertaining to the question *why* the

[1] See Robert K. Merton, George G. Reader, and Patricia L. Kendall (editors), *The Student-Physician: Introductory Studies in the Sociology of Medical Education*, Cambridge, Mass.: Harvard University Press, 1957; and *Journal of Medical Education* 31:515–565, 1956.

GMC Program did or did not achieve its aims would also be useful to medical education in general.

Since this research project was a pioneering effort, the third purpose was necessarily to explore and report on the problems inherent in this kind of psychological research. In the course of the project many such problems were encountered; some were solved satisfactorily; others were dealt with in ways that were perhaps not wholly satisfactory. For the information of other psychologists who may undertake this type of research at some future date, these problems and the measures taken to deal with them are discussed later in this chapter.

Finally, the fourth purpose of the research project was to determine the practicability and value of psychological research in medical education. Can such research be accomplished satisfactorily? Can it provide information of significance and use to medical educators? Does it make a contribution to basic psychological knowledge? The answers to these and similar questions should be of considerable importance.

Design of the Experiment

The first step in setting up the research project was to select a suitable design for the experiment. It appeared that the classical experimental design based on the use of experimental and control groups would best serve the purposes of the project as a whole. It proved feasible to divide each senior class so that half the students were in the GMC (the experimental group) and half in the usual senior medical clerkship (the control group). The students' schedules were arranged to allow time for the administration of pretests and posttests.

Experimental and control groups

Each of three classes (1954, 1955, and 1956) was divided into an experimental and a control group. Students were assigned to these groups at random. The groups were roughly matched for class standing in the following way: the class was divided into thirds on the basis of class standing, and an equal number of students from each third was randomly assigned to control and experimental groups. It should be noted that this design entailed a control group within the same medical school as the experimental group. This feature presented certain advantages and some disadvantages, which are discussed later in this chapter.

Curriculum and testing schedule

The curriculum in the senior year made it possible to arrange an experimental design which allowed more refined comparisons than a single pretest and posttest. As pointed out in Chapter 2, the control half of the class spent two quarters (three months each) on the medical clerkship (which included medicine, pediatrics, obstetrics and gynecology), one quarter on surgery, and one quarter free. The experimental group spent two quarters in the GMC, one quarter on surgery, and one quarter free. However, as Figure 10.1 shows, the sequence of these experiences was not the same for all students. For administrative reasons each group was further divided into two subgroups. This arrangement, shown in Figure 10.1, made possible an extremely interesting series of comparisons between the GMC and control groups:

1. Each of the eight groups of 10 randomly assigned students had a different sequence of experience. Thus, the most refined comparison that could be made was among eight groups.

2. Each experimental subgroup could be paired with a control subgroup which had an identical experience (except, of course, for the critical experience). Thus, E_1 matched C_1, E_2 matched C_2, E_3 matched C_3, and E_4 matched C_4. Thus, it was possible to make four comparisons.

3. It was possible to compare the combined groups E_1 and E_2

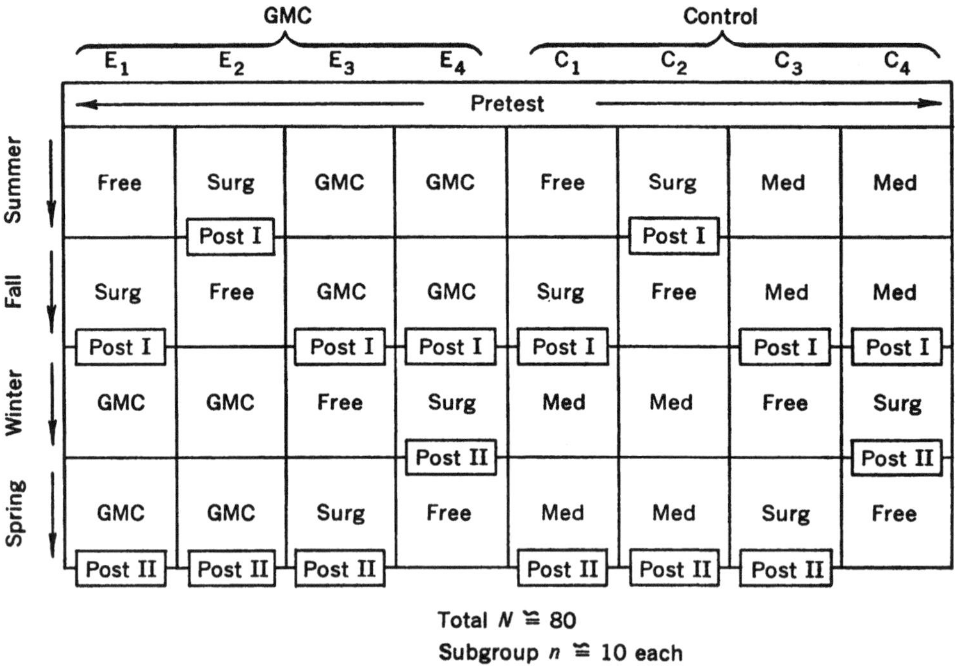

Figure 10.1. Curriculum and testing schedule for the GMC and control groups

with the combined groups E_3 and E_4 in order to discover whether the experience on the surgery clerkship affected the GMC experience, or vice versa. This comparison was possible because E_1 and E_2 took surgery prior to taking GMC, and E_3 and E_4 took GMC prior to surgery, and because Posttest I served as *pre*test for Posttest II. Similar comparisons could be made within the control group.

4. The combined groups E_1, E_2, E_3, and E_4 could be compared with the combined groups C_1, C_2, C_3, and C_4 in an over-all comparison.

Test administration

Two days were given over entirely to the Pretest administration. Approximately eight hours of that time were devoted to actual test taking. Two half-days each were allowed for Posttest I and Posttest II with the classes of 1954 and 1955, but with the class of 1956 one and a half days were allowed for each of these tests. Actual testing time averaged around six hours for each administration.

Besides the test administrations indicated in Figure 10.1, each student in the class of 1954 was interviewed for one hour during the same week in which the testing took place. Some of the students in the class of 1955 were interviewed twice, some three times. The students in the class of 1956 were not interviewed on a scheduled basis.

These curricula and testing schedules were maintained exactly as presented in Figure 10.1 for the classes of 1954, 1955, and 1956. No test administrations were missed or postponed.

Experimental variables

An important advantage of the design described above was that it drew attention to the three main sets of variables common to all experiments concerning behavior: independent variables, that is, those variables manipulated by the experimenter (in this case GMC vs. control medical clerkship); dependent variables, that is, those variables which appear as the results of such manipulation; and individual differences, that is, variations among individual subjects in their responses to the independent variables.

Independent variables. At the risk of oversimplification, it is important to point out the difference between the nature of independent variables in the usual laboratory experiment and the nature of the independent variables in the present study. In most laboratory experiments, in psychology or other disciplines, the nature of the independent variables is fairly obvious. For example, the experimental group is given some task to solve under certain conditions of noise, and the control group works on the same task during quiet. The experimenter describes the "noise" condition and "quiet" condition (the independent variable) in a simple way. The fact that these conditions are varied is ordinarily fairly obvious. In a study like the present one, however, the independent variables are not obvious. To be sure, a description may be available of the new and old programs by the people in charge of them, and the curriculum may describe how the student's time is allocated among various studies. But descriptions by the person in charge and statements about a curriculum only indicate how the programs should function—the experimenter must know how they actually function. Just what is the character of the independent variables of the experiment? Everything really hinges on the answer to this question, for unless the experimenter can state accurately which variables were manipulated (just how the experimental group differed from the control group), there is little point in trying to see what differences were produced. It is easy to see how erroneous conclusions might be drawn should the independent variables be incorrectly described. The efforts to describe the independent variables of this experiment are set forth in Chapter 14.

Dependent variables. In the present experiment the dependent variables were determined by the objectives of the GMC. For example, if the GMC was intended to inculcate positive attitudes in the student toward the psychological problems of patients, "attitudes toward psychological problems" would be a dependent variable, and some procedure for measuring this variable would have to be devised. In brief, dependent variables involved the "effects" of the experiment. These effects were measured by pretest and posttest comparisons, the details of which are presented in Chapter 13.

Individual differences. Those who devise experiments in human behavior must be prepared to find that although the independent variables may have the expected effect on the subjects, not all subjects behave as expected. There are always (or almost always) subjects in the control group who behave as experimental group subjects are expected to behave, and vice versa. In short, individuals in both the experimental and control groups are likely to differ from one another. In the present experiment it was important to identify the reasons for these individual differences. Such information should be of use in connection with the problem of selecting students for medical school and should promote further understanding of the effects of the independent variables. Therefore, a study of individual differences among the medical students was undertaken. Various personality measurement devices were administered during the pretest and posttest sessions. Details concerning the procedures for studying individual differences are set forth in Chapter 15.

Organization of the Project

The research project was organized around the three sets of variables, and responsibility for studying each set was allocated to a particular person. The project as a whole was under the direction of Kenneth R. Hammond. The section concerned with independent variables was under the direction of John Gyr; the section concerned with dependent variables was under the direction of Wayman Crow; and the section concerned with individual differences was under the direction of Byron Groesbeck. Thus, the organization of the project paralleled the logic of the design of the experiment. The responsibilities of each section are described below.

INDEPENDENT VARIABLES SECTION

The Independent Variables Section was responsible for studying the experimental group and control group situations in such a way as to be able to identify the "causes" of whatever "effects" were discovered by the Dependent Variables Section. The Independent Variables Section had to devise ways and means of observing and describing critical kinds of events in the senior medical students' experiences in both experimental and control programs.

At the outset the expectations regarding the ultimate achievement of this section were conservative, to say the least. The task seemed to present the experimenters with a choice of evils: either they might achieve realistic complexity at the sacrifice of objectivity; or they might achieve appropriate objectivity, but only at the cost of so simplifying the complex process under observation that the results would have no useful meaning. On the one hand—and this was the most frequently suggested solution—it would have been possible simply to engage an expert in the observation and description of human behavior to describe the two processes to be compared. This solution, though it might have resulted in a highly interesting description of suitable complexity, seemed likely to be unproductive, for the accuracy of such a description could not be tested objectively. If, for example, interested members of the medical faculty should challenge the expert's description, there would be no objective way of resolving such a difference of opinion. (Moreover, such differences of opinion were expected to arise, even though it could be pointed out that descriptions made by an expert observer were both sounder and less biased than the opinions of interested medical faculty members.) On the other hand, methods involving recording and counting seemed to require such a drastic reduction of scope and complexity that the results would have very little value when applied to the highly complex teaching process.

Nevertheless, there was great reluctance to abandon the independent variables phase of the project. In the first place, if this task could be performed with even a moderate degree of success, the results would be of very great value to the total research project. In the second place, even if this section of the project failed completely, the attempt to obtain this data would be justified; for the knowledge that this kind of research could or could not be done under the given conditions and with the given facilities would in itself be of value. For these two reasons, then, it was decided to proceed with this phase of the project. This proved a sound decision, for the results of this section's work far exceeded the original expectations.

Dependent variables section

The Dependent Variables Section was responsible for: (1) helping the faculty to make the objectives of the GMC explicit and testable; (2) developing procedures to discover to what extent the objectives were achieved and revising the procedures until they were technically sound; (3) administering tests to the experimental and control groups; and (4) analyzing the results.

Formulating the objectives of the GMC. It was necessary to formulate the objectives of the experimental program so that they were both susceptible to testing and meaningful to those concerned with the success or failure of the program. This was one of the most difficult tasks of the project because it required considerable understanding among members of different disciplines who were dealing with a problem new to all concerned. Furthermore, time was limited for this task; it had to be completed at a very early stage of the research so that procedures could be developed in time for the administration of pretests.

Developing tests. Once objectives had been formulated that were both meaningful and testable, procedures had to be developed for determining whether these objectives were achieved and how effectively. Because of the design of the experiment, the number of students (approximately 80) in each of the three classes studied, and the limited amount of student time available, only group, rather than individual, testing was considered.

It was not intended that small, subtle differences between the experimental and control groups be detected. New educational programs (especially those which are expensive, as this one was) cannot be regarded as successful unless they produce fairly marked changes; changes that can be detected only by highly refined procedures are not significant. Moreover, it seemed unlikely, in view of the pioneer nature of this research, that such highly refined procedures would be available or could be developed in time to be of use.

With respect to attitude measurement, it was expected that self-report techniques such as questionnaires and conventional attitude tests would be necessary but not sufficient. Some techniques in which the student was not aware of the implications of his responses would have to be evolved, as it would not be wise to assume that each student's self-report would always be sufficiently accurate. (The manner in which this expectation was borne out is discussed later in this chapter.)

Most importantly, it was necessary to develop almost all the procedures while the research was in progress. Tests for measuring medical knowledge, medical skill, attitudes toward medicine and medical education, etc., were not readily available. Therefore, once the objectives of the GMC were made explicit, it was necessary to develop new procedures for determining the extent to which these objectives were achieved.

Revising tests. Considerable trial-and-error research was anticipated because of unfamiliarity with the material and because previous research was lacking. For example, it was perceived that some provision would have to be made for testing medical knowledge in a fairly comprehensive way at the senior-year level. Although tests were routinely given to seniors at the University of Colorado, to establish the reliability and validity of a test of medical knowledge given to a (probably) fairly homogeneous group, empirical, trial-and-error, item analysis studies would have to be carried out.

Since new procedures had to be devised, revisions would obviously be needed to make sure that useful tests were developed. And since most of the data needed for revising and improving the tests could be obtained only from senior medical students, more than one class would have to be studied. That is, a test would have to be administered to one class, the data obtained analyzed so that the test could be revised, and the new test administered in order to check the value of the revision.

Analyzing results. Comparisons among groups (see Figure 10.1) were to be made by analyzing the differences between pretest and posttest performance. Because the research involved the development of new procedures and therefore required empirical analysis of the technical soundness of the procedures, an important problem arose. Once a test was administered, it had to be studied immediately in order to evaluate its reliability and validity for the purpose for which it was intended. For example, questions such as the following had to be answered: Is this attitude scale useful for measuring attitudes toward patients? Can we depend upon it to give accurate results, or should we drop it and attempt to devise a new one? This decision had to be made in time to devise a new procedure should it be necessary to do so. It can be seen in Figure 10.1 that only three months were available for this purpose. This unfortunate problem of "deadline research" seems unavoidable in a study of this sort.

Individual differences section

The Individual Differences Section of the project was responsible for studying differences among the students in an attempt to understand why their responses to the independent variables differed. Consequently, two major tasks were undertaken by this section: the analysis of the relation of individual attributes to *change* from pretest to posttest on the dependent variables tests and the analysis of the relation of individual attributes to performance in the GMC. Two kinds of data were used in these analyses: previous academic work and information obtained from personality tests administered at the pretest and posttest sessions.

Relation of individual attributes to change on dependent variables tests. There are several reasons why a student's attitudes, for example, might change from pretest to posttest. The change might be caused by the independent variables; that is, the experience of being in one program rather than the other might have been the decisive factor. Or, the change might be unrelated to the independent variables; that is, the student's personality might have produced the change during his senior year, irrespective of which program he participated in. Or, the change might result from an interaction between the independent variables and personality differences; that is, a particular educational program in conjunction with certain personality characteristics might produce a predictable attitude change. The questions investigated by the Individual Differences Section might be put this way: Is it possible to predict attitude change during the senior year? If so, is it sufficient to know whether the student was in the GMC or the control program; is it sufficient to know the student's personality test data; or is it necessary to know both?

Relation of individual attributes to performance in the GMC. The second task of the Individual Differences Section was to study the relation of personality characteristics to the student's performance in the GMC. This raised the question of the definition and measurement of performance. The only available measure of a student's performance was the rating of that student by the staff. Thus, it was not the student's performance per se which was under consideration, but the staff's evaluation of it. To put the matter even more strongly, this section of the project was attempting to study the behavior not only of the students but of the staff members as well. This complication is discussed in detail in Chapter 24.

The basic question the Individual Differences Section attempted to answer was: What measurable characteristics are associated with those students who are judged to be good performers in the GMC? Although it was natural to assume the student who had a good record in the first three years of medical school would continue to be judged a good student, this might not prove true. After all, the GMC required a different approach to patients, a different attitude toward medicine, a different relation with the ancillary services. There might even be an inverse relation between prior performance and GMC performance. Most important, if the GMC really required a different orientation to the practice of medicine, the study of individual differences should reveal it, for different personality configurations would then be related to adaptability to the new program.

The study of individual differences was also expected to supply useful information on the selection of medical students, a perennial problem. All studies so far published had been concerned principally with admission test scores and first- and second-year grades. The Colorado situation, however, provided an opportunity to study many personality variables in relation to specific ratings or evaluations of the students. Previous grade averages and admission test scores were also available. Thus, information concerning the relative utility of personality tests and previous performance measures would be forthcoming.

Value of this organization

The structure described above was found to be of great value to the project for several reasons. First, it made relative completeness possible. The Dependent Variables Section answered the question: What happened? The Individual Differences Section answered the question: To whom did it happen? The Independent Variables Section answered the question: Why did it happen? Second, the structure worked well both administratively and methodologically, for it defined duties and responsibilities clearly. Third, and most important, the administrative structure reflected the design of the experiment and pointed clearly to where integration of results took place. When the heads of the three sections met and discussed results, the data were integrated. To use a hypothetical example, suppose that the Dependent Variables Section had found that experimental students improved more than control students with respect to medical knowledge. The Individual Differences Section might then be asked to identify which experimental and/or control students improved and which did not, and to discover whether their changes could be accounted for by personality or ability variables, that is, general psychological characteristics of the individual. The question might then be pushed further, to the point of asking whether a given personality trait in conjunction with a given kind of experience accounted for the change. The Independent Variables Section of the research project was responsible for finding an answer to the last question. It takes only slight imagination to see the number of ways in which the data from the three sections of the project might be integrated.

In brief, the structure of the research project did not insure but did make possible completeness; it promoted easy definition of responsibilities; and it encouraged integration of the data.

CHRONOLOGICAL DEVELOPMENT OF THE RESEARCH PROJECT

The work of the research project began one year before the inauguration of the General Medical Clinic Program and lasted for five years. During this period three classes of senior medical students were studied. The work of the project was divided into five stages, as outlined below.

Stage 1 (1952–53): planning

The first was essentially a planning stage. The initial task was to familiarize the research personnel with the reasons for creating the GMC (which at this time was in the process of being established), with the aims of the GMC, and with the atmosphere of the medical school and the city hospital in which the GMC was to function. The second task was to assist the medical faculty in making the GMC objectives explicit and testable. The third task was to develop initial tests for determining whether the objectives of the GMC were achieved.

Stage 2 (1953–54): initial test administration

In the second stage the tests developed initially in stage 1 were administered for the first time, and some revision was accomplished. Also, studies of individual differences were begun, and the first steps were made in the study of the independent variables.

Stage 3 (1954–55): revising tests

The third stage was principally devoted to revision of tests. In addition, some data were analyzed in an effort to make certain comparisons between the GMC and control students. The staff was expanded to include three research associates, each of whom was in charge of one section of the research project; as previously described. The primary aim during this stage was to improve procedures to such an extent that the data collected during the following year (stage 4) could be regarded as definitive. During this stage the Independent Variables Section carried out the preliminary exploratory work necessary for the accomplishment of its task, and the Individual Differences Section studied measurements of performance in the GMC (the ratings of the students by the staff).

It should be pointed out that the GMC was in operation during stages 2 and 3. Thus, the definitive data concerned the *third* year of GMC operation and had the advantage of being collected after the research project had improved its procedures and after the staff had become familiar with the problems of teaching in the GMC.

STAGE 4 (1955–56): FINAL DATA COLLECTION

Although the procedures for the evaluation and study of the GMC were by no means beyond improvement, and although the GMC still faced many administrative problems, it was decided that this stage would be the "definitive" year. During this stage tests were administered in their final form.

STAGE 5 (1956–57): ANALYSIS AND WRITING

During this stage the data obtained from the class of 1956 were analyzed, and the present report was written.

One important advantage accrued from this plan of scheduling the work in definite stages: it helped to resolve the conflict between analysis and development. As research progresses, two pressures develop. One is the pressure to discover the results; in this case, whether the performance of GMC and control students differed, and in what ways. The other is the pressure to revise and improve tests on technical grounds (reliability and validity) and to develop new tests as they are needed, independent of the results in terms of experimental and control group performance. Logic is clearly on the side of the latter, human curiosity on the former's. The assignment of definite periods to specific tasks (especially in stage 3) enabled the research project to resist the pressure for early comparative analysis much more successfully than it probably would have been able to do otherwise.

PLAN FOR EVALUATING THE GMC

The primary task of the research project was to evaluate the General Medical Clinic Program. Basically, this was to be a comparative evaluation. The GMC Program was originally conceived as an improvement upon the traditional senior medical clerkship; it was expected that the GMC would fulfill certain needs in medical education better than the traditional program, and one of the tasks of the research group was to ascertain whether or not the GMC actually did this. However, to be adjudged successful, the GMC must not only fulfill these needs better than the traditional program, but it must do so *without sacrificing any of the values of the traditional program.* Therefore, evaluation required the answering of two questions: Did the GMC Program fail to attain any of the objectives attained by the traditional program, and did the GMC Program attain any objectives not attained by the traditional program? Obviously, the first step in the evaluation process was the clarification and classification of the objectives of the two programs and the selection of suitable tests by which the achievement of these objectives could be measured and compared.

Defining the Objectives of the GMC

Initially, an attempt was made to clarify the objectives of the two programs in the course of discussions and conferences between the medical faculty and the research staff. However, it quickly became apparent that the objectives articulated in these discussions were not precisely enough defined to permit accurate measurement or to be meaningful to both medical and research personnel.

These discussions were therefore abandoned, and another procedure was tried. A number of medical faculty members were asked to describe the most recent examples of "good" and "poor" medical practice that had come to their attention. The incidents reported were classified so as to show the kinds of behavior by physicians that the medical staff considered important. The main classes were: doctor-patient relations, doctor-doctor (professional) relations, community health problems and resources, relation of medicine and government, personal behavior, basic knowledge and technical competence. Although these data later proved useful in furthering understanding between the research and medical personnel, the procedure did not produce sufficiently precise definitions of objectives.

Therefore, a third method was attempted. The faculty members most familiar with the GMC (including GMC staff) were asked to state what they considered to be the GMC's objectives regarding three areas of medical education—knowledge, skills, and attitudes. (This three-area classification had been developed previously in general discussions between the research and medical staff.) The research staff grouped the objectives thus obtained into those that were testable and those that were not. After further consultation with the medical faculty, the researchers classified the testable objectives regarding knowledge, skill, and attitudes according to three more areas—medicine (in the traditional sense), psychology, and sociology. This combined classification is shown schematically in Figure 10.2. Each objective is discussed in turn below.

It should be noted here that throughout this book the terms psychology and sociology are used, for the sake of brevity, to mean "the psychological components of medicine" and "the social components of medicine." The GMC did not attempt to provide thorough preparation in either of these disciplines.

Medical knowledge

One objective of the GMC was to increase the student's medical knowledge. This, of course, was also a goal of the traditional program. However, this objective was of very great significance. If the GMC Program failed to increase the student's medical knowledge as effectively as the control program, it would mean that the new program involved sacrifice of the traditional goals of medical education. On the other hand, if the GMC increased the student's medical knowledge as well as or better than the control program, what was perhaps the most cogent objection to the new program would be disposed of. There is always considerable resistance to an educational innovation which involves extending the scope of medical education, on grounds that the teaching of medical knowledge will inevitably suffer. It is hardly too much to say, then, that the success or failure of the GMC as an experiment in medical education depended upon its achievement of this objective. Therefore, the research group planned to measure and compare the increase in medical knowledge of the experimental and control groups. Subsequent events proved this to be a fortunate step.

	Knowledge	Skill	Attitudes
Medicine	Objective i	Objective j	Objective k
Psychology	Objective l	Objective m	Objective n
Sociology	Objective o	Objective p	Objective q

Figure 10.2. Schematic presentation of the classification of GMC objectives

Medical skill

Another objective of the GMC Program was to enhance the student's acquisition of medical skill, that is, his ability to apply his knowledge in an effective fashion so that the patient derives maximum benefit. Special opportunities had, therefore, been provided for students to learn to apply their knowledge effectively, and it was expected that the GMC group would attain this objective more satisfactorily than the control group. However, it was possible that the GMC might have the reverse effect: so many difficulties (for the student) of a minor nature might be introduced that frustrations might occur which would impair the student's acquisition of medical skill. Therefore, the research group measured and compared the acquisition of medical skill by students in both the experimental and control groups.

Medical attitudes

Another objective of the GMC Program was to inculcate in the student certain attitudes toward the practice of medicine. The ultimate purpose of the GMC was to develop better physicians, better primarily in the sense that they practiced comprehensive medical care, as defined in Chapter 1. The medical faculty believed that the practice of comprehensive medical care required appropriate attitudes on the part of the physician, especially an attitude of responsibility toward his patients that included not only treatment of the immediate complaint but also concern for the total health of the patient. Although in the control medical clerkship attention was, of course, paid to the problem of the physician's responsibility to his patients, the new program was designed to increase the development of such attitudes. As in the case of medical skill, it was possible that this attempt might have the reverse effect. Again, therefore, the research staff planned to measure and compare the degree to which such attitudes were inculcated by the two programs.

Psychological knowledge

Because the GMC was established to acquaint the student with the principles and problems of comprehensive medical care, and because comprehensive medical care implies awareness of the psychological factors relating to illness, one of the objectives of the GMC was to increase the student's knowledge of the psychological components of medicine. Therefore, it was necessary to measure the acquisition of psychological knowledge in both the control and experimental groups in order to determine whether the GMC Program did enhance the student's acquisition of this kind of knowledge more than the control program, and if so to what degree.

Psychological skill

Another objective of the GMC was to enhance the student's acquisition of two kinds of psychological skills. The first was skill in establishing a good doctor-patient relation. Comprehensive care cannot be effectively applied without the full cooperation of the patient, and this cooperation cannot be obtained unless the physician is skillful in developing rapport with his patient. The second was the development of skill in applying psychological knowledge. The GMC was designed to provide opportunities for the student to learn how to use his knowledge of psychology effectively in dealing with the emotional problems related to illness. Again, it was possible that the attempt to develop these psychological skills would produce the reverse effect. Therefore, the researchers measured and compared the acquisition of psychological skill in the experimental and control groups.

Psychological attitudes

The term "psychological attitudes" here means the student's attitudes toward the psychological factors related to medicine. Inculcation of a favorable attitude toward the psychological aspects of medicine was an objective of the GMC Program for two reasons: (1) the medical faculty believed that the GMC student would not be likely to acquire psychological knowledge and skill (as described immediately above) unless he developed positive attitudes toward them, that is, unless he fully recognized their value in the practice of medicine; and (2) the medical faculty believed that even if a student acquired psychological knowledge and skill during his training, he would not use them fully in his later practice unless he had also acquired positive attitudes toward these important components of comprehensive medical care. Once more the possibility was recognized that the GMC's efforts to foster favorable attitudes toward the psychological aspects of medicine might produce the opposite effect, and the research group assumed the task of measuring and comparing the degree to which these attitudes were acquired by the experimental and control groups.

Sociological knowledge, skill, and attitudes

The last three objectives of the GMC were concerned with enhancing the student's understanding of the social components of medicine. The traditional concept of medical care was broadened to include not only psychological factors (the relation of the patient's behavior to his illness) but also social factors (the relation of the patient's social milieu to his behavior and his illness). Thus, the GMC Program attempted to impart to the student some knowledge of the social aspects of medicine and their relevance to medical practice. As with the psychological aspects of medicine, and for the same reasons, this sociological knowledge, to be effective, had to be supplemented by appropriate skill in application and by positive attitudes. Since it was possible that the attempt to enhance the student's sociological knowledge and skill and to foster positive attitudes might produce the reverse effect, the research group assumed three more tasks: to measure and compare in the experimental and control groups the degree to which sociological knowledge, skill, and attitudes were acquired.

In summary, then, it was decided that the General Medical Clinic aimed at the attainment of nine objectives; once these objectives had been defined and classified, the primary evaluative role of the research group became clear. It remained only to devise suitable pretests and posttests for measuring the changes in medical, psychological, and sociological knowledge, skill, and attitudes; to collect data; and to analyze and interpret these data.

Describing the Attainment of the Objectives

Each section of the research project was responsible for providing information concerning the attainment of the nine objectives of the GMC (Figure 10.3). For example, the first objective was to increase

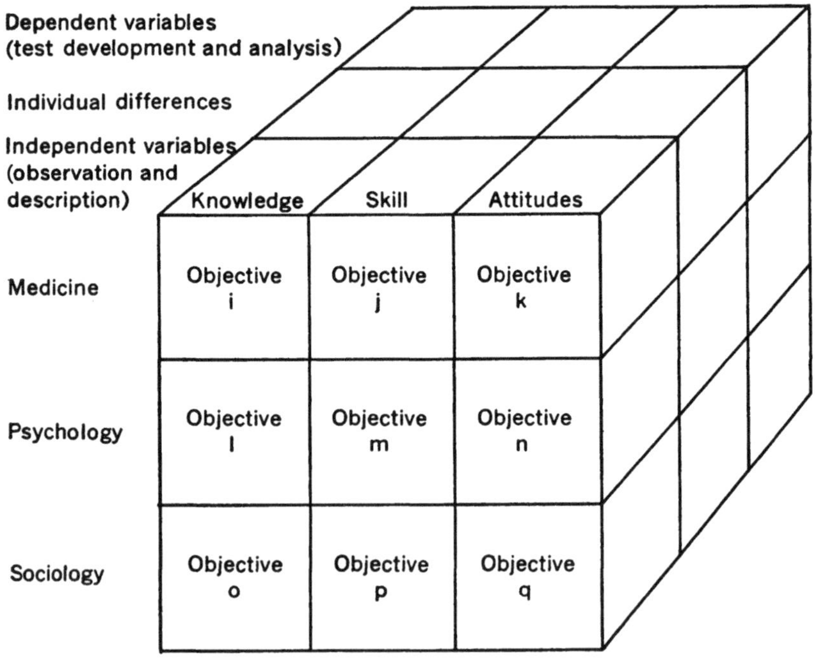

Figure 10.3. Schematic presentation of the plan for evaluating the GMC Program

the student's medical knowledge. The Dependent Variables Section had the primary task of evaluating the GMC in terms of the attainment of this objective. It had to develop tests of medical knowledge, administer the tests before and after the student's medical clinic experience, and compare the pretest and posttest performances of the experimental and control groups. The Individual Differences Section had to develop procedures to discover which students profited most from the two educational experiences and whether successful students were characterized by any special personality factors. This was important because students who were hostile to the GMC's concept of comprehensive medical care might fail to profit from their experience; if these students could be identified and described, it might be possible to predict, understand, and modify their reaction. The Independent Variables Section had to develop methods to observe and describe the techniques and processes of medical education in both programs in order to determine why the objective was (or was not) attained.

In short, each section asked a question. The Dependent Variables Section asked: Which group acquired the most medical knowledge? The Individual Differences Section asked: What are the characteristics of the individual students who acquired the most and the least medical knowledge? The Independent Variables Section asked: How were the students taught this medical knowledge? These same questions were asked concerning the attainment of each of the nine objectives.

LIMITATIONS AND PROBLEMS

It was apparent at the outset that certain limitations would be imposed on the scope of the research project and that a number of serious problems would arise in the course of its work. These difficulties and restrictions, though irksome at the time, were not without compensation, for one of the project's major contributions was expected to be the investigation of problems inherent in psychological research into medical education.

Some of the restrictions and problems were peculiar to this project. One of these was the lack of facilities for studying the actual teaching process. For example, no one-way vision rooms were available, and the work of recording student-staff conferences was somewhat hampered by the lack of suitable recording rooms. These limitations, however, were minor and did not seriously impair the research.

Another limitation was imposed by the fact that manipulation of the environment was precluded because the research concerned a functioning educational program whose procedures could not be manipulated for experimental purposes. Sometimes, for example, certain teaching procedures seemed to be producing certain effects. The only way to check these suspected cause-effect relations was to remove the suspected causes, that is, to change the teaching technique, and observe whether or not the effect remained. This, of course, could not be done, as it would have disrupted the medical training program.[2] In one sense, this restriction was peculiar to this particular project, but it would probably apply to any similar research endeavor in medical education—or in most other types of education.

Related to the preceding limitation was the problem of liaison between the GMC staff and the research group. More precisely, the problem was to maintain a balance between the demands of objectivity on the part of the research group and the necessity for close cooperation between the researchers and the medical school faculty. On the one hand, it was essential that the evaluation of the GMC Program be completely objective, and hence that the research project be independent of both the GMC and other departments of the medical school. On the other hand, members of the research group obviously had to work very closely with the medical school faculty, and the satisfactory solution of the many administrative problems that were anticipated depended on close cooperation between the two groups. These conflicting requirements presented a dilemma. The obvious solution was to establish a formal system of communication between the research group and the medical faculty through a nonpartisan body to which the research group could take administrative problems, from which it could seek advice, and to which both groups could appeal for arbitration should a serious conflict of purposes develop. To this end, a Research Advisory Committee was formed; it consisted of the director of the medical center, the dean of the medical school, the heads of several departments of the medical school, and a number of other prominent members of the medical school faculty. As it happened, except on one occasion (described below) this committee had no serious problems to solve because no serious conflicts arose between the faculty and the research group. However, the existence of the advisory committee was reassuring to the research group, since it signified that the principal authorities in the medical school stood behind the research; and its existence may also have prevented serious friction between the two groups. In short, the establishing of the

[2] If the research group was restricted in its activities by the requirements of the medical program, the converse was also true. For instance, when members of the GMC staff met with frustrations in teaching, it was natural for them to ask the psychologists close at hand for suggestions and assistance. These requests had to be refused, for granting them would have put the researchers in the position of having to evaluate their own educational predilections, and the objectivity of the evaluation would have been lost.

Research Advisory Committee appears to have been a wise step, for it permitted the research group to work closely with the medical school faculty without compromising its own independence and hence the objectivity of the project.

The amount of time which the students could and would make available for research purposes imposed further limitations on the project. The subjects were senior medical students, and the senior year in medical school is traditionally a time when the students "get all they can while they can." It is generally their last opportunity for formal training before they must undertake the responsibilities of internship; they are intensively acquiring the maximum amount of usable knowledge; and they are not much interested in devoting time to activities which are not directly helpful to them for this purpose, even though they realize that these activities do have a value for medical education. Senior medical students are concerned with improving themselves, not the process of medical education.[3] This somewhat resistant attitude on the part of the subjects, coupled with the facts that the curriculum for senior medical students was undeniably crowded and that heavy demands were made on them during this year, forced the research group to be conservative in its demands for students' time and to make the most of what time was allotted for research purposes.

The amount of time which members of the faculty could devote to this kind of research was likewise limited, not only by their research and teaching responsibilities, but also by their committee duties. This, however, proved a less serious disadvantage to the work of the research group than the restriction of students' time, though it did mean that only a very few members of the medical school staff became much involved in the research work.

The limited amount of both faculty and student time available did not prove detrimental to the project. Adequate time (approximately twenty-four hours per student in each class studied) was made available and utilized for testing, and numerous meetings with faculty members were arranged. Everyone concerned recognized that interference with already overloaded schedules could be tolerated only if absolutely essential, and acted accordingly. As with the problem of liaison, recognizing potential difficulties was tantamount to eliminating them.

Inextricably bound up with the psychological research in medical

[3] This does not mean that senior medical students are uncritical of the educational system in which they are involved; quite the reverse is true. But they are not interested in spending any *scheduled* time answering questions the import of which is not always apparent.

education is the question of the attitudes of both students and faculty toward the research. Successful completion of this type of project requires that these two groups cooperate intelligently with the research group. Either faculty members or students can, by non-cooperation, easily destroy the effectiveness of a research program. In this particular project faculty attitudes were not, in general, important limiting considerations, possibly because of the superb cooperation of the advisory committee. The committee did not refuse a single request made by the research group; administrative cooperation could not have been better. Individual staff members' attitudes toward the research, however, did limit one phase of the project. For example, some staff members occasionally balked at recording their teaching sessions with the students. In fact, our records indicate that they balked about half the time. The students, when criticized by the research group for not turning in the records, pointed out that it was the staff that was not cooperating; that in fact, they *preferred* to have the sessions recorded because the teaching was so much better!

On the whole, however, the attitudes of students caused far more difficulty in this research project than did faculty attitudes. Though it is unsound to generalize from a group of slightly over two hundred students, the inference of this research group, making all possible allowances for the irksomeness of spending valued time on psychological tests, is that the attitudes of medical students are not very satisfactory from the research worker's point of view.

All the researchers reported that the medical students, especially when they were met in groups, displayed a general lack of sympathy toward this project and toward psychological research in general. This attitude varied considerably: it varied from time to time, from individual to individual, and from class to class. Initially, most students seemed interested in the research program; they were curious about the tests they were being asked to take and asked questions about them. A few students maintained an intelligent interest throughout the program; the majority, when they could not immediately and easily perceive the purpose of a procedure, did what was required of them conscientiously enough, but without enthusiasm and occasionally with unconcealed hostility. That the students were annoyed at having to sacrifice time for a project that did not directly benefit them was understandable. In fact it had been anticipated that the students might be annoyed by the demands of the research program, and although this hostility turned out to be greater than expected, it did not really present a major problem.

Another more serious problem resulted from the design of the experiment. It will be discussed in considerable detail, for it produced the major crisis of the project. It is, moreover, a problem that is likely to be encountered whenever this type of research in medical education is undertaken.

The experimental design, it will be recalled, involved what may be termed an "inside" control group, one made up of students in the same medical school and class as those in the experimental group. The members of the two groups were in fairly close contact with one another, and it was expected that some partisanship would result which might prove detrimental to the research objectives. If too keen a sense of competition developed, each group identifying itself with a particular program (GMC or control), and if one group felt that it and its program were appearing to disadvantage, the members of that group might try to invalidate test results so as to "cover up" the supposed deficiencies of "their" program. Student partisanship did not develop in the classes of 1954 and 1955 (stages 2 and 3 of the project). It did, however, become apparent during stage 4, in the class of 1956, and it seriously endangered the work of the entire project. Fortunately, the difficulty was perceived immediately, and measures were at once taken to minimize the damage.

During stage 4 a group of about six students rendered the results of Posttest I worthless. This was apparent because their responses to certain personality tests were random, certain peer rankings were random, and responses to certain questions pertaining to the students' evaluation of previous clerkships were obviously false. The attempts to invalidate or falsify these tests were not uniform even among this small group. Some students made certain tests useless; others spoiled different tests. In some cases it was clear that the intention was to make the results misleading rather than meaningless. Although the data collected were not made totally useless, the entire project was seriously threatened by the behavior of these students, and it was necessary to take every possible precaution to protect it. As soon as the research staff noticed that something was wrong, they had to test every response of every student to determine the honesty of that response. In many instances techniques for testing the honesty of responses had to be devised, so that much time was consumed, and, therefore, certain additional lines of investigation could not be followed up.

Just why these students behaved in this manner never became entirely clear. The most significant facts were that all the uncooperative students were members of two control groups (C_3 and C_4) and that their responses, when not purely random, were such as to favor the control experience, to make it appear much better, in their evaluations, than it could possibly have been. After considerable investigation and extended discussions, three possible explanations emerged. It must be emphasized that these explanations are speculative and cannot be systematically supported by objective data.

The first explanation was that most medical students apparently do not fully understand research methods and are apt to be hostile to research which they do not understand, that is, psychological research in behavior. At the beginning of each year a representative of the medical faculty and the director of the research project spoke to the entire class and explained in general terms the nature and purpose of the research. However, it is the opinion of those observing the situation that the students were not interested in the explanations. At least this was true for both the classes of 1955 and 1956. There seems to be little doubt, however, that if the research project had been explained to the students in such a way as to engage their interest, their attitudes would have been more satisfactory.

The second explanation was that the class of 1956, to which the uncooperative students belonged, was noted for immature behavior in a variety of situations, not merely in the research context. The research episode could be regarded as simply one part of a larger pattern. That is, given the circumstances which might stimulate uncooperative behavior, this particular class was more likely than any of the other classes studied to behave in this way. However, it was primarily something in the conditions of the experiment that caused this behavior.

The third and most convincing explanation was that in 1956 the actual teaching processes in both the experimental and the control programs came under intensive observation for the first time. During stage 2 (1953–54) and stage 3 (1954–55) research activities, so far as the control group was concerned, had been limited to testing students; therefore, the fact that comparisons were being made was relatively unobtrusive. In stage 4 (1955–56), however, the comparisons were extended to include direct scrutiny of the teaching process; representatives of the research program were constantly visible, and the fact of comparison was thus more persistently evident than it had been previously. This situation undoubtedly stimulated partisanship among the students *in the control program.* Thus, although a strong negative attitude toward the research program existed in the classes of 1954 and 1955, this was merely a general resentment, an irritation at having to spend time doing something they did not understand or believed was useless; it was only in the class of 1956 that active non-cooperation appeared, aimed at thwarting the research and motivated by partisanship toward the control experience.

The third explanation is supported by the fact that the direct study of the teaching processes evidently encouraged partisanship among the staff in the control program as well as among the students. Although this cannot be systematically documented, considerable informal evidence came to light during the course of stage 4 indicating that some members of the control staff regarded the experiment as a contest between the two educational programs, the research group being equivalent to the referee. For example, one important member of the control staff, when asked about possible reasons for student partisanship, explained that it was "no more than natural," as the students who were associated with his particular staff group immediately prior to the testing period had been encouraged to "do well," in the competitive sense, on the tests. Even more revealing was a casual conversation that took place on one occasion between a member of the research staff and a member of the control teaching staff. The conversation went approximately as follows:

Researcher: By the way, I noticed that a teaching session of yours was recorded recently, and it seemed to me that it was quite long. Are your teaching sessions with students always that long?

Instructor: Oh, no. You see, when the student told me we were scheduled to record, I asked him why. He explained that it was part of the comparison of the GMC and the regular medical clerkship. So I decided that I would make the best impression I possibly could. Oh, no! I don't ordinarily take more than a third as much time as that.

Researcher: Would you tell me *why* you felt that you should make a good impression on the record?

Instructor: Well, I always identify rather strongly with the group I happen to be working with. It's a sort of "team feeling." When I was teaching at the GMC I identified strongly with the GMC. Now that I am up here I feel that I should do the best I can for this teaching program—and so I made the best impression I could on the record.

As this instructor continued to explain how he felt, he began to realize that his attitude, however commendable on other grounds, was not really a good one from the point of view of a research project whose purpose was to study two methods of medical education; and he finally remarked that he guessed what he did probably wasn't "fair." The researcher had the distinct impression that although the instructor was perfectly sincere, eager to help the research project, and anxious to know which method of education was better, he had not fully grasped the idea of the research as a study of educational method; the notion of team competition lingered.

To summarize, the uncooperative behavior of a small group of students in the control group during stage 4 probably stemmed from at least three roots: general hostility based on imperfect understanding of the research program; a larger number of immature, impulsive students in the class of 1956 than in previous classes; and the partisanship which developed toward the control program, stimulated by the constant presence of research personnel and apparently encouraged by the attitudes of some members of the control staff.

This episode demonstrated that there are dangers in using a control group in the same medical school as the experimental group. Those contemplating future research of this kind may wish to explore the possibility of using an "outside" control group, one in a separate institution. It is the opinion of the present authors, however, that the advantages of the "inside" control group outweigh the potential disadvantages, and that if the dangers inherent in the use of an "inside" control group are foreseen, unfavorable consequences can be prevented. In the present study the trouble that developed during stage 4 might have been avoided altogether if the relatively smooth conditions that prevailed during stages 2 and 3 had not engendered an unwary attitude in the research staff. It seems likely that certain fairly obvious precautions, such as using techniques which make the fact of observation and comparison less obtrusive, would make it possible to retain the advantages of an "inside" control group without undue risk. Of course, a great deal depends on the attitudes of faculty members in strategic positions and on the quality of the relations between the faculty members and the research staff.

Another problem inherent in the design of the experiment concerned "deadline research." The pretest-posttest design used in this study called for test administrations at three-month intervals. Since this was a pioneer project, the tests had to be evaluated and revised during the course of actual research. In practice this meant that a process involving scoring, item analysis, reliability checks, validity studies, and the devising and production of new tests had to be accomplished within a three-month period. The educational process could not be halted to give the research group time to perfect its techniques. "Deadline research" presents obvious difficulties and places a very heavy burden on the research staff. One method of dealing with this problem is to schedule the research in alternating years; that is, one year for development of tests, the next for data collection, the third for refinement of techniques, the fourth for data collection, etc. This plan would protract the study considerably. Another way to minimize the difficulties caused by "deadline research" is to allow ample time for preliminary work and to be certain that such work has been done as thoroughly as possible before data collection is begun. But "deadline research" will always cause some difficulty and should be taken into account whenever this type of project is contemplated.

A general question that continually faced the staff of the research project was how to maintain a balance between two sets of responsibilities: the specific responsibilities toward the medical school, which had requested the research project to provide fairly definite information for fairly definite purposes; and the more generalized responsibilities of research workers toward the science of psychology.

The responsibilities toward the medical school were fairly definite. First and most important was the task of evaluating the GMC Program: finding out whether it "worked," in terms of the knowledge, skill, and attitudes acquired by graduates of the GMC in comparison with those acquired by graduates of the control program. This was the raison d'être of the research project. In addition to performing this primary task, the research project was expected to produce certain other information of value to the medical faculty: information about students' attitudes toward medical education, about personality characteristics associated with different attitudes toward medicine, and about personality characteristics associated with success in medical school and the practice of medicine. This last item was of considerable interest to the medical faculty, for the selection of students has always been a serious problem, and data which could be used to predict success in medical school would be of great value.

The medical faculty, then, expected the research project to provide data on which decisions might be based. This last point is important: the medical school, which instigated the project, had to make certain decisions; the faculty and administration wanted these decisions to be based on data, not impressions or guesswork; and so far as the medical school was concerned, the research project was valuable only to the extent that it produced useful data. The research group therefore assumed the responsibility of making its reports fully *meaningful* to the medical faculty: meaningful both in the sense of being *understandable* and *pertinent* to the situations and problems under consideration and in the sense that the medical faculty *believed* in the data, that they understood and had confidence in the methods by which the data were obtained. Data procured by means that are incomprehensible are not fully meaningful and are therefore not likely to be as influential as they should be, especially when important practical decisions are the issue. This meant that during the planning stage the research group, in a series of conferences with a committee made up of various key members of the medical faculty, undertook the task of presenting and explaining the basic procedures to be used in the research program. If the faculty members did not understand a procedure after it was explained to them, the procedure was dropped, and one that could be understood was substituted.

This policy restricted the research project in the sense that it reduced the range of technical procedures available; on the other hand, it enhanced the potential effectiveness of the research by increasing the chances that whatever pertinent and useful data were produced would be *used* as the bases for decisions. In practice the limiting effect of this policy was slight, except very early in the planning stages. Once the research got underway, members of the advisory committee seldom questioned the meaningfulness of any proposed procedure.

Balanced against the responsibility of the research group to the medical school was its responsibility to psychology. The new program of medical education offered an opportunity to carry out psychological research on learning, motivation, attitudes, and personality in a "real-life" situation—an opportunity that presents itself all too seldom to psychologists. Moreover, this program was particularly interesting because a large part of the subject matter the students were studying and toward which they were forming attitudes was the behavioral, or psychological, aspects of illness. Thus, it was possible to study how psychological knowledge is imparted to and acquired by members of a related profession and to observe directly the development of attitudes toward psychology by these persons.

It might appear that the two responsibilities would conflict, that the research group would continually be forced to choose between producing meaningful data to apply to the practical problem and following out promising lines of research into more fundamental questions. To some extent this was true, but more often it was not. Basic and applied research frequently ran parallel with or complemented one another. For example, when it was decided that it was important to measure the accuracy with which the students could appraise the personality characteristics of patients, considerable basic research had to be carried out concerning interpersonal perception (see Chapter 13). Again, when it was decided to study the learning process in the experimental and control situations, considerable work of a purely theoretical nature was carried out (see Chapter 14). Thus, the problem of maintaining a balance between the two responsibilities of the research group never, in this case, became very acute. Most of the time, it was felt, the needs of the medical faculty were best served when the aims of psychology were being served.

Chapter 11

Summary of Findings and Conclusions

Because of the scarcity of research concerning higher education, the enormous interest in it, and the wide variety of more or less intensely held opinion about it, the present study must inevitably convey more than the conclusions drawn from a set of findings concerning one educational program at one medical school during a brief period of its history. The fact of scarcity of research implies that the methods and procedures developed will be of interest; the fact of considerable national concern over higher education implies interest in the broad, general nature of the findings over and above the comparison of two specific programs; and the fact of wide variety of opinion implies that, whatever the empirical findings may be, they will contradict some and confirm other philosophies of higher learning. This chapter, therefore, will address itself to larger issues as well as to reporting the method, procedures, and results of the research at the University of Colorado School of Medicine.

Method and Procedures

Organization of the Research Project

Undoubtedly the most important methodological feature of this research project was its general organization into three sections, each of which was concerned with one aspect of the experimental design. This division of effort and responsibility was important for several reasons. In the first place, it produced results: the Dependent Variables Section did discover "what happened" as a result of the new program; the Independent Variables Section did discover "why it happened"; and the Individual Differences Section did discover "to whom it happened." Not only did this organizational scheme promote easy definition of responsibility and integration of the data, but (and this was its main contribution) it led toward completeness. Although it is customary to compare the effects (dependent variables) of two different programs or to study individual differences within a single program, the writers know of no single evaluation project which has attempted to study the independent variables (the actual operational differences between the experimental and the control programs). Thus, besides facilitating the allocation of responsibility and the integration of data, the three-fold organization of the research project was a step in a new direction—empirical study of the nature of the two programs whose effects were to be evaluated.

Measures of dependent variables

Once the objectives of the GMC had been defined, the research staff had to develop procedures to measure the nine variables: medical knowledge, medical skill, medical attitudes, psychological knowledge, psychological skill, psychological attitudes, sociological knowledge, sociological skill, and sociological attitudes. These variables were measured in a number of different ways and with varying degrees of success. So that the reader may better understand the following summary account of the results, a brief description of each procedure is presented below. These procedures are described in detail in Chapter 13.

Most important of all the procedures used was a new one—the Sound-Film Interview. This procedure began with the presentation to the student of a six-minute sound-motion picture of a doctor interviewing a patient. At the conclusion of this presentation, the student opened a test booklet which provided him with certain factual medical information, such as laboratory findings, about the patient. On the basis of the information contained in the filmed interview and the test booklet, the student was required to answer multiple-choice questions about the patient. The questions required the student to apply his medical knowledge and skill, his psychological knowledge and skill, and his sociological knowledge and skill, and thus tested his ability in these areas.

Because it was important to measure the effect of the GMC on the student's skill in appraising patients' personal characteristics as well as on his attitudes toward patients, other procedures were employed in connection with the Sound-Film Interview. Particular attention was paid, for example, to the effect of the GMC on the student's skill in making accurate appraisals of patients' intelligence, vocabulary level, and personality characteristics, and on his tendency to perceive the individuality of each patient. The Sound-Film Interview also made it possible to discover the extent to which a student perceived the "overt," superficial aspects of patients' personalities to be different from the "covert," deeper aspects of their personalities; it was therefore used to study the effect of the GMC on the student's perception of patients. One important advantage of this technique was that it permitted measurement of certain variables without the student's being aware that these measurements were being made.

Films of 30 different patients were presented to the students—10 at the beginning of the senior year (Pretest), 10 after six months in the senior year (Posttest I), and 10 more at the end of the senior year (Posttest II).

Other procedures used to study the student's attitudes included the Medical Attitudes Test developed at the University of Utah by Neuman and Boswell. This test included five subscales: Attitudes toward Comprehensive Care, Attitudes toward Health Supervision, Attitudes toward Behavior Disorders, Attitudes toward Physician-Patient Relations, and Attitudes toward the Team Concept in Medicine (see Appendix 2).

To discover whether the GMC affected the student's image of himself, and whether his self-image changed so that he came to perceive himself as being more like a surgeon, a pediatrician or internist, or a psychiatrist, each student was required to fill out a self-description checklist and to use a similar checklist to describe typical members of the various specialties mentioned above (see Appendix 3).

A rather long and detailed questionnaire was also filled out by the students at each test administration. This questionnaire covered all nine objectives of the GMC Program (see Appendix 4).

Measures of independent variables

Besides attempting to measure the effects of the GMC Program, it was necessary to discover the reasons for these effects. Thus, the Independent Variables Section studied the control medical clerkship and the GMC in terms of the manner in which the students were taught in the individual student-staff teaching conferences. Recordings were made of almost two hundred of these conferences. These recordings were studied by means of a psychological procedure developed especially for this purpose. Special interview techniques were also used to study the individual student-staff conferences. Much of the questionnaire that each student filled out dealt with the student's general clinic experiences and his participation in various clinic and hospital activities. Both faculty and students were interviewed by members of the research staff, and sixteen students kept diaries in which entries were made three days per week during the entire senior year. Records of each student's participation in the various special educational features of the GMC were kept, and the relation between such participation and changes in test performance was studied.

The information from all these sources was considered in relation to the objectives of the GMC Program in the effort to discover the reasons why there were (or were not) differences in the attainments of the two programs.

The theory and special methods used to study the student-staff teaching conferences are set forth in detail in Chapter 14.

MEASURES OF INDIVIDUAL ATTRIBUTES

Because it was expected that students would vary in their reactions to the two programs, several tests designed to measure individual attributes were administered to the students in both the GMC and the control programs. It was hoped that the data provided by these tests would not only further the understanding of the effects of the experimental variables, but would provide information of general interest to both medical educators and psychologists.

Eight classes of individual attributes were assessed: aptitude for medical education, previous academic performance, peer-judged attributes (evaluations of one student by another), attitudes, values, social interaction, needs, background information and self ratings. The procedures used to assess these attributes are discussed in detail in Chapter 15.

The relations between these eight classes of attributes and the student's performance on all the dependent variables tests were studied. That is, the measures of individual attributes were correlated with both the student's pretest performance on the dependent variables tests and the change in his performance from pretest to posttest. This procedure made it possible to describe the type of student who had high (or low) scores on, for example, the Psychological Knowledge test, as well as the type of student who made the largest (or smallest) gain on this test.

More intensive studies of individual differences among students were carried out in connection with the staff's evaluation of each student's performance in the GMC. Detailed analyses of the adequacy of staff evaluations of students were also made. The study of students' performance in the GMC is reported in detail in Chapter 24; a brief summary of the findings of this study is included in the present chapter.

Findings

The over-all effect of the GMC Program can be summed up briefly: it had a positive effect on the student's attitudes; that is, it reduced the development of increasingly negative attitudes toward comprehensive care. This result was achieved without impairing the GMC student's acquisition of traditional medical knowledge and skill. The reason the

GMC student did not become increasingly antagonistic to the concept of comprehensive care was that his general experience with patients in the clinic made him increasingly aware of the importance of this concept. The more intelligent, independent, and mature student was the most responsive to the aims of the GMC. This very general statement must, of course, be qualified in many ways. A more detailed summary of the findings follows.

EFFECTS OF THE GMC PROGRAM

Medical knowledge and skill. Although increasing the student's medical knowledge and skill was not an objective peculiar to the GMC Program, it was of considerable importance to discover whether the new program's attempt to increase the scope of medical education involved any sacrifice of the traditional aims of medical education. Therefore, an attempt was made to compare the change in medical knowledge and skill in the experimental group with the corresponding change in the control group.

The evidence indicates that participation in the GMC did not impair the student's acquisition of medical knowledge and skill, although the GMC group was convinced that it did. The test data from all three classes studied were consistent; indeed, the data suggested that the GMC may have been even more effective in teaching medicine than the control clerkship. (See Chapters 16 and 17 for a detailed presentation of findings.)

Psychological knowledge and skill. Evidence concerning the effect of the GMC on the student's acquisition of psychological knowledge and skill is not so clear. There seems to have been a tendency for the GMC student to gain more psychological knowledge and skill than the control student, but this effect was apparently slight. Although the GMC student had more opportunity to become acquainted with the psychological problems of patients, and although this experience led him to feel he had developed greater knowledge and skill in this area, the test results indicated no clear differences between the two groups. The individual attributes of a student were found to be more definitely related to the development of psychological knowledge and skill than was participation in either educational program. (See Chapters 19 and 20 for a detailed presentation of these findings.)

Sociological knowledge and skill. Almost exactly the same results were obtained in connection with sociological knowledge and skill as with psychological knowledge and skill. (See Chapter 22 for a detailed presentation of these findings.)

Attitudes. The most definite effect of the GMC Program was to retard the growth of negative attitudes toward various aspects of comprehensive care. Whereas the control student developed increasingly negative attitudes toward every aspect of comprehensive medicine investigated by the research project, the attitudes of the GMC student tended to be the same at graduation as at the beginning of the senior year. Although the GMC student was much more aware of the difficulties involved in the actual practice of comprehensive care, more GMC than control students came to believe that comprehensive care was important. The GMC student also seemed more aware of psychological factors and seemed to attach more importance to them.

Persistent throughout the results, however, was a difference between the GMC student's attitude toward psychological *concepts* and his attitudes toward *patients*. That is, although the GMC student developed a greater appreciation of the significance of psychological factors in medical care, he was not more inclined to deal with psychological problems—or even to develop more fully his relations with patients. In short, the GMC did not much affect the student's attitudes toward those matters which directly concerned patients (health supervision and physician-patient relations).

When attitudes toward sociological factors were investigated, it was found that the GMC student developed a greater appreciation of the usefulness of ancillary staff members (social workers and the public health nurse) than did the control student. Nevertheless, the GMC student was no more impressed than the control student with the importance of the work of these staff members; in other words, he found the ancillary staff useful for unimportant purposes. (See Chapters 18, 21, and 23 for a detailed presentation of these findings.)

In brief, then, the GMC did not greatly affect the acquisition of either medical knowledge or knowledge of the psychological or social components of medicine. Nor did it apparently affect the student's acquisition of skill in applying such knowledge. The GMC did have some positive effects on the student's attitudes, however.

Scheduling effect. Certain phenomena were observed during the course of the research which, although secondary to the main purposes of the program, were important enough to warrant separate investigation. One such phenomenon was the fact that GMC seemed more successful in achieving its goals during the first half of the senior year than during the second half. This phenomenon, moreover, seemed to be particularly evident in connection with the special goals of GMC. It was referred to as the "scheduling effect."

Investigation of the scheduling effect led to the discovery of three important facts: (1) the GMC student considered learning traditional (organic) medicine to be much more important than learning the principles and techniques of comprehensive care; (2) the GMC student felt that his program presented inadequate opportunities for learning the traditional aspects of medicine; and (3) anxieties over learning traditional medicine increased as graduation and the responsibilities of internship approached. As a result of these three conditions, dissatisfaction and impatience with the special aims of the GMC became more pronounced during the second half of the senior year and seriously interfered with the learning process, particularly in those areas specifically related to comprehensive care. The GMC student felt he was being taught matters of secondary importance (psychological and social components of medical care) and being trained in skills in which he was already proficient (physician-patient relations), by professors who were neither especially well-informed nor especially skillful in these secondary areas, but who were well-informed and skillful in the very areas about which the student was eager to learn (traditional medicine). This situation apparently became more difficult to tolerate as graduation approached. This finding, of course, has serious implications for the timing of special educational efforts. (See Chapter 25 for a detailed presentation of these findings.)

In fact, the scheduling effect suggests that in the latter part of the senior year, the internship (or at least the student's expectation about it) has a greater influence on the student than his teachers do. The results suggest that the student's convictions about the importance of various activities in the senior year stem more from his motivation to conform to the requirements (and ideology) of internship than to the requirements (and ideology) of his faculty. And it seems probable that at this point in the student's career, expectations about residency and practice are also shaping his convictions about what he should be learning in medical school.

Therefore, any attempt to inculcate attitudes which are contrary to those the student expects to find in his immediate future is likely to result in eventual failure—even if it should succeed in the short run. Thus, efforts to develop certain attitudes among students should also include efforts to develop those attitudes in the group which constitutes the eventual frame of reference for the students. Most important, the effect of the future reference group is apparently more far-reaching than one might suppose. The scheduling effect shows that the future reference group (the internship) can "reach back" into the senior year of medical school and counteract the influence of the faculty. Because this conclusion has far-reaching theoretical and practical implications, and because this is not the first time such a conclusion has been reached in connection with the general problem of attitude change,[1] it deserves serious consideration.

Individual attributes and performance in the GMC. In a further attempt to understand the factors involved in teaching the principles of comprehensive care to senior medical students, a careful study was made to ascertain what, if any, individual attributes were correlated with staff ratings of students' performance in the GMC. It was hoped that this study would indicate what type of student would perform well in this type of educational setting.

The results showed rather clearly that, in the main, the GMC Program required of the student the same qualities of performance as did his first three years of training. It was the student with a high cumulative grade average who was rated highly by the GMC medical staff. Contrary to expectations, measures of a student's personality characteristics, attitudes, and values were essentially unrelated to medical staff evaluations. (Ratings made by the ancillary staff, however, were more highly related to the student's personality characteristics than to his previous academic performance.)

Although the conclusions summarized in the foregoing paragraph are in all likelihood quite firm, they were by no means immediately apparent, and were reached only after considerable detailed investigation of the manner in which the medical staff actually made the ratings. Indeed, the analysis of the ratings threw considerable doubt on the adequacy of staff ratings as a device for evaluating students. Each staff member, it was found, based his judgment of students on a single dimensioned and unique concept of what constitutes a good medical student.

The fact that the ratings made by the GMC staff were single dimensioned (that is, involved only the student's medical knowledge and skill) implies that the GMC staff did not take cognizance of the student's performance in the areas more directly related to the specific aims of the GMC Program. For this reason, the study of the staff's evaluations of students produced findings congruent with those obtained from test results—that there was equal emphasis in both programs on traditional medical knowledge.

The medical staff members differed widely among themselves in their appraisals of individual students. This uniqueness was sur-

[1] See Robert K. Merton and Alice S. Kitt, "Contributions to the Theory of Reference Group Behavior," in Robert K. Merton and Paul F. Lazarsfeld (eds.), *Continuities in Social Research: Studies in the Scope and Method of the American Soldier* (Glencoe, Illinois: Free Press, 1950); also Theodore M. Newcomb, "Attitude Development as a Function of Reference Groups: The Bennington Study," in Guy Swanson, Theodore M. Newcomb, and Eugene L. Hartley (eds.), *Readings in Social Psychology* (New York: Holt, 1952).

prising, since the staff members agreed rather well with one another in their verbal descriptions of what they considered to be desirable in the performance of a medical student. Of course, if staff members cannot agree among themselves which students are good ones and which poor ones, staff evaluation cannot be used as a criterion for appraising a student's performance, and questions concerning the attributes related to performance cannot be answered. If these findings serve to stimulate research into the nature of staff evaluations of students, they may well be the most important findings of the study. (See Chapter 24 for a detailed presentation of these findings.)

Reasons for the effect of the GMC

Seven sources of information were utilized in the effort to discover why the GMC had the effect it had: analysis of individual student-staff conferences in both programs; students' reports of their clerkship activities; students' reports of their general experience in their clerkships; records of students' participation in the special educational techniques of the GMC; faculty evaluations of students; interviews with students; interviews with GMC faculty. Analyses of data from all these sources showed a remarkable amount of agreement. Moreover, the general nature of the findings made the conclusions concerning the effects of the GMC entirely plausible.

Medical knowledge and skill. It would be reasonable to suppose that the effort to expand the scope of medical education would involve some sacrifice in the teaching of traditional medical knowledge. The data from all the sources mentioned above, however, indicate that equal emphasis was placed on traditional medical knowledge in both programs. For example, no differences were found in the individual student-staff conferences of the two programs—whether these conferences were studied by the psychological techniques designed specifically for this purpose, or evaluated by the physicians who analyzed each teaching conference. Except for the fact that far fewer GMC students reported that they had worked with patients presenting definite organic pathology, there were few important differences in the students' reports of their activities and their general clerkship experience. In general, interviews with both faculty and students confirmed the heavy emphasis on traditional medicine in the GMC as well as in the control program. Moreover, as pointed out above, it was found that the GMC medical staff evaluated the students almost entirely on the basis of their medical knowledge alone—not on the basis of other aspects of their performance more closely related to the special educational features of the GMC.

In general, the analysis of the two programs confirmed the conclusions drawn from the comparison of the performance of the two groups on the tests of medical knowledge and skill. That is, except for the fact that GMC students reported that they did not see enough patients with definite organic pathology or a wide enough variety of illnesses, the general experiences of the two groups regarding medical knowledge and skill were sufficiently similar to permit the conclusion that in this respect there should have been little difference between the two groups.

The students, however, were quite convinced that participation in the GMC impeded their efforts to acquire medical knowledge and skill. They therefore resented the program, and the resentment remained with the majority of GMC students for as long as two or three years after graduation, and possibly longer (data are available for this period only). Why did the GMC students believe that participation in the GMC handicapped them in their efforts to gain medical knowledge? The answer to this question was not difficult to discover because the students readily provided it: they definitely felt that they did not see a sufficient number of patients who were actually ill. "I don't see enough patients who are really sick—my patients are all crocks" was a constant complaint.

This discrepancy between students' impressions of the value of a special educational effort and the conclusion drawn from an analysis of research data is interesting because similar discrepancies were found throughout the data (see Table 11.1).

The data included in the chapters which follow indicate that the student's evaluation of the two programs was in all likelihood wrong. But the impression gained by the student would very likely be the impression of many persons observing the GMC Program. This impression might very plausibly come about in the following way. The GMC student, believing he was seeing far too few patients who were actually ill and far too limited a variety of illnesses, felt he was not learning enough organic medicine. At the same time, the GMC student believed he was seeing too many patients whose problems were entirely psychological and/or social in origin. Consequently, he felt he was gaining more than enough knowledge of, and skill in dealing

Table 11.1. Discrepancies between students' impressions and research conclusions concerning value of GMC Program in various areas of medical education

	Students' impressions	Research conclusions
Medical knowledge and skill	GMC hampered	GMC did not hamper
Psychological and sociological knowledge and skill	GMC helped a great deal	GMC helped somewhat
Students' attitudes	(Conflicting)	GMC improved

with, these latter problems. These impressions, although reasonable enough, rest on two assumptions—neither of which has been confirmed by empirical evidence.

The first assumption is that it is necessary to see a large number and a wide variety of patients with organic illnesses in order to acquire medical knowledge and skill. The second assumption is that the GMC student had the type of contact and experience with patients (and instructors) which necessarily increased his knowledge of the psychological and social aspects of medical care. The evidence throws considerable doubt on the assumption that it is necessary for a student, in order to acquire medical knowledge, to see a wide variety of patients with definite illnesses. In fact, the evidence tends to support the assumption that *intensive* experience with patients is more conducive to learning than *extensive* experience. And the evidence also indicates that the student's contact with patients and instructors has only slight effect on his acquisition of psychological and sociological knowledge.

The findings of this study do not provide definitive evidence concerning the validity of either assumption. But the findings do raise critical problems of immediate importance. The most obvious trend in medical education is to increase the scope of the student's knowledge. If the student holds the belief that in order to become a competent physician, his clinical experience in medical school must present him with concrete examples of each problem he is apt to meet in practice, then the faculty is, of course, faced with a hopeless problem. The awkward position of the faculty under these circumstances is illustrated nicely by these comments by one of the GMC staff:[2]

> The students feel they are not seeing enough problems to determine whether or not they know how to solve them. It is a grave problem for a student who is very insecure. He wants to see everything, in case he should miss something that he will need next week. He is afraid that next week he'll have a case of some exotic disease and he will not know how to handle it because he has never seen one. Perhaps this is a legitimate gripe on the student's part; perhaps it only really represents a manifestation of his own insecurity. He feels that if he sees everything in his medical school training, he will be able to handle everything. The uncertainties of medicine are a lot more prominent in his thinking at this time. Actually, what happens is that he cannot see everything, because disease, like everything else, changes; and when the time comes that he is presented with a problem, he may have had no concrete example of this problem with which he has dealt previously. Pedagogically speaking, I am sure that really teaching people how to solve problems in general is the best principle. On the other hand, it is less satisfactory for the student's peace of mind than if he knows he has coped with a lot of different problems. Since the student feels that

[2] This interview is presented in more detail in Chapter 16.

the GMC patients frequently do not have a wide variety of organic illnesses, he feels he is not being taught as well as if he saw many different organic problems. Actually, it is probably much better to learn how to solve problems in general. But, as far as the student is concerned, he wants to know he has handled specific things and has specific information, rather than general things and information. I think you could probably argue it both ways.

It is not unreasonable to suppose that until the medical schools execute with confidence a clear policy of teaching general principles in the clinical years, the student is likely to cling to a never-to-be-fulfilled hope of arming himself with increments of knowledge in direct proportion to the number of examples he actually sees. Should the teachers be uncertain which is the correct course to follow, as the above teacher was, one would expect the student's uncertainty to reach serious proportions.

It should be emphasized that it is far more profitable to gain an understanding of *why* students' conclusions about an educational program differ from conclusions reached by other procedures than it is to defend either conclusion against the other. (See Chapters 16 and 17 for a detailed presentation of the findings concerning medical knowledge and skill.)

Psychological and sociological knowledge and skill. As mentioned earlier, the conclusion was reached that although the GMC may have increased the student's psychological knowledge and skill, the findings were not definitive. However, if the GMC did increase the student's knowledge in this area, what caused this increase?

Again the evidence is not entirely unequivocal, but it seems doubtful that the efforts of the staff in the individual student-staff teaching conference had much effect. There was virtually no difference between the manner in which the GMC staff taught their students in these conferences and the manner in which the control clerkship staff taught their students. Nor were any of the special educational devices of the GMC related to gain in psychological knowledge and skill. Therefore, it must be assumed that general experience in the GMC (weekly psychosomatic conferences, preceptorial meetings, and informal chats with instructors—*which were not isolated for study by the research group*) and the increase in reading which the GMC students reported, accounted for any differences between the two groups which might have occurred but not been detected because of inadequacy of the testing procedure.

Except for the fact that on one occasion one group of GMC students gained far more sociological knowledge and skill than the control students, essentially the same explanation would apply to this area. (See Chapters 19, 20, and 22 for a detailed presentation of these findings.)

Attitudes. In general, it was found that the GMC student did not develop increasingly negative attitudes toward the concept of comprehensive care while the control student did. The most important reason for this difference seems to have been the nature of the student's relation to his patients. The GMC student had a greater sense of responsibility for his patients (even though he frequently disliked the patients) than did the control student, and this sense of responsibility seems to have led to a greater appreciation of the value of comprehensive care.

Furthermore, there was a definite tendency for those students in the GMC who had more direct experience with patients in their homes to attach increased importance to social components of medical care. Direct contact with the patients' environment seemed to lead to attitude change in this area. In fact, all the evidence indicates that those students who participated most in the special educational features of the GMC were affected most.

But the GMC student did not become more interested in his patients; he did not develop closer and better physician-patient relations—mainly because the psychological and social problems of patients were peripheral to the student's main interest, learning organic medicine. Not only did the GMC patients fail to provide the organic pathology the student wished to study, diagnose, and treat, but they presented the student with diffuse psychological and social problems which he did not want to study, diagnose, and treat—particularly in the senior year. In fact, if one takes the expressed hostility of the GMC group toward their patients (as a group) at its face value, it is remarkable indeed that the student was able to overcome his attitudes toward these agents of frustration sufficiently to be able to perceive the general significance of psychological and social factors. (See Chapters 18, 21, and 23 for a detailed presentation of these findings.)

These findings confirm the conclusions drawn earlier—that the medical student is affected primarily by concrete, first-hand experiences with patients. But the results also suggest that until the student (and instructors) perceive the learning situation to have more general purposes, patients such as those the GMC student studied are likely to be barriers, rather than aids, to education.

Individual attributes related to change in knowledge, skill, and attitudes

The findings discussed below were obtained by correlating measures of individual attributes (such as personality characteristics, attitudes, values, and previous academic performance) with changes in the student's performance from pretest to posttest (see Figure 10.1 for testing schedule).

Medical knowledge and skill. No important relations were discovered between measures of individual attributes and gain in medical knowledge and skill. This might be explained simply on the grounds that when selected students are in an intensive training situation in which their motivation to gain the requisite knowledge and skills to graduate is uniformly high, individual attributes such as personality characteristics, attitudes, and values are unimportant. Another explanation might be that the tests of medical knowledge and skill were technically deficient, in the sense that they were not very precise measures of *change* in knowledge and skill. It was found, however, that change in performance on these tests was related to measures of the characteristics of the individual student-staff teaching conferences. Therefore, if the tests were precise enough to detect the relation between teaching and gain in knowledge and skill, they should have been precise enough to detect substantial relations between individual attributes and gain in medical knowledge and skill, if there were any.

Thus, the following conclusion was drawn and is offered as a hypothesis worthy of further research: Individual attributes of a student are not related to the acquisition of medical knowledge and skill in the senior year. The kind of teaching the student receives from an instructor in the individual student-staff conference, however, is related to gain in medical knowledge and skill.

Psychological knowledge and skill. The results in this area were almost exactly the opposite from those presented immediately above. The individual attributes of a student were found to be related to gain in psychological knowledge and skill, whereas the kind of teaching was not. These findings, of course, lead to the formulation of a hypothesis exactly the reverse of the one stated immediately above: The acquisition of psychological knowledge and skill in the senior year is determined primarily by the individual attributes of a student. The kind of teaching a student receives in the individual student-staff conference is not related to gain in psychological knowledge and skill.

The student who was an "independent achiever," that is, interested more in academic achievement than in social acceptance, gained the most in psychological knowledge and skill. Factors involved in concern for social acceptance and factors involved in independent achievement were found to be interrelated in an interesting fashion. For example, when psychological skill was measured in terms of the number of correct answers made to multiple-choice questions about the psychological problems of patients seen in the Sound-Film Interview, it was the independent achiever who improved his score the most. However, when psychological skill was measured in terms of the student's ability to perceive accurately the personality characteristics of the patients in the Sound-Film Interview, the student who was more concerned with social acceptance made the greatest improvement in scores from pretest to posttest.

These problems deserve further research, for although the tests of psychological knowledge and skill were far from precise measures, it may well be that there are two types of students—those who "intellectualize" psychological problems, that is, understand and perceive them in a purely intellectual, logical sense, and those who perceive psychological problems in a more intuitive manner. The hypothetical existence of this polarity—not dichotomy—of types has often been discussed in both clinical medicine and clinical psychology, and in Jungian theory as well. The kinds of tests used in the present project might in the future be developed to the point where they could be used to test empirically the truth of this hypothesis and, in consequence, be used to identify students who function in these different ways (if they do).

Attitudes. In general, it was the student with a low academic standing and undesirable personality characteristics who developed negative attitudes toward the various facets of comprehensive care. The student who stood high in his class was more likely either not to have changed his attitudes or to have changed them in a positive direction. In the main, the intelligent, responsible student was the one who had positive attitudes toward comprehensive care at the beginning of the senior year, and who either did not change his attitudes in a negative direction (as the majority of the students did) or changed in a positive direction.

There was some evidence, however, which indicated that students with certain attributes were more likely to change their attitudes if they participated in one program than if they participated in the other. For example, in one control group almost all the poor students changed their attitudes in a negative direction. But in the GMC as many poor students changed positively (or did not change) as changed negatively. Both programs had about the same effect on the attitudes of the good students. Differential effects of this sort did not occur often. However, the findings suggest that future studies including larger numbers of subjects, larger differences between training programs, better measures of attitude change, and better measures of individual attributes, will discover marked differences in attitude change between those students who are mature, responsible, and capable, and those who are not. The most important problem will be to discover whether it is the poor student whose attitudes are more apt to be changed by an experience in a clinic like the GMC. The present study suggests that the good student is apt to develop positive attitudes toward comprehensive care in either type of clerkship.

To summarize, the entire set of findings fits together well. For example, if one were to look only at the findings of the analysis of the two programs, that is, the study of the individual student-staff teaching conferences, one would suppose that no large differences in gain of knowledge and skill between the two programs would be found. They were not found. Under these circumstances it is not surprising that those students who did acquire more psychological knowledge and skill were those who had the ability and motivation to seek it, irrespective of which program they were in. Nor would it be surprising to find that attitude change took place mainly as a function of the "institutional demand" which the GMC staff as a whole planned and created, rather than as a result of individual teaching.

Although many medical educators will be disconcerted to note that these senior medical students were tending to develop increasingly negative attitudes toward comprehensive care and its corollary concepts, others will find support for their hypotheses in these findings. For, indeed, it was upon the hypothesis that senior students were developing negative attitudes that the GMC Program was introduced at the University of Colorado. The findings of this study indicate that the GMC was a step in the right direction.

Reflections on the Research Project

The purpose of this section is to acquaint the reader with some of the afterthoughts which occurred to the psychologist who directed the research project. Since research in medical education is still in the pioneering stage, some comments on the project as a whole seem appropriate. These comments will be addressed to questions which, it has been found by experience, were apt to be asked at the end of a visit to the research project.

How did the project as a whole work out? In general, much better than expected. After all, there were serious doubts that research of this sort was at all feasible in institutions of higher learning—particularly in medical schools—which have earned, although perhaps have not deserved, a reputation for being impervious to ideas originating from nonmedical sources. The research went smoothly, with excellent rapport between members of the medical school faculty and the research group. The students were not quite so consistent in their cooperation, however, and although everyone will find it easy to understand and sympathize with the students' occasional departure from full cooperation, the researcher would do well to remain forewarned (see Chapter 10) of the potential catastrophe attendant on this lapse in sympathy with research.

The courage, patience, and stamina of the members of the medical school faculty and of the GMC staff in particular, who originated the suggestion that the GMC Program be studied and evaluated by research methods, was superb.

Do you think you really evaluated the GMC? Yes. The research group was able to identify and set forth the objectives of the GMC, to determine the extent to which these objectives were achieved and why they were or were not achieved, and to discover some facts about the attributes of individual students who did or did not achieve these aims. Moreover, these findings make sense.

However, the evaluation was certainly not very precise. The findings were obtained with imprecise tests, under rather poor testing conditions, with few opportunities for replication. Yet the findings achieved by various methods, crude and imprecise as they were, confirm one another. Thus, in spite of these defects, particularly among the measures of the effects of the GMC, there seems to be good reason to believe that the evaluation of the GMC was accomplished—although the reader, of course, must answer this question for himself.

Did you learn anything about this type of research? Yes. First of all, research of this type requires time. A project of this type should last for at least ten years. Replication is absolutely essential to prevent the drawing of conclusions from accidental combinations of student and staff personnel, etc. Moreover, it must be realized that although change implies progress and is therefore constructive, change is also destructive. That is, a change in theory, method, or technique normally means non-comparability of data and, therefore, subsequent reduction of opportunities for replication. One should anticipate a rather long period, say five years, before a research program is declared unchangeable. This is particularly true if "deadline research" is to be avoided (see Chapter 10).

Second, some arrangement should be made to give the researcher access to the student for a considerable quantity of time—perhaps forty-eight to seventy-two hours during a twelve-month year. This might not interfere with the student's academic work if some of the research study were carried out during the time the student was away from school.

Third, the student's career following graduation should be carefully studied. There are many obvious reasons for this, and the fact should not be overlooked that a long-term project is in an excellent position to carry out much-needed longitudinal studies of graduates.

Fourth, arrangements must be made for both basic and applied research. New theories, new methods, and new procedures will force new questions to be raised and new techniques to be tested. It may be necessary to carry out this basic research in a context separate from the applied research, perhaps in another medical school.

What was the most important contribution of each section?

DEPENDENT VARIABLES SECTION. Clearly the most important contribution of this section was the development of the Sound-Film Interview procedure, with its emphasis on interpersonal perception. The analysis of the manner in which one person perceives another promises to be an extremely important technique for quantifying various aspects of interpersonal relations, as well as for evaluating specific programs whose purpose is to improve skills in interpersonal relations. The methodological analysis undertaken in this project, it is hoped, was a definite step forward in this promising area.

INDEPENDENT VARIABLES SECTION. The most important feature of the work of the Independent Variables Section was its emphasis on *what the teacher and the student actually said to one another* in the individual student-staff conference concerning the problems of a patient. This point deserves some discussion.

It is perfectly apparent that the increasing organization and complexity of educational institutions has led to the development of complicated bureaucratic structures within them. As Merton has pointed out so well, bureaucratic structures lead to a situation wherein means become ends, and the original purposes of the institution become strangled in bureaucratic complexity.[3] No one who has talked to professors in schools of higher learning can fail to be impressed with their frustration as they try to avoid administrative entanglements in the effort to teach and to act like scholars rather than bureaucrats. And nowhere is this more apparent than in today's medical school. Because of the bureaucratic trend, research in higher education is likely to focus on practical questions posed by administrators, such as: Is this program (or curriculum) better than that one, or, how can we select students so as to decrease our rate of failures? Research, in short, is apt to be directed more at answering questions growing out of administrative problems (such as comparison of programs) than at questions growing out of problems of individual

[3] Robert K. Merton, "Bureaucratic Structure and Personality," *Social Forces* 18:560–568, 1940.

functioning (such as the teaching of students). That is not to say that administrative problems are not worthy of research. They are. However, the study of the actual teaching process—and by that is meant what the teacher says to the student and what the student says in return—is in danger of being overlooked because of the increasing bureaucratization of higher education. The emphasis which this section of the research project placed on the analysis of the interaction between student and teacher in the individual student-staff teaching conference was its most important contribution.

INDIVIDUAL DIFFERENCES SECTION. Perhaps the largest contribution of the Individual Differences Section of the research project came as a result of the study of GMC staff ratings. Discovery of the manner in which the medical staff of the GMC evaluated the students provided unexpected additional information about the nature of the experimental program itself. Careful attention to this possibility while planning for staff evaluation of students may well repay future research workers. In any event, the analysis of staff evaluations of students carried out in this study should direct more attention to the evaluation process than it has received heretofore.

Why did you include student opinion in your data? A substantial part of the data concerning the medical school environment was derived from students' reports (the questionnaire data). Consequently, conclusions concerning the nature of the independent variables of the experiment rest not only on objective analyses, but on students' reports as well. Was this good research strategy?

The answer to this question is a simple one—collection of such data cannot be avoided if the research worker has any pretensions to carrying out a study of an educational process. This question needs to be raised only because questionnaires have been misused and abused and because the function of students' reports has also been misunderstood. The reactions of the student, changes in his values, beliefs, and attitudes about his educational environment are important aspects of any educational environment. The beliefs and attitudes of the student are important because the teacher must somehow cope with them—whether he wants to or not. Attempting to ignore the student's attitudes may be the most difficult and ineffective of all ways of coping with them. Moreover, students' attitudes may occupy a central place in the aims of an educational program, as they did here.

Although few will deny the importance of the student's beliefs and attitudes, many will be dubious about the role of such beliefs and attitudes in a study which attempts to evaluate the effectiveness of an educational program. Are students really competent judges of the value of various educational experiences? many will wonder.

The answer to this question is clear—no, they are not (but neither are professors). However, it is extremely important to know what both parties believe to be true. For example, when the student reports that he does not believe his professors are proficient in a certain aspect of their profession, this must not be taken to mean that the professors are in fact not proficient. But if it is a fact that the student holds this belief, this fact is an extremely important piece of information about the educational program, for one can readily expect that the learning activities and general behavior of this student would differ from those of a student who held the opposite belief. The same is true of professors. They direct their teaching efforts toward those areas in which they feel the student most needs instruction. Of course, just as in the student's case, the professors may make incorrect appraisals of the student's proficiency—and they frequently do. Such mistakes often do not appear to the professors until they read final examination papers, and some professors never become aware of them. Student opinion, like faculty opinion, should be taken for what it is—subjective, informed appraisal of an educational program—very *important*, but not very *definitive*.

Did you, in the course of the research, develop any ideas about teaching comprehensive care—ideas resulting from your own experience rather than from the research itself? Yes, of course. First of all, it is of critical importance to make a distinction between *knowledge about human behavior* and *humanitarianism*.[4] Often it is assumed that the former is lacking and that there is a surfeit of the latter. And equally frequently the opposite assumption is made. Moreover, whichever seems to be lacking, it is often assumed that appeal to the one will decrease the deficiency of the other. Sometimes the concept "comprehensive care" implies mainly humanitarianism and sometimes mainly knowledge about human behavior.

What is needed first is a clear recognition that although there is a considerable relation between humanitarianism and knowledge of human behavior, they are not identical, and one is not necessarily the cause of the other. Humanitarian behavior does not require a scientific understanding of behavior, however much the latter may help. Nor do medical educators need to attempt to convince medical students of the practical value of a knowledge of behavioral science as an inducement for being a decent human being. Humanitarianism needs no defense—and physicians and medical students (and anyone else, including psychologists, atomic physicists, and politicians) should be censured for not practicing it in word and deed. Furthermore,

[4] The reader should be reminded that the viewpoint expressed here is that of the director of the research project and not that of the director of the GMC. For his viewpoint see Chapters 1 and 12.

it is futile to try to defend humanitarianism; it cannot be scientifically proved to be the most desirable attitude toward others. In attempting such a proof one rests his case on a weak science—the science of behavior; the empirical proof is often unconvincing simply because significant empirical laws of behavior are clearly lacking at this time. When the teacher attempts to demonstrate scientifically the value of the humanitarian viewpoint, the evidence is apt to be unconvincing, and as a result the student may reject the proposition that one should be humanitarian. The point is—it needs no proof: physicians and medical students should treat their patients in a humanitarian way, whether or not this philosophy can be empirically proved to be of immediate and direct value to the patient.

Nor is it necessary to urge that the medical student study psychology or sociology on the assumption that such study results in the development of humanitarian attitudes. It is the medical student's responsibility to study these subjects for whatever promise they hold as scientific disciplines relevant to the practice of medicine.

Failure to make the distinction between humanitarianism and the scientific understanding of behavior often causes the teacher and student to confuse the reasons for taking certain steps for the benefit of a patient. Consider the following example: patients, social workers, nurses, psychologists, psychiatrists, medical students, and physicians often criticize medical students and physicians for discussing a ward patient's illness in front of the patient in such a way as to markedly increase the patient's anxiety about his illness. How should the student learn to refrain from this kind of behavior? Should the internist or psychiatrist attempt to show on scientific grounds that this particular kind of inhumane behavior is inimicable to the patient's welfare? No, because the explanation often fails for perfectly good reasons: there are not sufficient data to establish empirical proof that this behavior is detrimental to the patient's welfare. Or, worse yet, the student refers to this kind of instruction as mere "common sense," and notes that he is often less foolhardy in this respect than his teachers; he may feel that his teachers are wasting their time and his in discussing so elementary a matter.

The student should learn that such behavior is inhumane and therefore not permissible on that ground alone. As a matter of fact, students seem to be quite convinced of this, in any case, and a change in their behavior seems to require only the assurance that humane behavior is appropriate. Moreover, the place to present whatever scientific information is available on what happens to patients under the conditions described in the example seems to be in basic courses in psycho-physiology.

The above illustration is admittedly an oversimplified one. But apparently it is necessary to point out to medical students and physicians the fact that they are often indifferent to human values in their work with patients. (Students should never, as one student did, regard their work as "veterinary medicine.") Let the medical schools unashamedly require humanitarian values for their own sake; and let the behavioral sciences stand or fall on scientific grounds. In those instances in which the behavioral sciences serve the cause of humanity, as medicine has so nobly done, let service be its own reward.

Distinguishing between these two concepts or definitions of comprehensive care raises the question of the implications of each concept. Implications of each point of view are discussed below with respect to two critical questions: Who is qualified to teach comprehensive care, and is comprehensive care to be taught by the clinical method, or in the context of a basic course in the behavioral sciences?

If the practice of comprehensive care signifies humanitarianism in action, then, of course, any decently motivated, conscientious instructor is capable of teaching in a comprehensive care clinic. Interviews with the faculty of the GMC (and many other physicians) leave the impression that to them comprehensive care implied humanitarianism rather than a body of knowledge, for they indicated that specific preparation is unnecessary as a prerequisite for teaching in a comprehensive care clinic (see Chapter 19).

If, however, the practice of comprehensive care requires familiarity with a body of knowledge and a series of techniques, it is natural to ask: Who is trained with respect to this knowledge and these techniques sufficiently well to teach them? The psychiatrist, of course, is assumed to be expert in this regard. To rely solely on the psychiatrist for the clinical instruction of medical students, however, would be to place a tremendous burden on an already overburdened specialist. Such reliance is impossible, for it would mean that the psychiatrist would have to see virtually all of the students' patients. It is clear that other teachers must assume responsibility for instruction in clinical psychiatry and psychology as well. But other members of the medical faculty are not sufficiently expert in psychiatry and psychology, as will be readily acknowledged by most members of a medical faculty. And it is interesting to note that the present study indicates that medical students feel they are more proficient than their instructors in working with the psychological problems of patients (see Chapter 19).

Thus, if comprehensive care signifies humanitarian attitudes, faculty members may be selected to teach comprehensive care simply on the basis of their attitudes. But if comprehensive care is to include a body of knowledge and a series of techniques, faculty members must be trained in this knowledge and these techniques, or specialists in the behavioral sciences must be added to the medical faculty. It is apparent that both these steps are presently being taken despite the fact that many physicians feel that comprehensive care does not include the application of the knowledge and techniques of the behavioral sciences.

In short, it is important to make a distinction between these conceptions of comprehensive care so that the instructor and student can perceive clearly the distinction between the application of the humanitarian values of the faculty and the application of scientific knowledge to a patient's problem. Failure to make this distinction is apt to lead to argument based on confusion of premises or failure to grasp the reasons for specific action.

On the assumption that comprehensive care signifies the application of knowledge, the next question is: Should comprehenive care be taught by the clinical method, or in the context of a basic course in the behavioral sciences? It will be instructive to consider first the different ways in which clinical medicine and psychology (or psychiatry) make contributions to the medical student's capacity to deal with a specific problem in the clinic. Consider how a student's training to deal with a specific organic disease helps him to cope with a patient's problem. Assume the ideal situation. The student begins with a series of facts, which at first have little structure and do not allow the student to take action. As the student (and his teacher) work with these facts, however, a certain structure begins to appear and the facts begin to develop meaning in relation to one another. As the organization of facts takes on more meaning and structure, the student finally arrives at a diagnosis. Now that a diagnosis has been achieved, the courses of action are opened up immediately, for (in the ideal case) a course of therapy is attached to the diagnosis. Thus, achievement of a diagnosis has moved the student closer to action. This, of course, is a highly gratifying situation for the medical student (and all concerned).

When a psychological problem is involved, however, exactly the opposite course of events is likely to take place; action is likely to be immediately apparent to the student, whereas organization of the facts may lead to inaction. For example, if a patient is found to be obese and the cause of the obesity is found to be in overeating, the action to be taken is direct and obvious—restriction of diet. Suppose, however, further facts are collected about the psychological aspects of the patient's problem, and a psychiatric diagnosis made. Because the diagnosis is likely to be much more complicated than "overeating," and because the student may discover that restriction of diet is exactly the wrong move, the student is now likely to find himself much further removed from action. The diagnosis is unlikely to be closely attached to therapy, as in the case of a strictly organic diagnosis, such as, say, appendicitis. Thus, a strictly organic diagnosis is much more apt to lead to action that enables the student to fulfill his role as a healer and is, therefore, far more likely to be satisfying than a psychiatric diagnosis which the student may find prevents him from fulfilling his role. If the above analysis is at all correct, it must be recognized that until psychological diagnosis and psychotherapy are on firmer scientific grounds, the clinical study of psychological factors in medicine will very likely require special motives on the part of the student (as in fact the present study indicates).

In short, because of the pressure on the medical student for action directly related to removing the patient's disease, the clinic appears to be a poor place in which to introduce the student to the role of psychological and social factors in medicine.

If the above conclusion is correct, it follows that the student should be introduced to the role of psychological and social factors in disease prior to participating in the clinic. Should this introduction take place in a basic course in the behavioral sciences in the already overcrowded medical school curriculum? The answer is obvious—if comprehensive care implies a knowledge of behavioral science, then medical students should learn behavioral science as a basic course. And behavioral science, it should be pointed out, is not identical with psychiatry any more than clinical medicine is identical with biology. But it must be recognized that it is an open question whether the behavioral sciences are, right now, developed to the extent that behavioral scientists are prepared to assume the responsibilities of a basic science course. However, if this question is answered in the negative, it is difficult to see what the term comprehensive care can signify at this time, aside from denoting the endorsement of humanitarianism.

Chapter 12

Implications of the GMC Program

In this chapter some of the implications of the General Medical Clinic Program will be explored—implications for medical education in general as well as at the University of Colorado. What is the value of this type of program? Was the GMC, from the educator's point of view, a success? What were the particular educational objectives and special techniques of the program? How did these relate to the over-all aims of medical education? Could the program have been made to function more effectively, and if so, how? Is it realistic to expect that the program could be improved? These questions are discussed in this chapter. In addition, certain aspects of the research project are considered: for example, its effect on the teaching program; whether the control group really functioned as such; the identification of the research group with the GMC; and the general validity of the findings of the research project. One specific phase of the research program, the Independent Variables Section, is criticized in some detail. Finally, there is a discussion of the present functioning of the GMC.

The Research Program

From the medical educator's viewpoint, the research project was of invaluable assistance in the conduct of the General Medical Clinic. In spite of a few criticisms that will appear below, it was generally regarded as a success.

The fact that the effects of the GMC and control programs were going to be measured and evaluated in a concrete, impersonal way by a separate group contributed greatly to the objectivity of the GMC staff. As a result the staff were able to focus their efforts on the efficient functioning of the program without being distracted by anxiety about how the program "looked" to the rest of the medical school staff and administration. Their energies could be concentrated on improving the program without being diverted to defending it. The only possible criticism of this aspect of the research is that there was some tendency for the research project to become too closely associated with the GMC Program. This statement should not be interpreted as casting any aspersions upon the objectivity of the research group itself—far from it. However, when the research workers first appeared in the medical school, their function was unfortunately labeled as "evaluating the GMC Program," and in the minds of a good many people they became identified with the GMC rather than with the medical school as a whole. This may have led to some unwarranted resistance to their presence and findings. In any future project of this kind, it would probably be advisable to make certain that the research group is identified with the entire medical school.

Were the results produced by the research program valid? This question is, of course, somewhat beyond the scope of the medical educators involved with the GMC Program; yet they could hardly avoid forming opinions on it. In general, they believed that the results were valid. One question, however, should be discussed in connection with this: the adequacy of the control group. Was it really a control? For one thing, there was a considerable amount of staff overlap; some people taught in both programs during the experimental period. Moreover, there was close contact between the two student groups, with consequent interaction. However, in some ways these apparent deficiencies were an asset: they meant that the organizational patterns and philosophies of the two clinics were the chief, if not the only, differences between the programs, and it was logical to attribute to these the different effects ascertained by the research team.

In working with and observing the researchers, the medical staff could not help being impressed with their thoroughness and objectivity. This also tended to promote confidence in the validity of the results.

Only one phase of the research program seemed to the medical staff to deserve serious criticism: the Independent Variables Section. The purpose of this section was to describe the actual operation of the clinic teaching program. However, its research was focused on only one phase of the teaching program: the student-staff conferences. Other aspects were not fully studied, including the fundamental organization which stressed student responsibility and continuity of care, and the weekly conferences—the family care conferences, the psychosomatic conferences, the preceptorial meetings. It was in these activities that the philosophy and attitudes of comprehensive medical care were repeatedly made explicit. Furthermore, most of the data on independent variables were processed for only one year (1956). Also, there can be little doubt that the use of visible recording machinery for collecting data had a selective effect on the data thus gathered. The fact that both the student and the staff physician knew the conference was being recorded undoubtedly made for somewhat atypical performances on these occasions. For these reasons, then, the medical staff was inclined to feel that the findings of the Independent Variables Section were quite incomplete. In extenuation, however, it should be stated that this section was attempting to do something new and very difficult, and complete success was not to be expected. It is encouraging that significant progress was made in this most important field of research.

The GMC Program

Probably the primary question in the reader's mind at this point is whether this type of program is worth while. Would it be advisable, in the opinion of the medical educators who conducted this program, to institute more such programs elsewhere? These questions cannot be answered with a categorical yes or no. Many subordinate questions must be considered separately. First, the special objectives of the program and the relation of these objectives to those of medical education in general must be considered.

A useful statement of the objectives of medical education was published by the Association of American Medical Colleges.[1] According to this statement (which must, the authors caution, "be considered a document still in development and under revision"), undergraduate medical education "should not aim at presenting the complete, detailed, systematic body of knowledge concerning each and every medical and related discipline. Rather, it must provide the setting in which the student can learn fundamental principles applicable to the whole body of medical knowledge, establish habits of reasonable and critical judgment of evidence and experience, and develop an ability to use these principles and judgments wisely in solving problems of health and disease."

The statement goes on to emphasize the importance of providing the student with incentive by giving him "definite responsibility in real day-to-day problems of health and disease," responsibility which "must, of course, be carefully graded to the student's ability and experience," and which "must be exercised under careful guidance by the faculty." The basic aims of undergraduate medical education are specified: "to help the student to: acquire basic professional knowledge; establish essential habits; attain clinical and social skills neces-

[1] "The Objectives of Undergraduate Medical Education" (eighth revision), *Journal of Medical Education* 28:57–59, March 1953.

sary to the best utilization of that knowledge; and develop those basic intellectual attitudes and ethical or moral principles which are essential if he is to gain and maintain the confidence and trust of those whom he treats, the respect of those with whom he works and the support of the community in which he lives."

In general, the special objectives of the GMC Program harmonized closely with the basic objectives outlined above. Most medical educators recognize that there are two competing types of education which the student must receive: (1) he must be taught principles of medicine—that is, he must learn a body of medical knowledge and acquire an understanding of the basic techniques used both in medical research and in the practice of medicine; and (2) he must receive a certain amount of training—that is, he must learn to practice medicine by applying his knowledge in the clinics and wards under appropriate supervision. These two aspects of medical education might be labeled the theoretical and the clinical (or practical). Both are, quite properly, recognized in the Association of American Medical Colleges' statement quoted above, and both were recognized in the GMC Program. If there was any important difference between the goals of the GMC and those of more traditionally oriented programs, that difference might be one of relative emphasis on these two competing types of education, with the curricular structure of the GMC making it possible to emphasize the clinical (or practical) aspect.

Such a difference, however, would be more apparent than real: the fundamental objectives of the GMC Program were identical with the over-all objectives of medical education; the difference was in educational technique only. It must be stressed again that the clinic (from an educational point of view) was a means only, not an end in itself. To clarify this point it will be necessary to review the distinction made in the preceding paragraph between theoretical and clinical medical education. Probably all medical educators recognize that their ultimate goal is to instill in the student an understanding of the fundamentals of medicine; without such theoretical knowledge the scientific practice of medicine would be impossible. It is also essential to motivate the student to acquire such understanding, and having the students engage in supervised clinical practice is the best method of motivation. Furthermore, theoretical understanding of medical principles, though fundamental, is not enough. It must be supplemented by the ability to apply that fundamental understanding in practice; again, supervised clinical practice in which the student feels responsible for "his" patients, is essential.

Thus, the relative value of the GMC type of program and those that are more traditionally oriented seems to depend on the answer to the question: Is it advisable to teach by giving the student the type and extent of responsibility he was given in the GMC Program? (It should be remembered that all the patients' medical and related problems were the responsibility of the student.) Since the ultimate goals were really the same, the question becomes a practical one: Did the attempt to teach comprehensive medicine in a general medical clinic where the student assumed definite and continued responsibility for his patients prove successful? Did the added responsibility and the emphasis on comprehensiveness stimulate the student to acquire the requisite understanding of medicine? Judging from the results of the tests of medical knowledge and medical skill developed by the research project, the answer was yes. However, a caveat should be entered at this point: it is possible that the apparent success of the program was due in part to the extra effort and enthusiasm of the staff and others participating in a new program. Any newly conceived and established venture is likely to arouse enthusiastic energy in those concerned in it, and the GMC was no exception to this generalization. However, the writers are still inclined to attribute the major part of the program's success to the special philosophy of the clinic: it was and is apparent to those directly involved that the operative factors in stimulating the student were the student's being given primary responsibility for "his" patients, frequent contact with patients over a six-month period, development of gratifying student-patient relations, and the emphasis on total care of the patients, including the Family and Home Care Program. Not only did these factors stimulate the GMC student to acquire (so far as could be ascertained) at least as much medical knowledge and skill as the control student, but, more importantly, they stimulated him to develop or maintain desirable attitudes toward his patients and the practice of medicine.

This last point concerning attitudes is felt to be important because as the program developed the medical educators in the clinic became increasingly convinced that the practice of comprehensive medicine is fundamentally a matter of an approach, a set of attitudes, on the part of the physician. It is a matter of what the physician believes his responsibility toward the patient to be. There is no concrete body of knowledge that can be labeled "comprehensive medicine." If there were, the techniques of the GMC Program might have been unnecessary. The appropriate way to impart a body of knowledge is through a curriculum of courses, not a clinical program. However, it was clear to the staff of the GMC that their function was not to convey facts about comprehensive medicine to the student, but rather to get the student to apply his knowledge of medicine and related disciplines to patient care in the best tradition. Thus, comprehensive medical care might be redefined as the sympathetic use of basic medical knowledge, intellectual curiosity, and honesty in the effort to help the patient with all the problems that he brings to his physician. It was never intended that the GMC should train the student in scientific psychology or sociology. Except for courses in abnormal psychology, the value for a physician of such training is not established. Physicians are not, nor can they be expected to become, sociologists or psychologists. They can and should be made aware of three facts: that there are psychological and social factors involved in the practice of medicine; that there are persons available, trained in these specialties, who can assist the physician in dealing with these factors; and that the physician should assume total responsibility for his patients' health, mental as well as physical. These and no others were the special goals of the GMC Program; otherwise its objectives were no different from those of any good program of medical education.

The above remarks do not imply that physicians would not profit by reading about psychology and sociology. Indeed, the opposite is strongly believed. Most physicians would benefit greatly by reading selectively in these social sciences and also in history. They could thus acquire a broadened view of human behavior that would probably promote the development of attitudes favorable to the practice of good medicine. Such reading would also promote increase in knowledge, but the knowledge so acquired would be general rather than specific. That is, these disciplines offer but few facts that the medical student or physician can be taught to apply to the treatment of an individual patient. Attempts to teach these facts usually result in the students' objecting that the information involved is "common sense."

A few questions about the operation of the clinic remain. One not yet fully answered (or possibly not answerable) is whether the senior year is the best time for such a program in the student's curriculum. The research project rather clearly revealed that the anxieties associated with the approaching responsibilities of internship disturbed some students and made them less receptive to the goals of the GMC. However, subsequent experience has shown that this effect was largely caused by the presence of the control group; now that all students are participating in the GMC Program, this type of dissatisfaction has been virtually eliminated. Possibly there would be advantages in placing the GMC Program earlier in the student's experience—the junior year for instance. However, there is some doubt that a student is qualified to obtain maximum benefit from this type of program before the senior year; moreover, the many other things that must be included in the early years of medical education make it extremely difficult to find room for such a program.

The answer to the question how the program could have been improved is threefold: it concerns the patients, the curriculum (or students), and the staff. In the first place, everyone connected with the program felt that it would have been more effective if the patients had been more satisfactory. The students were disturbed because they felt the patients did not present a concentration of specific disease entities such as they might see in a specialty clinic. The staff did not feel that this disadvantage was really as serious as the patients' lack of motivation to get well and the communication difficulties previously discussed. The high percentage of chronically, but not seriously, ill patients with insoluble psychological problems and hopeless social situations, together with the high missed appointment rate, definitely detracted from the effectiveness of the GMC as a teaching program. At present, therefore, the clinic patients are much more rigorously screened than they were during the experimental period. (This was made possible by the institution of another medical clinic and seven medical specialty clinics in July 1956.)

In the second place, many of the GMC staff felt that the program might have been more productive if it could have had a greater cumulative effect; that is, since its primary purpose was the inculcation of a set of attitudes, and since it takes a long time to change or develop attitudes, the program might have been more effective if it could have been extended over a longer period. The student's participation in the GMC should be prolonged to nine or twelve months.

Third, staffing a program of this kind is a major problem. Ideally, almost all the staff should be permanently associated with the program on a full-time basis; they should be skillful teachers, willing to devote long hours to working with students; and they should be highly competent in general medicine as well as the medical phases of psychology and sociology, and in their own medical specialty. Such people are not easy to find.

The difficulty is basic to medical education. Most qualified physicians tend to be interested either in medicine as a science or in the practice of medicine or both. They are not especially drawn to teaching per se, though many like the opportunities for research and teaching in their own specialties. A program designed to teach, in a clinical setting, the principles of comprehensive medicine calls for a rare combination of competence in scientific medicine and willingness to spend long hours working (sometimes to little apparent purpose) with patients whose problems are not amenable to scientific solutions. The problem is perhaps most apparent to the administrator who has to recruit staff for such a program. What are the rewards with which he can attract suitable people to participate in such a program? For the predominantly scientifically minded physician, the more conventional research and teaching situations are more enticing; for other physicians, the satisfactions of ordinary medical practice are greater. Moreover, the whole situation is complicated by the fact that the acceptance of almost any academic commitment means a serious financial sacrifice.

In view of the difficulties outlined above, it is perhaps somewhat unrealistic to expect a program of this type to be much more effective than the University of Colorado General Medical Clinic actually was. Certainly one fact clearly emerged from the present experiment: the success of this type of educational program depends upon the full support of everyone—participating faculty members, cooperating agencies, and the hospital staff. Without this support so many serious practical problems will arise that the effectiveness of the program will be seriously impaired.

It seems appropriate that this section should conclude with a description of the GMC Program as it has been functioning since the experimental period. Most of the basic features have been retained: the six-month continuity of student-patient contact, the same philosophy of total patient care, the same emphasis on the student's responsibility for his patients, the interest in family groups, and multiple department participation. However, partly as a result of what was learned during the experimental period, several changes have been made.

Since there is no longer any need of it, the control group has been eliminated. All students now participate in the GMC. This experience is, however, less concentrated. Students now attend the GMC two or three half-days per week instead of five or six half-days per week as they did during the experimental period. The extra time is spent in various specialty clinics at both teaching hospitals and in the Colorado General Hospital general medical and pediatric clinics.

The result of the foregoing changes has been the elimination of the students' dissatisfaction with the GMC. Most of this dissatisfaction had stemmed from the fact that the GMC students felt they were being deprived of specialty clinic experience which the control group had. Now that all students have both the specialty clinic and the GMC experience, they are highly satisfied with the GMC.

Two other changes have increased the effectiveness of the program. First, the family care conferences have been reinstituted, and thus the effectiveness of family care has been restored. Second, only about one fourth as many patients now participate in the GMC Program. This permits more rigorous screening of patients, and as a result many of the problems associated with poor teaching material have been eliminated.

Finally, it should be emphasized that the observations and conclusions of the research project were extremely useful in planning the senior curriculum after the experiment was completed. It is impossible to predict the conclusions the medical staff might have reached without the research, but the objective findings derived from the three years of study helped in the formulation of the present educational plan. The medical staff, of course, made their own observations, but were in the almost unique position of being guided by scientific data in making decisions about an educational program.

Part III

METHODOLOGY

Introduction to Part III

This section includes three chapters which describe the theories, methods, and procedures used in the research. Chapter 13 describes the manner in which the effects of GMC were determined, Chapter 14 describes the manner in which the two teaching programs—the (experimental) General Medical Clinic Program and the (control) medical clerkship program—were studied, and Chapter 15 describes the manner in which individual differences in response to the experimental and control programs were studied.

Chapter 13

Dependent Variables

How the Effects of the GMC Were Studied

The task of the Dependent Variables Section of the research project was to study the effects of the GMC Program. Once the objectives of the GMC were made clear, tests were developed to discover to what extent the objectives were met. These procedures were revised and improved as much as possible within the time limits of the research project. Because it was necessary to devise many entirely new procedures, considerable time and effort were devoted to test development and test revision. This chapter describes these efforts.

Owing to the nature of the objectives of the GMC (described in Part I and in Chapter 10), it was necessary to develop measures of the following variables: medical knowledge and skill, attitudes toward medicine, psychological knowledge and skill, attitudes toward the psychological components of medicine, sociological knowledge and skill, attitudes toward the social components of medicine. The traditional questionnaire and interview procedures and the traditional multiple-choice form of the attitude test were used. Besides these, several new procedures were devised. One of these, the Sound-Film Interview, provided a considerable amount of useful data and promises to be a valuable tool in the study of medical education. Because of the potential value of this procedure, the methodology involved in its development is presented in detail below. Descriptions of the other procedures follow in turn.

Sound-Film Interview

The traditional and primary function of the physician is to help sick patients, and students in the third and fourth years of medical school are learning to do just that. The senior medical student in particular is quite aware that his knowledge and skill are to be brought to bear on the problems of individual patients and he is keenly interested in patients and their illnesses. For this reason the research group wanted to develop a new type of test which would center on the problems presented by actual patients, rather than to rely entirely on more conventional testing procedures.

Because the design of the experiment was a comparative one, that is, it compared the performances of the GMC and the control students, and because the plan of the research involved studying more than one class of students, it was necessary for the *same* patients to be presented to each group in a rather well controlled way. Since the physician ordinarily interacts with the patient in the context of an interview, and since case records cannot include all the subtle, individual characteristics of a patient, it was decided to present the patients to the students by means of a sound-film interview.

Conducting the filmed interview. All interviews were conducted by a physician;[1] all followed the same general pattern; and all were six minutes in length. (Later developments in the administration of the tests indicated that six minutes is about the right length of time for a procedure of this sort.) Approximately the first minute and a half were devoted to the patient's medical problem, and the remaining time was spent discussing his personal and social history.

The patient sat at a table facing the interviewer. No attempt was made to conceal the camera; however, it was shielded by a heavy drape, and while the patient was being interviewed he could not see the cameraman or the observers behind the drape. The patient faced the camera and the picture was taken over the doctor's shoulder, showing part of his head and his left arm. The interviewer had access to the patient's history, from which he had prepared a series of interview questions. He had not met the patient previously. The doctor chatted with the patient until the patient's tenseness had disappeared; then he gave a secret signal to start the camera (which was noiseless). Within a few days after the film had been taken, a series of tests was administered to the patient. (The nature of these tests and the reasons for giving them are explained below.)

Selecting patients for filming. The success of this procedure, which involved presenting to students a series of patients, was critically dependent upon the method of selecting the patients. Patients might have been selected because they seemed interesting, challenging, or unusual; or because they seemed typical or classical. However, selection on the basis of these criteria was bound to be affected

[1] Approximately two thirds of the interviews were carried out by one physician and one third by another.

by the biases of the selectors. More important, unless patients were selected randomly it would be impossible to generalize the findings about students' responses to patients other than those presented in the films. It was, therefore, decided to select cases at random from the wards of the university's two teaching hospitals. (The technical aspects of the selection procedure are discussed below.) Complete randomness was not achieved, for certain restrictions had to be applied. Eliminated from the sample were patients who were too sick to be moved, patients who were senile, patients who were psychotic, and patients who did not speak English sufficiently well to be understood.

Films were made of thirty-six patients, but because of poor sound reproduction six were not used. Thus, thirty films were available, and ten different sound-film interviews were presented at each of the three test administrations, Pretest, Posttest I, and Posttest II.

Sound-film interview multiple-choice tests

Several tests were developed in connection with the Sound-Film Interview. Although it was not possible to develop tests relating to every objective of the GMC within the context of the Sound-Film Interview, tests were developed in connection with the medical, psychological, and sociological aspects of the patients' problems. Each of these is described below.

Medical Knowledge test. After the student saw a Sound-Film Interview of a patient he read a booklet which contained medical information about the patient, i.e., laboratory findings, pertinent physical findings, case history material, etc. (see Appendix 1). The student was then required to answer a number of questions involving medical knowledge related directly or indirectly to the patient's organic disease. Because this test was intended to measure medical knowledge (in the text book sense) rather than the ability to apply such knowledge to the problems of a particular patient, the medical knowledge questions could be answered without the information contained in the booklet or in the filmed interview. Questions 5, 7, 9, and 11 of Appendix 1 are examples of medical knowledge items. (Other questions related to the strictly medical aspects of the patient's problem which did require the student to utilize information presented in the interview or in the booklet constituted the Medical Skill test and are discussed below.) Test items were generally five-alternative, multiple-choice questions constructed by the GMC staff in consultation with the staff of the control clinic. There were 29 items in the Pretest, 26 in Posttest I, and 19 in Posttest II. The test was scored in terms of the percentage of items answered correctly. After administration to the class

Table 13.1. Corrected alternate-item reliability coefficients of scores on each test administration and of composite scores on all three administrations: medical knowledge (classes of 1954, 1955, 1956)

	Pretest		Posttest I		Posttest II		Composite	
	N	*r*	*N*	*r*	*N*	*r*	*N*	*r*
Class of 1954	79	.56	78	.55	56	.25	53	.75
Class of 1955	75	.54	55	.28	73	.44	55	.54
Class of 1956	65	.35	65	.17	65	.37	65	.45

of 1954, the questions were revised on the basis of the distributions of alternatives chosen, as well as of item reliability and item validity.

The reliability and validity of the Medical Knowledge test were investigated. Table 13.1 shows the alternate-item reliability coefficients of scores on each administration of the test, as well as of the composite scores on all three administrations, for each class of students. The reliability of the test as estimated by this procedure was low and appears to have decreased over the three years in spite of efforts to improve it. Table 13.2 presents the coefficients obtained when the students' scores on one administration were correlated with their scores on the other administrations. These correlation coefficients were also low.[2]

Reliabilities as low as those in Table 13.1 are generally considered inadequate. (As pointed out below, however, these tests were sufficiently accurate to detect group differences of the sort to be expected in this research.) What accounted for these low reliabilities? One might expect that poor test construction, inadequate attention to test format or test conditions, test heterogeneity, and group homogeneity would be pertinent factors. As a matter of fact, however, considerable attention was given to the construction of this test. Items were examined with respect to difficulty (percentage of students obtaining the correct answer[3]), reliability, and correlation between items and total test score. The questions were then revised by the medical staff. Little more could have been done in this way to improve test reliability. Although the test format seems to have been adequate, the testing conditions clearly decreased the reliability of this test to a definite, but unmeasured, degree. Fatigue, irritation, and other factors mentioned in Chapter 10 certainly reduced the reliability of this and other tests. Heterogeneity among various parts of the test also very likely was important in reducing alternate-item reliabilities. The total test concerning ten patients and their diseases essentially involved ten

[2] These correlations are not to be interpreted as test-retest reliability coefficients because different test-related educational experiences occurred between administrations of the test.

[3] The average item difficulty was approximately 50%, the range of item difficulty was from 20% to 80%.

Table 13.2. Correlation coefficients between scores on various test administrations: medical knowledge (classes of 1954, 1955, 1956)

	N	Pre–Post I	Pre–Post II	Post I–Post II
Class of 1954	75	.46	.42	.27
Class of 1955	55	.24	.15	.38
Class of 1956	65	.21	.26	–.05

subtests. The number of items relating to each patient was small (approximately two or three), and items were not equally difficult in all ten cases. Furthermore, senior medical students are quite homogeneous with respect to medical knowledge. If, for example, this test were given to juniors and seniors, these reliabilities very likely would reach adequate levels.

Results presented below, however, show that even these low reliabilities permitted useful discriminations to be made among groups. It should be recalled that this research project was not concerned with small, subtle differences which only highly reliable (highly accurate) tests would be able to detect. Also, it must be borne in mind that the statistical procedures used to detect differences between groups took account of the unreliability (statistical regression) involved in the change of scores from pretest to posttest.

The empirical validity of the Medical Knowledge Pretest proved to be substantial (see Table 13.3). In the classes of 1954 and 1955 scores on the Medical Knowledge Pretest substantially correlated with the staff's evaluations of students (grade averages) and students' evaluations of one another (peer judgments).[4] Moreover, the Pretest given to the class of 1955 correlated with Medical College Admissions Test scores administered three years earlier.

It is interesting to note that very low correlations between Medical Knowledge Pretest scores and grade averages were obtained in the class of 1956. It does not seem appropriate to attribute this finding to the invalidity of the test in view of the results obtained with the previous classes. Rather, the low correlations appear to reflect the attitudes of the faculty toward this class (see Chapter 10). In fact, given the history of this class and faculty attitudes toward it, the lack of relation between grade averages and Medical Knowledge Pretest scores might have been predicted.

Further evidence that the Medical Knowledge test possessed discriminating power is the fact that on five out of six occasions the test showed the students in both medical clerkships (GMC and control) to have gained more medical (as contrasted with surgical) knowledge than students in the surgery clerkship (see Table 16.2).

[4] See Chapter 15 for the complete list of peer judgments.

Table 13.3. Personal attributes correlated to a statistically significant degree ($p<.05$) with pretest of medical knowledge (classes of 1954 and 1955)

Class of 1954 (N=79)	Class of 1955 (N=70)
+.34 First-year grade average	+.35 Verbal Ability (MCAT)
+.52 Second-year grade average	+.29 Quantitative Ability (MCAT)
+.48 Cumulative grade average	+.30 Knowledge of Modern Society (MCAT)
+.36 Third-year grade average	+.34 Knowledge of Premedical Sciences (MCAT)
+.47 Competence as a physician (peer judgment)	+.35 Premedical grade average
+.36 Willingness and ability to work independently (peer judgment)	+.58 First-year grade average
+.59 Junior comprehensive examination	+.59 Second-year grade average
	+.44 Third-year grade average
	+.60 Cumulative grade average
	+.32 Grade in psychosomatics course
	+.29 Junior medical clerkship grade
	+.25 Junior pediatrics clerkship grade
	+.30 Junior OB-GYN clerkship grade
	+.34 Junior surgical clerkship grade
	—.28 Number of undergraduate credit hours in psychology
	+.30 Competence as a physician (peer judgment)
	+.41 Willingness and ability to work independently (peer judgment)
	+.27 Leadership (peer judgment)
	+.24 Sympathy to the concept of comprehensive care (peer judgment)
	+.31 Aesthetic value

In summary, the Medical Knowledge test was a useful procedure for ascertaining the extent to which students in the GMC and control groups acquired medical knowledge.

Medical Skill test. Because the GMC was intended to be a patient-oriented clinic, one of its objectives was to teach the student to apply his medical knowledge to his patient's problems more effectively than the traditionally trained student. Therefore, an attempt was made to develop a test to measure the student's skill in applying his medical knowledge to a patient's problem. Questions were written which required the student to relate his knowledge of the particular disease involved to specific information contained either in the booklet or in the filmed interview. (The reader will recall that correct answers to the Medical Knowledge test did not require the student to utilize information from either the booklet or the filmed interview.) Questions 1 and 3 of Appendix 1 are examples of medical skill items. In order to answer these questions correctly, the student had to apply his knowledge to the specific conditions presented by the patient's problems. Clearly, this procedure is only a rough approximation to

Table 13.4. Corrected alternate-item reliability coefficients of scores on each test administration: medical skill (class of 1956)

Pretest		Posttest I		Posttest II	
N	*r*	*N*	*r*	*N*	*r*
69	.44	65	—.10	65	.40

the measurement of a student's medical skill, but it was intended to be no more than that.

These questions were constructed by the same physicians and in the same manner as the medical knowledge questions. It was difficult, however, to obtain a sufficient number of medical skill questions because of the necessity of constructing them in connection with the content of the filmed interview and the information provided in the booklet. Moreover, the usual elimination of items occurred on the basis of item difficulty, reliability, and correlation between item and total test score. Thus, an adequate test was not ready until the class of 1956 was studied. There were 22 items in the Pretest, 21 in Posttest I, and 33 in Posttest II.

The alternate-item reliability of this test was low, and one reliability coefficient was slightly negative (see Table 13.4). This latter strange result may very well have been caused by the lapse in cooperation of the students (see Chapter 10). The reliability of the Medical Skill test was affected by factors in addition to those affecting the reliability of the Medical Knowledge test, for medical skill questions required that the student listen carefully to the not-always-adequate sound track of the film and read carefully the information contained in the test booklet. These conditions placed additional severe limitations on the reliability of this and the other measures of skill. The correlation coefficients between Medical Skill scores on various test administrations were also quite low (see Table 13.5).

Evidence for the empirical validity of the Medical Skill test is of necessity indirect, for there were no criteria readily available for assessing its validity (see Chapter 24). As hoped, however, the Medical Skill test did not correlate highly with the Medical Knowledge

Table 13.5. Correlation coefficients between scores on various test administrations: medical skill (classes of 1954, 1955, 1956)

	Pre–Post I		Pre–Post II		Post I–Post II	
	N	*r*	*N*	*r*	*N*	*r*
Class of 1954	75	.12	76	—.05	77	.13
Class of 1955	55	.12	72	.02	55	.08
Class of 1956	65	.24	65	.19	65	.00

Table 13.6. Corrected alternate-item reliability coefficients of scores on each test administration: psychological knowledge (class of 1956)

Pretest		Posttest I		Posttest II	
N	*r*	*N*	*r*	*N*	*r*
69	.35	64	.72	73	.41

test—the average correlation was +.40. Medical Skill Pretest scores (class of 1956) correlated highly with previous grade averages and students' evaluations (peer judgments) of one another with respect to medical knowledge. Also, on one of two occasions (change from December Posttest I to May Posttest II, class of 1956), the Medical Skill test discriminated between the students in the two medical clerkships (GMC and control) and the students in the surgical clerkship.

Psychological Knowledge test. The Psychological Knowledge test was constructed for the purpose of discovering whether participation in the GMC increased the student's knowledge of the psychological components of medicine more than did participation in the control clerkship. Like the medical knowledge items, questions in the Psychological Knowledge test could be answered by the student without reference to the information presented in either the film or the booklet. Questions 4, 8, and 12 of Appendix 1 are examples of psychological knowledge questions. (Questions which did require reference to information presented in the film and/or test booklet were included in the Psychological Skill test.) The Psychological Knowledge test consisted of five-alternative, multiple-choice questions constructed by the GMC psychiatrist in consultation with other members of the department of psychiatry of the medical school. The Pretest, Posttest I, and Posttest II each included 17 items. Questions concerning psychological knowledge were first introduced during the study of the class of 1955. After extensive revision, the test was used to compare GMC and control students in the class of 1956.

Reliability coefficients were quite low, as in the case of the other tests mentioned, and very likely for the same reasons: homogeneity of the group, too few items per patient, and test fatigue (see Table 13.6). Correlation coefficients between Psychological Knowledge scores on various test administrations are presented in Table 13.7.

Table 13.7. Correlation coefficients between scores on various test administrations: psychological knowledge (class of 1956)

Pre–Post I		Pre–Post II		Post I–Post II	
N	*r*	*N*	*r*	*N*	*r*
65	.58	65	.55	65	.64

The empirical validity of the Psychological Knowledge test is perhaps best substantiated by its consistent correlation with the Psychological-Mindedness scale of the CPI.[5] The Psychological Knowledge test and the Psychological-Mindedness scale were positively correlated to a statistically significant degree in the trial administrations with the class of 1955 and in the Pretest and Posttest I administrations with the class of 1956. Correlations between other measures and the Psychological Knowledge test are presented in Table 13.8. These suggest that a "psychological" component was present in the test, but that a general "ability to learn" factor was also present. The correlations should be noted between Psychological Knowledge scores and MCAT scores, grade averages, and peer judgments of ability (as well as self-ratings of interest in accomplishment).

The Psychological Knowledge test was combined with the Psychological Skill test and administered to fifteen members of the staff of the department of psychiatry (including residents) and to nineteen volunteer sophomore medical students. The difference between the mean scores of these groups, although not large, was statistically significant ($p<.01, t=3.16$).

The fact that positive correlations were obtained between the Psychological Knowledge test and a completely different type of test (Psychological-Mindedness scale) on three of four occasions, the indications that a general "ability to learn" component was present in the test, and the ability of the test to discriminate between groups, all lend credence to the conclusion that the test was capable of making appropriate discriminations—at least to the extent required by this research project.

Psychological Skill test. Questions designed to measure psychological skill required the student to apply his knowledge of psychology to a particular patient's problems. That is, correct answers to the questions required the student to recognize the significance of material contained in the interview and/or the test booklet. Five-alternative, multiple-choice questions were constructed by the GMC psychiatrist in consultation with other members of the department of psychiatry. For examples, see questions 6 and 10 in Appendix 1. There were 29 items in the Pretest, 18 in Posttest I, and 22 in Posttest II. The test was first administered to the class of 1955 and was revised extensively before administration to the class of 1956.

[5] This scale was designed to measure "the degree to which the individual is interested in, and responsive to, the inner needs, motives, and experiences of others," and its empirical validity has been demonstrated. See H. G. Gough, *Manual for the California Psychological Inventory* (Palo Alto: Consulting Psychologists Press, 1957).

Table 13.8. Personal attributes correlated to a statistically significant degree ($p<.05$) with tests of psychological knowledge (class of 1956)

Pretest ($N=65$)	Posttest I ($N=65$)	Posttest II ($N=65$)
+Amount of medical knowledge (peer judgment)	+Verbal Ability (MCAT)	+Verbal Ability (MCAT)
+General Anxiety scale	+Knowledge of Modern Society (MCAT)	+Quantitative Ability (MCAT)
+Psychological-Mindedness (CPI)	+Knowledge of Premedical Sciences (MCAT)	+Knowledge of Modern Society (MCAT)
+Achievement via Independence (CPI)	+First-year grade average	+Knowledge of Premedical Sciences (MCAT)
+Flexibility (CPI)	+Third-year grade average	+Third-year grade average
	+Cumulative grade average	+Cumulative grade average
	+Junior surgical clerkship grade	+Junior medical clerkship grade
	+Competence as a physician (peer judgment)	+Amount of medical knowledge (peer judgment)
	+Amount of medical knowledge (peer judgment)	+Liberal Attitude scale
	+Frequency of fantasy about intellectual and professional accomplishments (self-rating)	+Frequency of fantasy about intellectual and professional accomplishments (self-rating)
	+Psychological-Mindedness (CPI)	—Interest in minor surgery (self-rating)
	+Achievement via Independence (CPI)	—Amount of reward for ability to get along with others as an adolescent (self-rating)
		+Achievement via Independence (CPI)
		—Self-Control (CPI)
		+Need Aggression

The reliability coefficients of this test proved low (Table 13.9). As in the case of the Medical Skill test, the fact that the Psychological Skill test required careful attention to both the sound track of the film and the test booklet placed additional severe limitations on its reliability. The correlation coefficients between Psychological Skill scores on various test administrations are presented in Table 13.10.

There is only indirect evidence for the validity of the Psychological Skill test—mainly because there was no direct and obvious criterion available by which to assess the empirical validity of a measure of psychological skill. Two pieces of evidence were obtained, however, which concern the empirical validity of this measure. First, although Psychological Knowledge Pretest scores were found to be highly correlated with previous grades, Psychological Skill test scores were not.

Table 13.9. Corrected alternate-item reliability coefficients of scores on each test administration: psychological skill (class of 1956)

Pretest		Posttest I		Posttest II	
N	*r*	*N*	*r*	*N*	*r*
69	.25	65	.08	65	.47

This implies that in the pretest scores a knowledge component was not present in the Psychological Skill test. Second, the Psychological Skill items in combination with the Psychological Knowledge items were found to discriminate between medical school sophomores and members of the psychiatric staff. These results, it must be admitted, provide only weak empirical support for this test as a measure of skill. Perhaps its best claim to validity is not empirical, but rests on the care which went into the development of the items (two psychiatrists spent considerable effort on this) and the selection and revision of the items on the basis of item difficulty, reliability, and correlation between item and total test score. However, the technical deficiencies of this test are obvious. Fortunately, other tests of psychological skill (described later) were used to supplement this one.

Sociological Knowledge and Skill test. The purpose of the Sociological Knowledge and Skill test was to discover whether the GMC student's knowledge of the social components of medical care and his ability to apply such knowledge increased more than the control student's. Knowledge and skill were measured together because the social aspects of medical care were taught by the case method in the GMC, and in the case method there is no separation of knowledge and skill.

In order to measure the expected effects of the GMC, questions were asked about the personal and social problems of the patients presented in the Sound-Film Interview. Five-alternative, multiple-choice questions were constructed by a social worker, a sociologist, a psychiatrist, and an internist. For examples, see question 2 of Appendix 1. There were 10 items in the Pretest, 17 in Posttest I, and 16 in Posttest II.

Alternate-item reliability coefficients of scores on Posttest I and Posttest II were low (Table 13.11). Reliability of the Sociological

Table 13.10. Correlation coefficients between scores on various test administrations: psychological skill (class of 1956)

Pre–Post I		Pre–Post II		Post I–Post II	
N	*r*	*N*	*r*	*N*	*r*
65	.29	65	.04	65	.19

Table 13.11. Corrected alternate-item reliability coefficients of scores on each test administration: sociological knowledge and skill (class of 1956)

Posttest I		Posttest II	
N	*r*	*N*	*r*
69	.20	64	.54

Knowledge and Skill Pretest was not computed because the test contained only 10 items. Correlation coefficients between Sociological Knowledge and Skill scores on various test administrations were also low (Table 13.12).

As in the case of the previously discussed tests of skill, it was difficult to assess the empirical validity of the test of sociological knowledge and skill because no criterion for this type of skill was available (see Chapter 24). However, the empirical validity of this measure was supported by the fact that a statistically significant relation was found between Pretest scores and scores on the MCAT subtest, Knowledge of Modern Society.

Differential Memory test. In an effort to discover whether the GMC had an effect on the student's attitudes toward the importance of personal (as contrasted to medical) aspects of the patient's problems, a memory test was constructed in connection with the Sound-Film Interview. This test provided two measures: one concerned the student's memory for facts related to the medical aspects of the case presented in the Sound-Film Interview; the other concerned his memory for the personal aspects of the case. The rationale for this procedure was as follows: if a student remembered primarily medical information to the exclusion of personal information, it might be inferred that the former material was more important to him than the latter. Thus the extent to which one kind of information was remembered relative to another would provide an indication of the student's attitudes toward these two types of information.[6]

This test contained approximately forty questions relating to the medical aspects of the patient's problems and forty concerning personal aspects, for each of the three administrations. All items were five-alternative, multiple-choice questions, which were related to the content of the interview. For examples, see questions 35–42 in Appendix 1. The Differential Memory test was first administered to the class of 1954 and was revised for the class of 1955 because it was insufficiently difficult. It was revised again after the 1955 administrations for the same reason. The test was improved sufficiently by 1956.

[6] The psychological literature contains many experiments concerning selective memory in relation to attitudes. See, for example, C. E. Osgood, *Method and Theory in Experimental Psychology* (New York: Oxford University Press, 1953).

Table 13.12. Correlation coefficients between scores on various test administrations: sociological knowledge and skill (class of 1956)

Pre–Post I		Pre–Post II		Post I–Post II	
N	*r*	*N*	*r*	*N*	*r*
65	.04	65	.02	65	—.11

Alternate-item reliability coefficients are presented in Table 13.13. The correlation coefficients between scores on various test administrations are presented in Table 13.14.

Rather direct support was obtained for the hypothesis that differential memory (as measured by this test) was related to attitudes toward patients. After the difficulty of the test was increased, there was considerable evidence that the Memory for Medical Facts score was related to performance in medical school. Scores on this test were correlated significantly with grade averages on three of the last four administrations of the test (involving two different groups of students —the class of 1955 and the class of 1956). Scores on this test were also correlated significantly with MCAT scores of all three classes (including the class of 1954).

The Memory for Personal and Social Facts score was not correlated with grade averages, although it was occasionally correlated with MCAT scores. The best evidence for the empirical validity of the Memory for Personal Facts score is that it was positively correlated to a statistically significant degree with peer judgments concerning skill in developing good relations with patient and sympathy with the concept of comprehensive care.

To summarize, the multiple-choice tests used in connection with the Sound-Film Interview were, in the main, useful measures. Although these tests were not adequately reliable according to traditional standards, evidence of their validity (when obtainable) was satisfactory.

Should the Sound-Film Interview technique be used in the future to measure as many variables as requested in the present research, a much larger number of questions should be used in each subtest

Table 13.13. Corrected alternate-item reliability coefficients of scores on each test administration: differential memory (class of 1956)

	Pretest		Posttest I		Posttest II	
	N	*r*	*N*	*r*	*N*	*r*
Medical facts	65	.20	65	.36	65	.52
Personal and social facts	65	.54	65	.52	65	.68

Table 13.14. Correlation coefficients between scores on various test administrations: differential memory (class of 1956)

	Pre–Post I		Pre–Post II		Post I–Post II	
	N	*r*	*N*	*r*	*N*	*r*
Medical facts	65	.29	65	.07	65	.30
Personal and social facts	65	.46	65	.52	65	.50

(i.e., in connection with each patient) if adequate reliabilities are to be obtained. The fact that only two or three items were used in each subtest was undoubtedly one of the major causes of the low reliabilities of the present tests. Increasing the length of the test, however, increases the likelihood of test fatigue, which will in turn decrease reliability. Consequently, it will be necessary to make certain that the administration of tests is spread over several days so as to reduce test fatigue as much as possible.[7]

It should be pointed out that it is important to resist the temptation to reduce the number of patients presented in order to reduce the number of test hours. Fewer patients presented means greater likelihood that the inferences drawn about the students' responses will be in error. Indeed, it may well be that the primary cause of the unreliability of the measures described above is the relatively small number of patients (ten) presented to the students at each test administration. Stable, accurate tests of several aspects of students' performance will require enough time to ask students many questions about many patients.

Sound-film interview interpersonal perception tests

One of the most important objectives of the GMC concerned the nature of the relations between student and patient. That is, it was hoped that the GMC student, by virtue of his continued contact with patients, greater responsibility for patients' total care, etc., would develop more concern for, greater understanding of, and more skill in developing good physician-patient relations than would the control student. Thus, one of the tasks of the research project was to develop a test by which the nature of the relations between student and patient could be ascertained and measured. In 1952, at the very outset of the research project, it was decided to study the students' perceptions of their patients.

Previous research concerning interpersonal perception was found

[7] In the present project the student was required to answer questions concerning four patients (which took one and a half to two hours) before being given a rest period. This was clearly too fatiguing.

to contain little in the way of systematic theoretical work or methodological analysis. If the process of interpersonal perception was to be studied in the context of the evaluation of the GMC, considerable theoretical and developmental research would be necessary.

Such work was undertaken. This section presents the theory of the research, describes the solution of methodological problems, and indicates the application of the theory and the methodology to the practical problem. To accomplish this the presentation is organized as follows: first, the major components of the interpersonal perception situation are explained; each component is then discussed for the purposes of (1) identifying the major concepts, (2) presenting the methodological issues, and (3) indicating the significance of both (1) and (2) for the practical problem. It should be emphasized that our approach to this problem is an explication and application of the work of Egon Brunswik.[8]

Components of the interpersonal perception situation. The three major components of the interpersonal perception situation are the person about whom judgments are made (the person-object), the person who makes the judgments (the subject), and the mediation of information between the person-object and the subject (the cue situation). A model of the interpersonal perception situation is presented in Figure 13.1. On the right is the subject (the perceiver); on the left is the object (the person being perceived). Some trait or characteristic of the object (labeled "distal variable" and indicated by the circle inside the object) is perceived by the subject. The correspondence between the trait of the person-object and the subject's perception of it is indicated by the dotted line at the top of the figure. This correspondence, a type of achievement, is called "accuracy."[9] Achievement (accurate perception of the covert distal variable) is made possible by the presence of more or less valid cues on the surface (in the behavior) of the person-object.

PERSON-OBJECT COMPONENT

1. Covert distal variables. The covert distal variables include characteristics and traits of person-objects, such as intelligence and personality characteristics. They are *covert* in that they are inaccessible to

[8] See Egon Brunswik, "Organismic Achievement and Environmental Probability" (part of Egon Brunswik, Clark Hull, and Kurt Lewin, Symposium on Psychology and Scientific Method, University of Chicago, 1941), *Psychological Review* 50:255–272, 1943; "The Conceptual Framework of Psychology," *International Encyclopedia of Unified Science*, vol. I, no. 10 (Chicago: University of Chicago Press, 1952); and *Perception and the Representative Design of Psychological Experiments* (Berkeley: University of California Press, 1956).

[9] Functional achievement has been defined by Brunswik as "relationships better than chance existing between . . . an organism and variables in its . . . environment." See "Organismic Achievement and Environmental Probability."

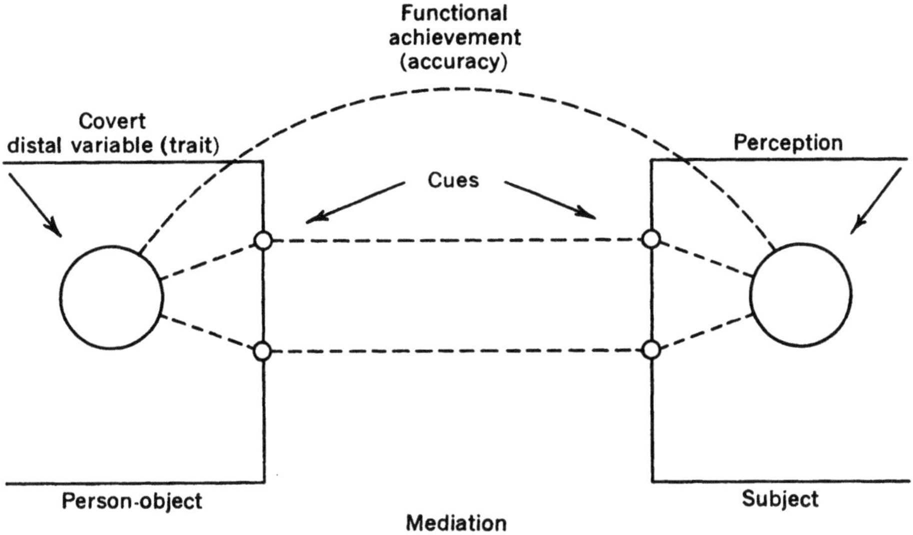

Figure 13.1. Schematic presentation of the interpersonal perception situation. Adapted from Egon Brunswik, *Perception and the Representative Design of Psychological Experiments* (Berkeley: University of California Press, 1956)

immediate and direct observation. They are *distal* in that they are defined independently of the sensory surface of the subject.

2. Methodological problems. The concept of covertness raises a methodological problem. This problem is illustrated in Figure 13.2, in which the perception of one person's intelligence by another has

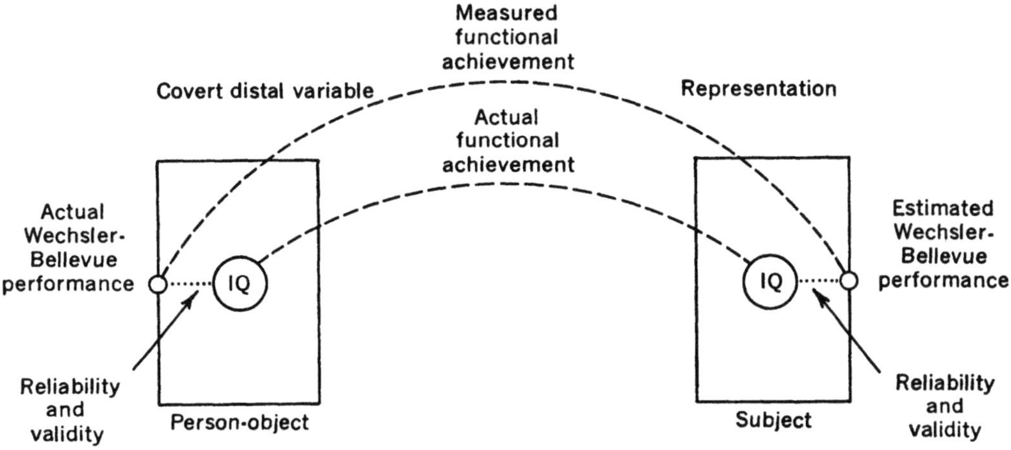

Figure 13.2. Schematic presentation of the functional achievement of a covert distal variable. Adapted from Brunswik, *Perception and the Representative Design of Psychological Experiments*

been used as an example. On the right is the subject (the perceiver); on the left is the person-object (the person whose intelligence is perceived). The mediational component (cue situation) is discussed below. The intelligence of the person-object is not directly observable by the experimenter, who therefore must use some device such as the Wechsler-Bellevue Intelligence Scale to obtain a measure of the person-object's intelligence.

The dotted line that connects the person-object's Wechsler-Bellevue performance with the trait "intelligence" inside the person-object, and the dotted line that connects the subject's perception of the object's intelligence with his *reported* estimate of it (his response) indicate that less-than-perfect relations exist in both cases. These less-than-perfect relations mean that there will be a less-than-perfect relation between *measured* functional achievement and the *actual* functional achievement of the subject.

Early attempts to study interpersonal perception were hampered because judgments of experts were used as criteria for the accuracy of judgments of the subjects. This procedure was inadequate not so much because it involved imperfect measurement, as because it merely pitted the perceptions of the judges against those of the subjects. Recently researchers have used immediately observable objective behavior of the object, rather than judgments of behavior, as criteria. For example, it is now customary to have the person-object take an intelligence test, and then to ask the subject to estimate the person-object's intelligence. The subject's accuracy is measured by the degree of correspondence between the person-object's measured intelligence and the subject's estimation of it. Although the relation between the person-object's intelligence and the objective measure of it remains imperfect, the principal difficulty of the criterion problem is eliminated by this procedure.

The significance of the less-than-one-to-one relation between the *subject's estimation* of the covert distal variable and his *perception* of it is explored below, in connection with the subject component.

3. Application. The concept of covert distal variables was particularly significant for the practical problem under consideration, for these variables serve as important orientation points when one person interacts with another. For example, estimations of such covert distal variables as the patient's intelligence and vocabulary level guide the physician when he gives instructions to the patient. And, of course, estimations of the patient's personality characteristics guide the physician in establishing and maintaining a good physician-patient relation. Since one of the principal objectives of the experimental program was to improve the student's ability to establish and maintain good physi-

cian-patient relations, it was important to study the extent to which the experimental and control programs improved the student's ability to perceive accurately covert distal variables such as intelligence, vocabulary level, and personality characteristics of patients.

MEDIATIONAL COMPONENT. The perception of some covert distal variable such as intelligence presupposes both the existence of cues indicating the variable and the accessibility of the cues to the subject. This is the second component of interpersonal perception—the mediation of cues. In Figure 13.3, on the left, the trait "intelligence" is indicated inside the object, and three examples of cues that might signify intelligence are indicated on the surface of the person-object.

1. Cue validity. Cue validity, or the expression value of a cue, is the degree to which a cue indicates the covert distal variable, in this case intelligence. Cues such as height have a general but very low correlation with intelligence. Cues such as the vocabulary used by the person-object have a much higher correlation with intelligence than height, and therefore have a higher expression value, or in other words, higher validity.

2. Cue utilization. Cue utilization, or the impression value of a cue, refers to the extent to which the cue is used by a subject. Cue utilization depends on the characteristics both of the subject and of the cues themselves. Subjects vary in their sensitivity to cues, the acuity with which they perceive them, and the manner in which they select

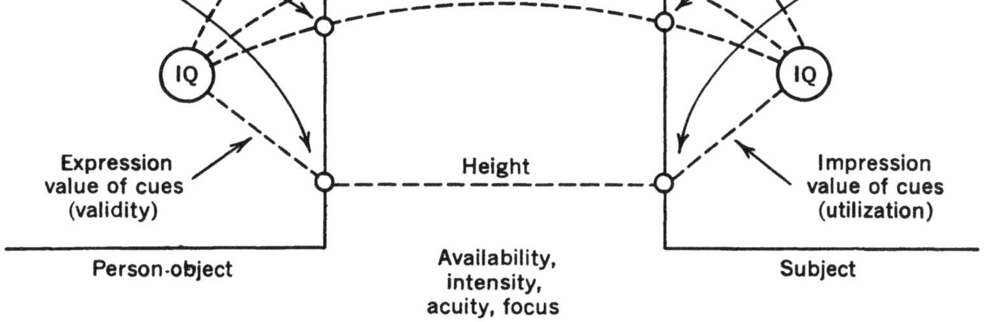

Figure 13.3. Schematic presentation of the cue situation. Adapted from Brunswik, *Perception and the Representative Design of Psychological Experiments*

or exclude cues from attention; cues vary in characteristics such as strength (e.g., deepness and extent of facial wrinkles).

3. Cue family-hierarchies. Cue family-hierarchies are important factors in the cue situation. All cues related to a given covert distal variable are considered to be in the same family. Cues within a family may be ordered into a cue validity-heirarchy according to the extent to which they indicate covert variables. Cues may also be ordered into a hierarchy corresponding to the degree to which they are utilized by the subject (a cue utilization-hierarchy). In a perceptually well-adjusted subject, the cue utilization-heirarchy should match the cue validity-hierarchy. That is, a well-adjusted subject who accurately perceives his environment relies more upon cues of high validity than upon cues of low validity.[10]

4. Methodological problems. There is an important methodological principle involved in the study of the mediational component. Only those interpersonal perception test situations in which the mediational component is *representative* of the situation to which the investigator wishes to apply his results permit such inductive generalizations. That is, the investigator must use interpersonal perception situations in which the mediational component contains the same cue family-hierarchies as the situation in which the subject and object interact.[11] In short, the principles of representative design must be considered in the development of measures of interpersonal perception.[12]

5. Application. Cue validity, cue utilization, and cue family-hierarchies are important in training the medical student (and physician) to become skillful in perceiving accurately the characteristics of patients. The student must somehow learn which cues are reliable and valid indicators of covert distal variables such as intelligence and personality characteristics.

These concepts were of direct importance to the research project, for they guided the development of the Sound-Film Interview. Interference with the natural cue situation in the interview between the

[10] See Kenneth R. Hammond, "Probabilistic Functioning and the Clinical Method," *Psychological Review* 62:255–262, 1955.

[11] It is necessary to make this point primarily because the long history of this problem indicates that, in the interest of greater control, investigators have ignored this methodological principle. See previously cited works by Egon Brunswik; also Wayman J. Crow, "The Need for Representative Design in Studies of Interpersonal Perception," *Journal of Consulting Psychology* 21:323–325, 1957; and the following articles by Kenneth R. Hammond: "Subject and Object Sampling: A Note," *Psychological Bulletin* 45:530–533, 1948; "Representative vs. Systematic Design in Clinical Psychology," *Psychological Bulletin* 51:150–159, 1954; "Probabilistic Functioning and the Clinical Method," *Psychological Review* 62:255–262, 1955.

[12] See Egon Brunswik, *Perception and the Representative Design of Psychological Experiments.*

physician and patient was minimized. That is, the mediational component was present in the interpersonal perception situation in its natural form and, therefore, was representative of the physician-patient situation.

SUBJECT COMPONENT

1. Intra-organismic variables. Central, or intra-organismic, variables, such as attitudes, sets, and motives, also form an important part of the interpersonal perception situation (see Figure 13.4). Two intra-organismic variables were studied rather carefully in this research project: the ability to perceive patients accurately (differential accuracy) and the tendency to perceive patients as similar to one another (adherence to stereotype). The subject's response (his estimation of the person-objects' self-ratings or scores), is a function of these, among other, intra-organismic variables. As illustrated in Figure 13.4, the subject's response unfortunately does not have a one-to-one relation with the central variable, differential accuracy, alone.

In the present study a procedure called the Random Comparison Method, discussed below, was developed to cope with the fact that a subject's response in the interpersonal perception situation is a multidetermined one.[13]

Both these methods are useful because they permit the relative contribution of each of the intra-organismic variables mentioned above to be ascertained. Although differential accuracy has held the primary interest of investigators, other variables promise to be of equal if not greater significance.

2. Methodological problems. Three methodological problems are involved in the study of intra-organismic variables. The first is the problem posed by the lack of a one-to-one relation between the subject's perception of an object and the investigator's measure of that perception (the subject's response). The second involves the functional significance of intra-organismic variables. The third concerns the type of experimental design which best permits investigation of these variables.

First to be considered is the problem posed by the lack of a one-to-one relation between the subject's perception of an object and the investigator's measure of that perception. Figure 13.4 represents an interpersonal perception situation in which the subject makes estimations about the intelligence of a number of person-objects. The circle on the right hand surface of the subject, labeled "estimate for each

[13] A method developed by L. J. Cronbach also takes multidetermination into account, see "Processes Affecting Scores on 'Understanding of Others' and 'Assumed Similarity,'" *Psychological Bulletin* 52:177–193, 1955. See also N. L. Gage, G. S. Leavitt, and G. C. Stone, "The Intermediary Key in the Analysis of Interpersonal Perception," *Psychological Bulletin* 53:258–266, 1956.

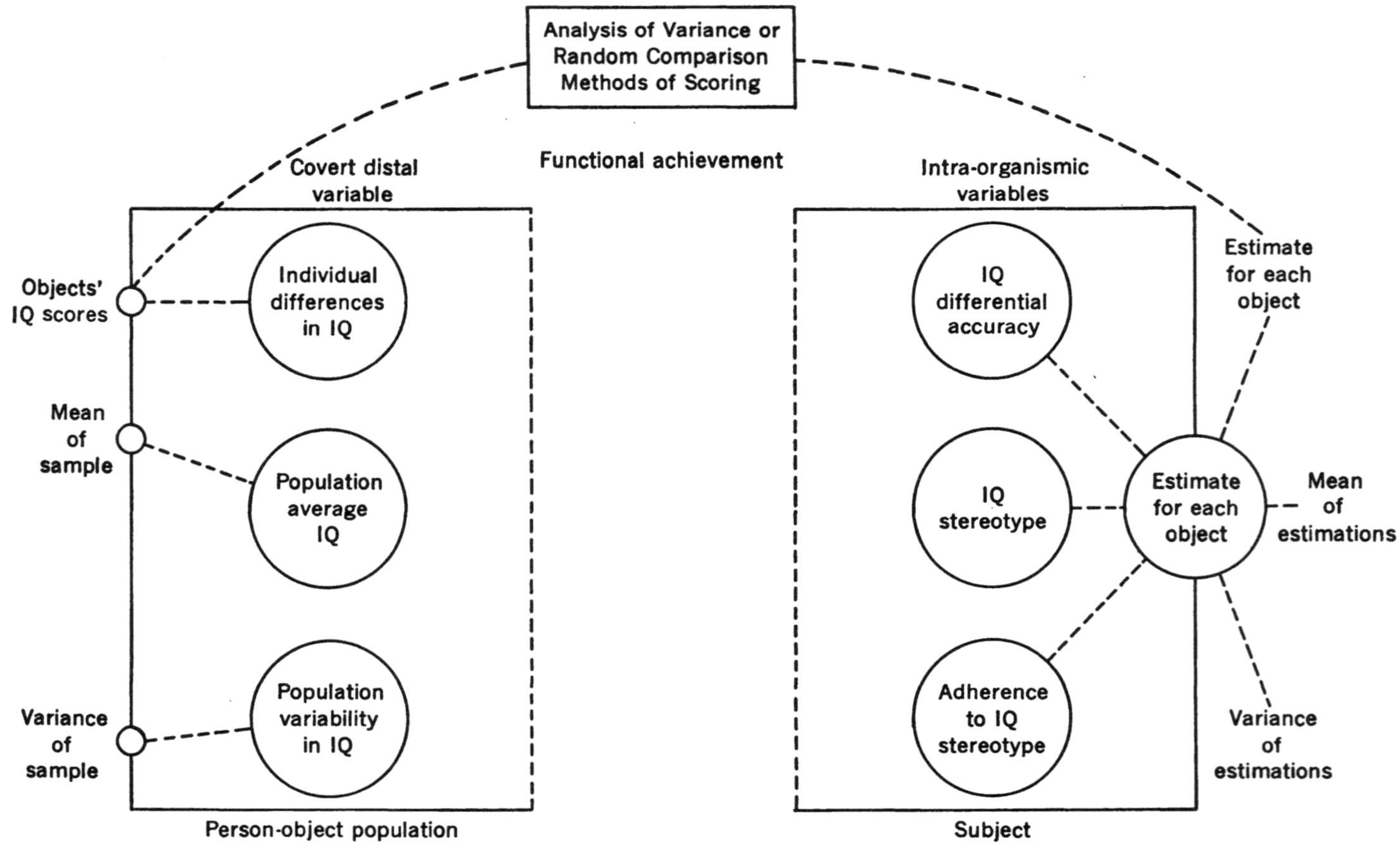

Figure 13.4. Schematic presentation of stabilization mechanisms. Adapted from Brunswik, *Perception and the Representative Design of Psychological Experiments*

object," is the subject's response. The dotted lines that connect this estimation with three intra-organismic variables—IQ differential accuracy (the extent to which objects are accurately differentiated), IQ stereotype (the average of the subject's judgments of the objects' IQ's), and adherence to IQ stereotype (the inverse of the amount of variability in the subject's judgments of the objects' IQ's)—indicate that all three may have contributed to the subject's estimation. In order to arrive at a correct measure of differential accuracy, it is necessary to eliminate the effects of all intra-organismic variables other than differential accuracy. This requires a statistical analysis of the subject's estimations and the objects' scores.

Two methods of statistical analysis which permit the computation of differential accuracy are indicated in the box at the top center of the figure—the (parametric) Analysis of Variance Method developed by Cronbach and the (nonparametric) Random Comparison Method developed at the Behavior Research Laboratory at the University of Colorado. In order to measure the content of a stereotype it is only necessary to use the mean of the subject's estimations. The variance of the subject's estimations provides a measure of the subject's adherence to stereotype; that is, the greater the variance, the less the adherence to stereotype. (The computation of differential accuracy is complicated and therefore is explained below.)

There is one further point to be made concerning intra-organismic determination of the subject's perception of the person-object. This point concerns the relation which the subject believes to exist among various personality traits. Cronbach refers to this as the subject's "implicit personality theory."[14] For example, a subject's estimations of objects' intelligence and leadership might be highly correlated. He would then be said to have an implicit personality theory that leadership and intelligence occur together (see Figure 13.5).

The *actual* intercorrelation of the traits in the population may be referred to as "ecological intertrait relations." The correspondence between implicit personality theories and ecological intertrait relations is also a form of functional achievement. This type of achievement certainly has considerable significance for the training of medical students and other clinicians.[15]

[14] Brunswik (following Thorndike) referred to these relations as "halo effects" (see "The Conceptual Framework of Psychology"). This term is not precisely correct, since halo effect refers specifically to high positive intercorrelations among socially desirable personality traits, whereas implicit personality theory implies intercorrelations of varying degrees.

[15] See F. J. Todd, "A Methodological Analysis of Clinical Judgment" (unpublished doctoral dissertation, University of Colorado, 1954); and J. Smedslund, *Multiple-Probability Learning* (Oslo: Akademisk Forlag, 1955).

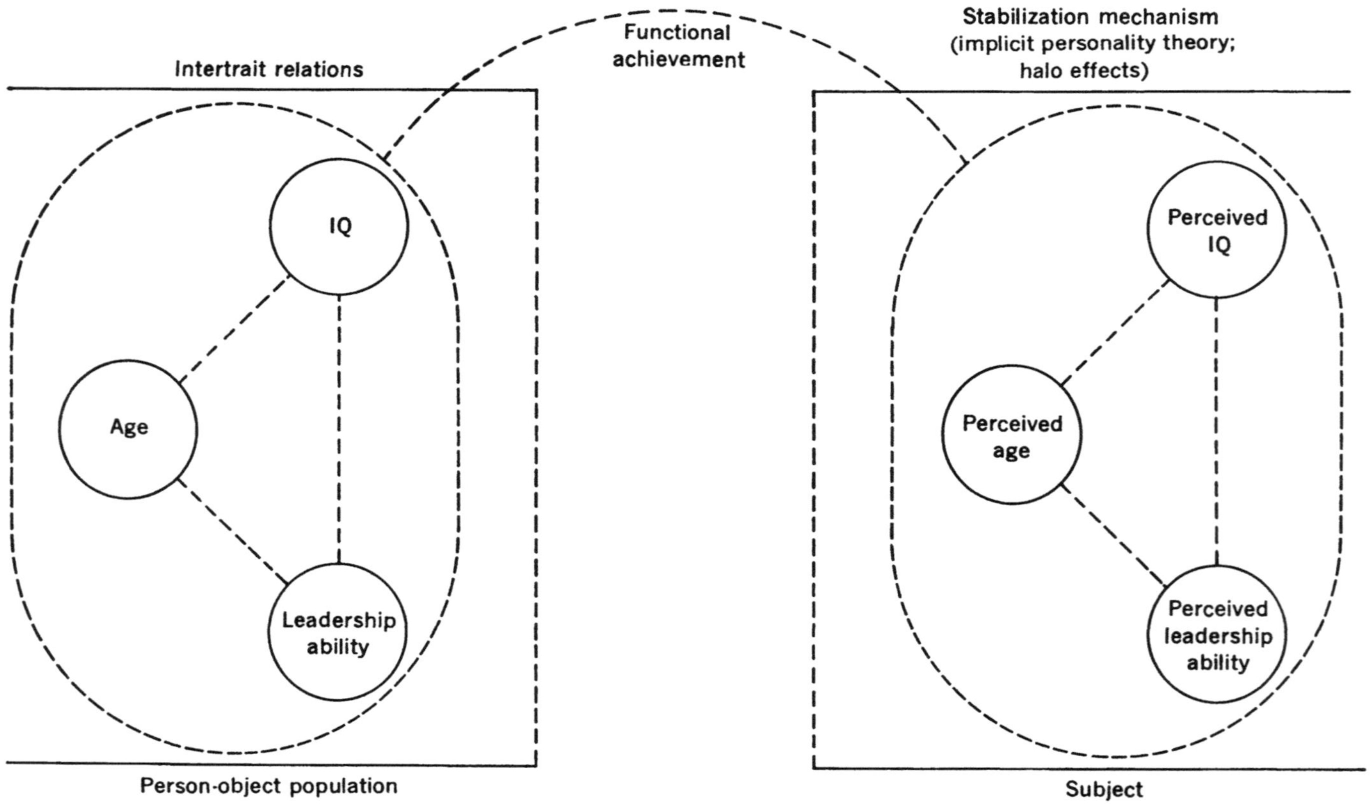

Figure 13.5. Schematic presentation of high-order stabilization mechanisms. Adapted from Brunswik, *Perception and the Representative Design of Psychological Experiments*

Both the lack of univocality between the subject's perception and his estimation of the person-object, and the importance of intra-organismic variables in determining his response, are significantly related to appropriate experimental design. In order to ascertain and measure the contribution of various intra-organismic variables to the subject's response, it is necessary for the subject to make estimations about a *number* of person-objects. Generalizations about a subject's performance with respect to person-objects are otherwise impossible. Therefore, a representative sample of person-objects must be presented to the subjects.

Equally important, however, is the fact that both the Random Comparison Method and Cronbach's Analysis of Variance Method are statistical (after the fact) operations performed upon the subject's responses. In this way passive, rather than active, control is applied by the experimenter.[16] The reader should note that each of the components of the interpersonal perception test situation mentioned above requires representative design.

3. Application. The application of these concepts in this research project can best be shown by presenting some results obtained in the study of students' interpersonal perceptions. It was expected that GMC training would increase the student's ability to perceive patients accurately (differential accuracy) more than the traditional training. It was found that the trend of the results was in the opposite direction; the GMC students seemed to become less accurate than the control students (see Chapters 21 and 25). Moreover, there were significant differences between the GMC and control groups in Adherence to Stereotype scores. The GMC group had lower Adherence to Stereotype scores after training than did the control group. This was interpreted to mean that, as a result of training, the GMC student's perception of individual differences among patients was increased. In other words, an intra-organismic variable (adherence to stereotype) was affected. Thus, because the theory focused attention upon the multidetermined nature of the student's perception of patients, important features of the student's performance (which might otherwise have been overlooked) were studied, with the result that further information was gained about the effect of the GMC Program.[17]

Random Comparison Method. The need for developing an appro-

[16] See Egon Brunswik, "The Conceptual Framework of Psychology," p. 8.

[17] For detailed discussion of Differential Accuracy and Adherence to Stereotype tests, see Wayman J. Crow, "The Effect of Training upon Accuracy and Variability in Interpersonal Perception," *Journal of Abnormal and Social Psychology* 55:355–359, 1957; and Wayman J. Crow and Kenneth R. Hammond, "The Generality of Accuracy and Response Sets in Interpersonal Perception," *Journal of Abnormal and Social Psychology* 54:384–390, 1957.

priate technique for scoring the interpersonal perception tests first arose in connection with the problem of determining when a subject's score reflected more than random performance. That is, when a subject is asked to estimate the intelligence of several person-objects, how is it possible to determine whether the subject's accuracy exceeds that which he would have obtained had he merely made random guesses?

A first step in the solution is to decide whether to create the distribution of responses which, in theory, would occur if chance alone determined the subject's responses, or whether to deal with the empirical distributions of person-objects' scores and subject's estimations of them. If a theoretical distribution is created, some assumption must be made about the distribution of the person-object's scores which the subjects are asked to estimate. The nature of this assumption is important, for the amount of error imputed to a subject's estimations depends directly on the assumption about the distribution of person-objects' scores. For example, Dymond had each of her subjects estimate the self-ratings of nine person-objects on twelve five-point scales.[18] Her assumption was that all points on the rating scale were equally likely to be used by the person-object; that is, the distribution of person-objects' self-ratings was rectangular. Thus Dymond's theoretical range of errors for subjects was from 0 to 432. A more tenable assumption would be that self-ratings are normally distributed. If this were actually the case, Dymond's theoretical range of equally likely errors of 0 to 432 would not be appropriate.[19]

The second step involves consideration of the nature of the subject's response. The subject's estimations of the person-object's self-ratings cannot be assumed to consist only of a "true score" component and a "random error" component. Empirical evidence has shown that these estimations include systematic error components such as response sets (predilections for odd or even numbers, tendencies to avoid extremes of the scale, etc.), which affect the subject's estimations to a significant degree.[20] Therefore, a statistical procedure which does not invoke either an assumption about the distributions of person-objects' scores or an assumption about true scores and random errors was devised. This procedure, called the Random Comparison Method of Chance Determination, took account of the specific distribution of person-

[18] Rosalind F. Dymond, "Personality and Empathy," *Journal of Consulting Psychology* 14:343–350, 1950.

[19] Similar criticisms have appeared in the recent literature. See, for example, Cohen's criticism of Nottcutt and Silva: E. Cohen, "The Methodology of Nottcutt and Silva's 'Knowledge of Other People': A Critique," *Journal of Abnormal and Social Psychology* 48:155, 1953; and B. Nottcutt and A. L. M. Silva, "Knowledge of Other People," *Journal of Abnormal and Social Psychology* 46:30–37, 1951.

[20] See Crow and Hammond, *op. cit.*

objects' scores (self-ratings) as well as the specific distribution of the subject's estimations. No assumptions were made.[21]

The Random Comparison Method of Chance Determination is based on the following reasoning. Consider the case of a single subject who predicts the scores of ten objects. If a subject makes an estimation about the score of a person-object, his estimation should be more accurate when compared with that person-object's score than when compared with another person-object's score (provided, of course, that he has some ability to perceive others accurately). If the subject's estimation of the score of person-object 1 is compared with the actual score of person-object 1, the difference provides a measure of his accuracy. If the subject's estimation for person-object 1 is compared with the actual scores of person-objects 2, 3, 4, 5, 6, 7, 8, 9, and 10, a set of difference scores is provided. If the subject blindly estimated the score of person-object 1, his estimation for person-object 1 should not correspond more closely to the actual score of person-object 1 than to the actual score of any other person-object. More precisely, if the subject has no ability to estimate correctly, his estimation for person-object 1 will correspond more closely to the actual score of person-object 1 than it does to the other person-objects' actual scores only by chance.

If each of a subject's estimations is compared with each of the 10 person-objects' scores, a total of 10 comparisons is provided. Because the number of person-objects is 10, and because the subject makes 10 estimations, 100 difference scores are provided. This distribution of 100 difference scores is obtained by comparing each estimation with every person-object's score. Now, if the subject possesses some real ability, his difference scores for a given person-object should be lower, as a result of this ability, than the difference scores obtained when every estimation is compared with every other person-object's score. The subject's 10 difference scores which were obtained by comparing his 10 estimations with the 10 person-objects' scores can be considered a sample of 10 drawn from the 100 difference scores. Therefore, the null hypothesis would assert that these 10 difference scores should differ only by chance from this distribution.

In some instances the random comparison score distribution may be normal in form, thus permitting the usual statistical tests of significance. In those instances where the random comparison score distribution departs markedly from normality, a distribution-free

[21] The authors wish to express their appreciation to Professor David Hawkins for his assistance in developing this procedure. For further reference, see Wayman J. Crow, "A Methodological Study of Social Perceptiveness" (unpublished doctoral dissertation, University of Colorado, 1954).

(nonparametric) statistical test is necessary. For example, if the subject's estimations are no more accurate than they would be by chance alone, one half of his difference scores would be expected to fall above the median of the (random comparison) difference score distribution and one half to fall below. Thus, the problem is reduced to an analogue of a coin-tossing situation.

A further point should be made about the use of this technique. In the above discussion only one subject's estimations were used in an attempt to simplify, and thereby clarify, the explanation of the Random Comparison Method of Chance Determination. However, this method also permits the utilization of the estimations of a group of subjects in computing the random comparison score distribution. The justification for this procedure is that the data from a number of subjects should provide better information concerning systematic error factors which might affect the subject's estimations. For example, should subjects in general have a tendency to seek or avoid the extremes of the scale, it would be difficult to demonstrate that fact with the data provided by only one subject.

The greatest asset of the Random Comparison Method of Chance Distribution is that it takes into account the specific distribution of the person-objects' scores and the specific distribution of the subjects' estimations. Its greatest limitation is that the procedures may be somewhat time consuming.

It should be pointed out that the Random Comparison Method is more than another method of chance determination or scoring. From the standpoint of the theory presented previously it is an ideal method of scoring interpersonal perception tasks. It involves none of the assumptions of the correlational or other parametric techniques, and it eliminates the effects of response sets.

Description and evaluation of the interpersonal perception tests. Each of the interpersonal perception tests is described below. The tests involve estimation of age, estimation of intelligence, estimation of vocabulary level, and estimation of personality characteristics.

ESTIMATION OF AGE. The students were asked to estimate the age of each patient presented to them in the films (see Appendix 1). This "easy" task was introduced for the class of 1956 when experience with other interpersonal perception tests indicated that they were very difficult.

The patients' ages were determined from their hospital records and were corrected for the period up to the time the films were made. The patients' ages were compared with the students' estimations using the Random Comparison Method to determine the students' accuracy. In addition, the students' Adherence to Stereotype scores

Table 13.15. Correlation coefficients between scores on various test administrations: differential accuracy and adherence to stereotype in estimating age (class of 1956)

	Pre–Post I		Pre–Post II		Post I–Post II	
	N	*r*	*N*	*r*	*N*	*r*
Differential accuracy	65	–.06	65	.21	65	.04
Adherence to stereotype	65	.31	65	.25	65	.28

were determined by computing the variance of each student's estimations. (The more variable a subject's estimations, the lower his Adherence to Stereotype score.)

Table 13.15 presents the correlation coefficients between Differential Accuracy scores and between Adherence to Stereotype scores on the three administrations of the test to the class of 1956. The correlations between Differential Accuracy scores were low, as were correlations between Adherence to Stereotype scores. However, because the test was too easy to discriminate sufficiently among students, low relations would be expected between Differential Accuracy scores. The low positive relations found between Adherence to Stereotype scores suggest that, for a relatively easy task such as estimating age, the subject's performance is not so highly determined by response sets as it is for more difficult tasks. As will be explained below, students' response sets were more stable in connection with such difficult tasks as estimating vocabulary level and personality characteristics.

Rather interesting evidence in support of the empirical validity of the Adherence to Stereotype scores was found. On two of three administrations there were significant negative relations between Adherence to Stereotype scores (in estimation of age) and the Flexibility subscale of the California Psychological Inventory. On the third administration this relation fell just short of significance.[22]

Although these results are not independent of one another (the same subjects were involved in all three studies), the fact that the Flexibility scale provides an entirely different type of data lends credence to the hypothesis that the Adherence to Stereotype score measures a general form of behavior.

Another interesting feature of the results was the close agreement between the students' mean age estimation and the mean age of the patients. On the Pretest (class of 1956) the mean age estimation of the entire class was 45.9 years, and the mean age of the ten patients was 46.0 years. On Posttest I the mean age estimation was 52.0 years, and the mean age of the patients was 50.7 years. On Posttest II the mean

[22] The CPI Flexibility scale was designed to indicate the degree of flexibility and adaptability of a person's thinking and social behavior, see Gough, *op. cit.*

Table 13.16. Correlation coefficients between scores on various test administrations: differential accuracy and adherence to stereotype in estimating intelligence (class of 1956)

	Pre–Post I		Pre–Post II		Post I–Post II	
	N	*r*	*N*	*r*	*N*	*r*
Differential accuracy	65	.31	65	.17	65	.03
Adherence to stereotype	65	.57	65	.32	65	.55

age estimation was 43.4 years, and the mean age of the patients was 41.5 years. In short, the mean estimations of the students agreed well with the actual mean ages of the three groups of patients.

Comparisons between the mean amount of variability of students' estimations and the actual amount of variability of the patients' ages again indicated good agreement. The mean variability of students' estimations for the Pretest, Posttest I, and Posttest II was 10.0, 14.1, and 13.4 years, respectively. The actual variability of the patients' ages was 10.2, 14.5, and 11.1 years, respectively.

It will be shown below that for other tests the students' mean estimations were often markedly different from the actual values in the patients. The significance of marked differences between mean estimations and the actual values was discussed above in the section on theory and is discussed further below.

ESTIMATION OF INTELLIGENCE. The students were asked to estimate the intelligence of each patient presented to them in the films. This test was first used with the class of 1956. An approximation to the patient's intelligence was computed from his score on the vocabulary section of the Wechsler-Bellevue Intelligence Scale.[23]

Table 13.16 presents the correlation coefficients between Differential Accuracy scores and between Adherence to Stereotype scores on the three administrations of the test to the class of 1956. Note that the correlations between Differential Accuracy scores were low, although those between Adherence to Stereotype scores were relatively high. These results indicate that Differential Accuracy scores were not so stable a component of the subjects' performance as Adherence to Stereotype scores.

As was found in connection with estimation of age, the Flexibility subscale of the CPI was negatively related to the Adherence to Stereotype scores, although the relation was not so strong. On each of the three test administrations for which results were available, the negative relation between Flexibility and Adherence to Stereotype fell

[23] See R. Lewinski, "Vocabulary and Mental Measurement: A Quantitative Investigation and Review of Research," *Journal of Genetic Psychology* 72:247–281, 1948.

just short of statistical significance. However, on two of the three test administrations, Adherence to Stereotype scores were significantly related (in a positive direction) to the Capacity for Status subscale of the CPI.[24]

As noted in connection with the students' estimations of age, there was a fairly close relation between the students' mean intelligence estimations and the mean intelligence of the patients. The students' mean scale estimations were 4.80, 4.73, and 4.55, while the comparable actual scores were 4.90, 3.80, and 4.10.[25] On two administrations the students systematically overestimated the patients' intelligence; this may indicate a general tendency of medical students to overestimate the intelligence of patients. A more definite departure of the students' mean estimations from the actual values occurred with respect to the variability of the patients' intelligence. The mean variability of the students' estimations was 1.4, 1.4, and 1.5, while the actual variability of the patients' scores were 2.3, 2.7, and 2.7. Thus the students tended to underestimate the amount of variability in intelligence among patients.

ESTIMATION OF VOCABULARY LEVEL. In order to communicate effectively with a patient a doctor must make some estimation of the patient's vocabulary level. It was felt that the increased contact with patients afforded the GMC student would not only emphasize this need but offer training in the ability as well. Consequently, it was hypothesized that GMC students would improve in the accuracy of their predictions of patients' vocabulary level from the pretest to the posttest more than control students.

The patients' vocabulary levels were determined from performance on the vocabulary section of the Wechsler-Bellevue Intelligence Scale. This graduated list of vocabulary words was administered to each patient following his filmed interview, and the first word each patient missed and the first three words he missed consecutively were determined.

After watching a Sound-Film Interview of a patient, the students were asked to estimate the first word the patient missed (task A), and the first three words missed consecutively (task B). The Differential Accuracy scores of the students were determined by the Random Comparison Method.

Table 13.17 presents the correlation coefficients obtained when Differential Accuracy scores on one administration were related to

[24] Subjects who score low on the Capacity for Status subscale are reported by Gough, *op. cit.*, to be seen as being stereotyped in thinking—a characteristic to be expected of subjects who adhere to their stereotypes.

[25] A score of five indicated an IQ score of 100; see Appendix 1 for example of test form.

Table 13.17. Correlation coefficients between scores on various test administrations: differential accuracy and adherence to stereotype in estimating vocabulary level (classes of 1954, 1955, 1956)

	Pre–Post I		Pre–Post II		Post I–Post II	
	N	*r*	*N*	*r*	*N*	*r*
Differential accuracy						
Task A						
Class of 1954	73	.01	73	.04	73	—.02
Class of 1955	73	.01	72	—.03	72	—.12
Class of 1956	65	—.16	65	.05	65	.11
Task B						
Class of 1954	77	—.13	77	—.11	78	.14
Class of 1955	73	.19	72	—.11	72	.04
Class of 1956	65	—.01	65	.10	65	.08
Adherence to stereotype						
Task A						
Class of 1954	73	.67	73	.46	73	.58
Class of 1955	72	.46	72	.27	72	.30
Class of 1956	65	.49	65	.46	65	.55
Task B						
Class of 1954	76	.45	76	.52	80	.50
Class of 1955	72	.20	72	.15	72	.42
Class of 1956	65	.56	65	.42	65	.70

Differential Accuracy scores on the other two administrations for both task A and task B. None of these correlations was significant. Table 13.17 also presents the correlation coefficients between Adherence to Stereotype scores; these indicate a strong relation between performances on two separate administrations of the tests. As was found with the two previously discussed measures, Differential Accuracy scores were not as stable a component of the students' performance as Adherence to Stereotype scores. On four test administrations for which results were available the Flexibility subscale of the CPI tended to be negatively related to Adherence to Stereotype scores for both task A and task B. The relations were significant ($p=.05$) on two administrations for task B and fell just short of significance on all other administrations for both tasks.

It should be noted that the students tended to overestimate the vocabulary level of the patients. As is shown in Table 13.18, the students' mean estimations were higher than the patients' actual mean in sixteen of the eighteen comparisons (see also Figure 13.6). However, no such consistent pattern was obtained with respect to the mean variability of the students' estimations and the actual variability among the patients. Students' communication with patients could, of course, be seriously hampered if the students consistently overestimated the vocabulary level of their patients.

Table 13.18. Students' mean estimations and variability in estimations of patients' vocabulary level compared with patients' actual performance on vocabulary test (classes of 1954, 1955, and 1956)

	Class of 1954			Class of 1955			Class of 1956		
	Pre	Post I	Post II	Pre	Post I	Post II	Pre	Post I	Post II
Mean estimations									
Task A									
Students' estimations	19.9	20.4	18.4	18.4	19.4	18.4	21.4	20.5	19.6
Patients' performance	18.0	16.2	13.5	18.0	16.2	14.9	18.0	17.9	14.0
Task B									
Students' estimations	27.0	26.4	24.4	26.5	25.4	24.8	27.6	26.0	25.5
Patients' performance	27.2	22.1	22.6	27.2	22.1	24.1	27.2	22.6	24.2
Mean variability									
Task A									
Students' estimations	7.3	7.8	7.7	7.4	7.8	7.1	7.4	7.4	7.5
Patients' performance	6.7	9.2	6.7	6.7	9.2	6.4	6.7	8.5	7.1
Task B									
Students' estimations	6.6	7.2	6.7	6.4	6.9	6.4	6.3	6.6	6.6
Patients' performance	7.1	8.7	9.7	7.1	8.7	9.9	7.1	8.9	9.9

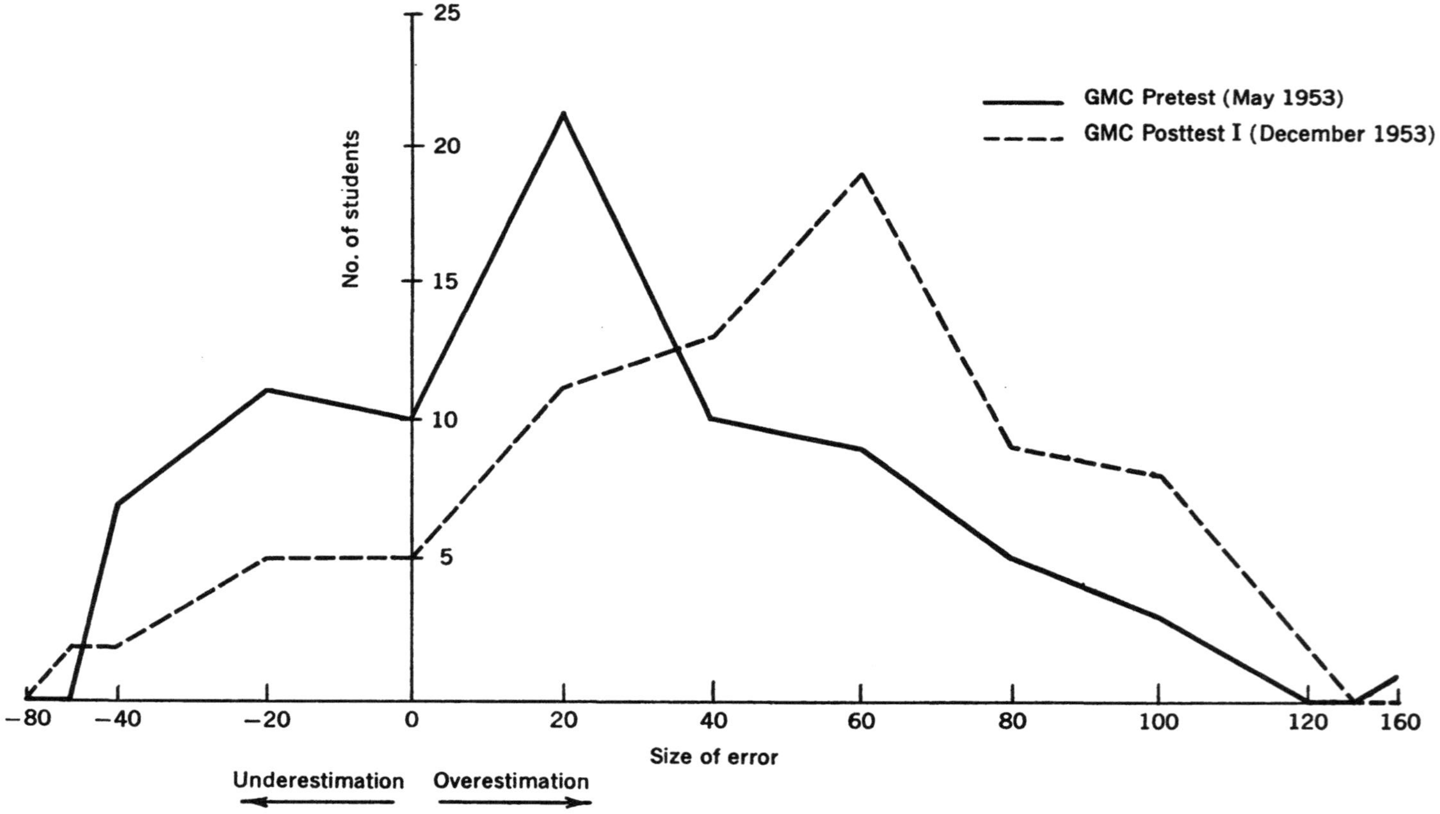

Figure 13.6. Students' errors in estimating patients' vocabulary levels (errors measured in terms of the algebraic sum of differences between students' estimates and patients' vocabulary scores)

ESTIMATION OF PERSONALITY CHARACTERISTICS. If an adequate physician-patient relation is to be developed, the physician must respond to the individuality of the patient—to the unique personality confronting him. Therefore a section of the Sound-Film Interview test was designed to measure the students' skill in assessing patients' personalities as revealed in brief interviews.

After watching a Sound-Film Interview of a patient, the students were asked to estimate where the patient would rate himself on each of seven personality variables, and what the patient's score "really was" on each of these variables. The test was administered in the same form (with minor changes of working to facilitate use of a score sheet) in all administrations.

The patients' scores on each of the scales were determined simply by asking each patient to rate himself on each scale. This procedure yielded the criterion of accuracy for students' estimations of the patients' self-ratings (task A). In addition, the Minnesota Multiphasic Personality Inventory (MMPI), card sort form,[26] was administered to the patients and their scores on comparable scales were used as criteria for the students' estimations of the patients' "real personalities" (task B).

The following seven-point scales (paraphrased from the MMPI) were used by the patients for the self-ratings; the corresponding MMPI scales are in parentheses:

Scale 1 (Lie Score). How much are you concerned with what the doctor thinks of you as a person: extremely concerned, very concerned, more than most people, about the same as most people, less than most people, unconcerned, don't care at all?

Scale 2 (K Score). Do you feel that you are: extremely critical of yourself, overly critical of yourself, more critical of yourself than most people, just as critical as most people, less critical than most people, not very critical of yourself, never critical of yourself?

Scale 3 (Hypochondriasis). How do you feel about your health and your past illnesses? Have you had: more trouble than anyone you know, far more than most people, more than most people, about as much as most people, less than most people, far less than most people, less than anyone you know?

Scale 4 (Paranoia). When you have had dealings with people, how have you found them to be? Was there: no one you could really trust, a few you could trust, some you could trust, you could trust about half the people, more than half you could trust, almost all could be trusted, no one you couldn't trust?

[26] See S. R. Hathaway and P. E. Meehl, *An Atlas for the Clinical Use of the MMPI* (Minneapolis: University of Minnesota Press, 1951).

Scale 5 (Psychasthenia). Some people are depressed, worry too much, have a lack of confidence, and are unable to concentrate. Would you say that you are usually: not at all like this, very little like this, some of it fits—most of it doesn't, some of it fits—some of it doesn't, most of it fits you, fits you well, fits you perfectly?

Scale 6 (Hypomania). How active a person have you been? Have you been engaged in: very many different activities, many activities, quite a few, some, not many, a few, very few different activities?

Scale 7 (Social Contact). Do you have your best times when you are: with a large number of strangers, with a large number of people —many of them strangers, with a large number of friends and strangers, with some friends and some strangers, with a small group of friends, with a few close friends, alone?

The Random Comparison Method of scoring was used to determine the students' differential accuracy in perceiving patients' self-ratings. The students' Adherence to Stereotype scores were determined by computing the variance of each subject's estimations for each scale. These variances were then summed and averaged for the seven scales. In addition, the fact that students estimated how a patient would describe himself (task A) and what the patient's true personality characteristics were (task B) made it possible to compute a new measure—assumed veridicality. That is, if a student perceived a patient to rate himself according to what the student thought were his (the patient's) true personality characteristics, the student would be assuming that the patient's self-report was a true (or veridical) one. Put in other words, the student would be perceiving little difference between the overt (self-ratings) and the covert (personality test scores) aspects of personality. Thus, if a student perceived small differences between self-ratings and "real scores," he received a high Assumed Veridicality score.

Table 13.19 presents the correlation coefficients between Differential Accuracy scores on three administrations of the test. Correlations are presented for both task A and task B for two classes. There appears to have been a positive relation between Differential Accuracy scores at one administration and Differential Accuracy scores at other administrations. This relation was particularly strong for task B for the class of 1956. Table 13.19 also presents similar correlation coefficients between the Adherence to Stereotype scores. All the relations were statistically significant ($p=.05$) and quite high. The same result was found for the Assumed Veridicality scores presented in Table 13.20. These results indicate a marked stability in the subjects' performance over six-month and one-year periods.

Although statistically significant relations were found between Ad-

Table 13.19. Correlation coefficients between scores on various test administrations: differential accuracy and adherence to stereotype in estimating self-ratings (classes of 1955 and 1956)

	Pre–Post I		Pre–Post II		Post I–Post II	
	N	*r*	*N*	*r*	*N*	*r*
Differential accuracy						
Task A						
Class of 1955	72	.19	72	.10	72	.24
Class of 1956	65	.41	65	.18	65	.09
Task B						
Class of 1955	72	.23	72	.28	72	.38
Class of 1956	65	.49	65	.51	65	.52
Adherence to stereotype						
Task A						
Class of 1955	72	.47	72	.55	72	.66
Class of 1956	65	.72	65	.44	65	.56
Task B						
Class of 1955	72	.53	72	.50	72	.74
Class of 1956	65	.61	65	.64	65	.59

herence to Stereotype scores and Flexibility and Capacity for Status scores on tests discussed previously, such relations were not found in connection with estimations of personality characteristics.

There was striking agreement among the three classes of medical students in their mean estimations of patients' personality characteristics. Results are presented in Figure 13.7 for the Pretest for task A, since the three classes had identical tests on this measure only. As can be seen from Figure 13.7, the mean estimations of the three classes are highly similar for all scales. The direction of the students' errors can be seen by comparing the students' mean estimations with the patients' mean actual self-ratings. Note, for example, the marked difference between the students' mean estimation and the patients' mean actual self-rating for scale 2. The students estimated that the patients had rated themselves as much less self-critical than the patients actually had rated themselves. On scale 3 the students estimated that the patients had rated themselves as much more concerned with their illnesses than the patients actually had. Since these errors were shared by three classes of medical students, it seems reasonable to assume

Table 13.20. Correlation coefficients between scores on various test administrations: assumed veridicality in estimating self-ratings and personality characteristics (classes of 1955 and 1956)

	Pre–Post I		Pre–Post II		Post I–Post II	
	N	*r*	*N*	*r*	*N*	*r*
Class of 1955	72	.64	72	.63	72	.76
Class of 1956	65	.76	65	.77	65	.85

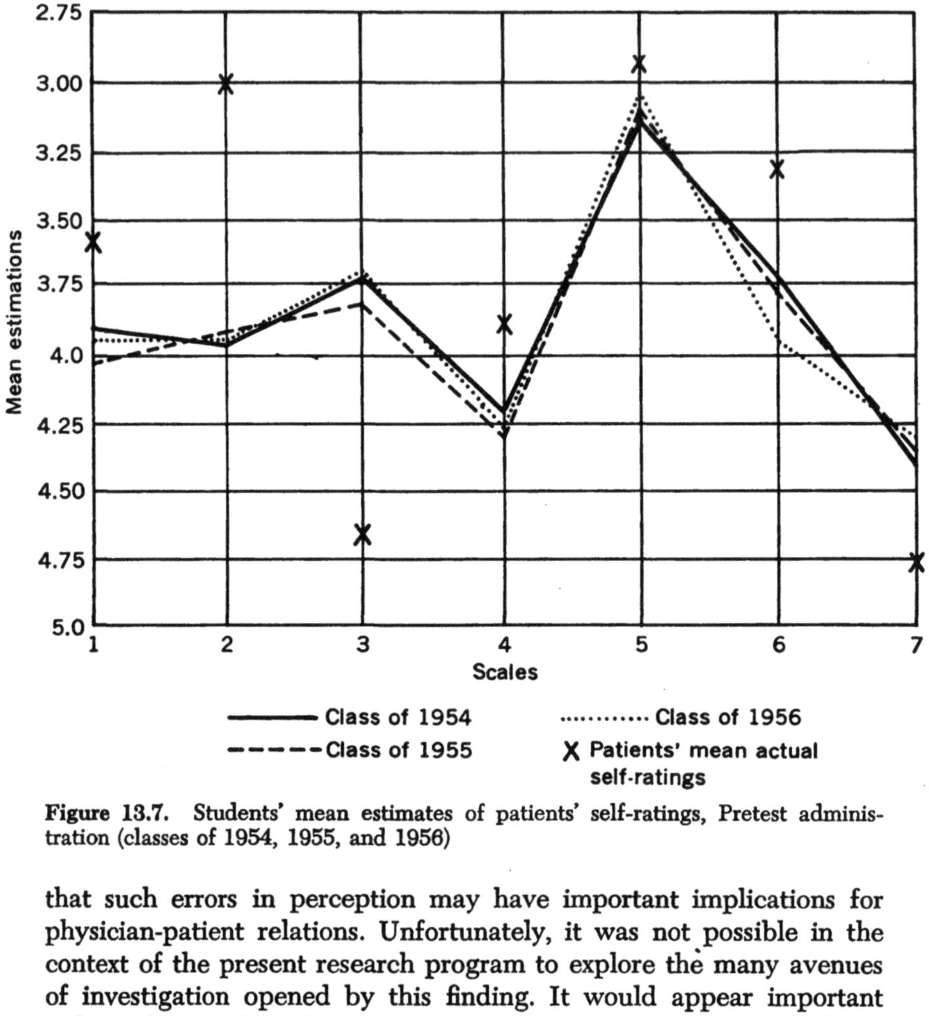

Figure 13.7. Students' mean estimates of patients' self-ratings, Pretest administration (classes of 1954, 1955, and 1956)

that such errors in perception may have important implications for physician-patient relations. Unfortunately, it was not possible in the context of the present research program to explore the many avenues of investigation opened by this finding. It would appear important to know how widely this orientation is shared within a medical school, how it develops, and how it affects the students' relations with their patients.

RELIABILITY AND VALIDITY OF THE TESTS. The traditional techniques for computing reliabilities are not applicable to tests of the accuracy of interpersonal perception when these tests are scored by means of the Random Comparison Method. This method is not dependent upon the "truth-error" postulate or upon its corollaries concerning the randomness of errors, equal variances, etc. The Random Comparison Method merely furnishes information about whether the subject's performance differs from random performance when the effects of response sets have been eliminated.

Table 13.21 shows the percentage of students whose Differential Accuracy scores were above chance levels. It also provides an indication of the relative difficulty of the various interpersonal perception tests. As might be expected (and as intended), estimation of patients' ages proved a relatively simple task for senior medical students; virtually every student performed better than chance at each test administration. This high degree of accuracy must be attributed to the high ecological validity of age cues such as hair color, skin wrinkles, etc. It is interesting to note that estimating personality characteristics proved easier than estimating vocabulary level, and that estimating accurately the *first three* words defined incorrectly by the person-object was less difficult than estimating the *first* word defined incorrectly. It should be relatively simple to order interpersonal perception tasks according to their difficulty by this method. Analysis of the availability, strength, ecological validity, and reliability of cues should make it possible to predict the rank order of difficulty of various types of interpersonal perception tasks.

The Sound-Film Interview technique was judged by the research staff to be a valuable procedure. It permitted the measurement of many variables (several of them rather subtle ones), it provided a method whereby certain measures could be taken without the subject's awareness, and it made possible the appraisal of a student's ability to cope with many aspects of a given patient's problem. Of course, many Sound-Film Interview tests had to be used in this project before they were adequately developed. However, the technique itself appears highly promising. In fact, because it is easily adaptable to many special problems as well as to many broad problems, this procedure is likely to be extremely useful. (See Figure 13.8 for a diagram of the rationale of the Sound-Film Interview.)

Table 13.21. Percentage of students whose Differential Accuracy scores were above chance ($p<.055$) on various interpersonal perception tests (class of 1956)

	Pretest	Posttest I	Posttest II
Estimation of age	92	98	100
Estimation of intelligence	49	58	68
Estimation of vocabulary level (first word missed)	29	11	15
Estimation of vocabulary level (first three words missed)	34	32	25
Estimation of overt personality characteristics—all scales	63	94	75
Estimation of covert personality characteristics—all scales	34	42	80

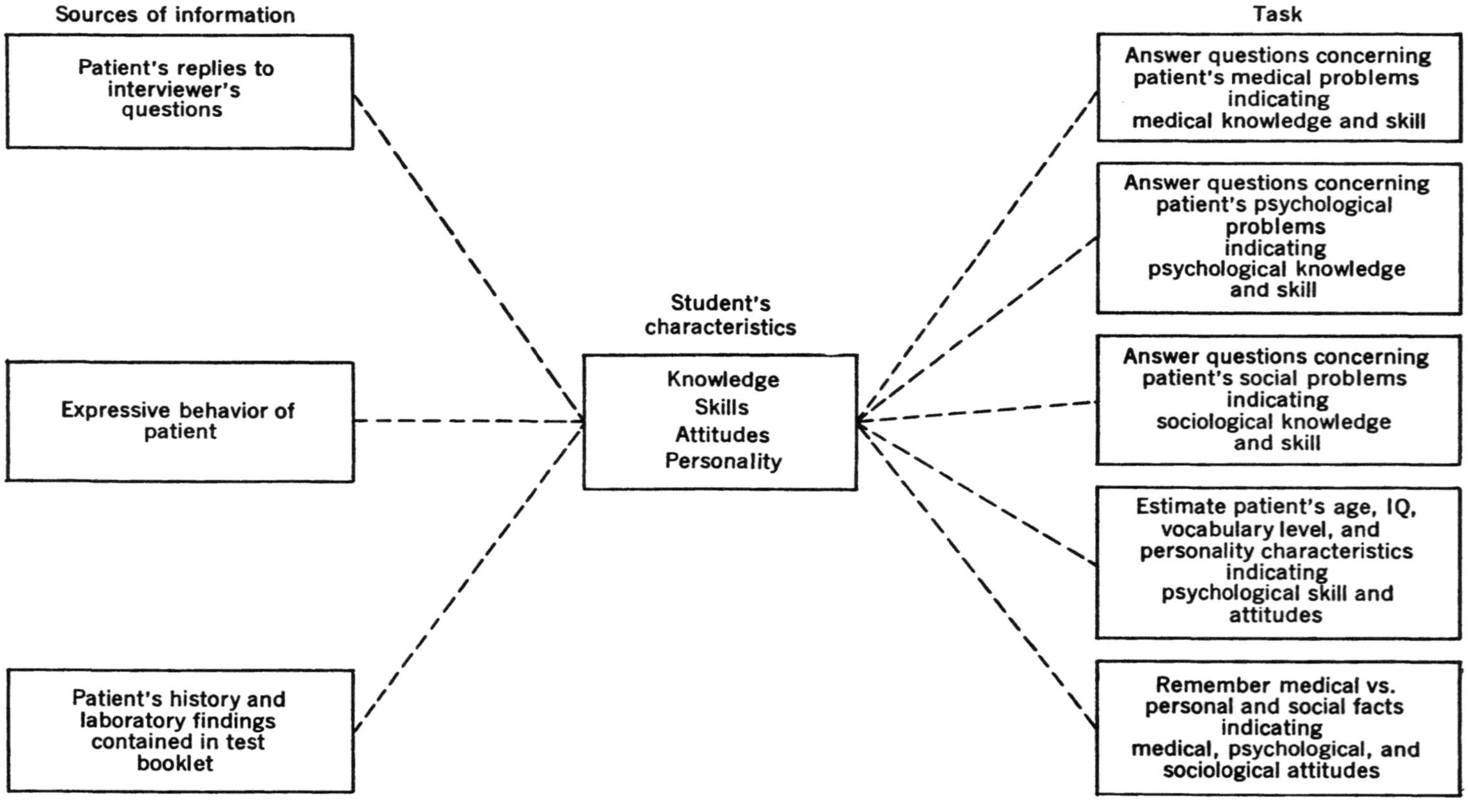

Figure 13.8. Schematic presentation of the rationale of the Sound-Film Interview

Other Procedures

MEDICAL ATTITUDES TEST

This procedure was developed at the University of Utah College of Medicine by Dr. Gerard Neuman and Dr. Reed Boswell. The Medical Attitudes test consists of five subscales: Attitudes toward Comprehensive Care, Attitudes toward Health Supervision, Attitudes toward Behavior Disorders, Attitudes toward Physician-Patient Relations, and Attitudes toward the Team Concept. All the items required the student to indicate the strength of his agreement or disagreement on a five-point scale. A copy of the test is presented in Appendix 2.

The Medical Attitudes test was developed in accordance with Guttman scaling procedures. Although reproducibility coefficients were not calculated in the present study, the coefficients reported by the research group at the University of Utah are uniformly rather high—the average for the five subscales being .88. Total test-retest correlations for two classes at the University of Utah were .60 and .77 for the classes of 1957 and 1958, respectively. The test-retest correlation for the total test score at the University of Colorado was .65. The correlation coefficients between scores on the various subtests are presented in Table 13.22.

It was originally intended that the Medical Attitudes test would be empirically validated against the staff's ratings of students' attitudes. This proved impossible because the study of staff ratings (see Chapter 24) indicated that the staff rated the students on medical knowledge only. However, several interesting correlations with various scales of the CPI were found, all of which provided empirical support for the validity of the Medical Attitudes test. For example, Health Supervision scores on Posttest I in the class of 1955 and on the Pretest in the class of 1956 were significantly related to the Tolerance scale of the CPI. Gough (*op. cit.*) describes the Tolerance scale as identifying persons with permissive, accepting, and nonjudgmental social beliefs and attitudes. (Tolerance was also significantly and positively related on at least two of four occasions to the Team Concept subscale, and to the total score on the Medical Attitudes test.) Health Supervision scores were significantly related to the CPI Responsibility scale on two occasions. Persons scoring high on the Responsibility scale are described by Gough as being alert to ethical and moral issues. Health Supervision scores were also positively and significantly related on at least two of the four occasions to the Good Impression and Sense of Well-Being subscales of the CPI. Persons scoring low on the Good Impression subscale are described by Gough as being self-centered and little concerned with the needs and wants of others. Those scoring low on the Sense of Well-Being subscale are described as being constricted in thought and action.

Table 13.22. Correlation coefficients between scores on Medical Attitudes subtests (classes of 1955* and 1956†)

	Comprehensive care	Team concept	Physician-patient relations	Behavior disorders
Team concept				
Class of 1955				
Posttest I	.41			
Class of 1956				
Pretest	.39			
Posttest I	.20			
Posttest II	.00			
Physician-patient relations				
Class of 1955				
Posttest I	—.03	.13		
Class of 1956				
Pretest	.30	.12		
Posttest I	—.12	.45		
Posttest II	.22	.30		
Behavior disorders				
Class of 1955				
Posttest I	.10	.43	.20	
Class of 1956				
Prettest	.11	.52	.32	
Posttest I	—.24	.11	.32	
Posttest II	—.11	.25	.53	
Health supervision				
Class of 1955				
Posttest I	.32	.31	.15	.27
Class of 1956				
Pretest	.46	.30	.49	—.05
Posttest I	—.20	.38	.47	.45
Posttest II	.23	.65	.20	.13

* Correlations are product-moment with $N=53$.
† Correlations are tetrachoric with $N=65$.

Students scoring high on the Physician-Patient Relation subscale of the Medical Attitudes test also scored high on the Good Impression and Sense of Well-Being subscales of the CPI on two of the four administrations.

Evidence from the questionnaire administered to the students indicated that self-ratings on Interest in the Welfare of the Patients' Family were also significantly related in a positive direction to Attitudes toward Health Supervision scores on the Pretest and Posttest II for the class of 1956.

Although empirical behavioral validation of these measures would have been welcomed, their internal consistency and their relations with measures obtained by a different type of test material supported their empirical validity.

Table 13.23. Correlation coefficients between scores on two test administrations: staff description checklist (class of 1956)

	Pre–Post II	
	N	*r*
Self-surgeon similarity	65	.19
Self-internist/pediatrician similarity	65	.65
Self-psychiatrist similarity	65	.62

STAFF DESCRIPTION CHECKLIST

This procedure was devised in order to discover whether the GMC student changed his conception of himself as a *medical* person. That is, an effort was made to discover whether the GMC student's self-concept changed so that he thought himself to be more like his conception of an internist, more like his conception of a psychiatrist, or more like his conception of a surgeon.

A modified version of the Gough Adjective Check-List[27] was used (see Appendix 3). The students were asked to fill out in four different ways a checklist consisting of 117 items. They were asked first to check those adjectives which they felt were descriptive of the typical surgeon, then to check those descriptive of the typical internist/pediatrician, and then to check those descriptive of the typical psychiatrist. At a later time in the testing period, they were asked to check adjectives descriptive of themselves. The test was administered twice to the class of 1956—at the Pretest and at Posttest II.

Thus, each student obtained a Self-Surgeon Similarity score, a Self-Internist/Pediatrician Similarity score, and a Self-Psychiatrist Similarity score. The student's Self-Surgeon score, for example, was computed by determining the proportion of all adjectives checked which was common to both surgeon checklist and self checklist.

Table 13.23 presents the correlation coefficients obtained when the students' scores on the Pretest were correlated with their scores one year later on Posttest II. The correlation coefficients between scores on the Internist/Pediatrician scale and on the Psychiatrist scale were very high, considering the fact that at least nine months (or one year) of medical school intervened between the Pretest and Posttest II. The correlation coefficients between scores on the Surgeon scale were, in contrast, quite low. This result was primarily due to the change in descriptions of the surgeon on the part of control students (see Chapter 18). Students clearly ascribe different personality characteristics to the various specialists (see, for example, Table 18.14).

[27] See H. G. Gough, *Reference Handbook for the Gough Adjective Check-List* (Berkeley: University of California Institute of Personality Assessment and Research, 1955).

Questionnaire

A questionnaire was developed which asked the student to divulge his opinions about many aspects of his education. Student reports of this kind must, of course, be used properly. Such reports could not be used directly as means of evaluation, for students were often asked to report their opinions about matters they were not qualified to judge. For example, students were asked to evaluate the proficiency of their teachers. Because the students were not qualified to make this judgment, their reports were not used to evaluate the quality of their instructors. However, it was important to know that the students did or did not gain the impression that they were being taught by proficient instructors. The students' opinions, right or wrong, are an important aspect of any educational situation. (See also Chapter 11 for a discussion of the use of student opinion.)

The questions were derived from a wide variety of sources. Many were written after interviews with students and with staff. In addition, the project was fortunate to have at hand the questionnaire used at the Cornell Medical College, which was made available by the Bureau of Applied Social Research of Columbia University. As the objectives of the GMC became clarified, however, the questionnaire was extensively revised to include only those items relevant to the specific aims of the program. A copy of the questionnaire is included as Appendix 4.

Conclusion

The most important technique developed in connection with the measurement of the effects of the GMC was the Sound-Film Interview. This technique made possible the measurement of several variables (knowledge, skill, and attitudes) in connection with a single patient in a given series of patients. The greatest advantage of this procedure is its potential flexibility. The Sound-Film Interview has, for example, already been recognized as an extremely important device for training students in the techniques of developing accurate appraisals of patients as well as evaluating the effects of training. It seems safe to say that the inherent possibilities of the Sound-Film Interview were only touched upon in this project.

There were serious deficiencies in the methods used by the Dependent Variables Section, however. Foremost among these deficiencies was the lack of coordination between theory and method. This lack of coordination was a direct result of the failure to give close attention to the role of theory in the early stages of the research. There was far too much reliance on the false hope of establishing the empirical validity of dependent variables measures within the context of the practical problem itself. Consequently, the validity of many of the dependent variables measures is questionable.

When it was discovered that the ratings made by the GMC staff would not provide adequate criteria for the evaluation of measures other than those of medical knowledge (for which the ratings were not needed), it was too late to seek new criteria. Had thoroughgoing consideration been given to the theoretical problems involved in the measurement of knowledge, skill, and attitudes at the outset of the research, and had it been possible to develop procedures in accordance with the theory so that the construct validity[28] of the tests was developed, the validity of many of these procedures would not be in doubt, as they are now.

In the early stages of the research, however, it was not certain that either the time or the resources would be available to carry out basic, developmental research. Nor was the notion of construct, as opposed to empirical, validity as clear in 1952 as it is in 1959. Thus it was quite in keeping with current research strategy to develop procedures on the basis of the best "informed guess" possible, and to make provisions for checking the validity of the procedures in the context of the research. Even though this line of reasoning is still the predominant one in much psychological research, it has two weaknesses: the criteria for checking the validity of the procedures may never become available (as in the present study and in many others), and even if such criteria do become available, in the form of behavior ratings, they are apt to raise more questions than they answer (see, for example, Chapter 24).

The problem of reliability (accuracy) of measurement was complicated not only by problems related to the development of tests but also by two conflicting requirements placed on the research project. On the one hand, because the aims of the GMC were quite broad, a large number of tests had to be employed; and the administration of the tests required considerable time. On the other hand, time is a precious commodity within a medical school. The result was an unfortunate compromise—too many tests taken by the students within too short a time period—which led to test fatigue and inadequate reliability of the tests.

[28] See L. J. Cronbach and P. E. Meehl, "Construct Validity in Psychological Tests," *Psychological Bulletin* 52:281–302, 1955; and R. Jessor and Kenneth R. Hammond, "Construct Validity and the Taylor Anxiety Scale," *Psychological Bulletin* 54:161–170, 1957.

Chapter 14

Independent Variables

How the Two Teaching Programs Were Studied

The primary task of the Independent Variables Section of the research project was to attempt to discover and analyze the reasons for the results of the new program; that is, to compare the GMC and control programs so as to discover what accounted for differences, or lack of differences, in their results.

Since both programs were essentially learning situations, it was obviously appropriate to focus this part of the research on the student-staff conference, where most of the senior medical student's learning about the facts and techniques of clinical medicine took place. However, once the student-staff conference had been selected as the focal point for the research of the Independent Variables Section, special difficulties became apparent. It should be pointed out that this was probably the first attempt to study the actual teaching process in higher education. There had, of course, been many studies of the effects of curricular changes; there had been formal studies of the teaching process at lower educational levels and informal commentaries on it at the graduate level; but so far as the present writers know, there had been no previous attempts at systematic study of the actual teaching process in medical schools. Virtually all previous work on the psychology of learning dealt with rather simple learning (motor skills, problem solving). The present study had to deal with a type of learning far more complex than had ever been studied before.

THE THEORY

Studying this type of learning posed a twofold problem. The demands of applied research required that the learning behavior of the medical student be studied as it actually occurred; to simplify the learning situation so that it could be analyzed by the usual laboratory experiment techniques would defeat the purpose of the applied phase of the research. On the other hand, the learning situation (the teaching conference) was so complex that unless some ordering principle was imposed the overwhelming amount of detail would make analysis impossible. It was at this juncture, then, that basic and applied research met: it was necessary to select or evolve an appropriate theoretical system (basic research) which would order the complex learning situation enough to permit solution of the practical (applied) problem *without oversimplifying the situation or removing the process from the context in which it actually took place,* since that context (environment) was an integral and functional part of the complex learning process to be studied.

What was needed was a theory of cognition which could be applied to the critical, change-producing situation (the student-staff conference) in all its complexity. In other words, the theory would have to take account of the complex processes involved in the acquisition and ordering of knowledge, in thinking, in problem solving, etc., in such a way as to enable the researchers to make quantified, objective comparisons of the cognitive aspects of the teaching-learning activities in the two programs—without the distortion consequent on oversimplification of these inherently complex activities. Only after such a suitable theory had been found or developed could the practical problem be attacked with some hope of success.

The theoretical system finally utilized was an adaptation of Zajonc's theory of cognition.[1] This system conceives of the "mind" as a changing structure of what are denoted cognitive elements (facts, or items of information) possessed by a person. These cognitive elements, which may be added to as the person perceives (or is "taught") new facts, are interrelated (structured), and this structure is subject to certain forces (potential for change). These forces result in changes in the cognitive structure; the new structure then produces new forces which lead in turn to new changes. This process of changing structural relations among cognitive elements, together with the addition of new cognitive elements (information from the patient or teacher), constitutes the complex learning process, which was the focal point of this part of the research project.[2]

[1] More specifically, the terms used to describe cognitive structures and their definitions were adapted from Zajonc's theory. See R. B. Zajonc, "Cognitive Structure and Cognitive Tuning" (unpublished doctoral dissertation, University of Michigan, 1955) and *Structure and Process in Cognition* (Ann Arbor: Research Center for Group Dynamics, 1955).

[2] This point of departure is roughly similar to that taken by many other psychological theorists. See, for example, George A. Kelly, *The Psychology of Personal Constructs,* vol. I (New York: Norton, 1955); David Krech, "Cognition and Motivation in Psychological Theory," in Wayne Dennis (ed.), *Current Trends in*

This theory, as the brief outline given above may suggest, possessed several significant advantages for the present study. It dealt with the precise aspect of cognition that was under consideration: namely, differences in cognitive structures brought about by the teaching conference. It not only took account of the quantity of factual information (cognitive elements); it also, and more significantly, provided a means for describing the relations (cognitive structure) existing among the cognitive elements in the cognitive structures of the students during the teaching conference. In order to indicate the application of the theory to the specific practical problem under study, the major concepts involved in the theory, its salient features, and the assumptions and hypotheses drawn from it, will be discussed in some detail.

Major Concepts

Three major concepts are involved in the theory: cognitive elements, cognitive structures, and cognitive processes.

1. Cognitive elements are the facts and items of information that compose the "mind." The cognitive elements of interest in the present study fall into two classes: facts or items of information about the patient (observations made during examination of the patient, laboratory findings, or data from the case history); and facts of medical knowledge, most of which have been acquired during the student's previous medical training. During the teaching conference, the student may add to his stock of cognitive elements through either direct perception or the mediation of the instructing physician.

2. Cognitive structures are the patterns of interrelations existing among the cognitive elements. By the time a senior medical student began his work in either the experimental or the control clinic, he had done more than merely accumulate a stock of facts (cognitive elements). He had come to see these facts as being related, the degree and nature of the interrelations varying considerably with the individual student. At the time of the teaching conference upon which the present study was focused, each student had evolved a pattern of relations (cognitive structure) involving both the facts he had gleaned about the patient and the pertinent elements of his previously acquired medical knowledge. From the point of view of the complex learning process, this structure is of more interest than are its component elements per se.

Psychological Theory (Pittsburgh: University of Pittsburgh Press, 1947); Kurt Lewin, "The Conceptual Representation and the Measurement of Psychological Forces," in *Contributions to Psychological Theory*, vol. I, no. 4 (Durham: Duke University Press, 1937); and Jean Piaget, *The Origins of Intelligence in Children* (New York: International Universities Press, 1952).

3. Cognitive processes are the changes that take place in the cognitive structure as a result of, among other things, complex learning. It is the emphasis on cognitive processes that made this theory particularly useful in the present study. In dealing with cognitive processes, the theory presented two major assumptions which, translated into hypotheses, were utilized in the research.

Assumptions and Hypotheses

The first assumption was that whenever a person's cognition (knowledge) of his environment is inconsistent with his perception of the environment, or whenever some of his cognitions are inconsistent with others that he has at the same time, a potential for work (which may produce change) results. The strength of the potential for work is a direct function of the extent to which the person's cognitive structure is involved in a state of inconsistency. The extent to which the cognitive structure is involved in a state of inconsistency depends in turn upon the degree to which the person's cognitive structure is integrated.

The application of this assumption may be illustrated by an example. A medical student is trying to arrive at a diagnosis of his patient's condition. Suppose the student at a given time perceives facts *a* and *b* in his patient. Suppose further that these facts lead him to suspect a diagnosis which can be made on the basis of facts *a*, *b*, *c*, and *d*. The student cannot assume that, having established facts *a* and *b*, he has arrived at a diagnosis. Doing so would set up an inconsistency between a medical precept that a diagnosis must be based on findings *a*, *b*, *c*, and *d*, and a new, ad hoc theory that a diagnosis can be based on findings *a* and *b* alone. Therefore, he will do work to try to reduce this inconsistency; that is, he will try to establish facts *c* and *d* or, alternatively, to find other facts that will lead to a different diagnosis. In this situation the strength of the potential for work depends on the extent to which the student's cognitive structure is involved in a state of inconsistency, and this depends on the degree to which his medical knowledge forms an integrated whole.

The potential for work can produce a change in the person's cognitive structure. That is, whenever there is an inconsistency which produces a potential for work, a potential for learning (change in cognitive structure) is present, and the strength of that potential is directly proportional to the extent to which the cognitive structure is involved in a state of inconsistency. The first principal hypothesis can now be stated:

Hypothesis 1: Given a setting in which a potential for learning is present, the student whose cognitive structure has a highly developed and extensive network of relations will have a greater potential for learning and will therefore learn more than a student whose cognitive structure has a less highly developed and extensive network of relations.

The second major assumption was that the strength of the potential for work is a direct function of the extent to which a person can anticipate a series of events which will resolve the state of inconsistency. The potential for work can also produce a change in the student's environment. That is, whenever there is an inconsistency which produces a potential for work, a potential for action by the student on the environment is present. In short, a cognitive state is also a motivational state. On the basis of the second assumption, the second hypothesis can be stated:

Hypothesis 2: Given a setting in which a potential for action on the environment is present, the student who can relate his cognition of anticipated future findings to all the available findings will be more highly motivated to work on the diagnostic problem than the student who cannot relate future and available findings.

Measuring Techniques

One of the advantages of the theory of cognition employed in this study is that it encouraged coordination of psychological and mathematical concepts. Translation of psychological concepts into mathematical terms means, among other things, that ambiguities are reduced, incorrect deductions are more readily discovered, and new and unexpected deductions are more likely to be made. The following section presents in mathematical terms the theory of cognition described above. For obvious reasons, a certain amount of verbal explanation supplements the formulae.

In order to test the hypotheses stated above it was necessary to obtain quantitative measures of the students' thinking about patients, of the instructors' contribution to the students' thoughts, and of the interaction between staff members and students. Two measuring techniques were used: the Teaching Conference Record and the Post-Conference Interview.

Teaching conference record

This technique was used to measure the dimensions of the student's thinking which developed during the teaching conference. In each of these conferences a student presented his findings and impressions of the patient whom he had examined just prior to the teaching session. The instructor then quizzed the student on certain problems of medicine, asked questions about the work-up, added new ideas, and pointed out the relevance or irrelevance of certain findings. Thus, in the teaching conference it was possible to distinguish the student's independent (prior) thinking about the case from the thinking which evolved as the staff began to interact with the student.

Recordings were made of a random sample of the teaching conferences attended by a random sample of approximately 50% of the GMC and control students. The data from a total of 13 GMC students and 10 control group students were used, and a minimum of four analyses of teaching conferences was available for each of these 23 students. These recordings were analyzed by a physician in accordance with a prearranged coding scheme designed to provide the data appropriate to the task of measuring cognitive dimensions.[3]

The student's thinking about the patient was measured in terms of his thinking about total diagnosis, organic diagnosis, psycho-social diagnosis, and total diagnosis including total therapy. The combined thinking of staff and student was measured in terms of the same four areas of thought (see Figure 14.1).

The recording of the student-staff conference did make possible the analysis of the cognitive interaction between instructor and student. However, it did not provide the research worker with an opportunity to resolve any doubts he might have had about the student's own thoughts concerning the patient. For this reason, the student was interviewed about teaching conferences.

Post-conference interview

This technique was used to measure the dimensions of the student's own thoughts and of the thoughts which the student reported he "learned from the staff," as well as the dimensions of the cognitive interaction between student and staff. Thinking was measured in terms of total diagnosis, organic diagnosis, and psycho-social diagnosis (see Figure 14.1).

As in the case of the Teaching Conference Records, Post-Conference Interviews were held with a random sample of approximately 50% of the GMC and control students with respect to a random sample of the teaching conferences. The data from a total of 17 GMC and 17 control students were used. Each of these 34 students was interviewed—once after his first visit with a patient and again after his final visit with that patient—on at least three diagnostic problems.

[3] Twenty-five of the Teaching Conference Records were analyzed independently by two physicians. These double analyses were used to determine the degree of inter-observer agreement and thus to check the reliability of the method (see page 259).

Figure 14.1. Staff's and student's thinking about patient, as measured by Teaching Conference Record and Post-Conference Interview

Measuring technique	Areas of thinking about patient: Total diagnosis	Organic diagnosis	Psycho-social diagnosis	Total diagnosis and therapy
Conference Record				
Student's thinking	x	x	x	x
Staff's and student's thinking	x	x	x	x
Post-Conference Interview				
Staff's and student's thinking				
After first and before second visit; thoughts about first visit	x			
After first and before second visit; thoughts about first and future visits	x			
After final visit; review of case	x	x	x	
Student's thinking				
After final visit; review of case	x	x	x	
Staff's thinking				
After final visit; review of case	x	x		

Definitions of Cognitive Dimensions

Differentiation

The student's thinking about a particular diagnostic problem is said to be highly differentiated if many "facts" are brought to bear in describing or discussing a diagnostic problem. For the purposes of this research a fact is considered to be any abnormal (or possibly abnormal) physical finding which student or staff thinks significant or potentially significant; a history of any symptom, diagnosis, or treatment which student or staff considers abnormal or significant; any projected therapy; any abnormal attitude or unusual socio-economic condition of potential significance.

Differentiation may be defined formally as follows (formula 1):

$$\text{dif}(C) = N$$

where C = any cognitive structure and where N = the number of cognitive elements in C.[4]

[4] Formula 1 and all consequent formulae are identical with Zajonc's operational definitions of cognitive dimensions. Reference to Zajonc's conceptual definitions of cognitive dimensions is omitted here. Those readers who are interested in the conceptual definitions of these dimensions are referred to Zajonc's *Structure and Process in Cognition.*

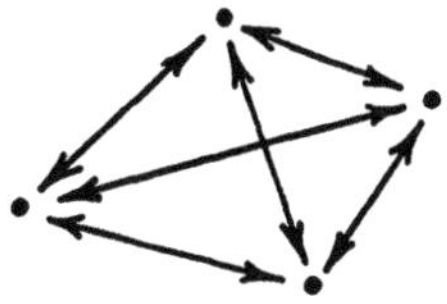

Figure 14.2a
High unity

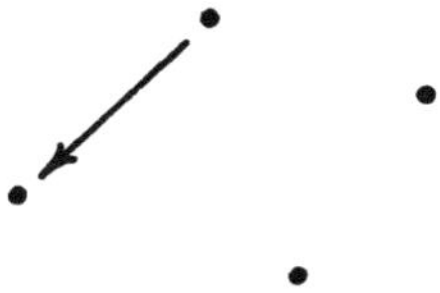

Figure 14.2b
Low unity

The concept of cognitive element used here corresponds to the concept of cognitive component used by Zajonc; the concept of cognitive structure corresponds to Zajonc's concept of cognitive complex. Inasmuch as there is no reference to Zajonc's conceptual definitions in this section, it was felt that terms should be used which had some common-sense meaning even though they were not as accurate as Zajonc's terms.

UNITY

The student's thinking is said to be highly unified if all the facts he brings to bear in discussing a diagnostic problem are highly "interrelated." The term interrelation has the following operational meaning: two facts, *a* and *b*, are said to be interrelated if the student sees fact *a* as "due to" fact *b*, or fact *b* as "due to" fact *a*, or both facts as "due to" one another. Stated differently, two facts, *a* and *b*, are said to be interrelated if fact *a* is "explained" by fact *b* (fact *a* is not present unless fact *b* is present), or if fact *b* is "explained" by fact *a*, or if fact *a* "explains" fact *b*, and vice versa. The term used by Zajonc to indicate a relation is dependence. If fact *a* is "explained" by fact *b*, fact *a* is said to depend on fact *b*, or *b* is said to determine *a*. If a fact is represented by a point, and a dependence relation between any two points by an arrow, Figure 14.2a represents thinking that is maximally unified, while Figure 14.2b represents thinking that is not highly unified.

The unity of a cognitive structure may be defined formally as follows (formula 2):

$$\text{uni}\,(C) = \frac{\sum_{i=1}^{N} \text{dep}\,(A_i, C - A_i)}{N(N-1)}$$

where A_i = the i-th cognitive element in C; dep $(A_i, C - A_i)$ = the number of dependences which exist between A_i and the remaining elements in C, that is, $C - A_i$. $\sum_{i=1}^{N}$ dep $(A_i, C - A_i)$ indicates that the dependence of any element, A_i, on other elements in C is computed for each A_i, that is, N times, and summed. N = the number of cognitive elements in C.

It follows from formula 2 that the unity of C is equal to the sum of the dependences of the i-th cognitive element, A_i, on all other cognitive elements in C, $C - A_i$, summed for all $i = N$ cognitive elements, and divided by the number of dependences which would exist if each cognitive element were dependent on all other cognitive elements in C, or N(N–1) dependences. (The dependence of a cognitive element on itself is excluded in Zajonc's system, hence the denominator in formula 1 is equal to $N(N-1)$ and not to N^2.) Unity is thus a relative dimension denoting the sum of all existing dependences between cognitive elements in the structure, divided by the maximum number of dependences which could exist in C if every element were dependent on all other elements.

Formula 2 is applied to Figure 14.2a as an example. Counting the arrows going each way between the points (elements) in C, it can be seen that the number of actual dependences in C,

$$\sum_{i=1}^{N} \text{dep}\,(A_i, C - A_i),$$

is equal to 12. The maximum number of dependences which could exist in C, $N(N-1)$, is equal to $4(4-1) = 12$. Thus, by formula 2, $\text{uni}(C) = 12/12 = 1$. C has maximum unity in Figure 14.2a.

Organization

The student's thinking is said to be highly organized if there is one fact in his thinking upon which all other facts depend. The student's thinking, therefore, is highly organized if the unity which characterizes it can be completely accounted for by the presence in the student's thought structure of one fact or concept. If a physician's cognitive structure is such that a particular diagnosis hinges primarily on one fact (or finding), if all other findings are explained by this one finding, and if in themselves these latter findings are sufficient evidence for the diagnosis only in conjunction with the one "governing" finding, then the physician's cognitive structure is highly organized.[5] Using the same notation employed in the previous figures, Figure 14.3a represents thinking that is maximally organized, and Figure 14.3b represents thinking that is not highly organized.

The organization of a cognitive structure may be defined formally as follows (formula 3):

$$\text{org}\,(C) = \frac{\text{det}\,(A_i, C - A_i)_{\text{MAX}}}{\text{uni}\,(C)}$$

[5] The reader should be cautioned to expect a certain arbitrariness in the application of such terms as "organization" to various cognitive states. Whether such arbitrariness occurs or not is unimportant so long as these terms are used consistently throughout, and so long as they are given operational specifications.

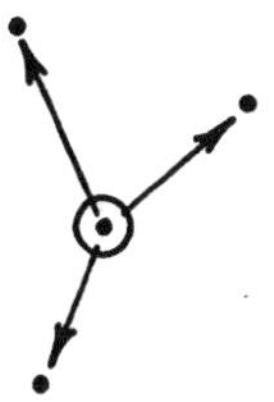

Figure 14.3a
High organization

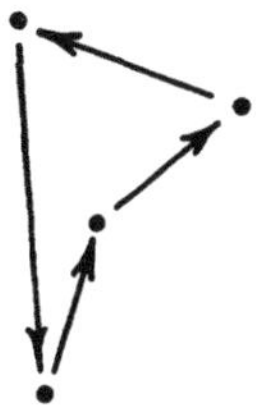

Figure 14.3b
Low organization

where det $(A_i, C - A_i)_{MAX}$ = that number of determinances, issuing from any one component, A_i, which is maximum for C. Thus, the organization of C is equal to the determinance of the cognitive element with highest determinance, relative to the unity which exists in C.

As an example, the organization of Figure 14.3a is computed below. The cognitive element with maximum determinance in Figure 14.3a is the ringed element. Its determinance equals 3 (there are three arrows going out from *a* to the other elements). Thus, det $(A_i, C - A_i)_{MAX} = 3$. The uni (C) now remains to be computed (see formula 2). The number of dependences in Figure 14.3a,

$$\sum_{i=1}^{N} \text{dep}\,(A_i, C - A_i),$$

is equal to 3. $N(N-1)$ is equal to $4(4-1) = 12$. Thus, uni $(C) = 3/12 = .25$. Referring to formula 3, it may be concluded that org $(C) = 3/.25 = 12$.

Maximum centrality

The concept of centrality is related both to the concept of organization and to the concept of unity. The student's thinking is said to be highly centralized if it contains a fact which is highly central; that is, if many facts in his thinking depend on that central fact and if the central fact itself in turn depends on some other facts in his thinking. The first variable is the more important, however. If a physician's cognitive structure is such that one finding is explained by a few others and it in turn explains all others, that finding is said to be highly central in the physician's medical thinking. Figure 14.4a represents thinking that contains one highly central fact, whereas Figure 14.4b represents thinking that does not contain any highly central fact.

The centrality of the cognitive element with maximum centrality may be defined formally as follows (formula 4):

$$\text{cen}\,(A_i)_{MAX} = \text{det}\,(A_i, C - A_i)^2_{MAX} + \text{dep}\,(A_i, C - A_i)$$

where det $(A_i, C - A_i)_{MAX}$ is defined in the same way as in formula

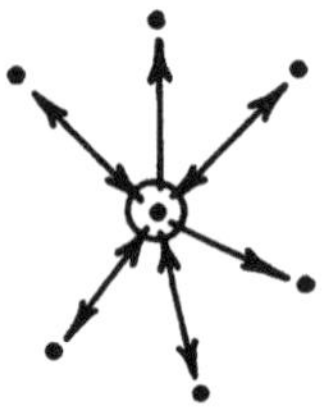

Figure 14.4a
One fact central

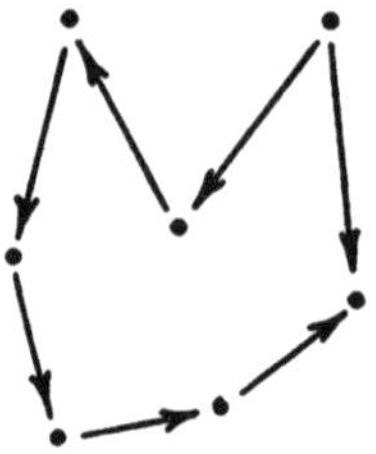

Figure 14.4b
All facts equally central

3, and where dep $(A_i, C - A_i)$ = the dependences which exist between the particular cognitive element A_i, which makes up the determinance term of the equation, and other elements in C. The determinance term is squared in order to weight it more heavily than the dependence term.

With the help of formula 4 the centrality of the element with maximum centrality can be computed for any C. In the case of Figure 14.4a, for example, the centrality of the circled point equals cen $(A_i)_{MAX} = (6)^2 + 3 = 39$.

Sum of the dependences

The sum of the dependences in the student's thinking about a diagnostic problem is said to be high if he considers many facts in arriving at a diagnosis and if these facts are highly interdependent. The concept of the sum of the dependences is like the concept of unity except that, unlike unity, it is measured in absolute rather than relative terms. Figure 14.5a represents thinking where the sum of the dependences is high. Figure 14.5b represents thinking where the sum of the dependences is low.

The formal definition of the sum of the dependences (formula 5) is the numerator of the formula for unity (formula 2):

$$\Sigma \text{ dep } (C) = \sum_{i=1}^{N} \text{dep } (A_i, C - A_i)$$

In Figure 14.5a it can be seen easily that Σ dep (C) = 20.

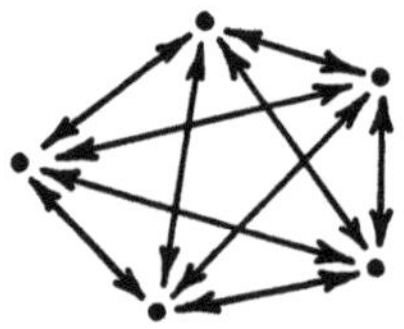

Figure 14.5a
Sum of dependences high

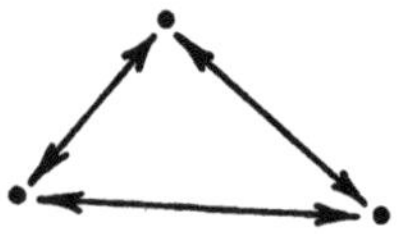

Figure 14.5b
Sum of dependences low

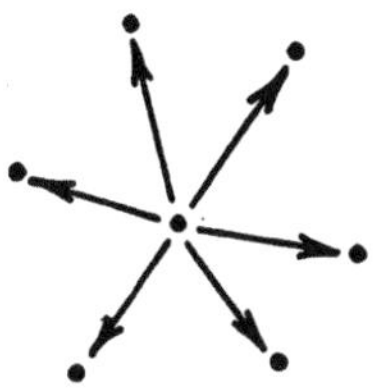

Figure 14.6a
One fact has high determinance

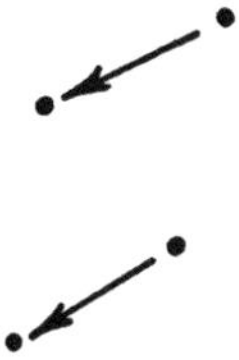

Figure 14.6b
No fact has high determinance

Maximum determinance

A fact in the student's thinking is said to have high determinance if the student can differentiate many facts and if one fact determines all other facts. The concept of the maximum determinance equals a concept of organization which is not relative to the unity. Figure 14.6a represents thinking where one fact has relatively high determinance. Figure 14.6b represents thinking where no fact has a great deal of determinance.

The formal definition of the maximum determinance of a cognitive structure (formula 6) is the numerator of the formula for organization (formula 3):

$$\text{det}\ (A_i)_{MAX} = \text{det}\ (A_i, C - A_i)_{MAX}$$

In Figure 14.6a the det $(A_i)_{MAX} = 6$.

Segmentation

The student's thinking is said to be segmented if, even though the unity of his thinking is relatively high, this unity is due to a high interdependence between facts within clusters of facts and a low interdependence between the clusters.[6] Thus, a physician who relates social and psychological facts to one another, and who relates organic facts to one another, but who keeps these two sets of facts completely independent, is said to have a cognitive structure which is segmented in terms of the organic and psycho-social aspects of medicine. Figure 14.7a represents thinking that is highly segmented, whereas Figure 14.7b represents thinking that is less highly segmented.

Segmentation, as computed in this study, is the average independence between the elements in each segment and all other elements in C but not in that particular segment. First the notion of the independ-

[6] These clusters, or segments, were generally found to consist of those elements which pertained to the organic symptoms and those which pertained to the psycho-social aspects of the case. Hence, segmentation was generally an inverse function of the degree to which the student integrated the organic and other aspects of the case into the total diagnosis.

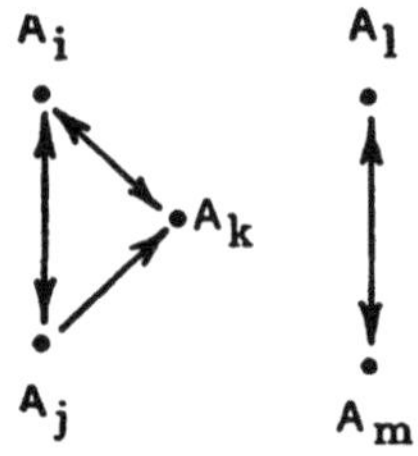

Figure 14.7a
High segmentation

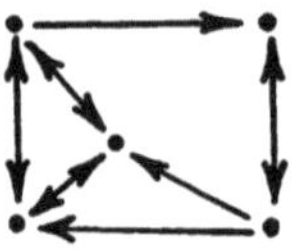

Figure 14.7b
Low segmentation

ence of a segment must be defined. Let elements A_i, A_j, and A_k constitute a segment labelled $U_{A_iA_jA_k}$. The independence of this segment is then defined as (formula 7a):

$$\text{indep}\left(U_{A_iA_jA_k}\right) = \frac{\text{indep}\left(A_i, U'_{A_iA_jA_k}\right) + \text{indep}\left(A_j, U'_{A_iA_jA_k}\right) + \text{indep}\left(A_k, U'_{A_iA_jA_k}\right)}{n(N-n)}$$

or in a more general form (formula 7b):

$$\text{indep}(U) = \frac{\sum_{1}^{n} \text{indep}(A_U, U')}{n(N-n)}$$

where n = the number of cognitive elements in segment $U_{A_iA_jA_k}$, N = the total number of cognitive elements in C, and $U'_{A_iA_jA_k}$ = all those cognitive elements which are members of C but not of the particular segment $U_{A_iA_jA_k}$. In formula 7b, U = any segment, A_U = any element in segment U, U' = all elements in C but not in U, and n = the number of cognitive elements in U.

The segmentation score is equal to the sum of the independence of each of the segments in C (computed by formula 7a above) divided by the number of segments in C. Formally, the segmentation can be written as (formula 7c):

$$\text{seg}(C) = \frac{\sum_{i=1}^{M} \text{indep}(U_i)}{M}$$

where U_i = the i-th segment in C and M = the number of segments in C.[7]

Formulae 7a or 7b and 7c may be applied to Figure 14.7a. In Figure

[7] This formula for the segmentation differs somewhat from the formula presented by Zajonc.

14.7a it is easy to separate two segments, one consisting of elements A_i, A_j and A_k, and one of elements A_l and A_m.
By formula 7a:

$$\text{indep}\left(U_{A_iA_jA_k}\right) = \frac{\text{indep } A_i\ (A_l, A_m) + \text{etc.}}{n(N-n)}$$

$$= \frac{2+2+2}{3(5-3)} = \frac{6}{6} = 1.0$$

$$\text{indep}\left(U_{A_lA_m}\right) = \frac{3+3}{2(5-2)} = \frac{6}{6} = 1.0$$

By formula 7b:

$$\text{seg }(C) = \frac{1.0 + 1.0}{2} = 1.0$$

The segmentation of C is maximal, as can be seen from inspection of Figure 14.7a.

It should be added that in this study the two segments considered were the segment composed of all organic findings and the segment composed of all psycho-social findings. That is, since the study involved an investigation of the effectiveness of a comprehensive care program, it was of interest to discover the extent to which the staff and/or the students were able to combine organic and psycho-social variables into an integrated whole when they discussed a patient's problem. (See Chapters 1 and 2 for a discussion of the aims of GMC.)

Homogeneity

The student's thinking is said to be homogeneous if the findings considered by him can all be classified within one narrow class of phenomena. For example, according to the classification scheme employed in this study, the thinking of the student is homogeneous when, in making a diagnosis, he restricts himself to facts pertaining exclusively, say, to the heart. It is heterogeneous if the student, in a like problem, considers not only facts pertaining to the heart, but facts pertaining to the chest or to the patient's psychological make-up as well.

Homogeneity may be defined formally as follows (formula 8):

$$\text{hom }(C) = \frac{\sum_{i=1}^{n} (2^{m_i} - 1 - m_i)}{2^N - 1 - N}$$

where m_i = the number of elements in the i-th class of phenomena, N = the number of elements in C, and n = the number of classes in C.

Formula 8 is derived in the following way. All the elements in a given class have, by definition, .a given dimension or property in common. In set theoretical terms, each element is said to intersect with all others. It can be shown that if a given class of phenomena, i, in C includes m_i cognitive elements, there will be $2^{m_i} - m_i$ intersections between the elements. Accordingly, the maximum possible number of intersections occurs in C when all the elements in C form one class of N elements, where $N > m_i$.

Thus, according to formula 8 the homogeneity of C is a relative dimension in which the number of intersections which does occur between elements of C is divided by the maximum number of intersections which could occur between the elements in C. The more coding categories which can be constructed to classify the elements in C, the smaller each value of m_i and the smaller the homogeneity.

Relations ratio

This ratio was developed for the analysis of the Teaching Conference Records. Since the participants in the teaching conference were not always explicit about all facts and relations they actually used in their thinking, it was not always possible for the physician observer to assign relations between pairs of explicitly mentioned facts. Therefore, the physician observer indicated which relations were directly mentioned (direct relations), and which were implied (indirect relations). The "relations ratio" is the sum total of all direct relations (Σ dep (C), see formula 5) plus the number of relations which were present but could not be assigned to particular elements (indirect relations) divided by the number of elements in the cognitive structure. The relations ratio may be defined formally as follows (formula 9):

$$\text{relations ratio} = \frac{\Sigma \text{ dep } (C) + \Sigma \text{ indirect relation}}{N}$$

where N is the number of elements in C.

Although the concepts described above are complex and their application in practice was by no means easy, the analysis of individual student staff conferences was carried out in these terms. A discussion of the value of the analysis is presented later.

METHOD AND PROCEDURE

The discussion that follows describes the methods and procedures employed by the Independent Variables Section: how the cognitive dimensions outlined above were ascertained in practice; which areas of the thinking of students and staff (and of both combined) were studied; how students were selected for study; how many students were studied by these techniques, and how often; and what the problems of data collection, processing, and analysis were.

As explained above, the Independent Variables Section focused its attention on the teaching conference and employed two techniques to measure the dimensions of the staff's and students' thinking: direct analysis of the conferences and interviews with the students concerning the conferences. These two techniques are described in detail below.

Teaching Conference Record

Recordings of a number of the teaching conferences were analyzed in order to measure the dimensions of the students' thinking and of the combined thinking of the staff and students which developed in the course of the staff's teaching. Initially, data were collected by a researcher who attended the conferences and observed the teaching situation. However, owing to the speed of the discussion and the complexity of the dimensions to be measured, this technique of direct observation had to be abandoned. Instead, recordings were made of teaching sessions. These recordings were then analyzed by a physician in accordance with a prearranged coding scheme designed to isolate certain cognitive dimensions.

Below, the text of an actual recording is presented in full. This sample recording is then used to illustrate the method of analyzing and coding the Teaching Conference Record and the method of computing the desired cognitive dimensions.

TEXT OF SAMPLE TEACHING CONFERENCE

Student: This is Mr. John Doe, sixty-six-year-old, white, retired typewriter repairman, and he comes in with a chief complaint of skin trouble. His skin was clear until late 1954, shortly after he retired from his work. At this time he noticed a reddened, scaling, pruritic rash, which first appeared in the skin fold behind the right knee, and over the course of three or four weeks extended down onto the calf and a little bit on the posterior aspect of the leg, and was followed in four or five weeks by a similar rash in the skin fold behind the left knee, which proceeded to extend in the same manner. This has progressively grown worse since that time. Two weeks ago he noticed that the back of his neck had become similarly involved. This condition has been treated with salves and calomine lotion which he has applied, and he has had six shots of ACTH from his present doctor, and he has applied cortisone ointment to the rash area. The ACTH gave him a transient improvement, and the cortisone ointment which he has been applying for only two weeks seems to relieve the condition, and he feels that the condition is not as bad now as it was two weeks ago.

Staff: What's he doing here? How did he happen to come to this hospital?

Student: I don't know—he's been here before—I don't know whether his private physician suggested that he come here or whether he came here by himself. He's been here before. He had infantile eczema, and he had eczema all through childhood and early adult life until fifteen years ago when he said that he learned to relax. This was a scaling, itching, lesion similar to the involvement that he has now, but it was generalized. He volunteers the information that after retiring from his typewriter repair work, which he had to do because his eyesight had grown so bad—he's had his lenses removed bilaterally, and his vision has just grown so bad that he had to give up—and he volunteers the information that this made him very nervous, that he had nothing to do, and he feels that this was related to the breaking out of the skin.

Staff: In other words, he had eczema all his life until he was about forty-five?

Student: Yes, it would be about fifty, I guess, fifteen years ago and he's sixty-six now.

Staff: It went away for fifteen years and came back?

Student: Came back in a localized . . .

Staff: Similar lesions?

Student: Yes, yes. Only I don't believe it was ever as severe as it is now, small areas. He's had chronic bronchitis for many years and chronic bronchial asthma since the age of about thirty. As I said, he's had both lenses removed for cataract, one was removed some fifteen or twenty years ago and the other was removed just three years ago. He had a coronary thrombosis in 1950, and in 1943 a hemorrhoidectomy.

Staff: What about the coronary thrombosis?

Student: He describes it as a not very severe coronary thrombosis. He was treated at home, he did have a serial electrocardiogram and was bedfast for a month. No activity. He said no angina; he said that he had perceived no angina. Systems review: the eyes I mentioned. ENT: has sinus trouble which he has had for many years; and he's had three nasal polyps removed. Cardio-respiratory: he has no chest pain; he has no exertional dyspnea; he can climb approximately three flights of stairs; he has no paroxysmal nocturnal dyspnea, but he does have some orthopnea and he uses one very large pillow which he says is equivalent to two or three regular pillows; he coughs up one or two ounces of a thick yellow sputum each day, but he's never had any hemoptysis; he had no edema before this rash appeared, and now that it extends down to the leg his ankles are slightly swollen and he feels that this is a skin involvement.

Staff: What do you think?

Student: I think that it probably is. He has some heartburn and takes baking soda. No other abdominal pains. He's never had any GI studies.

Staff: How much baking soda does he take?

Student: He takes it infrequently. He takes—when his stomach bothers him he'll take it two or three times a week—a teaspoonful of baking soda which he sometimes mixes with aspirin.

Staff: Can you draw any . . . does that suggest anything to you about his edema?

Student: Well, if this were on a cardiac basis you would have a high sodium intake, particularly if he were taking more. I think those one or two teaspoons a week would be undesirable, but . . .

Staff: What about a third possibility? So that cardiac, cardiac disease, but what else?

Student: Stasis dermatitis? Is that what you mean?

Staff: Medication.

Student: Cortisone, yes, which would cause him to retain sodium.

Staff: It's possible, though, that many people have to be taken off salt and put on completely salt poor diet, or intake, when they are getting any of the steroid hormones, you know.

Student: Yes, sure. He has nocturia at times too, but he's never had any burning or pyuria. The systems review is negative. Physical examination shows that his eyes . . . bilaterally, his lenses are removed. The retina and the nerve head seem normal. He appears somewhat emphysematous and he is moderately obese so he is not particularly resonant, but there is a lot of wheezing inspiratory and expiratory musical knock heard throughout the whole entire chest. There is no dullness to percussion. The diaphragm doesn't move well, the area of dullness seems to move about a centimeter posteriorly. His heart is difficult to count because of his emphysema, and the impulse diffusion can be felt in the precordium, but most of the impulse is really abdominal, epigastric. And his heart is difficult to hear, but it's a normal sinus rhythm with the exception of an occasional extra systole, and he had quite a few at one period but then he seemed to settle down and didn't have more and I felt that these were clinically probably ventricular, extra systole.

Staff: Why?

Student: Because they occurred on time as you tapped them out, the next beat was right on time.

Staff: There wasn't any compensatory pause, in other words.

Student: Well, there was the compensatory pause, but the next beat was on schedule. I mean it wasn't a true extra systole. It was a premature contraction with a compensatory pause so that the next beat came on time. . . . I think that I can feel the tip of the spleen.

Staff: Hmmm.

Student: And the liver is down four to five fingerbreadths. It is real difficult to feel, but I seem to get an idea of where the edge is and it percusses down that far, and the upper border of liver dullness is almost coincident with the costal margin there, so I suppose if his liver is down rather than enlarged, it's non-tender. The abdomen is soft, and there are no other masses of viscera palpable. The back and extremities aren't remarkable, with the exception of the rash which is pretty much as I've already described it, weeping, crusting, erythematous eruption centered around the fold behind the knee and extending down almost to the ankle and up five or six centimeters from that fold on the posterior aspect of both legs, and he has a little bit on his chest and quite a bit on the back of his neck with some cracking and excoriation. Neurologically he's unremarkable with the exception that he has very active knee jerks and no ankle jerks.

Staff: This is sometimes true because of edema. What about his blood pressure?

Student: I didn't take his blood pressure.

Staff: What's your opinion about him? What do you think his diagnosis is?

Student: Well, I think he's got what you'd call a chronic eczematoid dermatitis, and then he's got a—I don't believe—he's emphysematous, and I'm sure that he has a chronic bronchial asthma with emphysema.

Staff: In other words, he's had this asthma since he was a child, too. . . .

Student: Since he was thirty.

Staff: Thirty. OK.

Student: I don't know about that spleen. If I did feel it, it must be enlarged. I don't believe—is the spleen ever down so far that it can be felt without enlargement?

Staff: No. You mean due to emphysema?

Student: Yes.

Staff: I don't think so, no. Livers are, but not spleens. Any palpable spleen is an indication of pathology.

Student: He's got a real ruddy complexion which I didn't mention, and I'm sure that he's got some secondary polycythemia.

Staff: Probably so. Did you notice anything else unusual about his laboratory work?

Student: I might look at it. Looks like he's got a little urinary infection here . . . 20 to 40 WBC's in his urine. He's got 10,900 WBC. He's got 55% hematocrit, which is just in the upper limits or a little above the upper limits. He's got 10 eosinophils which I suppose might fit in with his allergic type.

Staff: Allergic state, yes. That's a little bit more evidence for both eczema and asthma.

Student: His asthma, however, seems to be the intrinsic or infectious type asthma. There is no seasonal variation, and he notices that it's worse when he has a respiratory infection and if anything it's worse in the winter than in the summer.

Staff: Well, that's the natural history of asthma in general, isn't it? As people get older it gets to be more chronic and more of a bronchitic type of asthma, doesn't it?

Student: I'm sure that he does have some bronchitis or possible bronchiectasis, coughing up yellow sputum.

Staff: Well, let's go see him.

[A joint examination of the patient by both student and staff intervened here.]

Staff: What do you think now about him?

Student: Well, we decided that that probably wasn't a spleen.

Staff: That's right.

Student: I guess it's pretty much . . .

Staff: The main thing now, here's what I want you to tell me. Edema of the legs, liver down, do you think he has a congestive heart failure?

Student: No, I don't. I don't think it's a heart failure.

Staff: Why not?

Student: Well, his liver isn't tender, and the upper margin is down as well as the lower margin, so I think it's just secondary to his emphysema. . . .

Staff: That's right.

Student: . . . that you feel his liver. Although he has all kinds of noises in his chest, he doesn't have any of the fine moist rales that you would expect in a pulmonary edema.

Staff: That's right.

Student: And although his ankles are slightly swollen there, it isn't the typical pitting edema.

Staff: Pitting edema with congestive heart failure? They're not like that at all.

Student: No.

Staff: What else, what other signs did he fail to exhibit? He was lying there pretty comfortably, flat on his back, wasn't he?

Student: Yes. Yes. Although he sleeps with the pillow I think it's largely his pulmonary . . .

Staff: Veins were not . . .

Student: No, he has no—his neck veins aren't even visible.

Staff: The basic trouble right now, he has two really basic problems and what are they?

Student: Well, I think if you asked him his basic trouble he'd tell you it was his skin disease.

Staff: Yes, that's right.

Student: And I'm sure that's true.

Staff: Yes, it would drive anybody crazy, wouldn't it?

Student: He's got a very extensive, real serious eczema, there.

Staff: What was his blood pressure, by the way?

Student: It was 110 over . . . . [Record not clear]

Staff: What about his dorsalis pedis and posterior tibial?

Student: I thought I felt his dorsalis pedis.

Staff: Did you think he was sclerotic in any of these other . . .?

Student: No, his retinas looked real normal so I don't think . . . We have good evidence that his coronary arteries are involved, but as far as other arterial involvement, I don't think there's much of it.

Staff: Why is that important in this situation?

Student: In this situation?

Staff: Yes.

Student: You mean with the treatment you would give him?

Staff: No, not the treatment but with the hazards associated with lesions on his calves like that?

Student: Well, if . . .

Staff: How about varicose ulcers in old people versus young people? Sclerotic people versus nonsclerotic people—what are the differences between diabetics versus nondiabetics?

Student: Well, unless you get a good blood supply your chances of healing any infectious lesion in particular are . . .

Staff: Are very poor.

Student: Are very, very small.

Staff: Yes, very poor, and you are especially afraid of infection in a leg that has very poor blood supply. Why you're just continually worrying about it and you're continually worrying about the healing if they do break down and ulcerate or get infected.

Student: I didn't think this had any stasis basis or lack of good arterial . . .

Staff: No, the outlook greatly depends on whether there is stasis or not.

Student: I see.

Staff: Many of these old people with varicose ulcers get a secondary allergic type of reaction around their ulcers or on their legs, things like that. They're the people who complain about burning and itching, like diabetics. It's a serious sign of pruritis, burning itself, though I don't think you have to worry about that in this situation. What do you think the skin people will do for him?

Student: Oh, gosh, I suppose they'll give him soaks.

Staff: What kind of soaks?

Student: Potassium permanganate, probably, because it's wet now and . . .

Staff: His legs can't be wet right now!

Student: Well, when I put my hands underneath his legs to test his patellar tendon reflexes I got some water in my hands so I think he probably has some . . .

Staff: The stuff on his face is all lichenified. That's old stuff.

Student: Yes. Yes, I think so.

Staff: Is there any way you can soften that up?

Student: Oh, gee, I don't know, I don't think you'd worry about it, as long as . . .

Staff: Might not worry a man and all that, but a lot of women worry very badly about that, don't they?

Student: Yes.

Staff: They give them salicylates, local salicylic acid, things like that . . .

Student: Yes, clear it away.

Staff: Grease to get it soft again, and there are all sorts of . . .

Student: Put on aquaphors like lanolin . . .

Staff: Yes, aquaphors. That would be good for his neck, I think. Now what's his second problem?

Student: Well, his second problem is his pulmonary problem which is bronchial obstructive emphysema.

Staff: More than that, isn't it? Don't you think he has true asthma?

Student: Yes.

Staff: True bronchial asthma.

Student: Yes, yes. I think he's got emphysema too.

Staff: That's the end result, the end result of a lifelong, fairly mild asthmatic—that he should live so long is evidence that he wasn't a severe asthmatic, but it's taken its toll and done its damage now, emphysema and bronchioles that are not smooth and not equal caliber and things like that. He's probably got a degree of bronchiectasis which undoubtedly contributes somewhat to his current allergic state. Some of these people we treat with antibiotics for two or three weeks, things like that, to try to change their flora, their respiratory tree, and it gives them a lot of relief, although it's certainly not permanent. He should be treated for every upper respiratory infection he gets pretty vigorously with antibiotics. What are you going to do with him now as far as your working him up further?

Student: Well, he has this inhaler and he feels that his asthma is pretty controlled with that. You might think of putting him on one of the longer acting bronchodilators.

Staff: Like what?

Student: Like ephedrine.

Staff: We kind of want to check the status of his coronary first, don't we, before we want to do things like that? He's got a pretty rapid pulse now which we usually see and associate with people who inhale a lot of Isuprel.

Student: He has these extra systoles. Did you . . .

Staff: I didn't hear any. You probably read it right after you got him undressed or something like that.

Student: Like I said, I thought they were ventricular, which would probably mean more than if they were . . .

Staff: Let's order an EKG on him, and I'd rather not treat his legs until he can be seen by the skin people—tomorrow probably, and I think that's time enough for him to . . . tell him we would rather not do anything until they saw him and prescribed treatment.

Student: I think that this is a man where you might consider some barbiturates or something along that line because he says that he is nervous and he has his eczema, and you might imagine that his asthma would be helped.

Staff: What about some of the other drugs that we have?

Student: Well, we have combinations of the ephedrine barbiturates . . .

Staff: What about the so-called "tranquilizing drugs"?

Student: Serpasil, Miltown, and so forth, you mean?

Staff: Chlorpromazine, Thorazine.

Student: Antibiotic . . .

Staff: Thorazine is very effective for itching skin.

Student: I've heard that, that's right. That might be a good idea. I was thinking along the line of a phenobarbital.

Staff: Phenobarbital is a lot cheaper, certainly. What about antihistamines?

Student: Well . . .

Staff: They've been pretty disappointing on skin diseases.

Student: I think you might say that they would deserve a try, but I wouldn't expect too much of a result.

Staff: What about antihistamine creams and lotions?

Student: I don't think the local antihistamines turn out so good.

Staff: They're about out of business, aren't they? They were just completely unsuccessful, many people were made worse with them.

Student: Same as the local antibiotics.

Staff: That's right. So let's send him to the skin clinic and order an electrocardiogram, have him come back in about ten days, and if the skin people haven't put him on the track, why we will. He's basically a skin problem with a certain amount of cardiac and pulmonary difficulties that we want to sort of help him out with, but he's bothered mostly by his skin now and we'd better not prescribe chlorpromazine or anything like that until the skin people have a chance to get a regular program going for him.

Student: What is chlorpromazine?

Staff: Chlorpromazine is Thorazine.

Student: Oh, I see, it's the chemical name for that?

Staff: OK. It takes that long to get an EKG, that's the only reason I'm having him wait that long.

Student: OK.

Staff: He'll be busy as a bird dog with his skin treatment when he gets started so that will keep him plenty occupied—all these soaks, you know. OK?

Student: Yes. Thank you very much.

METHOD OF ANALYSIS

Noting each fact. Each fact reported by either the student or the staff was noted on an individually numbered card. A fact was considered to be any abnormal (or possibly abnormal) physical finding which student or staff thought significant or potentially significant; a history of any symptom, diagnosis, or treatment which student or staff considered abnormal or significant; any projected therapy; any abnormal attitude or unusual socio-economic condition of potential significance. Facts were itemized as they were verbalized. For example, the student might say, "There is an old history of an irregular *fever* preceded by *sore throat* caused by *streptococcus* and followed by joint *swelling, tenderness,* and *redness,* with questionable *heart findings* and an abnormal *electrocardiogram,* causing extreme *maternal concern,* particularly in view of a *cousin's illness* and the high *cost of his hospitalization.*" This statement would be considered to contain 11 facts (the italicized items). An attempt was made not to use any presently considered diagnosis as a fact; a diagnosis was considered to be a set of facts rather than a single fact.

The facts noted by the physician analyst concerning the sample conference are shown in Table 14.1. It will be recalled that the patient discussed in this conference was found to be suffering from chronic eczematoid dermatitis (primary diagnosis) and chronic bronchial asthma (secondary diagnosis).

Coding facts. Each fact was coded according to a prearranged numerical scheme covering the patient's physical examination; laboratory findings; psychological examination; personal and family history of medical, psychological, social, and economic conditions; and treatment (see Table 14.2). This coding was done for the purpose of computing homogeneity and proved helpful also in the classification of facts into organic and psycho-social categories. The code numbers assigned to the seventy-eight facts listed in Table 14.1 are given in Table 14.3.

Classifying facts according to primary or secondary diagnosis. The primary and secondary diagnoses written by the student on the envelope containing the recording were used if at all appropriate. The staff's diagnosis was used if it differed materially from the student's. Each fact was classified according to whether it concerned the primary or secondary diagnosis. Facts that concerned neither were labeled "unused." Table 14.4 shows how the facts listed in Table 14.1 were classified.

Classifying facts according to diagnostic or therapeutic category. Each fact was classified according to whether it concerned diagnosis or therapy. Classification was based on the coding scheme presented

Table 14.1. Facts noted in analysis of sample teaching conference. (Numbers indicate order in which facts were verbalized)

1. Sixty-six years old
2. White
3. Male
4. Patient has a rash, beginning in 1954, right leg
5. Patient is retired
6. Rash extended to left knee and leg
7. Rash also extended to back of patient's neck
8. Patient has used salves to cure rash
9. Patient has used calomine lotion
10. Patient once had 6 shots ACTH
11. Patient also received cortisone, which seems to have some effect
12. Staff question: Why did patient come here? Student replies: Patient was here before
13. Patient had infantile eczema and all through childhood until 15 years ago
14. Patient learned to relax
15. Patient has poor vision
16. Patient's lenses have been removed
17. Patient has been very nervous
18. Patient has had "bronchitis" for years
19. Patient had a coronary thrombosis in 1950
20. Patient had a hemorrhoidectomy in 1943
21. The patient was given serial EKG's
22. Patient was bedfast for a month
23. Patient has had sinus trouble for years
24. Patient has had 3 polyps removed
25. Patient has dyspnea when walking up 3 flights of stairs
26. Patient's orthopnea is dubious
27. Patient has a history of edema
28. Patient coughs up 1–2 oz. of sputum per day
29. Patient takes baking soda 2–3 times per week
30. Patient has heartburn
31. Staff question: Could edema be brought about by baking soda, cortisone? Student replies to the effect that this may be so
32. Patient may have to be put on salt free diet
33. Patient has nocturia at times
34. Patient has bilateral aphakia, but nerve heads are normal
35. Patient looks emphysematous
36. Patient has musical rales over-all
37. Patient has a 1 cm. or so diaphragm move
38. Patient's heart is hard to evaluate
39. Normal sinus rhythm except for occasional extra systole
40. Patient's extra systoles believed to be ventricular
41. Staff question: Why are extra systoles ventricular? Student explains his reason
42. Believe I can feel patient's spleen
43. Patient's liver is down
44. Patient has a weeping, scaling, erythematous rash, with cracking and excoriation
45. Patient has very active knee jerks and no ankle jerks
46. Patient has a history of asthma since thirty years of age
47. Patient's spleen is definitely enlarged
48. Patient has a ruddy complexion as in original physical
49. I suspect polycythemia
50. Patient had 20–40 white blood cells in his urine
51. 55% hematocrit on laboratory test
52. 10 eosinophils on laboratory test
53. There is an infectious basis for asthma and skin rash
54. There is the non-seasonal history
55. The basis of the asthma could be the bronchiectasis
56. Patient has non-tender liver
57. There is suspected coronary arteriosclerosis
58. There is stasis
59. Patient will most likely get potassium permanganate soaks from the skin clinic
60. Omitted (on later analysis not considered a fact)
61. Patient has lesions on face (lichenified)
62. Salicylates
63. Softeners
64. Emphysema is a result of chronicity of asthma
65. The bronchioles are of uneven caliber
66. Treat upper respiratory infection with antibiotics
67. And each future URI with antibiotics
68. The patient has his inhaler
69. We might try cautiously bronchodilator
70. Get another EKG
71. Patient must first be seen by skin clinic
72. Give patient phenobarb
73. Give patient Serpasil
74. Antihistamines have been disappointing
75. Local antibiotics have also been disappointing
76. Patient will be kept busy as a bird dog with his skin therapy
77. Give patient Chlorpromazine
78. Give patient Miltown

Table 14.2. Numerical scheme for coding facts according to patient's physical examination; laboratory findings; psychological examination; personal and family history of medical, psychological, social, and economic conditions; and treatment

History of present complaint and physical examination

1. Name, age, sex
2. Race
3. Head
4. Skin and appearance
5. Ears
6. Eyes
7. Nose
8. Oro-pharynx
9. Neck
10. Thyroid
11. Trachea
12. Nodes
13. Chest
14. Lungs
15. Blood pressure
16. Heart
17. Vascular system
18. Abdomen
19. GI system
20. GU system
21. Spleen
22. Liver
23. Rectum
24. Back
25. Extremities
26. Neuro-muscular system
27. Temperature
28. Time at which significant events occurred
29. Weight
30. Activity

Psychological examination

31. Patient's attitudes toward relatives
32. Relatives' attitudes toward patient
33. Patient's attitudes toward human environment
34. Human environment's effect on patient
35. Mental states
36. Sexual adjustment
37. Doctor-patient relations

Personal and family history of medical, psychological, social, and economic conditions

38. Congenital defects
39. Infectious illnesses
40. Medical history
41. History of traumatic events
42. Surgical history
43. Allergies
44. Metabolic disturbances
45. Neoplastic surgery
46. OB and GYN
47. Socio-economic condition
48. Birth and development
49. Education
50. Occupation
51. Habits
52. Family
53. Human environment
54. Physical environment

Laboratory findings

55. CBC
56. Urine
57. Sedimentation rate
58. Chemistry
59. Bacteriology
60. X-ray (diag)
61. Biopsy
62. Morphology
63. Metabolism
64. EKG
65. Miscellaneous

Treatment

66. Treatment
67. Dietary
68. Medical
69. Physical
70. Surgical
71. Radiological
72. Socio-economic
73. Psychological

Referrals

74. Medical
75. Surgical
76. Psychological
77. Socio-economic
78. Dietician

in Table 14.2. Facts with code numbers 1–65 were classified as diagnostic; those with code numbers 66–78 were classified as therapeutic. There was one major exception to this rule: past therapies noted by student or staff were regarded as part of history work-up and were classified as diagnostic. Thus, only therapies being considered at present were classified as therapeutic.

Classifying facts according to organic or psycho-social category. Each fact was classified according to whether it concerned organic or psycho-social conditions. Again, classification was based on the coding scheme presented in Table 14.2. Facts with code numbers 1, 3–30, 38–46, 48, 52, 55–71, 74, 75, and 78 were classified as organic; those with code numbers 2, 31–37, 47, 49–51, 72, 73, 76, and 77 were classified as psycho-social; and those with code numbers 51, 53, and 54 might be in either classification, depending on the nature of the habit or environment involved.

If a habit was concerned primarily with the intake of toxic agents or other such factors it was classified as organic. For example, the habit of smoking a pack of cigarettes a day was considered an organic fact. However, if a habit was concerned primarily with the expression of interests, attitudes, and the like, it was classified as psycho-social. Thus, the habit of watching television most of the day was considered a psycho-social fact.

The rules for classifying facts about environment were the same as for those about habit. If the physical or human environment in-

Table 14.3. Code numbers assigned to facts of sample teaching conference

Fact number	Code number	Fact number	Code number	Fact number	Code number	Fact number	Code number
1	1	21	64	40	16	59	68
2	2	22	66	41	16	60*	
3	1	23	40	42	21	61	4
4	40	24	42	43	22	62	68
5	50	25	30	44	4	63	68
6	40	26	30	45	26	64	43
7	40	27	40	46	43	65	14
8	68	28	40	47	21	66	68
9	68	29	68	48	4	67	39
10	68	30	40	49	17	68	68
11	68	31	68	50	55	69	68
12	37	32	67	51	55	70	64
13	43	33	40	52	55	71	74
14	35	34	6	53	39	72	68
15	51	35	13	54	40	73	68
16	42	36	14	55	14	74	68
17	35	37	13	56	22	75	68
18	40	38	16	57	17	76	30
19	40	39	16	58	17	77	68
20	42					78	68

* Omitted (on later analysis not considered a fact).

Table 14.4. Facts of sample teaching conference, classified according to whether they concerned primary or secondary diagnosis, or were not used

Fact number	Diagnosis concerned		Fact unused	Fact number	Diagnosis concerned		Fact unused
	Primary	Secondary			Primary	Secondary	
1			x	40			x
2			x	41			*
3			x	42			x
4	x			43			x
5	x			44	x		
6	x			45			x
7	x			46		x	
8	x			47			x
9	x			48	x		
10	x			49		x	
11	x			50			x
12			*	51		x	
13	x			52	x	x	
14	x			53		x	
15			x	54		x	
16			x	55		x	
17	x			56			*
18		x		57			x
19			x	58	x		
20			x	59	x		
21			x	60			*
22			x	61	x		
23			x	62	x		
24			x	63	x		
25			x	64			*
26			x	65		x	
27	x			66		x	
28		x		67		x	
29			x	68		x	
30			x	69	x		
31			*	70			x
32	x			71	x		
33			x	72			x
34			x	73			x
35		x		74	x		
36		x		75	x		
37		x		76			x
38				77	x		
39			x	78	x		

* These items were unused because they did not qualify as facts.

volved the intake of toxic agents or other such factors it was classified as organic. For example, "living in the goiter belt" was considered an organic fact; "living on a farm" was considered a psycho-social fact.

Classifying facts according to contributor (student or staff and student). Each fact was classified according to whether it was contributed spontaneously by the student or contributed by the staff or by the student in response to the staff's teaching. Table 14.5 shows how the facts listed in Table 14.1 were classified.

Table 14.5. Facts of sample teaching conference, classified according to contributor (student or staff and student)

Fact number	Contributed by student	Contributed by staff and student	Fact number	Contributed by student	Contributed by staff and student
1	x		40	x	
2	x		41	x	
3	x		42	x	
4	x		43	x	
5	x		44	x	
6	x		45	x	
7	x		46		x
8	x		47		x
9	x		48	x	
10	x		49		x
11	x		50		x
12	x		51	x	
13	x		52		x
14	x		53		x
15	x		54		x
16	x		55		x
17	x		56		x
18	x		57		x
19	x		58		x
20	x		59		x
21		x	60		x
22		x	61		x
23	x		62		x
24	x		63		x
25	x		64		x
26	x		65		x
27	x		66		x
28	x		67		x
29	x		68		x
30	x		69		x
31	x		70		x
32		x	71		x
33	x		72		x
34	x		73		x
35	x		74		x
36	x		75		x
37	x		76		x
38	x		77		x
39	x		78		x

Eliminating facts. All items listed as facts but not actually qualifying as facts were eliminated. (1) The physician analyst often wrote down on cards not only the facts of the case which were brought out by the student or staff but also questions asked by either student or staff. Such questions were usually followed by answers containing facts. The answers were included and the facts recorded; the questions, however, were eliminated as being elicitors of facts but not facts themselves. (2) The analyst often noted relations which were drawn between facts by the student or staff. These relations did not meet the definition of fact and were therefore eliminated. (3) Owing to the original definition of fact (an *abnormal* or significant physical finding; a history of any symptom, diagnosis, or treatment considered to be *abnormal* or significant; or any *abnormal* attitude or unusual socio-economic condition), negative (normal) findings were not considered facts and were not included in the early analyses. As the study proceeded, it became evident that significant negative findings were part of the student's thinking about the patient's diagnosis. However, at that stage no alteration in the analyzing procedure could be made. Fortunately, the number of significant negative findings mentioned by the student or the staff in connection with any particular case tended to be rather low. (4) Facts not relevant to the diagnostic problem were also eliminated. The question of relevance in each case was decided by the analyst.

In the analysis of the sample Teaching Conference Record, facts 12, 31, 41, 56, and 64 were eliminated (see Tables 14.1 and 14.4). Facts 12 and 41 did not contribute significant information; facts 31 and 64 indicated relations between already noted facts, and the relations were not considered facts. Fact 56 was a significant negative finding.

Noting relations between facts. Relations were indicated separately for the part of the conference concerned with the student's presentation of the case and the part concerned with the staff-student discussion.

When the staff or student stated that a fact was due to another fact, or by close association in speech implied this, a direct relation was noted—regardless of whether the relation seemed to the analyst close or tenuous, certain or impossible, medically reasonable or not. When the context in which a fact was mentioned indicated that the fact was part of a diagnostic category, but the relation could not, by the above criteria, be termed direct, it was noted as an indirect relation. However, when such a relation involved two facts, both of which had been noted, the relation was usually considered direct. Duplication of relations was avoided as much as possible. For example, in the sentence, "Patient has a sore throat followed by fever, headache, and cough; was found to have a red throat; and was treated with sulfa, nose drops, and cough syrup," the fever, headache, and cough would be due to sore throat, which would be due to red throat; sulfa would be due to red throat (and not due to each of four complaints singly). Cough syrup would be due to cough. Note that fever is not considered due also to headache and cough, or cough due also to fever and headache, or headache due also to fever and cough. The treatment "nose drops" pertains to this diagnostic category, but the relation would be considered indirect, as no symptom or finding stated is directly treated with nose drops. Therefore, an indirect relation, "diagnostic-therapeutic" would be noted.

The students appeared to think of the relation between historical facts and the findings of the physical examination in at least two ways. Some students seemed to feel that the historical facts depended on the physical findings. Others seemed to group historical facts and physical findings independently. The physician analyst tried to relate the facts in whatever way it seemed the student intended. If the student seemed to group facts in several different ways, sometimes by placing a new interpretation on a fact or hypothesizing an intermediate fact, the additional relations were also indicated.

Computation of cognitive dimensions

The method of analysis described above made it possible for the researchers to compute various dimensions of the student's thinking and of the combined thinking of staff and student. Again, the sample teaching conference concerning the patient with chronic eczematoid dermatitis (primary diagnosis) and chronic bronchial asthma (secondary diagnosis) is used as illustration.

Student's thinking. The student's thinking about the patient was defined as all the facts presented by the student in discussing the patient's problem with the staff. It was measured in terms of his thinking about total diagnosis, organic diagnosis, psycho-social diagnosis, and total diagnosis including therapy.

TOTAL DIAGNOSIS. The student's thinking about total diagnosis included all the facts he considered in his presentation of the patient's diagnostic problem. The problem might concern either primary or secondary diagnosis, or both. In the computation, each diagnosis was considered separately. The illustration below concerns the primary diagnosis of the patient discussed in the sample teaching conference.

Facts 4–11, 13, 14, 17, 27, 44, and 48 made up the student's thinking about total diagnosis. To these were added fact 15 (classified as unused) and facts 35 and 36 (classified as concerning the secondary diagnosis chiefly), since these determined some of the facts concerning the primary diagnosis. Of the seventeen facts composing this student's thinking about his patient's total diagnosis, facts 4, 6–11, 13, 15, 27, 35, 36, 44, and 48 were classified as organic; facts 5, 14, and 17 were classified as psycho-social. Figure 14.8 indicates the direct relations between these facts. No indirect relations were noted. In this and similar figures a tally (1) indicates a relation between two facts. The dependences of a fact can be seen by reading from left to right along a row of the matrix. The determinances can be seen by reading from

		(Organic facts) Depends on													(Psycho-social facts)			
	Fact	4	6	7	8	9	10	11	13	15	27	35	36	44	48	5	14	17	
(Organic facts) Determines	4	x							1					1		1		1	4
	6	1	x																1
	7	1		x															1
	8				x														0
	9	1				x													1
	10	1					x												1
	11	1						x											1
	13								x										0
	15									x									0
	27	1									x								1
	35											x	1						1
	36												x						0
	44													x					0
	48											1	1		x				2
(Psycho-social facts)	5									1						x			1
	14	1							1								x		2
	17															1		x	1
		7	0	0	0	0	0	0	2	1	0	1	2	1	0	2	0	1	17

Figure 14.8. Relations between facts composing student's thoughts concerning total diagnosis

top to bottom along a column of the matrix. For example, fact 4 depends on facts 13, 44, 5, and 17; fact 4 determines facts 6, 7, 9, 10, 11, 27, and 14.

The dimensions computed for this area of the student's thinking were: differentiation, centrality of the fact with maximum centrality, unity, organization, sum of the dependences, determinance of the fact with maximum determinance, and segmentation. The operational definitions (formulae) for these dimensions were applied:

$$\text{dif}\ (C) = N = 17$$

$$\text{cen}\ (A_i)_{MAX} = \text{det}\ (A_i, C - A_i)^2_{MAX} + \text{dep}\ (A_i, C - A_i) = 7^2 + 4 = 53$$

(where A is fact 4)

$$\text{uni}\ (C) = \frac{\sum_{i=1}^{N} \text{dep}\ (A_i, C - A_i)}{N\ (N - 1)} = \frac{16}{17\ (17 - 1)} = .059$$

$$\text{org (C)} = \frac{\text{det }(A_i, C - A_i)_{MAX}}{\text{uni (C)}} = \frac{7}{.059} = 118.64$$

$$\Sigma \text{ dep (C)} = \sum_{i=1}^{N} \text{dep }(A_i, C - A_i) = 16$$

$$\text{det }(A_i)_{MAX} = \text{det }(A_i, C - A_i)_{MAX} = 7$$

$$\text{seg (C)} = \frac{\dfrac{\sum_{1}^{n} \text{indep }(A_u, U') \text{ organic}}{n\,(N - n)} + \dfrac{\sum_{1}^{N-n} \text{indep }(A_u, U') \text{ psycho-social}}{(N - n)\,(n)}}{2}$$

$$= \frac{\dfrac{1+3+3+3+3+3+3+3+3+3+3+3+3+3}{14\,(17-14)} + \dfrac{13+12+14}{3\,(17-3)}}{2}$$

$$= \frac{.952 + .928}{2} = .940$$

ORGANIC DIAGNOSIS. The student's thinking about organic diagnosis included all the facts classified as organic that he considered in his presentation of the patient's diagnostic problem. In the case used as illustration these were facts 4, 6–11, 13, 15, 27, 35, 36, 44, and 48. The direct relations existing between these organic facts are shown in Figure 14.8. No indirect relations were noted. The dimensions computed for this area of the student's thinking were: differentiation, centrality of the fact with maximum centrality, unity, organization, sum of the dependences, determinance of the fact with maximum determinance, and homogeneity. Computation of all dimensions except homogeneity has been given above. The computation of homogeneity follows. All facts classified as organic were coded according to the numerical scheme (Table 14.6). Only the facts originally classified as pertaining to the primary diagnosis were included in the computation of homogeneity (facts 15, 35, and 36 were excluded).[8] It can be seen from Table 14.6 that four facts were coded as 40, four as 68, two as 4, and one as 43. The operational definition of homogeneity was applied:

$$\text{hom (C)} = \frac{\sum_{i=1}^{n} (2^{m_i} - 1 - m_i)}{2^N - 1 - N} =$$

$$\frac{(2^4 - 1 - 4) + (2^4 - 1 - 4) + (2^2 - 1 - 2) + (2 - 1 - 1) + (2 - 1 - 1)}{2^{11} - 1 - 11}$$

$$= .011$$

[8] A better procedure would have been to consider all the facts in computing the homogeneity.

Table 14.6. Code numbers assigned to organic facts classified as concerning primary diagnosis

Fact number	Code number
4	40
6	40
7	40
8	68
9	68
10	68
11	68
13	43
27	40
44	4
48	4

PSYCHO-SOCIAL DIAGNOSIS. The student's thinking about psycho-social diagnosis included all the facts classified as psycho-social that he considered in his presentation of the patient's diagnostic problem. These were facts 5, 14, and 17. The direct relations existing between the psycho-social facts are indicated in Figure 14.8. No indirect relations were noted. The dimensions computed for this area of thought were the same as those computed for organic diagnosis.

TOTAL DIAGNOSIS INCLUDING THERAPY. The student's thinking about total diagnosis including therapy consisted of all the facts he considered in his presentation of the patient's diagnostic and therapeutic problems. Unused facts, facts pertaining to secondary diagnosis, and facts pertaining to primary diagnosis were included. These were facts 1–11, 13–20, 23–30, 33–40, 42–45, 48, and 51. Since the student in the sample teaching conference did not report on present therapy, no therapeutic facts are listed here. Figure 14.9 shows the direct relations existing between these facts. In addition, four indirect relations were noted by the physician analyst. The dimensions computed for this area of thought were the same as those computed for total diagnosis. In addition, the relations ratio was computed as follows:

$$\text{relations ratio} = \frac{\Sigma \text{ dep (C)} + \Sigma \text{ indirect relations}}{\text{N}} = \frac{28 + 4}{41} = .78$$

(where the quantity 4 is the number of indirect relations noted by the analyst)

Combined thinking of staff and student. The combined thinking of staff and student was defined as all the facts considered by staff and student in the course of the staff's teaching. Facts mentioned by the student in his initial presentation were included only if they were specifically noted during the teaching. Combined thinking was measured in terms of thinking about total diagnosis, organic diagnosis, psycho-social diagnosis, and total diagnosis including therapy.

Depends on

Determines: Fact	1	2	3	4	5	6	7	8	9	10	11	13	14	15	16	17	18	19	20	23	24	25	26	27	28	29	30	33	34	35	36	37	38	39	40	42	43	44	45	48	51	
1	x																																									0
2		x																																								0
3			x																																							0
4				x	1							1				1																						1				4
5					x																																					1
6				1		x																																				1
7				1			x																																			1
8								x																																		0
9				1					x																																	1
10				1						x																																1
11				1							x																															1
13												x																														0
14				1								1	x																													2
15														x																												0
16														1	x														1													2
17					1											x																										1
18																	x								1						1											2
19																		x																	1							1
20																			x																							0
23																				x																						0
24																				1	x																					1
25																						x																				0
26																							x																			0
27				1																				x																		1
28																									x						1											1
29																										x	1															1
30																											x															0
33																												x														0
34																													x													0
35																														x	1											1
36																															x											0
37																															1	x										1
38																														1			x									1
39																																		x	1							1
40																																			x							0
42																																				x						0
43																																					x					0
44																																						x				0
45																																							x			0
48																														1	1									x		2
51																																									x	0
	0	0	0	7	2	0	0	0	0	0	0	2	0	2	0	1	0	0	0	1	0	0	0	0	1	0	1	0	1	2	5	0	0	0	2	0	0	1	0	0	0	28

Figure 14.9. Relations between facts composing student's thoughts concerning total diagnosis including therapy

TOTAL DIAGNOSIS. The combined thinking about total diagnosis included all facts considered by staff and student in the course of the staff's teaching. As in the computation of the student's own thinking, primary and secondary diagnoses were considered separately. The illustration below concerns the primary diagnosis.

Facts 11, 27, 44, 48, 52, 58, 60, and 61 (classified as pertaining to the primary diagnosis) made up the combined thinking about the patient's total diagnosis. To these were added Facts 1, 29, 39, 49, and 57 (classified as pertaining to the secondary diagnosis), since these determined some of the other facts. All facts were classified as organic. The direct relations between these facts are shown in Figure 14.10. No indirect relations were noted.

ORGANIC AND PSYCHO-SOCIAL DIAGNOSES. Since all the facts making up the combined thinking of staff and student about the total diagnosis were classified as organic, their thinking about the organic diagnosis is the same as their thinking about the total diagnosis. They did not think about the psycho-social diagnosis.

Depends on (columns); Determines (rows)

Fact	1	11	27	29	39	44	48	49	52	57	58	60	61	
1	x													0
11		x												0
27		1	x	1	1	1								4
29				x										0
39					x									0
44						x			1					1
48							x	1						1
49								x						0
52									x					0
57										x				0
58	1					1				1	x			3
60											1	x		1
61													x	0
	1	1	0	1	1	2	0	1	1	1	1	0	0	10

Figure 14.10. Relations between facts composing combined thoughts of student and staff concerning total diagnosis

TOTAL DIAGNOSIS INCLUDING THERAPY. The combined thinking about total diagnosis including therapy included all the facts considered by staff and student concerning the patient's diagnostic and therapeutic problems. These were facts 1, 11, 17, 19, 21, 22, 27, 29, 32, 35–37, 39, 42–63, and 65–78. The direct relations between these facts are shown in Figure 14.11. In addition, five indirect relations were noted by the analyst.

PROBLEMS OF ANALYSIS

This description of the analysis of the Teaching Conference Record will be concluded with a discussion of some of the problems encountered by the two physicians who made the analyses.[9]

Noting each fact. Although the definition of fact (given above) seems fairly precise, uncertainty about whether an item of information qualified as a fact existed in every analysis and was particularly troublesome in certain areas. First, since a presently considered diagnosis did not qualify as a fact, confusion resulted each time a student or instructor used a diagnostic term to mean a pathological entity and involved it with other facts, for example, "Patient's bronchiectasis [diagnostic term] and subsequent pooling of secretions caused her shortness of breath." Confusion also resulted when the nature of a lesion was discussed in anatomic terms, since in such instances the anatomic term was used to mean the diagnostic term. Second, there was uncertainty about whether an item of information mentioned more than once should be considered a new fact each time. For example, was the recurrence of a certain finding through past and present physical examinations to be considered a new fact each time, or did presenting it as a new fact each time constitute duplication? No satisfactory criterion for making these decisions was found. The rule used was as follows: whatever the student or staff appeared to consider a fact was noted and used as a fact. A third problem encountered in noting facts occurred in records of conferences concerning well-baby visits. Owing to the definition of fact, normal physical examination findings, diets, procedures, etc., were not considered facts. In retrospect, this seems to have been a mistake; each change of diet, weight, etc., even though within normal limits, should have been noted in a conference concerning a well-baby visit.

Coding facts. Uncertainty arose regarding the coding of facts which could be assigned equally well to several different code numbers. For example, "history of hypertensive retinal hemorrhages," could be coded as "blood pressure," "vascular," or "eye." It was decided

[9] This information is taken from a report by the two analysts, Gerald J. Conlin, M.D., and E. Michael Flaherty, M.D.

Depends on

Determines

Fact	1	11	17	19	21	22	27	29	32	35	36	37	39	42	43	44	45	46	47	48	49	50	51	52	53	54	55	56	57	58	59	60	61	62	63	65	66	67	68	69	70	71	72	73	74	75	76	77	78	
1	x																																																	0
11		x																																																0
17			x																																															0
19				x																									1																					1
21					x																																													0
22					1	x																																												1
27		1					x	1					1			1																																		4
29								x																																										0
32		1					1		x																																									2
35										x																																								0
36											x													1	1											1														3
37												x																																						0
39													x																												1									1
42												1		x					1																															2
43													1		x																																			1
44																x								1																										1
45							1										x																																	1
46											1							x																																1
47																			x																															0
48																				x	1																													1
49										1	1										x		1																											3
50																						x																												0
51																							x																											0
52																								x																										0
53	1																								x	1	1																							3
54																										x																								0
55																											x																							0
56																												x																						0
57																													x																					0
58	1															1													1	x																				3
59																1															x																			1
60																														1		x																		1
61																																	x																	0
62																																	1	x																1
63																																	1		x															1
65																		1																		x														1
66											1																										x	1												2
67																																						x												0
68											1																												x											1
69											1																													x										1
70																																									x									0
71																																										x								0
72			1								1					1																											x							3
73																																											1	x						1
74																1																													x					1
75																1																														x				1
76																																															x			0
77																																											1					x		1
78																																											1						x	1
	2	2	1	0	1	0	2	1	0	1	6	1	2	0	0	6	0	1	1	0	1	0	1	2	1	1	1	0	2	1	0	0	2	0	0	1	0	1	0	0	1	0	3	0	0	0	0	0	0	45

Figure 14.11. Relations between facts composing combined thoughts of student and staff concerning total diagnosis including therapy

arbitrarily that in such cases the highest numbered code would be favored. Another question concerned whether findings resulting from the student's previous examinations of the patient should be considered history or present findings. Since the student usually seemed to consider these present findings, they were so coded. Experience suggests that in future studies, the following additional codes should be used: history of psychiatric conditions, marital history, organic disease in the family, psychiatric diseases in the family, and, in the laboratory findings section, serology.

Determining primary and secondary diagnoses. In most cases the primary and secondary diagnoses decided on by the student were written on the envelope containing the record, and these were used by the physician analysts in classifying facts. If the staff's diagnoses differed materially from the student's, they were used. This happened only rarely, since the student's diagnoses were arrived at after consultation with the staff. In a few instances, usually when the diagnoses were psychological or social, rather than organic, the student did not write the diagnoses on the envelope. In these cases, the physician analysts used the diagnoses that seemed to have been decided on in the course of the conference.

Noting relations between facts. No matter how simple the case, connections between facts were often difficult to assign. Whenever a staff man heckled a student throughout his presentation, for instance, asking questions out of context, not only were fewer facts noted, but the relations between them became nebulous, except for answers to specific questions. As explained earlier, each fact was noted on a card, and relations between facts were determined by grouping cards. It was frequently found easier to work from the last card of a group toward the first. This leads to the suspicion that the student sometimes thinks from the physical examination back toward the history, and this seems consistent with the observation frequently made by medical educators that students who are in a hurry will often mention the salient physical findings before beginning a history.

Post-Conference Interview

The principal inadequacy of the Teaching Conference Record as a technique for measuring cognitive dimensions was that the physician analyzing the record often could only infer what the student was actually thinking. To permit a more accurate analysis of their cognitive activity, the students were interviewed concerning the teaching conferences. Ordinarily, interviews were conducted after the teaching conference concerning the patient's first visit and after the final teaching conference concerning that patient.

Since these interviews were not recorded, no verbatim account is available. The interviewing procedure, the method of analyzing the information obtained, and the method of computing the desired cognitive dimensions are described below.

INTERVIEWING PROCEDURE

The questions addressed to the student after the conference concerning the patient's first visit were designed to ascertain the facts that made up the student's own thinking about the diagnosis as well as the facts the student reported he had "learned" from the staff. The questions also distinguished facts which formed part of the student's knowledge about the patient at the time of the first visit (those on which he based his possible diagnoses) from facts that he planned to acquire in the future (in order to confirm or deny the diagnoses). The following questions were asked:

1. List *all* of the positive organic, psychological, and sociological aspects of this case that you know of. List these facts on these cards, listing only one aspect on each card. (Number cards 1, 2, etc.)
2. Which of these aspects do you consider as having a bearing on the diagnosis and future management of the patient?
3. Are any of these facts due to your discussion with the staff? If so, indicate which ones.
4. Do any findings, previously considered relevant by you, now seem irrelevant as a result of your discussions with the staff?
5. Did your discussion with the staff add any further facts not listed under 2 above? If so, which findings are these?
6. Now these facts are probably related in some way. As for your own patient, can you say that fact 1 is due to fact 2, 3, etc.?
7. Are there additional facts which you want to establish—that is, facts necessary in order to confirm a new, or establish a present, diagnosis?
8. Are there additional facts which, while they are not related to the diagnosis, are nevertheless needed for the management of the patient? *That is, what future activities, excluding therapy, do you expect to carry out with this case?*
9. Is the need for the additional or new facts a result of your discussion with the staff?
10. Did the staff discourage you from ascertaining further facts previously considered relevant by you?
11. Did your consultation with the staff add any further facts not mentioned by you?
12. Would additional or new fact x be due to fact 1, etc.? Would fact 1 be due to additional or new fact x, etc.?

13. What are your present diagnoses?
14. Are any of these diagnoses due to the discussion which you had with the staff, or are any diagnoses previously considered relevant by you now considered irrelevant as a result of your discussion with the staff?
15. Did your discussion with the staff add any further diagnoses not listed by you under 13? If so, what are these diagnoses?
16. Are these diagnoses complementary or incompatible?[10]
17. Which of the facts given by you are relevant to diagnoses 1, 2, etc.?

The student was then asked with respect to each diagnosis: How strongly are you motivated at this time to pursue this particular line of diagnostic inquiry (as opposed to other lines of diagnostic inquiry which might seem possible)?

After the final teaching conference concerning that patient, the student was given a list of all the diagnostic facts from the first interview and was asked the following questions:

1. Did any further findings become relevant since you last talked to us?
2. Are any of the findings listed in the original cards no longer considered relevant?
3. Are any of these changes due to your contact with the staff?

The student was then asked to interrelate all the facts as in the first interview. The original diagnosis was pointed out to the student, and he indicated whether there had been any changes in diagnosis.

Method of analysis

Noting each fact. In answer to the second question of the first interview and the first question of the second interview, the student listed all facts about the patient that he considered relevant to diagnosis. Table 14.7 presents the diagnostic facts listed by a student in both interviews concerning a patient with cardiac pain due to hysteria.

Classifying diagnostic facts. The coder classified each diagnostic fact according to the possible diagnosis to which the student indicated it pertained. The coder also noted which facts formed part of the student's present knowledge about the patient and which he planned to acquire in the future; and which facts were part of the student's own thinking and which resulted from the staff's teaching.

[10] Occasionally a student arrived at two or more diagnoses which were not incompatible. In such a case, the student's thinking with respect to each diagnosis was treated separately, as primary and secondary diagnostic areas were treated separately in the case of the Teaching Conference Record. If the student held two or more incompatible diagnoses, his thinking about these was assumed to be a whole, and the analysis proceeded as if he were concerned about one diagnosis only.

Table 14.7. Facts listed in sample Post-Conference Interview

Interview after first teaching conference
1. Atypical attacks of chest pain, 1 year
2. Divorced female with history of:
   a) first husband committed suicide
   b) second husband in penitentiary for raping his stepdaughter
3. Normal EKG
4. No tachycardia or change in blood pressure during attack
5. Emotional
6. Immature
7. Evidence of concern about her heart
8. Withdrawn
9. On welfare
10. Tenderness on chest wall with history of rib fractures

Interview after final teaching conference
11. X-ray reveals lungs, bones, and heart within normal limits
12. History that she has visual and auditory revelations from God
13. Now states she is blind in right eye—doubtful as she blinks with attempted quick movements
14. Feel that patient is progressively withdrawing from her environment because of:
    a) the stress of remembering her environment
    b) the lack of reasons to want to relate to her environment
15. Upon subsequent visits she has not had any emotional tearing heart pains in my office
16. She communicates more easily and has developed a teasing manner of speech
17. Patient desires to have friends
18. She asserts disinterest in her friends as a defense mechanism
19. Patient is unable to talk freely about herself to friends for fear of being hurt

Classifying facts according to organic or psycho-social category. Each diagnostic fact was classified according to whether it concerned organic or psycho-social conditions. Decisions were made on the basis of the rules outlined in the section on the Teaching Conference Record.

Noting relations between facts. The coder noted the relations between facts indicated by the student in response to questions concerning which facts on his list were due to other facts. These relations were, by definition, direct.

Computation of cognitive dimensions

The method of analysis described above made it possible for the researchers to compute various dimensions of the student's thinking and of the combined thinking of staff and student. The case of a patient with possible diagnoses of either cardiac pain due to hysteria or intercostal neuralgia is used as illustration. The student ultimately decided in favor of the former diagnosis. The facts listed by the student as relevant to the problem of diagnosis are shown in Table 14.7. The mathematics involved in computing cognitive dimensions is the same as that described in connection with the Teaching Conference Record.

Combined thinking of staff and student. The combined thinking of staff and student was defined as all facts (his own and those he learned from the staff) considered by the student in making the diagnosis. It was measured in terms of thinking about total diagnosis, organic diagnosis, and psycho-social diagnosis.

Combined thinking about patient's first visit, based on interview conducted after first teaching conference

TOTAL DIAGNOSIS. The combined thinking of staff and student about the total diagnosis in relation to the patient's first visit included all facts the student considered relevant to the diagnostic problem at the time of the patient's first visit. Table 14.7 shows that facts 1–10 made up the combined thinking about the total diagnosis of the patient used as illustration. The relations between these facts are shown in Figure 14.12. The dimensions computed for this area of thought were: differ-

Determines ↓ / Depends on →		(Organic facts)				(Psycho-social facts)						
	Fact	1	3	4	10	2	5	6	7	8	9	
(Organic facts)	1	x	1		1	1	1		1			5
	3		x	1	1	1						3
	4		1	x	1	1	1					4
	10	1			x							1
(Psycho-social facts)	2					x	1					1
	5			1		1	x	1				3
	6					1	1	x				2
	7								x			0
	8					1	1			x		2
	9					1					x	1
		1	2	2	3	7	5	1	1	0	0	22

Figure 14.12. Relations between facts composing combined thoughts of student and staff concerning total diagnosis, after first teaching conference

entiation, centrality, unity, organization, sum of the dependences, determinance, and segmentation.

Combined thinking about patient's first and future visits, based on interview conducted after first teaching conference

TOTAL DIAGNOSIS. The combined thinking about total diagnosis in relation to the patient's first and future visits included all the facts the student considered relevant to the diagnostic problem at the time of the patient's first visit plus all the facts he wanted to establish in future visits in order to arrive at a diagnosis. In the sample case these were facts 1–10. The relations between these facts are shown in Figure 14.12. The dimensions computed were: differentiation, centrality, unity, organization, sum of the dependences, determinance, and segmentation.

Combined thinking about review of case, based on interview conducted after final teaching conference

TOTAL DIAGNOSIS. The combined thinking about total diagnosis in relation to the review of the case included all the facts the student considered relevant to the diagnostic problem at the time of the patient's final visit. In the sample case, these were facts 1–4, 7, and 11–19. Fact 16 was contributed by the staff. The relations between these facts are shown in Figure 14.13. The dimensions computed were: differentiation, centrality, unity, organization, sum of the dependences, determinance, and segmentation.

ORGANIC DIAGNOSIS. The combined thinking about organic diagnosis in relation to the review of the case included all the organic facts the student considered relevant to the diagnostic problem at the time of the patient's final visit. These were facts 1, 3, 4, 11, 13, and 15. Figure 14.13 shows the relations between these facts. The dimensions computed were the same as for total diagnosis.

PSYCHO-SOCIAL DIAGNOSIS. The combined thinking about the psycho-social diagnosis in relation to the review of the case included all psycho-social facts the student considered relevant to the diagnosis at the time of the patient's final visit. These were facts 2, 7, 12, 14, and 16–19. Relations between these facts are shown in Figure 14.13. The dimensions computed were the same as for total diagnosis.

Student's thinking. The student's own thinking was defined as all the facts considered by the student in making the diagnosis, excluding those facts he reported he had learned from the staff. It was measured in terms of thinking about total diagnosis, organic diagnosis, and psycho-social diagnosis.

Student's thinking about review of case, based on interview conducted after final teaching conference

TOTAL DIAGNOSIS. The student's thinking about total diagnosis in relation to the review of the case included all facts the student consid-

Depends on: (Organic facts) 1, 3, 4, 11, 13, 15; (Psycho-social facts) 2, 7, 12, 14, 16, 17, 18, 19

Determines: (Organic facts) 1, 3, 4, 11, 13, 15; (Psycho-social facts) 2, 7, 12, 14, 16, 17, 18, 19

Fact	1	3	4	11	13	15	2	7	12	14	16	17	18	19	
1	x	1	1	1			1	1		1					6
3		x	1	1			1	1							4
4		1	x	1			1	1							4
11		1	1	x			1	1							4
13					x		1			1					2
15						x									0
2							x						1	1	2
7	1						1	x		1					3
12							1		x	1					2
14					1		1		1	x			1	1	5
16						1					x				1
17							1				1	x			2
18							1			1			x	1	3
19							1			1			1	x	3
	1	3	3	3	1	1	11	4	1	6	1	0	3	3	41

Figure 14.13. Relations between facts composing combined thoughts of student and staff concerning total diagnosis, after final teaching conference

ered relevant to the diagnostic problem at the time of the patient's final visit. These were facts 1–4, 7, 11–15, and 17–19. Facts 1, 3, 4, 11, 13, and 15 were classified as organic; the remaining facts were classified as psycho-social. The relations between these facts are shown in Figure 14.14. The dimensions computed were: differentiation, centrality, unity, organization, sum of the dependences, determinance, and segmentation.

ORGANIC DIAGNOSIS. The student's thinking about organic diagnosis in relation to the review of the case included all organic facts the student considered relevant to the diagnostic problem at the time of the patient's final visit. These were facts 1, 3, 4, 11, 13, and 15. The relations between these facts are indicated in Figure 14.14. The dimensions computed were the same as for total diagnosis.

PSYCHO-SOCIAL DIAGNOSIS. The student's thinking about psycho-social diagnosis in relation to the review of the case included all psycho-social facts the student considered relevant to the diagnostic problem at the time of the patient's final visit. These were facts 2, 7, 12, 14, 17, and 19. The relations between these facts are shown in Figure 14.14. The dimensions computed were the same as for total diagnosis.

Staff's thinking. The staff's thinking was defined as the facts the student reported he had learned from the staff. It was measured in terms of total diagnosis and organic diagnosis. The interest here was in determining the student's estimate of the staff's contribution to his thinking.

Staff's thinking about review of case, based on interview conducted after final teaching conference

TOTAL DIAGNOSIS. The staff's thinking about total diagnosis in relation to review of the case included all facts the staff contributed to the student's thinking. In the sample case this was fact 16, a psycho-social fact.

ORGANIC DIAGNOSIS. Since the one fact that the staff contributed to the student's thinking was classified as psycho-social, no computations could be made concerning the staff's thinking about organic diagnosis.

		(Organic facts)						(Psycho-social facts)							
		Depends on													
Determines	Fact	1	3	4	11	13	15	2	7	12	14	17	18	19	
(Organic facts)	1	x	1	1	1			1	1		1				6
	3		x	1	1			1	1						4
	4		1	x	1			1	1						4
	11		1	1	x			1	1						4
	13					x		1			1				2
	15						x								0
(Psycho-social facts)	2							x					1	1	2
	7	1						1	x		1				3
	12							1		x	1				2
	14					1		1		1	x		1	1	5
	17							1				x			1
	18							1			1		x	1	3
	19							1			1		1	x	3
		1	3	3	3	1	0	11	4	1	6	0	3	3	39

Figure 14.14. Relations between facts composing student's thoughts concerning total diagnosis, after final teaching conference

Undoubtedly the foregoing explanation of the analysis of the techniques used to measure the dimensions of the staff's and students' thinking in the teaching conferences will raise many questions of definition, classification, procedure, and logic in the mind of the reader. There is no claim, however, that ours were perfectly finished theory or techniques. The principal task which confronted the research group was to study systematically the actual teaching process in a fashion which would do justice to the complexity of the situation. It should be pointed out that after one year of exploratory work with these procedures, the research group, in the summer of 1955, had the choice of accepting these procedures as adequate (although admittedly imperfect) or postponing the definitive study of the teaching process for another year in order either to refine further the procedures described above or to develop an entirely new method. Because the choice of the latter alternative would have meant lengthening the research project by one year, and because the procedures described above had been developed to a point where they were deemed workable, it was decided that they should be used in the study of the class of 1956. As it turned out, data from empirical studies indicated rather unexpected points of strength and weakness in the theory and techniques, but definitely indicated that the procedure was a useful one.

The Sample

SAMPLING FOR THE CONFERENCE RECORD

Recordings were made of the teaching conferences of a random sample of students. For each student selected a random sample was drawn of his conferences with the staff concerning outpatients. Excluded were consultation sessions taking place in those outpatient clinics in which the staff consulted with a group of students at a time rather than with students individually. Consultations taking place in the neurology, hematology, and skin clinics were therefore excluded.

In the GMC Program a random, approximately 50%, sample of students was selected. For each student thus selected a random sample was drawn of his conferences with the staff. To sample consultation sessions, a random sample was drawn of the days on which the student was scheduled for medicine and pediatrics. In this way a number of recording appointments was made for each student. The student was provided with a list of dates and times and was asked to record a consultation session with the staff on each of the dates and times. He was asked to record, if possible, the conference concerning the first patient seen by him on that day and time. If he could not record the first conference he was asked to record his consultation with regard to the second patient seen by him that day and time, etc. The consultations sampled in this way might concern initial visits or revisits.

Table 14.8. Number of GMC and control students who participated in recording teaching conferences, and number of first and revisit recordings provided by each student

Students	First visit recordings	Revisit recordings
1956 I		
1. GMC	0	3
2. GMC	3	0
3. GMC*	5	7
4. GMC*	3	6
5. GMC*	2	4
6. GMC*	1	3
7. GMC*	7	13
8. GMC	3	0
9. GMC	0	3
10. GMC	1	2
1. Control*	5	0
2. Control	2	0
3. Control*	3	1
4. Control*	6	1
5. Control	2	0
6. Control	2	0
7. Control	1	0
8. Control	2	0
9. Control	2	0
1956 II		
1. GMC*	2	3
2. GMC*	4	0
3. GMC*	3	1
4. GMC*	4	1
5. GMC*	1	0
6. GMC*	3	1
7. GMC*	6	3
8. GMC*	3	1
9. GMC*	7	4
10. GMC	2	0
1. Control*	10	0
2. Control	2	0
3. Control	2	0
4. Control*	3	1
5. Control*	4	2
6. Control*	7	0
7. Control	3	0
8. Control*	4	0
9. Control*	4	0
10. Control*	8	0
	132	60

* Indicates students used in the analysis reported on later.

In the control group also a random, approximately 50%, sample of students was chosen for observation, and for each student selected a random sample was selected of his consultations with the staff. The sampling rate applied to his consultations in general medicine, the medical specialty clinics, the pediatrics clinic, and the pediatrics specialty clinics, and were in accordance with the frequency with which he attended each of these clinics. Dates were also sampled. Each student was provided with a list of dates, and the instructions to the control group were identical with those to the GMC group.

The number of GMC and control students in the sample and the number of records concerning first visits and revisits obtained for each student are indicated in Table 14.8. Asterisks indicate students included in the analysis to be reported later in this chapter. These were students for whom recordings of at least four different consultation sessions were made. The total sample, with the exception of two students, was used in the GMC–control group comparisons. The major reasons for the inadequate number of recordings for some students included lack of cooperation on the part of some students and some staff members, unavailability of the staff at certain times, and unavailability of a room in which to make a recording. The latter problem was especially severe at times in the case of the control group.

Sampling for the post-conference interview

Interviews were obtained for a random, approximately 50%, sample of the GMC and control students. Appointments were made with students for certain interview times which were convenient to the student and the interviewer. At the appointed time the interviewer had the student select randomly one of the new outpatient contacts he had had that day. The interview then focused on that patient's diagnostic and therapeutic problems. If the student had not seen any new patients on the day of the interview, he was asked to select his most recent new patient. A first interview on a patient was always followed up by a final interview after the student's final contact with that particular patient.

In Table 14.9 are presented the number of GMC and control students in the sample, and the number of first interview–final interview pairs obtained per student.

EMPIRICAL STUDIES OF COGNITIVE STRUCTURE AND LEARNING

The first section of this chapter described the theoretical approach to the study of the teaching conferences. The second section described the methods and procedures used to analyze the cognitive structure of staff and student in the conferences. The present section discusses the

Table 14.9. Number of first interview–final interview pairs for each student, by type of diagnosis

1956 I		1956 II	
Students	No. of interview pairs	Students	No. of interview pairs
	Total and organic diagnoses		
1. GMC	6	9. GMC	12
2. GMC	5	10. GMC	6
3. GMC	4	11. GMC	5
4. GMC	7	12. GMC	8
5. GMC	6	13. GMC	6
6. GMC	5	14. GMC	6
7. GMC	10	15. GMC	7
8. GMC	4	16. GMC	12
		17. GMC	8
1. Control	6	7. Control	7
2. Control	3	8. Control	5
3. Control	3	9. Control	6
4. Control	3	10. Control	6
5. Control	3	11. Control	9
6. Control	6	12. Control	6
		13. Control	6
		14. Control	12
		15. Control	5
		16. Control	4
		17. Control	5
	Psycho-social diagnosis		
1. GMC	1	10. GMC	4
2. GMC	1	11. GMC	3
3. GMC	1	12. GMC	3
4. GMC	1	13. GMC	1
5. GMC	2	14. GMC	1
6. GMC	1	15. GMC	2
7. GMC	1	16. GMC	3
8. GMC	3	17. GMC	1
9. GMC	1		
1. Control	1	6. Control	1
2. Control	1	7. Control	1
3. Control	1	8. Control	3
4. Control	3	9. Control	3
5. Control	2	10. Control	1
		11. Control	4
		12. Control	3
		13. Control	1
		14. Control	4

Table 14.10. Reliability coefficients of dimensions of student's cognitive structure and combined cognitive structure of student and staff, as measured by the Teaching Conference Record

	Differentiation		Sum of the dependences		Relations ratio	
	N	*r*	*N*	*r*	*N*	*r*
Student's cognitive structure						
Total diagnosis	37	.75	37	.74		
Organic diagnosis	36	.75	36	.75		
Total diagnosis including therapy					25	.38
Student-staff cognitive structure						
Total diagnosis	29	.47	29	.61		
Organic diagnosis	27	.54	27	.47		
Total diagnosis including therapy					23	.29

N in most cases is larger than 25 because each record might contain not only a cognitive structure regarding a main diagnostic problem, but also a cognitive structure regarding a secondary diagnostic problem.

studies that were undertaken in order to discover whether the theory, method, and procedures employed actually provided useful data. The accuracy (reliability) of certain measures; the intercorrelations among measures; and the relations between various measures of cognitive structure and changes in knowledge, skill, and attitudes will be explained and evaluated. The results of these studies indicated that the reliability coefficients of the measures were somewhat low, and the correlation coefficients between measures were disappointingly high. In the main, however, very encouraging relations were obtained between cognitive measures and other measures of change in knowledge, skill, and attitudes.

Accuracy of the Measures of the Teaching Conference Record[11]

Because twenty-five of the Teaching Conference Records were analyzed independently by two physicians, it was possible to compute inter-observer agreement in these cases. For these twenty-five records, the following dimensions were computed: differentiation, sum of the dependences, and relations ratio. Reliability coefficients (Pearson *r*'s) were obtained by comparing the computations resulting from the two analyses. Owing to an insufficient number of psycho-social diagnoses in the set of twenty-five recordings, reliability coefficients were computed only for total and organic diagnoses (see Table 14.10).

It may be seen from Table 14.10 that reliability coefficients were

[11] Reliability coefficients were not computed for the Post-Conference Interview because there was no opportunity for a reinterview with which to compare the original.

generally higher for the measures of the student's cognitive structure than for measures of the combined cognitive structure of staff and student. This may be because in the latter instance the physician observers had to analyze an interaction between two persons which included considerable questioning and involved very complex material. In general, although the reliability coefficients were not satisfactory, they were encouraging in view of the extremely difficult nature of the physician observers' task.

Correlations between Cognitive Dimensions

It was important for the purposes of this research project to know whether the nine dimensions of cognitive structure postulated in our theory of cognition were actually (as well as theoretically) different from one another. For example, far more relations between cognitive measures and measures of knowledge, skill, and attitudes would have had to be computed if all cognitive dimensions had been uncorrelated than if the cognitive dimensions had been highly correlated. Correlation coefficients were therefore computed between the cognitive dimensions as measured by the Teaching Conference Record and the Post-Conference Interview.

Teaching conference record

The correlation coefficients between various dimensions of the student's cognitive structure and between the dimensions of the combined cognitive structure of staff and student are shown in Table 14.11. In the main, these intercorrelations were disappointingly high, although there were encouraging exceptions. (The dimensions used in further analyses are those italicized in Table 14.11.)

The relatively high negative correlation between unity and both the sum of the dependences and the maximum determinance should be noted. This negative correlation is particularly strong in the area of the student's own thoughts concerning organic diagnosis. The negative correlation in this case can be explained by the fact that unity is a relative measure, whereas sum of the dependences and maximum determinance are absolute measures. That is, according to formula 2, high unity can be obtained with either a small absolute number of relations between cognitive elements or with a large absolute number of relations. One would not expect, therefore, a high correlation between unity and the absolute measures. In fact, one would expect a random relation. (A random relation did in fact tend to occur between these dimensions as measured by the Post-Conference Interview, as will be shown later.) As measured by the Teaching Conference Record, however, the correlation between these dimensions was

Table 14.11. Correlation coefficients between dimensions of student's cognitive structure and combined cognitive structure of student and staff, as measured by the Teaching Conference Record

Student's cognitive structure: total diagnosis (N* = 23)

	1	2	3	4	5	6	7	8
1. Maximum centrality		.85	.92	.97	—.35	.68	.08	—.20
2. Organization			.92	.92	—.78	.96	.45	—.45
3. Sum of the dependences				.96	—.68	.92	.60	—.20
4. *Maximum determinance*					—.45	.78	.60	—.35
5. Unity						—.92	—.35	.60
6. Differentiation							.20	—.35
7. *Relations ratio*†								—.85
8. *Homogeneity*								

Student's cognitive structure: organic diagnosis ($N = 23$)

	1	2	3	4	5	6	7
1. Maximum centrality		.96	.97	.97	—.68	.85	—.35
2. Organization			.97	.92	—.85	.96	—.35
3. Sum of the dependences				.97	—.77	.92	—.46
4. *Maximum determinance*					—.78	.92	—.20
5. Unity						—.85	.08
6. Differentiation							—.35
7. *Homogeneity*							

Combined student-staff cognitive structure: total diagnosis ($N = 23$)

	1	2	3	4	5	6	7	8
1. Maximum centrality		.68	.85	.77	.05	—.45	.96	.45
2. Organization			.45	.61	.30	—.68	.68	—.35
3. *Sum of the dependences*				.61	—.20	—.45	.97	.45
4. *Maximum determinance*					.17	—.61	.61	.30
5. *Segmentation*						—.05	—.20	—.46
6. *Unity*							—.45	.08
7. Differentiation								.45
8. *Relations ratio*†								

Combined student-staff cognitive structure: organic diagnosis ($N = 23$)

	1	2	3	4	5	6	7
1. Maximum centrality		.92	.92	.78	—.45	.92	—.60
2. Organization			.85	.45	—.60	.88	—.68
3. *Sum of the dependences*				.45	—.35	.97	—.68
4. *Maximum determinance*					—.60	.46	—.20
5. *Unity*						—.30	.35
6. Differentiation							—.46
7. *Homogeneity*							

* The N is equal to the number of students studied by means of the Teaching Conference Record which was used to test hypotheses 1 and 2.

† The relations ratio from the student's and the staff-student over-all cognitive structure for diagnosis and therapy is entered also.

strongly negative. This finding implies that a cognitive structure with a high differentiation and a high absolute number of relations between elements, has a network of relations which is less complete than a cognitive structure with a lower differentiation and fewer relations. In this instance, the reason for this finding seems to be that all or most relations are due to the presence of a single element. It can be shown mathematically that under such conditions there should be a negative correlation between the unity and both the sum of the dependences and the maximum determinance.

Post-conference interview

The correlation coefficients between various dimensions of the combined cognitive structure of staff and student are shown in Table 14.12.

Table 14.12. Correlation coefficients between dimensions of combined cognitive structure of student and staff, as measured by the Post-Conference Interview

	Total diagnosis ($N = 34$)					
	1	2	3	4	5	6
1. Maximum centrality		.67	.95	.99	.13	.86
2. Organization			.61	.73	.00	.80
3. Sum of the dependences				.93	.38	.80
4. *Maximum determinance*					.19	.89
5. *Unity*						.26
6. Differentiation						
	Organic diagnosis ($N = 34$)					
	1	2	3	4	5	6
1. Maximum centrality		.47	.87	.97	—.10	.73
2. Organization			.45	.75	.09	.74
3. Sum of the dependences				.84	.27	.74
4. *Maximum determinance*					—.10	.84
5. *Unity*						—.09
6. Differentiation						
	Psycho-social diagnosis ($N = 31$)					
	1	2	3	4	5	6
1. Maximum centrality		.92	.97	.92	.60	.90
2. Organization			.92	.92	.60	.60
3. Sum of the dependences				.92	.76	.76
4. *Maximum determinance*					.63	.90
5. *Unity*						.38
6. Differentiation						
	Organic compared with psycho-social diagnoses					
	1	2	3	4	5	6
1. Maximum centrality	—.09					
2. Organization		.00				
3. Sum of the dependences			.00			
4. Maximum determinance				—.03		
5. Unity					.00	
6. Differentiation						.00

These correlations indicate fewer empirical dimensions than theoretical dimensions. (Those dimensions used in further analyses are italicized in Table 14.12.) Similar correlations existed between various dimensions of the student's own cognitive structure, as shown in Table 14.13.

The fact that the intercorrelations reported above are quite high seems discouraging and somewhat embarrassing to a theoretical system which postulates nine dimensions of cognition. Few psychologists would hesitate to dismiss a theoretical system which postulates many different dimensions, but empirically demonstrates a high rate of redundancy among these dimensions. However, such a dismissal at this point might well be short-sighted. First, the empirical relations presented in the tables are based on small numbers (*N*'s = 23 to 34) of subjects not representative of the general population. Second, the technical as well as the conceptual aspects of the theory have not had the benefit of extensive application and reformulation. Finally, the high intercorrelation between, for example, maximum determinance and sum of the dependences does not necessarily prove that one of these dimensions is generally redundant. It is recognized explicitly in the

Table 14.13. Correlation coefficients between dimensions of student's cognitive structure, as measured by the Post-Conference Interview

Total diagnosis (*N* = 34)	1	2	3	4	5	6
1. Maximum centrality		.85	.93	.98	.09	.81
2. Organization			.85	.80	.09	.90
3. Sum of the dependences				.85	.09	.95
4. *Maximum determinance*					.19	.75
5. *Unity*						.00
6. Differentiation						

Organic diagnosis (*N* = 34)	1	2	3	4	5	6
1. Maximum centrality		.85	.96	.98	.45	.96
2. Organization			.80	.82	.60	.90
3. Sum of the dependences				.92	.68	.93
4. *Maximum determinance*					.18	.99
5. *Unity*						.37
6. Differentiation						

Psycho-social diagnosis (*N* = 31)	1	2	3	4	5	6	7
1. Maximum centrality		.99	.99	.95	.78	.68	.45
2. Organization			.99	.99	.79	.68	.45
3. Sum of the dependences				.99	.78	.68	.45
4. *Maximum determinance*					.78	.68	.45
5. Unity						.13	.13
6. *Differentiation*							.34
7. *Segmentation*							

theory that there can be a high correlation between maximum determinance and sum of the dependences, given the appropriate conditions (as when the cognitive structure is highly organized).[12] In fact, under conditions of maximal organization, the sum of the dependences becomes identical with the maximum determinance.

Nevertheless, in light of the evidence presented, the purposes of the present research were obviously best served by restricting the number of dimensions employed in further analysis.

Relations between Cognitive Dimensions and Learning

There were two reasons for investigating the relations between cognitive dimensions and changes in knowledge, skill, and attitudes. First, the theory was an untried one. Although Zajonc[13] had carried out some experiments based on his theory and had achieved encouraging results, it could hardly be said that the results had been proved to be generally useful. Second, the present research was breaking new ground. There had been no previous attempts to study the teaching conference, or indeed to study so intensively any learning situation as complex as this one. And, of course, these particular methods and procedures had not been tried before. In short, the value of the theory, method, and procedures was unknown.

Two hypotheses derived from the theory were tested. If the tests had indicated that the theory had no basis in empirical fact, data provided by the methods described above would not have been used to describe the teaching conferences in the two programs. As it turned out, the theory seemed to have considerable basis in empirical fact, despite the high intercorrelations between various measures. The hypotheses tested were:

Hypothesis 1: The more highly developed and extensive the network of dependence relations in the student's cognitive structure, the greater the student's change in knowledge, skills, and attitudes.

This hypothesis is the most important one for it deals directly with the problem of change, which, of course, was the most important aspect of the research project. The second hypothesis deals with the problem of the student's motivation to pursue a particular diagnostic hypothesis.

Hypothesis 2: The strength of the student's potential for work (for pursuing a diagnostic hypothesis) is a function of the extent to which he perceives future findings to be related to present findings.

A description of the data included in the empirical tests of the

[12] The reader will remember that high organization means that the relations existing in the cognitive structure are due to one element.

[13] "Cognitive Structure and Cognitive Tuning."

above hypotheses follows. Generally, and unless otherwise indicated, only the data from students who were interviewed a number of times, or for whom a number of recordings were available, were used. Data from Teaching Conference Records were included for students for whom recordings of at least four different conferences were available. The number of students whose data were included varied from 13 to 22 (the median was between 20 and 21)—this variation occurring for statistical convenience. A total of 156 teaching conferences was analyzed for the purpose of testing hypothesis 1. Data from Teaching Conference Records were not used in tests of hypothesis 2.

Data from Post-Conference Interviews were used in tests of hypothesis 1 which involved cognitive dimensions regarding total and organic diagnoses. Data were included from 34 students who had been interviewed with respect to at least three different diagnostic problems. In tests of hypothesis 1 which involved cognitive dimensions regarding psycho-social diagnoses, data were included from all students who had been interviewed and who had psycho-social material to report. It was necessary to abandon the more stringent rules for inclusion because of the relatively few instances in which students reported psycho-social diagnostic material. The data from a total of 31 students were thus included. A total of 220 interviews was analyzed.

Interviews from 16 students were used in tests of hypothesis 2. These were students who were still engaged in establishing a diagnosis after the first visit with a patient.

STUDIES OF HYPOTHESIS 1[14]

Cognitive dimensions as measured by the Teaching Conference Record compared with dependent variables measures

STUDENT'S THINKING. Analysis of the student's thinking about total diagnosis revealed that the following conditions were conducive to learning: the presence in the student's cognitive structure of a concept which determined (explained) many others (high maximum number of determinants), and the presence in the student's cognitive structure of only one such concept (low unity). The data shown in Tables 14.14 and 14.15 indicate that students with the foregoing cognitive structures gained more on the Medical Knowledge test from pretest to posttest than students whose cognitive structures were not characterized by such conditions.

[14] The negative relation noted between unity and maximum determinance as measured by the Teaching Conference Record now became important. Hypothesis 1 stressed, among other things, the *extensiveness* of the network of dependence relations, i.e., the absolute number of relations which existed. If hypothesis 1 was correct, a strong negative relation should have been found between unity and learning in the case of the Teaching Conference Record data.

Table 14.14. Relation between cognitive determinants and gain in medical knowledge

		Gain in medical knowledge		
		Low	High	
Cognitive determinants	High	3	8	11
Cognitive determinants	Low	8	1	9
$p = .009$*		11	9	20

* Where $N < 30$, p is derived from Fisher-Yates 2 x 2 contingency tables. See D. J. Finney, "The Fisher-Yates Test of Significance in 2 x 2 Contingency Tables," *Biometrika* 35:149–154, 1948. Unless otherwise indicated, one-tailed tests of significance are used throughout this chapter.

Relations between dimensions of thinking about the total diagnosis and gain in tests of medical skill, psychological knowledge and skill, and sociological knowledge and skill were not statistically significant, although with few exceptions the relations were in the expected direction.

When that part of the student's cognitive structure which was concerned only with the organic aspects of the patient's problem was considered, the results were similar to those reported above in connection with the total diagnosis.

Analysis of the student's thinking about total diagnosis including therapy indicated that the student who interrelated his findings and plans for the patient's therapy (high relations ratio) tended to gain more on the Medical Knowledge test from pretest to posttest than the student who did not interrelate findings and therapy (see Table 14.16).

There was no relation between the dimensions of the student's thinking about the psycho-social aspects of the patient's problem and gain on the tests of psychological knowledge and skill or sociological knowledge and skill.

It is of particular interest to note that students whose total cognitive structures contained high determinacy relations tended to become less accurate perceivers of patients' personalities and to become more aware of individual differences among patients. The relation between cognitive determinance and interpersonal perception measures, however, became more apparent when the psycho-social aspects

Table 14.15. Relation between cognitive unity and gain in medical knowledge

		Gain in medical knowledge		
		Low	High	
Cognitive unity	High	7	2	9
Cognitive unity	Low	3	8	11
$p = .035$		10	10	20

Table 14.16. Relation between relations ratio and gain in medical knowledge

		Gain in medical knowledge		
		Low	High	
Relations ratio	High	3	8	11
Relations ratio	Low	5	2	7
$p = .10$		8	10	18

of the student's thoughts were analyzed. It was found that if the psycho-social part of the student's cognitive structure contained a concept which determined (explained) many others, the student was likely to perceive greater individuality among patients at the posttest than at the pretest (see Table 14.17).

The empirical relations discovered between various dimensions of the student's cognitive structure and the dependent variables measures of knowledge, skill, and attitudes support the hypothesis that such relations should exist.

Apparently, dimensions of the student's thinking about the total and organic diagnoses are related to the student's ability to acquire medical knowledge. These cognitive dimensions also seem to be positively related to the student's ability to increase his awareness of individual differences among patients, and negatively related to the student's ability to perceive accurately patients' personality characteristics.

Dimensions of the student's thinking about the psycho-social diagnosis, however, were unrelated to change in psychological knowledge and skill. There was a relation between cognitive dimensions regarding the psycho-social diagnosis and the student's increased awareness of individual differences among patients—as in the case of the total and organic diagnosis. However, the relation in connection with the psycho-social diagnosis was more definite—a finding which seems reasonable, inasmuch as the student's thoughts about the psycho-social diagnosis are more relevant to the task of perceiving individual differences among patients' personalities than are his thoughts about

Table 14.17. Relation between cognitive determinants and perception of patients

		Perception of patients		
		Less individuality	More individuality	
Cognitive determinants	High	1	7	8
Cognitive determinants	Low	9	4	13
		10	11	21
$p = .017$				

Table 14.18. Relation between sum of the dependences and gain in medical knowledge

		Gain in medical knowledge		
		Low	High	
Sum of the dependences	High	2	7	9
Sum of the dependences	Low	8	3	11
$p = .035$		10	10	20

the organic diagnosis. An increase in the awareness of individual differences among patients is apparently more probable when a student is able to integrate his cognitions regarding the psychological characteristics of people. And the perception of individual differences among others seems to be related to effectiveness in establishing good relations with them (see Chapters 20 and 21).

COMBINED THINKING OF STAFF AND STUDENT. The conversation between the staff and student was analyzed by the same method used in analyzing the student's thoughts. Relations between the various cognitive dimensions and measures of knowledge, skill, and attitudes, were investigated with the following results: first, when the instructor and student succeeded in interrelating many findings (high sum of dependences), the student gained on the Medical Knowledge test from pretest to posttest more than did the student who did not participate in such a conference (see Table 14.18). Second, when the instructor and student interrelated organic and psycho-social findings (low segmentation) the student gained on the Medical Skill test (see Table 14.19).

Analysis of the staff-student interaction which involved the psycho-social aspects of the patient's problem resulted in a somewhat different set of findings. When the staff-student interaction touched upon many different aspects of the person's psychological and social problems (low homogeneity), the student showed less improvement in his attitudes toward behavior disorders (see Table 14.20).

When the staff-student interaction involving the psycho-social diagnosis invoked a single concept which explained many others (high maximum number of determinants), the student showed less gain on

Table 14.19. Relation between cognitive segmentation and gain in medical skill

		Gain in medical skill		
		Low	High	
Cognitive segmentation	High	9	2	11
Cognitive segmentation	Low	2	8	10
$p = .007$*		11	10	21

Table 14.20. Relation between cognitive homogeneity and attitudes toward behavior disorders

		Attitudes toward behavior disorders		
		Low	High	
Cognitive homogeneity	High	4	10	14
Cognitive homogeneity	Low	8	0	8
$p = .004$ * †		12	10	22

* The use of a two-tailed statistical test is not really correct here, since the theoretical hypothesis is a unidirectional one, i.e., results which are the reverse of those to be expected are to be considered random, no matter how large the reversal is. However, the two-tailed test is applied here because these results may have interest over and beyond their purely theoretical relevance. For example, although the results in Table 14.21 are to be interpreted as evidence for the acceptance of the null hypothesis with respect to the *theory*, the results also indicate that a purely "common-sense" hypothesis might be accepted rather than the null hypothesis. This "common-sense" hypothesis suggests that teachers' efforts lead to less rather than more knowledge in the sociological area. The probability level is included here merely for the convenience of those who wish to consider the statistical acceptability of this hypothesis in contrast to the null hypothesis. Because this hypothesis may carry as much significance as the theoretical one, the practice of presenting two-tailed tests where the results may have practical significance is continued throughout this chapter. Such tests will be indicated by †.

the tests of sociological knowledge and skill, and less improvement on the test of attitudes toward the team concept (see Tables 14.21 and 14.22). This finding was opposite to the results obtained in connection with medical knowledge. In that case, high determinacy relations led to greater, not less, gain in medical knowledge.

The experimental hypothesis was supported by the fact that the cognitive dimensions of the staff-student interaction concerning the total diagnosis were related to change in medical knowledge, and, in this instance, even to change in medical skill. Data from the study of the psycho-social diagnosis, however, did not support the hypothesis.

Aside from theoretical implications, the finding of a negative relation between cognitive dimensions of the psycho-social diagnosis and change in sociological knowledge, although the same cognitive dimensions of the total and organic diagnoses were positively related to change in medical knowledge, raises an interesting question about the differences between the cognitive structures possessed by students and staff concerning these disciplines, as well as about possible differences between organic and psychological phenomena themselves. This difference was discussed in Chapter 11.

A comparison of the characteristics of the student's thoughts and of the combined thinking of staff and student indicates that, in both instances, the presence of a cognitive structure in which concepts were interrelated was conducive to change in medical knowledge. In the case of the student's thoughts, the presence of one concept which determined many others seemed to be of primary importance, whereas in the case of the staff-student combined thoughts, the absolute number of dependence connections seemed to be of importance. This difference may have had a bearing on the two different roles performed by the student in presenting the case, and by the staff and the student combined in discussing and learning from the case. These findings are quite similar to findings obtained by Zajonc in studying the process of "cognitive tuning." Zajonc hypothesized that there should be differences between the cognitive structures of the person who transmits information and the person who receives information.

Cognitive dimensions as measured by the Post-Conference Interview compared with dependent variables measures

COMBINED THINKING OF STAFF AND STUDENT AFTER FINAL VISIT. It will be recalled that the analysis of the Teaching Conference Record suggested that when the student (or student and staff) invoked a single concept which determined (explained) many findings, the student gained medical knowledge and became a less accurate perceiver of patients' personalities—although he tended to perceive more individuality among patients. The results from the corresponding analysis of the Post-Conference Interview confirm this result. When the interaction between the instructor and student, as shown in the analysis of the Post-Conference Interview, involved a single concept that explained many others (high maximum number of determinants), the student gained more medical knowledge and medical skill from pretest to posttest than when this condition was not present (see Tables 14.23 and 14.24). The student also improved his attitudes toward comprehensive care under the above condition (see Table 14.25). Furthermore, when the segmentation between organic and psycho-social concepts was low, the student gained relatively more on the test of sociological knowledge and skill (see Table 14.26).

The analysis of the staff-student interaction concerning the organic aspects of the patient's problems provided results similar to those reported above for the total diagnosis.

In contrast to the results reported for the total diagnosis and the organic diagnosis, which showed relations between cognitive dimensions and gain in medical knowledge and skill, no relation appeared

Table 14.21. Relation between psycho-social cognitive determinants and gain in sociological knowledge and skill

		Gain in sociological knowledge and skill		
		Low	High	
Cognitive determinants	High	6	1	7
Cognitive determinants	Low	5	9	14
$p = .09$*†		11	10	21

Table 14.22. Relation between psycho-social cognitive determinants and attitudes toward team concept

		Attitudes toward team concept		
		Low	High	
Cognitive determinants	High	6	1	7
Cognitive determinants	Low	5	10	15
$p = .06$*†		11	11	22

Table 14.23. Relation between cognitive determinants and gain in medical knowledge

		Gain in medical knowledge		
		Low	High	
Cognitive determinants	High	6	9	15
Cognitive determinants	Low	12	7	19
$p = .09$		18	16	34

Table 14.24. Relation between cognitive determinants and gain in medical skill

		Gain in medical skill		
		Low	High	
Cognitive determinants	High	5	10	15
Cognitive determinants	Low	11	8	19
$p = .08$		16	18	34

Table 14.25. Relation between cognitive determinants and attitudes toward comprehensive care

		Attitudes toward comprehensive care		
		Low	High	
Cognitive determinants	High	5	10	15
Cognitive determinants	Low	12	7	19
$p = .04$		17	17	34

Table 14.26. Relation between cognitive segmentation and gain in sociological skill

		Gain in sociological skill		
		Low	High	
Cognitive segmentation	High	10	4	14
Cognitive segmentation	Low	4	10	14
$p = .05$		14	14	28

between cognitive dimensions of the psycho-social diagnosis and gain in psychological knowledge and skill or sociological knowledge and skill. However, when the staff-student interaction involved a single concept which determined (explained) many others (high maximum number of determinants), the student improved his attitudes toward physician-patient relations (see Table 14.27).

The above results in general tended to confirm the hypothesis that dimensions of cognitive structure (as measured by both techniques described above) are related to learning. Cognitive dimensions were related to gain in medical knowledge and medical skill. Moreover, when the total diagnosis was not sharply separated into two components (organic and psycho-social) more gain in sociological knowledge and skill was found to occur than when the total diagnosis was separated into two components.

The analysis of the cognitive dimensions of the psychosocial diagnosis based on the Post-Conference Interview provided results similar to those found in connection with the analysis of psycho-social diagnosis based on the Teaching Conference Record: greater cognitive complexity did not lead to positive change in knowledge and skill.[15]

Cognitive dimensions as measured by the Teaching Conference Record compared with grade averages. Despite the well-known disadvantages of using grade averages as indicators of proficiency in learning, the relation between cognitive dimensions and grade averages was investigated because of the general positive relations discovered between cognitive dimensions and various tests of knowledge and skill reported above. The hypothesis that cognitive dimensions should be correlated with grade averages was borne out by the data.

There was a relation between the dimensions of the student's thinking about total diagnosis as measured by the Teaching Conference Record and cumulative grade average. Both homogeneity (the extent to which the student's thinking was restricted to one narrow class of phenomena)[16] and unity (the extent to which "everything was [indiscriminately] related to everything else") were negatively related to cumulative grade average (see Tables 14.28 and 14.29). However, there was a positive relation between the relations ratio and fourth-year grade average (see Table 14.30).

Unity seemed to be the cognitive dimension with the most endur-

[15] This conclusion was supported by data derived from an independent source (see Chapters 16, 17, 18, and 19) which indicated that participation in the special features of the GMC did not lead to gain in knowledge and skill in the psychological and sociological areas.

[16] Note that the reverse effect was obtained between homogeneity and attitude change. See Table 14.20 above.

ing effect; for the unity of the student's thoughts concerning the organic diagnosis was negatively related to first-, second-, and third-year grade averages as well.

Cognitive dimensions as measured by the Post-Conference Interview compared with grade averages. The extent to which a student invoked a single concept which determined (explained) many findings (maximum number of determinants) as indicated by analysis of the Post-Conference Interview was found to be related to first-, second-, and third-year grade averages as well as to the cumulative grade average. This relation was found in connection with the total diagnosis and

Table 14.27. Relation between cognitive determinants and attitudes toward physician-patient relations

		Attitudes toward physician-patient relations		
		Low	High	
Cognitive determinants	High	5	10	15
Cognitive determinants	Low	11	5	16
$p = .03$		16	15	31

Table 14.28. Relation between cognitive homogeneity and cumulative grade average

		Cumulative grade average		
		Low	High	
Cognitive homogeneity	High	8	2	10
Cognitive homogeneity	Low	2	9	11
$p = .005$		10	11	21

Table 14.29. Relation between cognitive unity and cumulative grade average

		Cumulative grade average		
		Low	High	
Cognitive unity	High	8	2	10
Cognitive unity	Low	2	9	11
$p = .005$		10	11	21

Table 14.30. Relation between relations ratio and fourth-year grade average

		Fourth-year grade average		
		Low	High	
Relations ratio	High	3	8	11
Relations ratio	Low	8	3	11
$p = .03$		11	11	22

Table 14.31. Relation between maximum determinants and first-year grade average

		First-year grade average		
		Low	High	
Maximum determinants	High	8	10	18
Maximum determinants	Low	8	6	14
$p > .05$		16	16	32

the organic diagnosis. (Tables 14.31–14.34 present the data with respect to the organic diagnosis.) These findings provide additional support for the hypothesis that cognitive dimensions are related to learning.

STUDIES OF HYPOTHESIS 2

This hypothesis was tested by investigating the relation between a single cognitive dimension and the students' rating of their motivation to establish a particular diagnosis.

The cognitive dimension involved the dependence of the present findings on the findings expected in the future. If the expected findings were seen to be highly related to those already established, it was hypothesized that the student would be highly motivated to establish this (tentative) diagnosis. The strength of the student's motivation was measured simply by asking him: How strongly are you motivated at this time to pursue this particular diagnostic line of inquiry? The student then rated his motivation on a seven-point scale.

The findings supported the hypothesis. When the dependence of thoughts regarding the present visit on thoughts regarding future visits was high, the student rated himself as being more highly motivated to pursue the particular diagnostic problem (see Table 14.35). The reverse was not true, however; there was no relation between the dependence of thoughts regarding future visits on thoughts regarding the present visit and motivation to pursue the particular line of diagnostic inquiry (see Table 14.36).[17] Hypothesis 2 seems to have been supported by the data. Due to the number of subjects, however, this conclusion must be accepted with reservation.

Other Methods

In addition to the methods described above, the Independent Variables Section utilized data collected by means of a questionnaire

[17] It should be mentioned that the median number of findings considered by the student when he thought about the first visit was 7.5 (the range was from 13 to 3). The median number of findings included in his thoughts about future visits was equal to 2 (the range was from 1 to 7). It also appeared that there was no difference between the highly motivated students and the less motivated students in the number of facts which they wanted to ascertain for their patients during future visits.

Table 14.32. Relation between maximum determinants and second-year grade average

		Second-year grade average		
		Low	High	
Maximum determinants	High	6	12	18
Maximum determinants	Low	10	4	14
$p = .02$		16	16	32

Table 14.33. Relation between maximum determinants and third-year grade average

		Third-year grade average		
		Low	High	
Maximum determinants	High	8	10	18
Maximum determinants	Low	9	5	14
$p > .05$		17	15	32

Table 14.34. Relation between maximum determinants and fourth-year cumulative average

		Fourth-year cumulative average		
		Low	High	
Maximum determinants	High	4	11	15
Maximum determinants	Low	13	6	19
$p = .01$		17	17	34

Table 14.35. Relation between dependence and motivation

		Motivation to pursue diagnostic problem		
		Low	High	
Dependence of thought about present visit on thoughts about future visits	High	1	7	8
Dependence of thought about present visit on thoughts about future visits	Low	7	1	8
$p = .005$*		8	8	16

Table 14.36. Relation between dependence and motivation

		Motivation to pursue diagnostic problem		
		Low	High	
Dependence of thought about future visits on thought about present visit	High	4	4	8
Dependence of thought about future visits on thought about present visit	Low	4	4	8
		8	8	16

(which also supplied data for the Dependent Variables Section and the Individual Differences Section). Students and faculty were also interviewed, and two other special techniques were utilized. Because of their special nature they are described briefly below.

Students' diaries

Sixteen students in the class of 1956 (eight in the control group and eight in the GMC group) kept diaries for the research project. Diaries were written by the students three days per week during the entire nine months of the senior year. Although the diaries provided useful information, a good, workable method for analyzing them in a quantitative way was never developed, although many attempts were made. As a result, the diaries were scanned for material which was relevant to various aspects of the general trend of the results and were used where appropriate.

Relation between the special educational techniques used by the GMC and change in test scores

Records were kept of the extent to which the GMC student participated in the various educational techniques emphasized by the GMC. For example, records were kept concerning the number of patients seen, the average number of visits per patient, amount of contact the student had with patients' families, the number of times the student consulted the psychiatrist and/or the social worker about his patients, the number of home visits the student made, etc. Also, the student was asked on the questionnaire about his attitudes toward these special educational features. The complete index of participation is presented in Appendix 6.

CONCLUSION

The Independent Variables Section placed heavy emphasis on the study of the student-staff teaching conferences. This policy was based on the conviction that the most important aspect of any educational program is the exchange of knowledge between teacher and student. It would, of course, have been desirable to study the teaching in the seminars and the group conferences also. However, the resources (including the conceptual and methodological resources) of the project did not permit this. In any event, the primary emphasis was placed on what was felt to be critical—the individual teacher's efforts to teach the student how to study a patient.

Whether the theoretical approach undertaken here is a good one remains to be seen. Certainly it was a valuable approach for this project, and when all the results are taken into consideration, the results of the analyses carried out in terms of this theory made good sense. Furthermore, in view of the fact that this theoretical approach was tested in the field, rather than under laboratory conditions, the results seem definitely encouraging.

It should be noted that, in retrospect, the time, energy and money that went into the collection of diary material would have been more wisely expended in making sociological analyses of the medical school environment. Although diary material is almost always intriguing, its very mass and unsystematic nature are severe barriers to analysis. Sociological analyses of the behavior of students and professors in the two educational programs (in addition to detailed analyses of the teaching process itself) very likely would have thrown far more light on the nature of a medical school environment than did the material in the students' diaries.

The most important positive feature of the Independent Variables Section, insofar as the comparison of the two educational programs is concerned, was that information was drawn from several sources. The fact that the teaching conferences were analyzed in three different ways (the Teaching Conference Record, the Post-Conference Interview, and physicians' ratings), that students' reports of their activities and general experiences were taken from the questionnaire, that both faculty and students were interviewed, and students' diaries scanned, that student participation in the special educational features of GMC was recorded, made it possible to draw important conclusions about the reasons for the differences and lack of differences between the experimental and control groups.

Chapter 15

Individual Differences

How the Variations in Response to the Two Programs Were Studied

The task of the Individual Differences Section of the research project was to study differences among students in an attempt to understand the reasons for variations in responses to the GMC and control programs. In all, eight classes of attributes were assessed by means of psychological tests: aptitude for medical education, previous academic performance, peer-judged attributes, attitudes, values, social interaction attributes, needs, and background information and self-ratings. This chapter describes the measurement of these attributes and explains their relevance to the purposes of the research program. The technical characteristics of the measuring instruments are discussed, and statistical descriptions of the student groups are given. A list of all measures of individual attributes (and the occasions upon which they were administered) is presented in Appendix 5.

Aptitude for Medical Education

The aptitude test on which scores were readily available for all medical students was the Medical College Admission Test (MCAT). This instrument, commonly used in selecting medical students, provided quantitative estimates of four attributes relevant to performance in medical school: verbal ability, quantitative ability, knowledge of modern society, and knowledge of premedical sciences.

The two abilities are measured by the usual general scholastic aptitude test. Items requiring the subject to choose the correct definition of a word or the proper verbal analogy are used in the Verbal Ability test, while items requiring comprehension of arithmetic and algebraic principles make up the Quantitative Ability test. In the test of Understanding Modern Society questions are asked about basic principles of economics, sociology, and political science, and the candidate's general knowledge of history is evaluated. Understanding of fundamental principles is also stressed in the test of Knowledge of Premedical Sciences (biology, chemistry, and physics).

The MCAT is produced by the Educational Testing Service and is administered to virtually all applicants to medical schools in the United States. It is revised at intervals, and reports on its development and modifications have been published.[1]

Relevance

A measure of intelligence, or something near it, was obviously desirable. The Verbal Ability test was the best estimate of general ability or "intelligence" available to the research group; verbal ability had been shown to be highly correlated with general ability.[2] Moreover, this Verbal Ability test had been standardized on all the applicants to medical schools in a given year, thus providing an accurate estimate of individual differences in a population already selected with respect to intelligence.

The research group was also interested in knowing the value to the *senior* medical student of his knowledge of the premedical sciences as well as his knowledge of modern society and his quantitative ability. And of course, the opportunity to measure the relation between MCAT scores and such seldom studied criteria of student performance as the third- and fourth-year grade averages was welcomed.

Technical characteristics

The reliability and validity of the MCAT subtests have been published on occasion,[3] although these data were not available for the particular tests administered to our subjects. The published figures are quite reassuring regarding the technical adequacy of this instrument. Reliabilities near .90 have been reported, and studies of the item types

[1] See J. M. Stalnaker, "Medical College Admission Test," *Journal of the Association of American Medical Colleges* 25:428–434, 1950 and "Other Psychometric Instruments: D: Medical College Admission Test," in A. Weider (ed.), *Contributions toward Medical Psychology* (New York: Ronald Press, 1953).

[2] See A. Anastasi and J. P. Foley, Jr., *Differential Psychology* (New York: Macmillan, 1949), p. 487.

[3] See Stalnaker, *op. cit.* and "Validation of Professional Aptitude Batteries: Tests for Medicine," *Proceedings of the 1950 Conference on Test Problems*, (Princeton: Educational Testing Service, 1951), pp. 46–51; R. A. Dykman and J. M. Stalnaker, "The History of the 1949–50 Freshman Class," *Journal of Medical Education* 30:611–621, 1955; and C. W. Taylor, "Check Studies on the Predictive Value of the Medical College Admission Test," *Journal of the Association of American Medical Colleges* 25:269–271, 1950.

mentioned above indicate that the content validity of the subtests is high.

STATISTICAL DESCRIPTION

Each class mean score on the MCAT was slightly above the national mean score for applicants to medical schools. There were some rather large differences between the means of the two GMC groups within each of the three student classes. For example, the 1954 I GMC group had a mean Verbal Ability score of 529.5, while the 1954 II GMC group had a mean score of 461.1, a difference of 68.4 score points. The amount of variability around these means was also markedly different for the two student groups, the second group showing less variability than the first. The implications of these differences for the studies of the General Medical Clinic is pointed out in Chapter 24.

The correlation coefficients between scores on the four subtests for the classes of 1955 and 1956 are presented in Table 15.1. Verbal ability and knowledge of modern society were correlated above .70 in both the 1955 and 1956 classes. Quantitative ability tended to be correlated about .40 with each of the other subtests. It is apparent in Table 15.1 that all four subtests are measuring a common factor, something basic to both the ability and the knowledge tests.

As indicated above, the test results presented here were obtained four years before the students became seniors and subjects of the present research. It is important that this discrepancy in time be kept in mind in interpreting some of the results to be presented later, because the MCAT scores will be studied in conjunction with scores obtained from the students *as seniors*. Thus, for example, verbal ability cannot be said to be related to another student characteristic (measured when the student is a senior) unless it is assumed that the four-

Table 15.1. Correlation coefficients between scores on MCAT subtests (classes of 1955 and 1956)

	1	2	3
Class of 1955 (N = 70)			
1. Verbal Ability			
2. Quantitative Ability	.44		
3. Knowledge of Modern Society	.71	.43	
4. Knowledge of Premedical Sciences	.48	.49	.39
Class of 1956 (N = 62)			
1. Verbal Ability			
2. Quantitative Ability	.37		
3. Knowledge of Modern Society	.72	.38	
4. Knowledge of Premedical Sciences	.50	.57	.57

year-old score is a valid index of current verbal ability, that is, that the attribute is relatively stable over a four-year period. However, some studies will be carried out in which interest will be centered on students' verbal abilities at the time of entry into medical school. No assumption of stability need be made in these latter studies.

Previous Academic Performance

Several indices of previous academic performance both in medical school and in an undergraduate college were obtained. From students' undergraduate records, the following data were selected: premedical grade average, number of courses (or credit hours) in psychology, number of courses (or credit hours) in sociology, number of courses in philosophy. From students' records in medical school, the following data were selected: first-year grade average, second-year grade average, third-year grade average, fourth-year grade average, eight-quarter cumulative grade average, over-all cumulative grade average, psychiatry course grade, psychopathology course grade, psychosomatics course grade, functional psychoses course grade, public health course grade, junior medical clerkship grade, junior pediatrics clerkship grade, junior obstetrics-gynecology clerkship grade, junior surgical clerkship grade, junior comprehensive examination scores.

The premedical grade average was computed on the basis of grades received in all undergraduate courses. Number of undergraduate credit hours in the departments listed above was obtained for one class of students, while number of courses in the departments was obtained for another class. No attempt was made to analyze individual grades in these courses, since grading criteria presumably varied widely from one course to another.

All the medical school grade averages were based on course grades weighted by the number of clock hours assigned to the course. The first-year curriculum consisted primarily of basic courses in human biological and physical sciences. During the second year, the medical sciences, pathology, physical diagnosis, and other subject matter including psychiatry and public health were studied. These first two years are commonly termed the "preclinical" or "academic" years of medical education. Evaluation of the student during this time usually is accomplished by means of achievement tests. The third-year curriculum involved the ward clerkships in medicine, pediatrics, obstetrics-gynecology (OB-GYN), and surgery. The fourth year was spent in clinical clerkships which have been described in detail in Chapter 2. Evaluation of the student during these latter two, or "clinical," years usually depends more upon human judgment than upon objective test scores. Thus, the third- and fourth-year grade averages are probably influenced by personal interaction to a greater degree than are the first- and second-year grade averages.

The eight-quarter cumulative grade average was computed because it represents the quality of the student's performance during two and a half years of medical training (almost his entire experience before entering the experimental or control group of this research study). The over-all cumulative grade average represents the student's entire performance in medical school.

The course grades in medical school listed above need no further description. The junior comprehensive examination was a general achievement test in medicine. It was administered to only one class of subjects and then discontinued.

Relevance

The desirability of obtaining indices of previous academic performance for studies of individual differences was obvious. As indicated earlier, a study of medical school performance was planned for which grade averages would be used as measures of performance and the premedical grade average would be used as a predictor of performance. Moreover, there was strong interest in the differential effects of the GMC and the control clinic on superior students. In addition, the grade averages were expected to serve as measures against which certain dependent variables tests, such as the Medical Knowledge test, would be validated.

The GMC was designed to put greater emphasis on training in the areas of psychological and social medicine. Therefore, indices of prior interest and performance in these areas were sought and were provided by the measures of interest in undergraduate psychology and sociology and by the grades in relevant courses in medical school, for example, psychiatry and public health.

The junior clerkship grades were selected because of the similarity between the junior and senior clerkship experiences. That is, in the junior clerkships the student saw patients and had some opportunity to apply his knowledge in a role like that of a doctor. Because of this similarity, it was of interest to compare grades in the junior medical clerkship with those in both the experimental and the control senior medical clerkships.

The only objective evaluation of medical school achievement obtainable was the junior comprehensive examination. It was administered to only one student class in the subject sample (the class of 1954) and was thereafter discontinued. An attempt was made to obtain student scores on the National Board Examination, but this request was not granted.

Technical characteristics

Reliability statistics are usually not computed for grade data. However, it is very likely that grade averages are more reliable measures of performance than are grades in single courses.

Validity of these grade data derives from the assumption that the teachers responsible for the development of the student are the best available "measuring instruments" of the student's achievements in the several content areas.

Statistical description

There were no large differences between means or between standard deviations within any student class or between classes. However, the medical school grade averages for the 1956 class were slightly lower than those for the other two classes.

Correlation coefficients between grade averages for each of the three classes of students are presented in Table 15.2. The majority of the correlation values are significant beyond the .01 level of confidence. When correlations between the annual grade averages (first, second, third, and fourth years) are observed, it is clear that the first- and second-year averages were more highly related than any other pair of

Table 15.2. Correlation coefficients between grade averages (classes of 1954, 1955, 1956)

	1	2	3	4	5	6
Class of 1954 (N = 78)						
1. Premedical grade average						
2. First-year grade average	.33					
3. Second-year grade average	.25	.55				
4. Third-year grade average	—.02	.11	.35			
5. Fourth-year grade average	.02	.17	.33	.44		
6. Cumulative (8-quarter) grade average	.14	.55	.71	.56	.61	
Class of 1955 (N = 70)						
1. Premedical grade average						
2. First-year grade average	.54					
3. Second-year grade average	.51	.68				
4. Third-year grade average	.38	.62	.72			
5. Fourth-year grade average	.22	.33	.60	.60		
6. Cumulative (8-quarter) grade average	.54	.88	.87	.88	.55	
7. Over-all grade average	.47	.79	.87	.88	.77	.95
Class of 1956 (N= 62)						
1. Premedical grade average						
2. First-year grade average	.35					
3. Second-year grade average	.35	.73				
4. Third-year grade average	.32	.52	.58			
5. Fourth-year grade average	—.02	.15	.37	.36		
6. Cumulative (8-quarter) grade average	.38	.89	.86	.78	.27	
7. Over-all grade average	.29	.78	.85	.79	.65	.89

averages ($r = .55$, .68, and .73 in the classes of 1954, 1955, and 1956, respectively). Apparently students' performance in the preclinical years was more consistent (or more reliably evaluated) than performance in the clinical years. The correlation between first-year and fourth-year performances tended to be relatively low ($r = .17$, .33, and .15 in the three classes, respectively).

The correlations between premedical grade average and medical school grade averages are of great interest to persons concerned with the selection of medical students. These results will be discussed as part of the study of medical school performance (see Chapter 26).

Peer-Judged Attributes

One valuable source of information about a student's attributes is what his peers think of him. The medical students in this study were asked to make two types of judgments about their peers: they were asked to rank other students on various attributes, and to *nominate* the "five best" students in the class on various attributes. The attributes on which peer judgments were made were:

A. leadership (peer ranking, peer nomination)
B. likeability (peer ranking, peer nomination)
C. cooperativeness (peer ranking, peer nomination)
D. competence as a physician (peer nomination)
E. skill in developing good relations with patients (peer ranking)
F. willingness and ability to work independently (peer ranking)
G. sympathy to the notion of comprehensive medical care (peer ranking)
H. responsibility and maturity (peer ranking)
I. amount of medical knowledge (peer ranking)

Because new attributes on which rankings were to be made were added from time to time throughout the course of the project, a chart showing the times at which judgments on each attribute were made is presented in Table 15.3. It should be noted that two different forms were used to collect peer-ranking data. Form 1 was used when all the students in a ten-man group were seated in a circle and each student was identified by a letter. The task under these conditions was to rank the other nine students on each of several attributes. There were eight such groups in a student class. Form 2 differed from Form 1 in that the names of the ten students in a group were written on the form. It was possible for a student to rank his peers during the regular testing period because it was found that students knew each other well enough so that the more cumbersome procedure could be dispensed with.

Table 15.3. Administration chart for peer judgment forms

		Class of 1954			Class of 1955				Class of 1956		
Attribute	Form	Pre	Post I	Post II	Pre	Post I Aug.	Post I Dec.	Post II	Pre	Post I	Post II
A (ranking)	1	x	x		x	x					
	2								x	x	x
A (nomination)		x	x				x	x	x		x
B (ranking)	1	x	x		x	x					
	2								x	x	x
B (nomination)		x	x				x	x	x		x
C (ranking)	1	x	x		x	x					
C (nomination)		x	x				x	x			
D (nomination)		x	x	x	x	x	x	x	x		x
E (ranking)	2			x	x	x	x	x	x	x	x
F (ranking)	2			x	x	x	x	x	x	x	x
G (ranking)	2			x	x	x	x	x	x	x	x
H_1 (ranking)	2						x	x			
H_2 (ranking)	2								x	x	x
I (ranking)	2							x	x	x	x

The same form was used to collect peer-nomination data in all classes.[4]

Relevance

Data bearing on the social structure of the subject population are a source of information that is usually valuable in individual differences studies. Obviously, the nature of the interaction between a subject and his human environment determines to some extent his satisfactions, his changes in attitude, and perhaps his gains in knowledge. This is especially true in the case of a subject like a medical student, whose behavior is largely dependent upon the stimulation of social intercourse. It is also likely that the impressions a student makes on his peers are not greatly different from those he makes on staff members. For these reasons and others, peer judgments of subjects on several attributes were used in studies carried out by the Individual Differences Section.

Technical characteristics

Because the technical characteristics of the judgment data did not affect the decision to use them, no reliability coefficients were computed. However, a cursory review of the data suggested that students agreed fairly well among themselves in their peer judgments.

[4] On occasion, use was made of student rankings (collected in ten-man groups) in studies which involved an entire class. In such cases a student's rank obviously only approximated the rank he might have had if *all* the students in the class had judged him.

STATISTICAL DESCRIPTION

The correlation coefficients between peer-judged attributes for the classes of 1955 and 1956 are presented in Table 15.4. The wider spaces in the table separate three clusters of attributes. The first includes three traits: likeability, skill in physician-patient relations, and sympathy to the concept of comprehensive care. (Cooperativeness is also included in this cluster in the class of 1955 data.) These attributes, which are highly correlated among themselves, are related to a noticeably lesser extent to the second cluster of attributes. This second cluster includes: ability to work independently, competence as a physician, and amount of medical knowledge (in the 1956 class). Thus, students were able to discriminate to some degree between one cluster of attributes (which could be designated "facility in interpersonal relations") and another cluster (which could be designated "professional competence").

Two other peer-judged attributes listed in Table 15.4, leadership and (in the 1956 class) responsibility and maturity, were strongly correlated with *both* clusters of attributes described above. Thus, students who were judged by their peers to be leaders also tended to be judged capable in interpersonal relations, capable in academic endeavor, and responsible and mature.

The correlations in Table 15.4 are fairly high (near .50 or above), with a few exceptions. In other words, the students did not make many

Table 15.4. Correlation coefficients between scores on peer-judged attributes (Pretest, classes of 1955 and 1956)

	1	2	3	4	5	6	7
Class of 1955 (N = 70)							
1. Likeability (PR)							
2. Skill in physician-patient relations (PR)	.78						
3. Sympathy to comprehensive care (PR)	.62	.78					
4. Cooperativeness (PR)	.79	.72	.70				
5. Ability to work independently (PR)	.18	.45	.42	.28			
6. Competence as a physician (PN)	.28	.51	.46	.38	.72		
7. Leadership (PR)	.61	.80	.65	.51	.73	.65	
Class of 1956 (N = 62)							
1. Likeability (PR)							
2. Skill in physician-patient relations (PR)	.83						
3. Sympathy to comprehensive care (PR)	.65	.76					
4. Ability to work independently (PR)	.34	.46	.42				
5. Competence as a physician (PN)	.29	.48	.47	.53			
6. Amount of medical knowledge (PR)	.08	.29	.40	.72	.60		
7. Leadership (PR)	.60	.69	.54	.67	.56	.56	
8. Responsibility and maturity (PR)	.59	.73	.70	.72	.54	.59	.66

clear-cut distinctions among one another, at least in regard to the attributes on which they were asked to make judgments.

Attitudes

Five attitude scales were administered to the medical students: the California F scale, the Liberal Attitude scale, the General Anxiety scale, the ACL Self-Acceptance scale, the ACL Self-Criticality scale. The latter two scales consist of items from the Adjective Check-List (ACL).[5]

The California F scale, hereafter referred to as the F (Authoritarian) scale, is usually described as a measure of authoritarian attitudes.[6] One feature of "authoritarianism" as defined by this scale is a two-valued orientation. For example, authoritarians are likely to perceive other people as strong or weak, as leaders or followers, etc. They are uncritical and deferential toward the strong, whereas they are likely to have an aggressive, critical attitude toward the weak. This intolerance of ambiguity or complexity extends to values. A rigid, exaggerated adherence to conventional, middle-class values about home, sex, religion, and the state, characterizes authoritarianism. Any deviation from the conventional arouses a hostile, punitive, intolerant attitude. Minority groups are usually seen as deviant and therefore "legitimate" objects of aggressive action.

The authoritarian attitude treats intellectual, thoughtful endeavor as of little importance. Instead, superstitious, paranoid beliefs and concern for the "practical" things are of major importance. "Science has its place, but . . . " characterizes authoritarian belief. More detailed expositions of this typology are available elsewhere,[7] but this summary should clarify the meaning attached to the term "authoritarianism" in this book.

The Liberal Attitude scale was adapted from the Politico-Economic Conservatism scale developed in the California study of the "authoritarian personality."[8] It consists of thirty items to be answered "agree" or "disagree." For example, one item is, "There should be more labor

[5] See H. G. Gough, *Reference Handbook for the Gough Adjective Check-List* (Berkeley: University of California Institute of Personality Assessment and Research, 1955).

[6] The short version (Form 45) was used in this study. One item about the use of postwar authorities in the occupation of Germany was deleted because of its probable unfamiliarity to some of the students. Hence, the 28-item form was used.

[7] See R. N. Sanford, "The Approach of the Authoritarian Personality," in J. L. McCary (ed.), *Psychology of Personality* (New York: Logos Press, 1956); and T. W. Adorno, E. Frenkel-Brunswik, D. J. Levinson, and R. N. Sanford, *The Authoritarian Personality* (New York: Harper, 1950).

[8] See Adorno, Frenkel-Brunswik, Levinson, and Sanford, *op. cit.*

newspapers, published by the labor unions, for the general public to read."

The General Anxiety scale, developed by Mandler and Sarason,[9] consists of forty statements dealing with general anxiety symptoms on which each subject rates himself. The content of the statements includes inability to fall asleep, inadequacy of social adjustment, inability to concentrate on studies, and tendencies to bite nails or to have headaches. Several of the individual items have been used separately in individual differences studies. These latter items will be discussed with other self-ratings in a subsequent part of this chapter.

The other two attitude scales concern the self. One scale measures self-acceptance (or perhaps more accurately, self-approval); the other measures self-criticality. The meaning of these terms will be clearer if the procedures followed in obtaining the scores are briefly explained. The Adjective Check-List, from which the scales were derived, was developed by Gough.[10] It consists simply of 300 adjectives. Thirty-four judges were asked to choose the most favorable and the most unfavorable adjectives, and the 75 favorable and 75 unfavorable adjectives most often chosen were noted. A subject's ACL Self-Acceptance (or Self-Approval) score is the ratio of the number of favorable adjectives checked to the total number of adjectives checked. The ACL Self-Criticality score is the ratio of the number of unfavorable adjectives checked to the total number of adjectives checked.

Relevance

The medical staff of the GMC thought that the complexity and ambiguity of medical problems and clinic duties would frustrate the student and interfere with his performance in the clinic. This expectation seemed well founded, and it was further suspected that the more authoritarian student would be thus affected to a greater degree than the less authoritarian student. It was also expected that the authoritarian student would perceive patients with behavior disorders as being blameworthy, an orientation that might affect his willingness to change his attitudes about behavior disorders.

The potential importance of another attitude was also suggested by the description of the GMC conditions. This was general anxiety. A student easily made anxious might have a difficult time adjusting to the many demands made upon him by his GMC duties. The Mandler-Sarason test of general anxiety was chosen to measure this attribute, partly because it had been used with medical students in previous

[9] See G. Mandler and S. D. Sarason, "A Study of Anxiety and Learning," *Journal of Abnormal and Social Psychology* 47:166–173, 1952.

[10] *Op. cit.*

studies.[11] The effect of liberal attitudes and of attitudes toward oneself upon psychological change and performance was also of considerable interest. This was particularly true of the ACL Self-Acceptance test and the ACL Self-Criticality test because attitudes toward oneself are often overlooked in research of this type.

Technical characteristics

The development of the F (Authoritarian) scale is reported in detail in *The Authoritarian Personality;* reliability estimates of the equivalence type reported there were high, the most typical equivalence value equalling .90.[12] When a similar estimate was computed for some of the data in the present study, the equivalence coefficient equalled .82 ($N = 80$), and a stability coefficient, which was also computed, equalled .80 ($N = 65$) for a one-year period. Thus, it seems safe to say that the F (Authoritarian) scale is a reliable instrument. Both the evidence presented in *The Authoritarian Personality* and that obtained since then indicate that the scale is also valid.[13] However, criticisms of the test, e.g., its susceptibility to response set, have not been answered satisfactorily.[14]

An equivalence estimate of the reliability of the Liberal Attitude scale based on 81 subjects was .76. And a stability estimate (one-year interval) was .83 ($N = 78$). No validity studies have been undertaken on this test.

Statistics obtained during the development of the General Anxiety scale showed it to be technically sound as a personality measure.[15] A reliability estimate (stability type) computed on data collected during the present study extended previous findings ($r = .80$, $N = 65$, six-month interval).

Reliability and validity coefficients have not been computed for the two measures of attitude toward oneself. It is regrettable that test-retest correlations (stability coefficients) were not obtained, but con-

[11] See L. D. Eron, "Effect of Medical Education on Medical Students' Attitudes," *Journal of Medical Education* 30:559–566, 1955.

[12] See Adorno, Frenkel-Brunswik, Levinson, and Sanford, *op. cit.*, especially p. 258.

[13] See J. Block and J. Block, "An Investigation of the Relationship between Intolerance of Ambiguity and Ethnocentrism," *Journal of Personality* 19:303–311, 1951; J. Fisher, "The Memory Process and Certain Psychosocial Attitudes with Special Reference to the Law of Prägnanz: I. Study of Non-Verbal Content," *Journal of Personality* 19:406–420, 1951; and H. E. Titus and E. P. Hollander, "The California F Scale in Psychological Research, 1950–55," *Psychological Bulletin* 54:47–64, 1957.

[14] See R. Christie and M. Jahoda (eds.), *Studies in the Scope and Method of the Authoritarian Personality* (Glencoe: The Free Press, 1954); and Titus and Hollander, *op. cit.*

[15] See Mandler and Sarason, *op. cit.*

ditions of testing (described in Chapter 10) made such computations impossible.

Statistical description

The typical class mean score on the F scale was near 84. Only roughly 5% of each class agreed with scale items as often as they disagreed with them. However, a relatively wide range of scores was obtained, which permitted the use of this scale in individual differences studies.

At Pretest time students in the 1956 I GMC group had relatively low General Anxiety scores (mean = 136.33) while students in the 1956 II GMC group had relatively high scores (mean = 168.24) at the time they entered the GMC (at Posttest I time).

A final comment on these data concerns the ACL Self-Acceptance and ACL Self-Criticality scales. The ACL Self-Acceptance scores tended to fall near .50. That is, although only one quarter of the 300 adjectives were favorable, one half of the adjectives checked by subjects tended to be favorable. In other words, subjects checked a large number of favorable adjectives relative to other adjectives in describing themselves. When ACL Self-Criticality scores were studied, however, a different condition was found. Only 8% of the self-descriptive adjectives checked tended to be unfavorable, despite the fact that one quarter of the 300 adjectives were unfavorable. A numerical estimate of the degree to which medical students have positive, not negative, self-concepts is thus presented.

Correlation coefficients between scores on the five attitude scales are shown in Table 15.5. The strong negative correlations between the Liberal Attitude scale and the F (Authoritarian) scale ($r = -.39$ and $-.47$) provide some reassurance of the validity of the former measure, since authoritarianism has been shown to be correlated with conserva-

Table 15.5. Correlation coefficients between scores on various attitude scales (classes of 1955 and 1956)

	1	2	3	4
Class of 1955 (N = 53)				
1. F (Authoritarian) scale (Pretest)				
2. Liberal Attitude scale	—.39			
3. General Anxiety scale	.30	—.18		
4. ACL Self-Acceptance scale	—.07	—.05	—.25	
5. ACL Self-Criticality scale	—.02	.12	.24	—.85
Class of 1956 (N = 62)				
1. F (Authoritarian) scale (Pretest)				
2. Liberal Attitude scale	—.47			
3. General Anxiety scale	.23	.04		
4. ACL Self-Acceptance scale	—.10	—.09	—.50	
5. ACL Self-Criticality scale	.03	—.04	.35	—.81

tism.[16] Table 15.5 also shows that the General Anxiety scores bear a moderately positive relation to the F (Authoritarian) scale scores ($r = .30$ and $.23$), although the ACL Self-Criticality scale is not positively related to either of the scales in question to a very high degree. Finally, the very high negative correlation between Self-Acceptance and Self-Criticality ($r = -.85$ and $-.81$) means that these two scales cannot be treated as independent measures, but should be thought of as the opposite poles of one dimension—favorability of attitude toward oneself.

Values

A standardized instrument, the Allport-Vernon-Lindzey Study of Values scale, was employed to assess student values. Value strength in the following six areas was assessed by this test: theoretical, aesthetic, economic, political, social, religious.

These areas of values were derived from the concepts of "ideal types," as set forth in Spranger's *Types of Men.*[17] Their meaning may most conveniently be indicated by means of the following brief descriptions of the content of the six scales, derived in large part from characterizations of the six personality types discussed in the manual of this test.[18]

Theoretical value. "The dominant interest of the theoretical man is the discovery of *truth.* . . . Since the interests of the theoretical man are empirical, critical, and rational, he is . . . frequently a scientist or philosopher. His chief aim in life is to order and systematize his knowledge."

Aesthetic value. "The aesthetic man sees his highest value in *form* and *harmony.* He regards life as a procession of events; each single impression is enjoyed for its own sake. . . . He tends toward individualism and self-sufficiency."

Economic value. "The economic man is characteristically interested in what is *useful.* . . . This type is thoroughly 'practical' and conforms well to the prevailing stereotype of the average American business man."

Political value. "The political man is interested primarily in *power.* His activities are not necessarily within the narrow field of politics; . . . There are . . . certain personalities . . . who wish above all else for personal power, influence, and renown."

[16] See Adorno, Frenkel-Brunswik, Levinson, and Sanford, *op. cit.*

[17] E. Spranger, *Types of Men* (Halle: Niemeyer, 1928); now available from Hafner Publishing Company, New York.

[18] See G. W. Allport, P. E. Vernon, and G. Lindzey, *Study of Values: A Scale for Measuring the Dominant Interests in Personality* (Boston: Houghton Mifflin, 1951, revised edition).

Social value. "The highest value for this type is *love* of people. In the Study of Values it is the altruistic or philanthropic aspect of love that is measured. . . . The social man . . . is kind, sympathetic, and unselfish."

Religious value. "The highest value of the religious man may be called *unity*. He is mystical, and seeks to comprehend the cosmos as a whole, to relate himself to its embracing totality." Many of the scale items represent an interest in some form of organized religious activity.

Relevance

The selection of a test of values for inclusion in this research was based primarily on the hypothesis that the values one esteems as being a significant aspect of human personality should affect a student's acquisition of knowledge and his performance in medical school. This particular value measure was selected because of its extensive use in research on values.[19]

Technical characteristics

Since the Study of Values is a standardized test, the reliability of each of the six scales is fairly high. The equivalence coefficients range between .73 and .90, and the stability coefficients (one-month interval) between .77 and .92.[20]

A fairly large number of studies provide indirect validation of separate value scales. In particular, several studies of perceptual and cognitive correlates of values have been done.[21] The reader is referred to the test manual for this information.[22]

A notable feature of this instrument is the interdependence of the scores; a high score on one value requires offsetting low scores on other values. Thus, the measured strength of any one value is relative to the measured strengths of others. Because of this feature the several scales tend to be negatively correlated with each other (see below).

Statistical description

The Study of Values test was administered at the following times: Posttest II (class of 1954), Pretest (class of 1955), and Posttest I (class of 1956). For the purpose of comparing the class mean scores

[19] See W. F. Dukes, "Psychological Studies of Values," *Psychological Bulletin* 52:24–50, 1955.

[20] See Allport, Vernon, and Lindzey, *op. cit.*, pp. 7, 8.

[21] See E. McGinnies, "Personal Values as Determinants of Word Association," *Journal of Abnormal and Social Psychology* 45:28–36, 1950; and J. M. Vanderplas and R. R. Blake, "Selective Sensitization in Auditory Perception," *Journal of Personality* 18:252–266, 1949.

[22] See Allport, Vernon, and Lindzey, *op. cit.*, pp. 10–12.

with the undergraduate normative data, these means have been plotted on standard profile forms (see Figure 15.1). It can be noted that all three classes had fairly high mean scores on the Theoretical scale (mean scores = 47, 48, and 47, respectively). A similar result for medical students is reported in the manual. Presumably the interest in science, which in part attracts students to medical school, accounts for this finding.

Correlation coefficients between scores on value tests, presented in Table 15.6, were generally negative, as pointed out above. However, economic and political values tended to be positively correlated, as

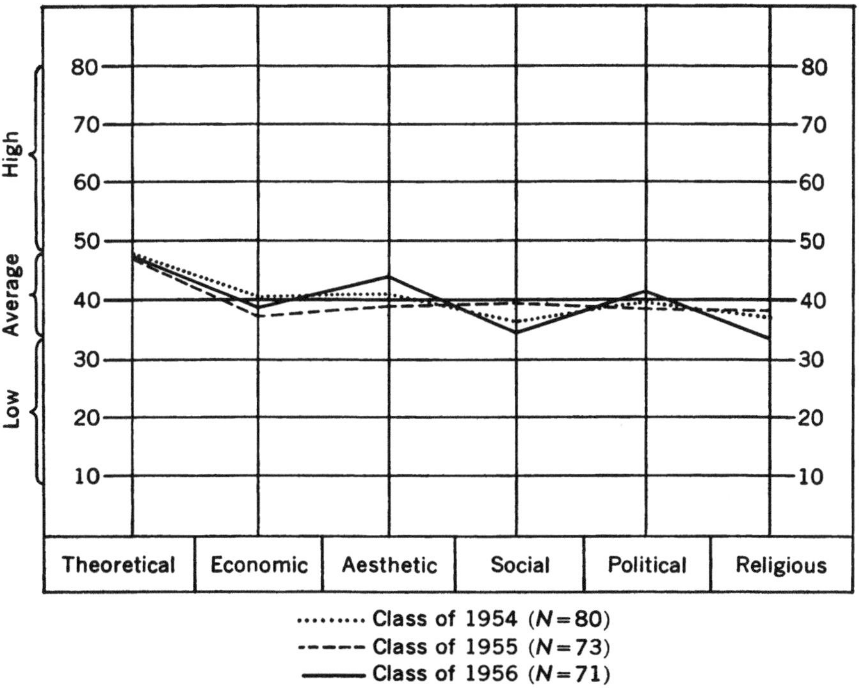

Figure 15.1. Profiles of class mean scores on Study of Values scale (classes of 1954, 1955, and 1956)

High and low scores. A score on one of the values may be considered definitely high or low if it falls outside the following limits. Such scores exceed the range of 50% of all scores for that value, i.e., 1 probable error. (These ranges are approximate since each probable error is rounded to the nearest whole number.)

Theoretical	34–46	Social	35–45
Economic	34–46	Political	35–45
Aesthetic	34–46	Religious	33–47

Outstandingly high and low scores. A score on one of the values may be considered very distinctive if it is higher or lower than the following limits. Such scores fall outside the range of 82% of all scores for that value, i.e., exceed 2 probable errors.

Theoretical	29–51	Social	30–50
Economic	29–51	Political	31–49
Aesthetic	27–53	Religious	25–55

Table 15.6. Correlation coefficients between scores on Study of Values test (classes of 1955 and 1956)

	1	2	3	4	5
Class of 1955 (N = 70)					
1. Theoretical value					
2. Aesthetic value	.01				
3. Economic value	—.13	—.39			
4. Political value	—.38	—.17	.26		
5. Social value	—.09	—.32	—.29	—.25	
6. Religious value	—.24	—.32	—.38	—.37	.14
Class of 1956 (N = 62)					
1. Theoretical value					
2. Aesthetic value	.01				
3. Economic value	—.09	—.46			
4. Political value	.05	—.24	.23		
5. Social value	—.22	—.26	—.31	—.25	
6. Religious value	—.48	—.21	—.30	—.45	.11

did social and religious values. The same tendency, to a lesser extent, is shown in the theoretical-aesthetic value correlations. These findings parallel those reported in the manual and appear to be characteristic of the general population.

Social Interaction Variables

It was desired to assess one class of personality characteristics which described the normal functioning of an individual in his social milieu. The standard test best suited to this purpose was judged to be the California Psychological Inventory (CPI). Its eighteen scales are "intended to provide a comprehensive survey of an individual from the social interaction point of view."[23] The scales are: Good Impression, Self-Control, Sense of Well-Being, Socialization, Responsibility, Achievement via Conformance, Dominance, Sociability, Self-Acceptance (not to be confused with the ACL Self-Acceptance scale), Social Presence, Capacity for Status, Tolerance, Intellectual Efficiency, Psychological-Mindedness, Achievement via Independence, Flexibility, Femininity, Communality. The following brief descriptions of the purpose of each scale are adapted from the manual.[24]

Good Impression. The purpose of this scale is to identify persons who are capable of creating a favorable impression and are concerned about how others react to them.

Self-Control. The purpose of this scale is to assess the degree and adequacy of self-regulation and self-control and freedom from impulsivity and self-centeredness.

[23] H. G. Gough, *Manual for the California Psychological Inventory* (Palo Alto: Consulting Psychologists Press, 1957), p. 7.
[24] *Ibid.*, pp. 12–13.

Sense of Well-Being. The purpose of this scale is to identify persons who minimize their worries and complaints and who are relatively free from self-doubt and disillusionment.

Socialization. The purpose of this scale is to indicate the degree of social maturity, integrity, and rectitude which the individual has attained.

Responsibility. The purpose of this scale is to identify persons of conscientious, responsible, and dependable disposition and temperament.

Achievement via Conformance. The purpose of this scale is to identify those factors of interest and motivation which facilitate achievement in any setting where conformance is a positive behavior.

Dominance. The purpose of this scale is to assess factors of leadership ability, dominance, persistence, and social initiative.

Sociability. The purpose of this scale is to identify persons of outgoing, sociable, participative temperament.

Self-Acceptance. The purpose of this scale is to assess factors such as sense of personal worth, self-acceptance, and capacity for independent thinking and action.

Social Presence. The purpose of this scale is to assess factors such as poise, spontaneity, and self-confidence in personal and social interaction.

Capacity for Status. The purpose of this scale is to serve as an index of an individual's capacity for status (not his actual or achieved status). The scale attempts to measure the personal qualities and attributes which underlie and lead to status.

Tolerance. The purpose of this scale is to identify persons with permissive, accepting, and nonjudgmental social beliefs and attitudes.

Intellectual Efficiency. The purpose of this scale is to indicate the degree of personal and intellectual efficiency which the individual has attained.

Psychological-Mindedness. The purpose of this scale is to measure the degree to which the individual is interested in, and responsive to, the inner needs, motives, and experiences of others.

Achievement via Independence. The purpose of this scale is to identify those factors of interest and motivation which facilitate achievement in any setting where autonomy and independence are positive behaviors.

Flexibility. The purpose of this scale is to indicate the degree of flexibility and adaptability of a person's thinking and social behavior.

Femininity. The purpose of this scale is to assess the masculinity or femininity of interests. (High scores indicate more feminine interests, low scores more masculine.)

Communality. The purpose of this scale is to indicate the degree to which an individual's reactions and responses correspond to the modal ("common") pattern established for the inventory.

RELEVANCE

The traits manifested by a subject in interpersonal relations (e.g., dominance, tolerance, and flexibility) are often believed to influence judgments made about that subject in social situations. Because a study of performance utilizing ratings made by the teaching staff was planned, it was expected that measures of these traits would aid in understanding the evaluation of student performance. In addition, the development of a measure of responsibility was planned, and this inventory provided an already validated scale with which the experimental device could be compared.

TECHNICAL CHARACTERISTICS

The eighteen scales of the CPI each consisted of between 22 and 56 items to be checked by the subject as either applicable or not applicable: for example, "I get excited very easily"; "People often expect too much of me." Reliabilities of these scales have been studied by means of the stability coefficient (one-year interval).[25] The coefficient values (for high-school males) ranged from .38 to .75, median = .645. Only three values were less than .60.[26]

The empirical validity of each scale has been established by several independent studies.[27] A frequently used procedure is to correlate ratings and the inventory scores on the same attribute.

STATISTICAL DESCRIPTION

The CPI was administered at Posttest I time to the class of 1955 and at Pretest time to the class of 1956. It was not administered to the class of 1954.

The class mean values on each CPI scale have been plotted on profile sheets so that the profiles of both the 1955 and 1956 classes can be compared with the subject sample on which the test was standardized (see Figure 15.2). The profile of the college undergraduate male sample is also drawn on the figure. It can be seen that the medical student profiles (both classes) are closer to the undergraduate male sample than to the total standard sample. The largest differences between medical students' and undergraduates' CPI profiles were the

[25] *Ibid.*

[26] *Ibid.*

[27] For some scales up to four studies are reported. All evidence is drawn from cross-validation studies. Typically, validity coefficients fall in the .40 range. See *Ibid.*, pp. 23–27.

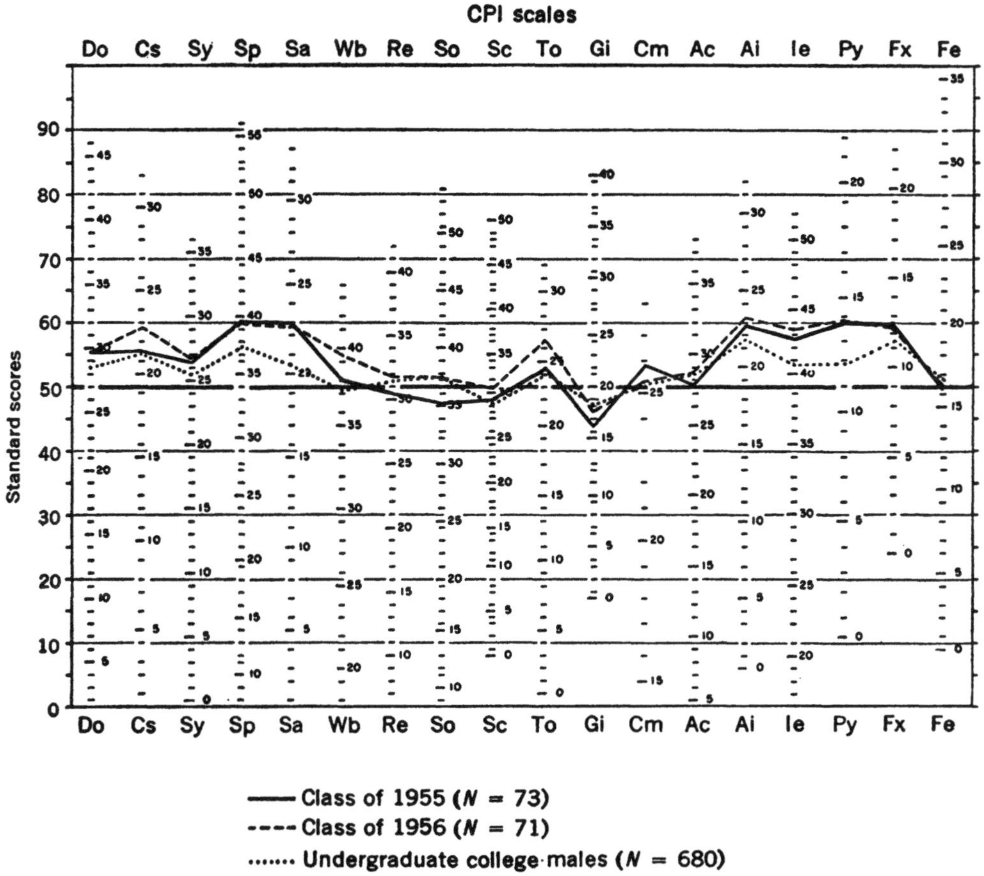

Figure 15.2. Profiles of class mean scores on California Psychological Inventory (classes of 1955, 1956, and undergraduate college males). Profile sheet reproduced from H. G. Gough, *Manual for the California Psychological Inventory* (Palo Alto: Consulting Psychologists Press, 1957)

former's higher scores on the Psychological-Mindedness and Self-Acceptance scales. The class of 1955 also had higher scores on the Intellectual Efficiency scale than did either the undergraduates or the class of 1956. Although none of the differences was very large, it appears that the two classes of medical students tended to be more responsive to others and to have a greater capacity for independent thinking and action than either undergraduate males or the standard sample of males.[28]

Correlation coefficients between scores on the eighteen CPI scales are shown in Table 15.7. Several of the scales are related to a fairly

[28] The publishers of the CPI make no claim that their "standard sample" is representative of the general population of males.

Table 15.7. Correlation coefficients between scores on the California Psychological Inventory (classes of 1955 and 1956)

	1	2	3	4	5	6	7	8	9	10	11	12	13	14	15	16	17
Class of 1955 (N = 53)																	
1. Good Impression																	
2. Self-Control	.78																
3. Sense of Well-Being	.62	.66															
4. Socialization	.36	.42	.26														
5. Responsibility	.44	.48	.51	.17													
6. Achievement via Conformance	.59	.57	.59	.37	.67												
7. Dominance	.39	.05	.28	–.02	.42	.51											
8. Sociability	.36	.13	.28	.02	.33	.48	.50										
9. Self-Acceptance	–.09	–.29	.03	–.02	–.02	.05	.52	.30									
10. Social Presence	–.03	–.22	.21	–.36	.02	.17	.41	.35	.38								
11. Capacity for Status	.21	.04	.25	–.05	.24	.29	.48	.33	.18	.40							
12. Tolerance	.55	.56	.65	.44	.48	.06	.39	.39	.04	.37	.30						
13. Intellectual Efficiency	.30	.26	.45	–.02	.44	.40	.46	.32	.30	.47	.46	.62					
14. Psychological-Mindedness	.22	.15	.38	–.29	.37	.42	.49	.29	.18	.56	.43	.53	.54				
15. Achievement via Independence	.24	.45	.47	–.01	.43	.42	.11	.11	.01	.43	.23	.61	.52	.44			
16. Flexibility	–.02	.03	.25	–.30	.04	.05	.09	.07	.07	.56	.32	.40	.37	.47	.55		
17. Femininity	.15	.36	–.01	.25	.26	.24	–.18	.06	–.25	–.47	–.27	–.15	–.15	–.17	.02	–.18	
18. Communality	.09	.07	.05	.14	.05	–.05	.00	.15	–.01	–.14	–.23	–.16	–.26	–.32	–.29	–.30	.21
Class of 1956 (N = 62)																	
1. Good Impression																	
2. Self-Control	.71																
3. Sense of Well-Being	.70	.64															
4. Socialization	.35	.53	.40														
5. Responsibility	.46	.47	.55	.57													
6. Achievement via Conformance	.53	.44	.49	.53	.58												
7. Dominance	.16	–.25	.20	–.06	.28	.36											
8. Sociability	.21	–.21	.24	.03	.21	.31	.74										
9. Self-Acceptance	.02	–.36	.08	–.14	.00	.17	.64	.77									
10. Social Presence	.07	–.23	.25	–.23	–.10	.08	.49	.61	.54								
11. Capacity for Status	.43	–.02	.35	.04	.19	.30	.55	.65	.53	.65							
12. Tolerance	.45	.30	.67	.29	.53	.48	.44	.42	.22	.42	.38						
13. Intellectual Efficiency	.51	.32	.57	.25	.43	.60	.38	.45	.28	.47	.50	.71					
14. Psychological-Mindedness	.25	.07	.27	–.05	.17	.19	.28	.23	.23	.36	.34	.43	.44				
15. Achievement via Independence	.25	.17	.26	.04	.24	.25	.21	.07	–.01	.26	.20	.62	.58	.58			
16. Flexibility	–.06	–.17	–.03	–.25	–.36	–.21	–.09	–.08	–.06	.38	.19	.18	.19	.40	.55		
17. Femininity	.15	.07	–.04	.21	.22	–.04	–.12	–.15	–.13	–.43	–.09	–.12	–.23	–.27	–.14	–.20	
18. Communality	–.02	.13	.05	.27	.31	.40	.09	.02	–.08	–.08	–.12	.04	.17	–.08	–.16	–.30	.01

high degree. The wider spaces in the table mark off groups of scales which are fairly highly correlated with one another. This pattern of grouping differs somewhat from that suggested in the manual.[29] The first six scales all appear to be concerned with adherence to socially desirable goals of behavior. The second group of scales represents a less conforming, more independent orientation toward social behavior. Self-confidence and initiative seem to characterize these five attributes. The third group of scales, Tolerance, Intellectual Efficiency, Psychological-Mindedness, and Achievement via Independence, tend to be correlated to a fairly high degree with both the groups mentioned above. The other three scales are not related to any of the three groups previously distinguished to any large extent, although in the 1955 class, Flexibility was rather highly correlated with scales in the third group.

Needs

The Edwards Personal Preference Schedule (EPPS) is a standardized psychological measuring instrument which yields scores on fifteen personality characteristics, or, more specifically, needs. The statements which make up the several scales were suggested by the work of Murray and others.[30] The names of the needs are: n(eed) affiliation, n(eed) nurturance, n(eed) succorance, n(eed) endurance, n(eed) order, n(eed) deference, n(eed) abasement, n(eed) dominance, n(eed) aggression, n(eed) achievement, n(eed) exhibition, n(eed) autonomy, n(eed) intraception, n(eed) change, n(eed) heterosexuality.

The outstanding feature of the EPPS is that the social desirability of an item, usually a substantial factor in personality inventories, is controlled. This is done by presenting the subject with two statements, each representing a different need but of equal social desirability, and asking him to choose one or the other. Thus, the subject is not permitted to use an irrelevant cue in deciding which alternative he will endorse. For example, one test item is: A—I like to help my friends when they are in trouble; B—I like to do my very best in whatever I undertake. There follows an adaptation of the partial listing of statements associated with each of the EPPS variables which appears in the manual.[31]

N(eed) Affiliation. This term designates the need to be loyal to friends, to participate in friendly groups, to form new friendships.

[29] *Ibid.*, p. 7.

[30] See H. A. Murray and others, *Explorations in Personality* (New York: Oxford University Press, 1938).

[31] A. L. Edwards, *Manual for the Personal Preference Schedule* (New York: Psychological Corporation, 1954).

N(*eed*) *Nurturance.* This term designates the need to help friends when they are in trouble, to assist others less fortunate, to treat others with kindness and sympathy.

N(*eed*) *Succorance.* This term designates the need to have others provide help when in trouble, to seek encouragement from others, to have others be kindly.

N(*eed*) *Endurance.* This term designates the need to keep at a job until it is finished, to work hard at a task, to work at a single job before taking on others.

N(*eed*) *Order.* This term designates the need to make plans before starting on a difficult task, to have things organized, to keep things neat and orderly.

N(*eed*) *Deference.* This term designates the need to get suggestions from others, to follow instructions and do what is expected, to let others make decisions.

N(*eed*) *Abasement.* This term designates the need to feel guilty when one does something wrong, to accept blame when things do not go right, to feel that personal pain and misery suffered does more good than harm.

N(*eed*) *Dominance.* This term designates the need to argue for one's point of view, to be a leader in groups to which one belongs, to persuade and influence others to do what one wants.

N(*eed*) *Aggression.* This term designates the need to attack contrary points of view, to tell others what one thinks about them, to blame others when things go wrong.

N(*eed*) *Achievement.* This term designates the need to do one's best, to be successful, to accomplish tasks requiring skill and effort.

N(*eed*) *Exhibition.* This term designates the need to say witty and clever things, to tell amusing jokes and stories, to be the center of attention.

N(*eed*) *Autonomy.* This term designates the need to be able to come and go as desired, to say what one thinks about things, to be independent of others in making decisions.

N(*eed*) *Intraception.* This term designates the need to analyze one's motives and feelings, to understand how others feel about problems, to judge people by why they do things rather than by what they do.

N(*eed*) *Change.* This term designates the need to do new and different things, to meet new people, to experience novelty and change in daily routine.

N(*eed*) *Heterosexuality.* This term designates the need to go out with members of the opposite sex, to be in love with someone of the opposite sex, to be regarded as physically attractive by those of the opposite sex.

Relevance

Needs represent still another aspect of personality, different from attitudes, values, and social interaction attributes, yet a potential determinant of performance and of change in knowledge, skill, and attitudes. For example, medical educators have often remarked that aggressive students probably do not perform well in senior clinics. By assessing need for aggression, it was possible to test the accuracy of this statement. In addition, it was of considerable interest to ascertain whether a measure of general need for achievement was related to indices of achievement in medical school.

Technical characteristics

Reliability coefficients of both the equivalence and the stability type are presented in the manual.[32] Values for the equivalence coefficient vary from .60 to .87; the median value is .78. Values for the stability coefficient (one-week interval) vary from .74 to .88; the median value is .81. In other words, the reliability of the several scales of this test is satisfactory.

Statistical description

The EPPS was administered to the class of 1956 only; this administration took place at Posttest I time. Figure 15.3 presents the profile of mean scores for this class and for the entire standardizing sample. Although there is little difference between the two profiles, it can be seen that the medical students have higher n Endurance and lower n Succorance scores than the normative population. These findings are consistent with the ones reported by Schlag on a medical student sample.[33] The relatively low n Dominance found in this 1956 class was not found in Schlag's data, however.

The correlation coefficients between scores on the EPPS for the class of 1956 are presented in Table 15.8. The fact that few high correlations appear there indicates that the variables measured are relatively independent. The highest correlation value, −.57 between n Dominance and n Abasement, may be explainable by the tendency of these variables to represent opposite poles of a "need to influence—need to be influenced" dimension. In view of the positive, accepting attitude toward others implicit in the definitions of both n Affiliation and n Nurturance, the .52 correlation between them was not surprising. Thus, the largest correlations between EPPS variables were not unexpected.

[32] *Ibid.*, p. 12.

[33] See M. R. Schlag, "The Relationship between the Personal Preference Schedule and the AVL Study of Values: A Personality Study of a Group of Medical Students" (unpublished master's thesis, University of Washington, 1954).

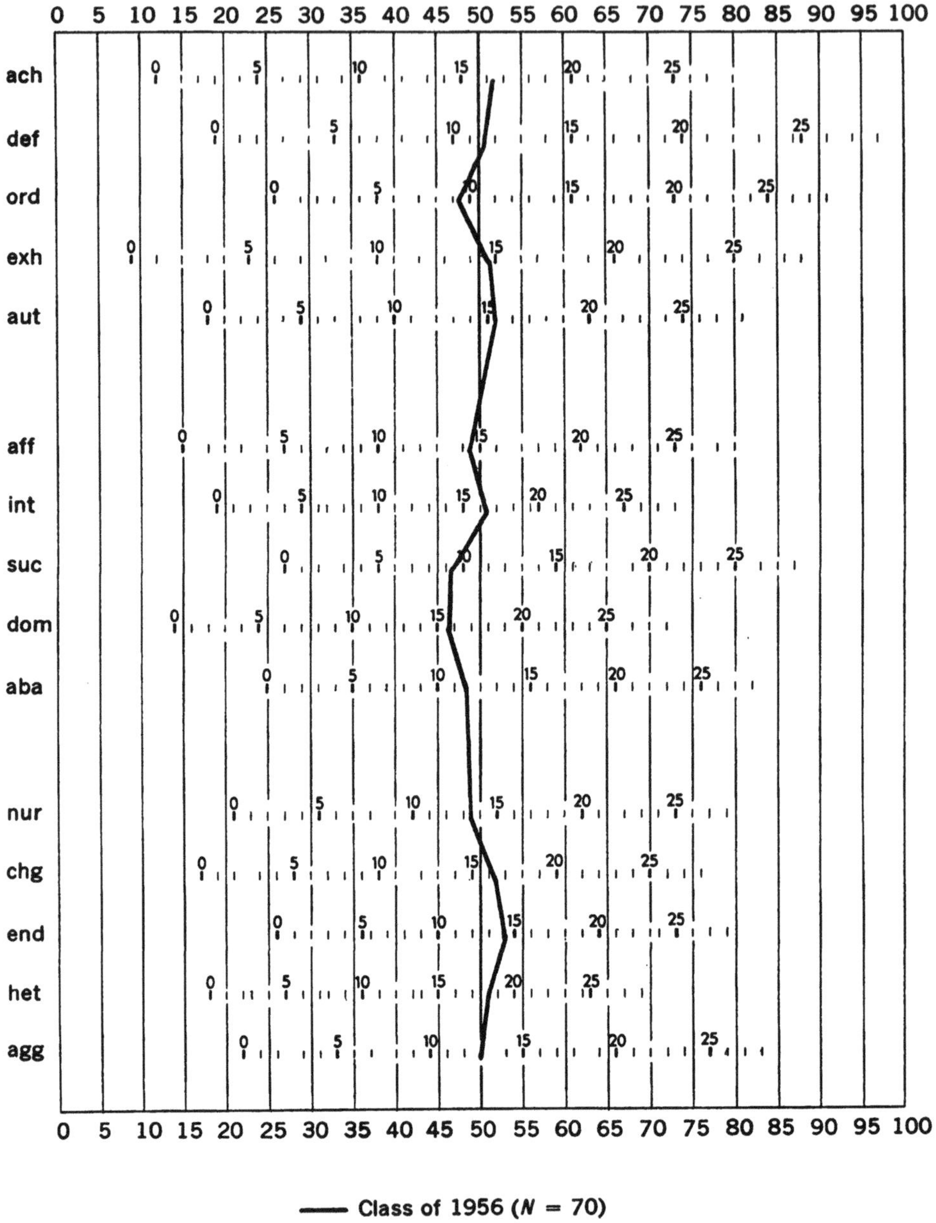

Figure 15.3. Profile of class mean scores on Edwards Personal Preference Schedule (class of 1956). Profile sheet reproduced from A. L. Edwards, *Manual for the Personal Preference Schedule* (New York: Psychological Corporation, 1954)

Table 15.8. Correlation coefficients between scores on the Edwards Personal Preference Schedule (class of 1956)

	1	2	3	4	5	6	7	8	9	10	11	12	13	14
Class of 1956 (N = 62)														
1. n Affiliation														
2. n Nurturance	.52													
3. n Succorance	.16	.16												
4. n Endurance	—.18	—.07	—.20											
5. n Order	—.09	—.24	—.02	.39										
6. n Deference	—.22	—.22	—.15	.33	.26									
7. n Abasement	—.08	—.14	.15	.06	.28	—.02								
8. n Dominance	—.10	.02	—.20	—.11	—.39	.04	—.57							
9. n Aggression	—.16	—.26	—.02	—.30	—.23	—.36	—.16	.19						
10. n Achievement	—.30	—.04	—.15	.13	—.17	.10	—.26	.23	.11					
11. n Exhibition	—.13	—.30	—.15	—.27	—.12	—.18	—.07	.02	.07	.01				
12. n Autonomy	—.11	—.27	—.21	—.26	.16	—.11	—.08	—.16	.14	—.21	.15			
13. n Intraception	—.03	—.13	—.48	—.02	—.17	.11	—.22	.15	—.16	.06	.14	.21		
14. n Change	.09	—.07	—.14	—.27	—.41	—.26	—.04	—.15	.06	—.10	.18	.08	—.03	
15. n Heterosexuality	—.28	—.17	.10	—.29	—.13	—.20	.07	—.07	.12	—.32	—.04	—.12	—.25	.08

The relatively large number of negative correlations was due, in large part, to the nature of the test. As stated before, each item requires the subject to choose between two alternative statements, each of which represents a different need. Thus, a preference for one statement is also a rejection of another statement. That is, the score on one need scale is dependent upon the scores on all other need scales. (It will be remembered that this feature also characterized the Study of Values test.) Because of this feature of the test, negative correlations among need scales are more likely to occur than if the scores on the scales were determined independently. However, the large number of scales (fifteen) minimizes the distorting influence of this feature.

Background Information

Questions pertaining to family relations, amount of reward for significant behaviors, peer relations, activities, etc., were asked in addition to the routine items of age, sex, and marital status. Moreover, items which had been found to discriminate among Ph.D.-seeking graduate students in terms of their personal soundness[34] were used in this part of the questionnaire.

The chief purpose of obtaining students' responses to the biographical items of information was to seek relations between the items and performance in medical school. A certain amount of folklore about these relations exists (e.g., that sons of physicians perform better than other medical students), and Deitrick and Berson have pointed out the need for this type of study.[35]

Self-Ratings

Another section of the questionnaire required the medical student to rate himself according to the degree of his interest in several aspects of a physician's role: research, performing minor surgery, and hospital administration. These self-ratings, together with others from the questionnaire and eight self-rating items from the General Anxiety scale, constituted the self-ratings used in various studies made by the Individual Differences Section. Four of the Anxiety scale items were part of the original 40-item test, and four (nos. 41–44) were new ones written especially for medical students. All the self-ratings (identified

[34] See F. X. Barron, *Personal Soundness in University Graduate Students*, University of California Publication in Personality Assessment and Research, no. 1 (Berkeley: University of California Press, 1954).

[35] J. E. Deitrick and R. C. Berson, *Medical Schools in the United States at Mid-Century* (New York: McGraw-Hill, 1953).

by questionnaire (Q) or Anxiety scale (A) item number) are listed below:

Q 4	(For those who work) How many hours per week do you work?
Q 25–1	Amount of reward for scholastic success as an adolescent
Q 25–2	Amount of reward for showing initiative as an adolescent
Q 25–3	Amount of reward for ability to get along with others as an adolescent
Q 25–4	Amount of reward for showing responsibility as an adolescent
Q 25–5	Amount of reward for being influential (among friends) as an adolescent
Q 32–a	Amount of interest in research
Q 32–b	Amount of interest in considering the patient's social circumstances
Q 32–c	Amount of interest in working with social service or public health nurse
Q 32–d	Amount of interest in consideration of the welfare of the patient's family
Q 32–e	Amount of interest in minor surgery
Q 32–f	Amount of interest in major surgery
Q 32–g	Amount of interest in taking an administrative position in a hospital
Q 33	How early in life did you feel confident in your ability to develop satisfying relationships with others?
A 5	In comparison with other people that you know who are of approximately the same age as yourself, how would you rate yourself in terms of the importance you attach to intellectual and professional accomplishments?
A 9	When you fantasy or day-dream, how frequently do they concern intellectual or professional accomplishments?
A 14	When you are in a situation in which you are competing with someone who is also present, to what extent is your efficiency interfered with by the fear that you are not doing or will not do well?
A 17	To what extent is the adequacy of your social adjustment a source of worry to you?
A 41	To what extent do you find yourself worrying about whether or not your fellow students accept you as a friend?
A 42	How often do you experience some anxiety when a patient presents an ambiguous problem in diagnosis?
A 43	When you think of the responsibilities you will have for

your patients when you are practicing medicine, to what extent do you experience fear or anxiety?

A 44 To what extent do you find yourself worrying about the adequacy of your knowledge of differential diagnosis?

The above items were selected for use in individual differences studies because they appeared to fill gaps in the array of individual attributes already chosen. No other measures of interests or worries specific to medical students were obtained. The reason for including items pertaining to social adjustment was that the degree of a student's concern about acceptance by his peers has been demonstrated to be relevant to graduate school performance,[36] and it was suspected that the amount of reward a student could remember having received for certain behaviors as an adolescent (desirable in medical students, see Q 25–1 through Q 25–5) would be at least one sign which would predict the exhibition of these traits in medical school.

Technical characteristics

The reliability and validity of these data were not checked empirically. It is suspected that the self-ratings are not highly reliable. Since interest was centered in the subjects' responses per se, there was no question of the validity of their responses.

[36] See B. L. Groesbeck, "Personality Correlates of the Achievement and Affiliation Motives in Clinical Psychology Trainees" (unpublished doctoral dissertation, University of Michigan, 1956).

Part IV

FINDINGS AND CONCLUSIONS

Introduction to Part IV

Part IV presents the findings of this research project concerning the students' acquisition of medical, psychological, and sociological knowledge, skill, and attitudes. A summary at the beginning of each chapter presents the findings and conclusions concerning all three aspects of the study: the effects of the GMC, the reasons for those effects, and the individual differences among students. Details are given within each chapter.

The introductory summaries also indicate the extent to which the test and other procedures allow confidence in the conclusions. Therefore, each single result is discussed in the text with a minimum of qualification, in order to avoid repetition. More important, however, is the fact that, owing to the organization of the research, conclusions mentioned in the summary are often *structural* in nature. That is, they depend more on the relations among the data drawn from all sources than on the dependability of any single result. Thus, the degree of confidence placed in any conclusion is a function of the extent to which data from several sources confirm one another.

Because Chapters 16 through 23 present the detailed results of the research project, it is in these chapters that the problem of addressing two different audiences most keenly makes itself felt. The critical aspect of this problem lies in the presentation of the basic data. Many readers, more interested in results than procedures, will doubtless feel that the significance of a finding is often lost because too many data are provided; others, more interested in procedures, will feel that too often results are reported without adequate supporting data—in spite of the fact that there are over three hundred tables in this book. The compromise which was reached will, of course, be as satisfactory to the reader as it reflects his special interest.

The following rules were adopted regarding the inclusion of data.

All basic data pertaining to the effects of the GMC are presented. The rules for including data concerning the study of the characteristics of the two programs (the independent variables) were more complex, however. The only basic data regularly presented are those concerning the physician observer's ratings of the individual teaching conferences. The basic data concerning the psychologist's analyses of the conferences are not presented because statistical analysis of these data indicated that there was no difference in the teaching provided in the two programs. The physician observer's ratings, although not susceptible to statistical test, are presented in detail because they provide interesting and informative material. The basic data concerning students' responses to questionnaire items are always presented because of the relative ease of reproducing such questions for comparative purposes. The basic data concerning the effects of special educational techniques employed by the GMC are not included simply because of the large number of tables this would require. All relations between the special educational techniques of the GMC and students' responses were analyzed by means of 2 x 2 tables with (ordinarily) median breaks. Only those relations which met a .05 probability level are discussed in the text. The frequency distributions relating to the special educational techniques of the GMC are presented in Appendix 6.

The rule concerning inclusion of the basic data pertaining to individual differences was that only those relations which reached the .05 probability level are presented—although certain results which do not meet this criterion are discussed as *tendencies*. Basic data in the form of correlation coefficients, or tables, are provided only when an important point requires the data as a part of the explanation (see, for example, the discussion of the relations between academic ability, participation in the GMC, and attitude change, in Chapter 18). It would have been preferable to report the basic data for all findings presented. However, some selection had to be made in order to keep the size of the book within appropriate limits.

A word should be said about tests of significance. *No claims of inductive generality can be made for any of these findings.* Generality can be established only on the basis of random sampling. The subjects in this study cannot be thought of as random samples of any population or universe. If, however, one considers a given class to be a population, and the members of the four subgroups to be selected at random within this finite population (which they were), then it is possible to test any set of results to discover whether it could reasonably be accounted for on the basis of random sampling within the class. This reasoning was applied to the results of the comparison of the four subgroups—the (experimental) GMC group, the (control) medical clerkship group, and the two surgery groups—and appropriate significance tests were used in the class of 1954. However, on subsequent occasions the usual tests of significance (without correction for further sampling) were applied. This procedure resulted in a bias in the direction of accepting the null hypothesis when it was in fact false. However, as stated in Chapter 10, there is little interest in educational innovations which produce only minor effects, detectable only by refined statistical procedures. More important is the fact that the organization of the project with its three forms of inquiry made it possible to interrelate several different types of results. Thus, the confidence placed in any interpretation was not a function of the likelihood of replication of any single result, but rather a function of the plausibility of such an interpretation. As mentioned above, however, tests of significance were used, but these were considered simply screening devices—used merely through force of tradition, not necessity.

Chapter 16

Medical Knowledge

Summary

This chapter is concerned with the question of what effect the General Medical Clinic Program had on the students' acquisition of traditional medical knowledge, why the GMC had the effect it did, and which individual attributes of students were associated with the acquisition of medical knowledge.[1]

Any effort to increase the scope of the education of the senior medical student will inevitably raise the question of whether the change will adversely affect his acquisition of traditional medical knowledge. It is quite clear that participation in the GMC did not adversely affect acquisition of medical knowledge, although students were quite convinced that they were penalized in this respect. Analysis of the teaching conferences indicates that the GMC student learned as much about medicine as the control student because medical knowledge was given equal emphasis by the staff in each program. Moreover, the activities of the two groups of students (as reported by them) were highly similar. In fact, if one were not looking for differences between the two programs, the similarities would be striking.

The GMC student's impression that he received inadequate training in medicine stemmed directly from his feeling that he saw too few patients with specific organic illnesses, and instead saw too many patients with vague complaints. Apparently the GMC student did see fewer patients with specific diagnoses than the control student did, but the fact remains that the GMC student's acquisition of medical knowledge was not impaired. To what extent a senior medical student should see patients with acute illnesses is evidently a matter which needs

[1] The explanation in this chapter is somewhat more detailed than in those which follow. The outlines of all chapters are identical.

further study; faculty, students, and test data presently provide different answers to this question.

This study indicates that a student's individual attributes were not significantly related to gain in medical knowledge. Although it is quite clear that previous academic performance was closely related to initial (Pretest) scores, gain in medical knowledge was not found to be related to measures of individual attributes. On the other hand, it will be recalled that characteristics of the teaching conference were found to be related to gain in medical knowledge (see Chapter 14). Thus it appears that the acquisition of medical knowledge in the senior year is mainly a function of the teaching the student receives from his instructors. Since the teaching as well as the students' activities in the two programs were found to be similar, it is not surprising that both groups of students gained the same amount of medical knowledge.

Because the results from independent operations confirm one another, the above conclusions seem to be firm ones.

Dependent Variables (Effects of the GMC)

One of the most important questions—possibly the most important single question—that the research group was called on to answer was whether or not the GMC Program, in aiming at goals broader than those of the traditional medical program, involved any sacrifice of the student's acquisition of knowledge about medicine.

In attempting to answer this question, the research group utilized two approaches. The first approach was objective: quantitative tests of medical knowledge were devised and administered to both the experimental and the control groups, before and after their respective clerkship experiences. In this way objective data for six pairs of groups were obtained. It was felt, however, that to limit this phase of the investigation to the compilation and analysis of objective test data reflecting quantitative change in medical knowledge would be a somewhat superficial method of treating a complex problem of major importance. Therefore, questionnaires were developed to ascertain the students' subjective evaluations of their own proficiency in medical knowledge, of the effectiveness of the two programs in enhancing this proficiency, and of certain other related factors.

OBJECTIVE TEST DATA

Table 16.1 summarizes the principal results of the pretest-posttest comparisons between the GMC and control groups with respect to the acquisition of medical knowledge. Of the six comparisons between the GMC and control students, three show the GMC group to have made the greater gain, and three show the control group to have made

Table 16.1. Mean percentage increase in Medical Knowledge scores from pretest to posttest, and difference in gain (classes of 1954, 1955, and 1956)

	1954 I	1955 I	1956 I	1954 II	1955 II	1956 II
GMC	7.32	7.35	7.39	5.61	10.89	0.25
Control	3.28	3.33	5.23	7.45	13.50	1.17
Difference in gain	4.04*	4.02*	2.16	1.84	2.61	0.92

* *t*-test significance $< .05$.

the greater gain.[2] However, in two of the instances in which the GMC group made the greater gain (1954 I and 1955 I) the differences in gain were markedly larger than in the other four. The 1954 I GMC group's gain was 4.04 percentage points more than that of the corresponding control group, and the 1955 I GMC group's gain was 4.02 percentage points more than that of the corresponding control group. All other differences were less than 3 percentage points.

The data summarized in Table 16.1 to facilitate presentation of the comparisons between the GMC and control students are given in greater detail in Table 16.2, where the mean increase in Medical Knowledge scores from Pretest to Posttest I (first-half groups) and from Posttest I to Posttest II (second-half groups), the standard deviations, and the number of students in each of the twelve groups (four clerkship groups in both halves of the three years) are presented. The question arises of whether the differences among the means of the four clerkship groups are merely the result of random sampling, or whether they indicate real differences among the groups with respect to gain in medical knowledge. To evaluate the role of chance in the differences obtained among the means, a statistical test (t) was made of the hypothesis that the differences would occur by chance. Whenever the results of the statistical test indicated that random sampling could not account for the differences in gain among the four groups (as in the 1954 I and 1955 I groups) the differences between particular *pairs* of means were evaluated by the t-test. Thus it was found that the differences between the mean increase for the GMC 1954 I group and the other 1954 I groups were significant at the .05 level of confidence. It was concluded, therefore, that the GMC students' greater gain in medical knowledge was not an accident due to random sampling. The same result was obtained for the 1955 I groups; the GMC students' greater gain was not due to mere sampling fluctuations. The remaining differences among the clerkships could have occurred by chance.

[2] It should be noted that the GMC I groups lead in all three years, whereas the reverse is true for all the GMC II groups. This phenomenon is discussed in Chapter 25.

Table 16.2. Means and standard deviations for increase in Medical Knowledge scores (classes of 1954, 1955, and 1956)

	1954			1955			1956		
	No.	Mean increase	Standard deviation	No.	Mean increase	Standard deviation	No.	Mean increase	Standard deviation
First-half									
GMC	19	7.32	8.17	20	7.35	9.55	18	7.39	10.40
Control	20	3.28	5.82	18	3.33	9.97	13	5.23	14.13
Surgery I	19	0.16	5.30	*	*	*	17	5.65	11.00
Surgery II	21	1.68	8.12	17	0.59	11.50	17	0.53	9.74
Second-half									
GMC	19	5.61	8.78	9	10.89	10.05	16	0.25	20.56
Control	21	7.45	6.60	8	13.50	11.01	18	1.17	15.98
Surgery I	20	0.71	7.25	19	0.32	12.19	15	5.60	14.25
Surgery II	19	3.00	7.42	19	4.79	11.92	16	5.62	14.51

* Data not available due to test revisions.

The intention of the GMC staff to broaden the traditional disciplinary limits of medicine, then, did not result in penalizing the GMC students with respect to their acquisition of medical knowledge. In fact, on the two occasions when non-chance differences occurred between the two groups, these differences favored the GMC.

QUESTIONNAIRE DATA

In addition to objective test data, the answers to three questions were analyzed in order to discover how the students evaluated the effectiveness of the experimental program. Specifically, an effort was made to learn how the GMC and control students rated their clerkships, how they rated their own proficiency, and how important they thought it was to acquire more of the basic facts of clinical medicine.

It is interesting to learn that the GMC students' evaluation of the helpfulness of their clerkship with regard to the acquisition of the basic facts of clinical medicine was at variance with the results obtained from the objective test data reported above. Table 16.3 shows the percentage of students who rated their clerkship as extremely or very helpful in acquiring medical knowledge. In all comparisons a larger percentage of control students than GMC students rated their

Table 16.3. Percentage of students rating their clerkship as extremely or very helpful in acquiring medical knowledge (classes of 1954, 1955, and 1956)

	1954 I	1954 II	1955 I	1955 II	1956 I	1956 II
GMC	38	32	*	30	45	12
Control	*	*	*	55	77	77

* No data.

Table 16.4. Change in percentage of students rating themselves above average in medical knowledge (1955 II, 1956 I and II)

	1955 II			1956 I			1956 II		
	Post I	Post II	Change	Pre	Post I	Change	Post I	Post II	Change
GMC	*	65	*	17	45	*28*	37	25	*—12*
Control	*	33	*	15	38	*23*	39	39	*0*
Surgery I	*	*	*	0	30	*30*	53	67	*14*
Surgery II	*	47	*	0	47	*47*	31	38	*7*

* No data.

clerkship as extremely or very helpful. However, there were no significant differences between the groups with respect to change in the percentage of students who rated themselves above average in proficiency in medical knowledge (see Table 16.4), nor were there significant differences in the ratings of the importance of medical knowledge (see Table 16.5).

To summarize, the results indicate that the intention of the GMC staff to broaden the educational program did not result in penalizing the GMC students with respect to their acquisition of medical knowledge. GMC and control students made virtually equal scores on the test of medical knowledge. However, the GMC students thought they had been penalized (they would have said the test results were wrong). But, although they were unaware of it, the GMC students' evaluations of their own proficiency supported the test results.

Independent Variables (Reasons for the Effects of the GMC)

This section deals with the problem of why the GMC Program affected the students' medical knowledge as reported above. The GMC students were in an educational situation intended to introduce psychological and sociological material in addition to and, to a certain extent,

Table 16.5. Change in percentage of students rating acquisition of more of the basic facts of clinical medicine as extremely or very important (1955 II, 1956 I and II)

	1955 II		1956 I			1956 II		
	Post II	Change	Pre	Post I	Change	Post I	Post II	Change
GMC	82	*	94	83	*—11*	88	82	*—6*
Control	66	*	77	69	*—8*	89	73	*—16*
Surgery I	*	*	89	83	*—6*	80	80	*0*
Surgery II	99	*	89	94	*5*	75	69	*—6*

* No data.

in place of traditional medical material. Yet the GMC students learned as much about traditional medicine as the control students. Why? Both groups of students, however, felt that the GMC students did not acquire as much medical knowledge as the control students. Why?

In an effort to answer these questions, analyses were made of the following: student-staff conferences in both programs; students' reports of their clerkship activities; students' reports of their general clerkship experience; the relation between the special educational techniques employed by the GMC and scores on the test of medical knowledge; the staff's evaluation of students; interviews with students, and diaries kept by students; and interviews with the faculty.

Results from all the above studies point in the same direction—both groups of students received essentially the same education with respect to traditional medical knowledge. The principal difference between the two clerkships (insofar as medical knowledge is concerned) occurred with respect to the GMC students' evaluation of the patients they saw; GMC students were highly dissatisfied with the teaching value of their patients.

Analysis of the teaching conferences

One major effort in the research project was to study the interaction between the student and his teacher in the conference in which the student presented his work-up of the patient to the instructor. Approximately two hundred teaching conferences were sound-recorded and analyzed by one of the research psychologists. Also, 34 students were interviewed concerning particular student-staff conferences on at least three occasions. (The procedure by which these recordings and interviews were analyzed has been presented in Chapter 14.) Comparisons were made between the 1956 I GMC students and the 1956 I and II control students, as well as between the combined 1956 I and II GMC and control groups. Statistical tests of the differences between groups were made by means of the Chi-squared test. The number of students included in the Post-Conference Interview and Teaching Conference Record analyses is presented in Table 16.6.

Table 16.6. Number of students included in Teaching Conference Record and Post-Conference Interview comparisons (class of 1956)

	1956 I		1956 II		Total	
	GMC	Control	GMC	Control	GMC	Control
Teaching Conference Record	10	8	9	10	19	18
Post-Conference Interview	8	6	9	11	17	17

In the main, no differences were discovered between the teaching of the GMC staff and of the control staff in the teaching conferences. This result suggests that insofar as teaching has any effect on the acquisition of medical knowledge (and in Chapter 14 it was demonstrated that teaching did have an effect) one would not expect differences between the GMC and control groups with respect to gain in medical knowledge from pretest to posttest. Consistent differences were not obtained.

The minor differences which were noted in the staff's teaching suggested that the teachers in the control clinic tended to introduce more new facts about the patients and to be more exact about the specific relation of these facts to others.

There were no differences between the experimental and control groups with respect to the manner in which the students thought about their patients' (strictly medical) problems and presented them to their teachers. The students (on the average) presented the same number of medical facts and interrelated these facts to the same degree.

As pointed out in Chapter 14, the physician who carried out the initial steps in the analysis of the Teaching Conference Records also rated each conference on several scales. Ninety-nine GMC and 76 control teaching conferences were rated. The physician rating the conference was not told from which teaching program the record was obtained. The mean rating of students on medical knowledge was identical for both programs: 3.9 on a seven-point scale. In virtually all conferences (97.8% GMC and 100% control) the physician observer found that the staff devoted attention to knowledge of the basic facts of clinical medicine. Only slight differences were found between the two groups with respect to the depth to which the teacher carried the problem (see Table 16.7). Moreover, the ratings of the conferences concerning the teaching value of the patients were virtually identical for the two programs (see Table 16.8). And, although there seemed to be somewhat more variability in the ratings of the helpfulness of GMC teaching than control teaching, these ratings also indicated that

Table 16.7. Rating of staff with respect to their analysis of problems associated with basic facts of clinical medicine

	Percentage of conferences		
	Staff only recognized problem	Staff explored problem	Staff went to core of problem
GMC ($N = 90$)	34.4	53.3	12.2
Control ($N = 75$)	32.0	48.0	20.0

Table 16.8. Rating of teaching conferences with respect to degree to which patients' medical problems were potentially stimulating to students

	Percentage of conferences						
	Negative effect on stimulation	Stimulating	Slightly	Somewhat	Moderately	Very	Extremely
GMC ($N = 90$)	2.0	5.1	18.2	39.4	31.3	4.0	0.0
Control ($N = 76$)	2.6	3.9	19.7	32.9	36.8	3.9	0.0

the teaching in the two programs was highly similar (see Table 16.9).

In brief, analysis of the Teaching Conference Records and Post-Conference Interviews by the research psychologist, and ratings of the conferences by the physician observer, confirm one another and serve to explain why the two groups of students did not differ with respect to the acquisition of medical knowledge: teaching of medical knowledge in the student-staff conferences was essentially identical.

STUDENTS' REPORTS OF ACTIVITIES ENGAGED IN

Students in the class of 1956 were presented with a list of 59 different "activities" (see Appendix 4) and asked to indicate on a seven-point scale the extent to which a particular activity was "present" in the clerkship just completed. For example, students were asked to indicate whether following patients for several months was an activity that was "never present, seldom present . . . always present" in the clerkship just completed.

Comparison of the responses of the GMC and control students provided an interesting insight into the GMC students' dissatisfaction with the GMC as a situation in which to gain (traditional) medical knowledge. Moreover, this comparison suggested the reason for the GMC students' underestimation of their medical knowledge. Table

Table 16.9. Rating of teaching conferences with respect to their helpfulness to students' learning about organic medicine

	Percentage of conferences						
	A hindrance	Not helpful	Slightly	Somewhat	Moderately	Very	Extremely
GMC ($N = 99$)	0.0	6.1	25.2	30.3	27.3	10.1	1.0
Control ($N = 76$)	0.0	3.9	18.4	43.4	22.4	7.9	3.9

Table 16.10. Percentage of students indicating that certain activities were very frequently or always present in their clerkship (class of 1956)

	1956 I		1956 II	
	GMC	Control	GMC	Control
Working with diagnostic problems	28	54	6	44
Seeing a wide variety of illnesses	17	77	0	50
Seeing unusual pathological conditions	6	62	0	45
Having patients with definite pathology	12	46	6	39

16.10 presents the percentage of students indicating that certain activities were frequently or always present in their clerkship. Far fewer GMC students than control students felt that they very frequently worked with diagnostic problems, saw a wide variety of illnesses, saw unusual pathological conditions, or had patients with definite pathology. These data indicate why the students felt that the GMC group learned less than the control group; the activities which the GMC students felt were not frequently present are also the activities which both groups felt were important. (Data concerning the latter point are presented in Chapter 25.)

The data in Table 16.11 suggest that the students performed equally well on the test of medical knowledge because they engaged in highly similar activities.

Table 16.11. Percentage of students indicating that certain activities were very frequently or always present in their clerkships (class of 1956)

	1956 I		1956 II	
	GMC	Control	GMC	Control
Having responsibility for diagnosis of patients	45	62	32	39
Having responsibility for treatment of patients	50	46	44	33
Having opportunities for consultation with medical specialties	62	70	25	61
Having staff supervision time readily available	39	30	44	44
Having a high quality of staff supervision	72	61	56	50
Having specific staff suggestions for the interpretation of symptoms and treatment	67	61	57	55
Learning the amount and dosage schedule for specific therapies	50	62	50	77
Learning the principles of therapy	66	61	32	55
Developing physical examination skills	50	77	76	67
Developing skill in history taking	61	69	88	61
Handling medical problems of patients	72	93	63	50
Doing laboratory procedures	17	8	25	6
Following the latest medical advances in books and journals	50	39	57	44
Handling routine medical problems	78	54	44	39

Table 16.12. Percentage of students rating their staff as extremely or very proficient in medical knowledge (1955 II, 1956 I and II)

	1955 II	1956 I	1956 II
GMC	88	84	32
Control	78	76	72
Surgery I	—	47	87
Surgery II	64	70	69

STUDENTS' REPORTS OF GENERAL CLERKSHIP EXPERIENCE

Students in all four clerkships were asked to evaluate their teachers' proficiency in medical knowledge and helpfulness in acquiring medical knowledge. Regarding proficiency, a larger percentage of GMC than control students in the 1955 II and 1956 I groups rated their staff as extremely or very proficient, but the reverse was true for the 1956 II group (see Table 16.12). Regarding helpfulness, in the 1956 I group a larger percentage of students in the GMC than in any other clerkship rated their staff as extremely or very helpful, but in the 1956 II group a smaller percentage of students in the GMC than in any other clerkship rated their staff as extremely or very helpful (see Table 16.13).

It is quite evident that the 1956 I GMC students' evaluations of their teachers were different from the evaluations of the 1956 II GMC group. In only one other clerkship (Surgery I) was such a marked variation noted. This difference in students' attitudes between first and second halves is discussed in Chapter 25.

It should be noted also that a far smaller proportion of GMC than control students believed that their patients were helpful teaching material (see Table 16.14). The patients in the GMC did differ from those in the control clinic. A comparison of patients in the two clinics revealed that GMC patients were older, came from lower socioeconomic backgrounds, and displayed fewer clear-cut disease entities that would respond positively to therapy. These characteristics of patients were among those most frequently listed as descriptive of patients that students disliked to deal with. There were, in short, important differences between the patient populations, and these differences ap-

Table 16.13. Percentage of students rating their staff as extremely or very helpful in acquiring medical knowledge (class of 1956)

	1956 I	1956 II
GMC	78	19
Control	61	67
Surgery I	30	73
Surgery II	53	44

Table 16.14. Percentage of students rating their patients as extremely or very helpful in acquiring medical knowledge (class of 1956)

	1956 I	1956 II
GMC	39	19
Control	85	77
Surgery I	64	94
Surgery II	82	82

parently led GMC students to believe they were not being provided with good teaching material. (See Chapters 4 and 5 for a description of GMC patients.)

The data shown in Table 16.15 support this contention. A larger percentage of GMC than control students reported "quite a lot" and "very much" reading about internal medicine—particularly during the second half of the year. If the GMC students did indeed feel (as they reported) that their clerkship did not provide them with adequate learning experience, it is reasonable to suppose they would try to supplement their clinic experience by additional reading.

The GMC students' evaluations of their staff and patients with respect to helpfulness in acquiring medical knowledge indicate that it was the GMC students' dissatisfaction with their patients (and their staff during the latter half of the year) which led them to believe that they were not as proficient as the control students.

Special educational techniques of the GMC

The GMC included various techniques intended to help students become good physicians: the Family and Home Care Program, continuity of care, large responsibility for patients, comprehensive study of individual patients, stress on the "clinic team" approach, ready access to psychiatric consultation about patients, ready access to consultation with social workers and public health nurse, and emphasis on the physician-patient relation.

Records were kept of the extent to which each GMC student participated in each of the above activities (see Appendix 6), for participation depended to a large extent on the volition of the student. Re-

Table 16.15. Percentage of students reporting "quite a lot" or "very much" reading about internal medicine (class of 1956)

	1956 I	1956 II
GMC	66	75
Control	61	39
Surgery I	18	40
Surgery II	6	0

lations between the amount of participation and change in knowledge, skill, and attitudes were studied in the classes of 1955 and 1956. No positive relations were discovered between participation in any of the special educational techniques and gain in medical knowledge within the GMC group. On the other hand, there was no indication that participation in these activities retarded the students' acquisition of medical knowledge. Consequently, these results are congruent with the finding that the two groups did not differ in acquisition of medical knowledge.

Staff's evaluation of students

The medical staff intended to evaluate the GMC students' performance with respect to knowledge, skill, and attitudes in relation to the psychological and social, as well as the purely medical, aspects of medical care. It is significant that the results of a special study (presented in detail in Chapter 24) show that the staff did not do so. The medical staff evaluated students solely on the basis of the students' medical knowledge. This finding is congruent with the fact that GMC students did not differ from the control students with respect to gain in medical knowledge, that the GMC and control teaching conferences were highly similar, and that both groups of students reported similar activities.

Interviews with students

All students (with the exception of the class of 1956) were interviewed by members of the research staff at each testing period. Most of the class of 1956 were interviewed at various times throughout the school year. The interview material makes it clear that both GMC and control students definitely believed that GMC students did not see enough patients who were "really" sick. Whatever the source of their information, a larger number of control than GMC students were convinced of this. Moreover, both groups had the impression that other departments of the hospital acted to aggravate what they believed to be an already serious lack of good teaching material. For example, one student asserted that certain members of the hospital staff "deliberately referred old crocks" to the GMC. Another student remarked: "I would like to supply you with a direct quote from a surgical resident in the emergency room, 'This patient is an old crock. Let's send him over to the General Medical Clinic; that's all they want over there.'"

Another student reported that "the residents and the interns on the wards consider GMC a clinic they only send people to when you can't do anything for them anywhere else. This attitude, which persists on the ward, is the reason why this clinic hasn't done as well as I think it should have done. These residents take a patient, and if the patient has a good heart condition, they will send a patient to a cardiac clinic. If this patient—and I've seen both of these things happen, by the way—if this patient happens to be a patient with multiple complaints of nervousness or anxiety, he gets shoved to General Medical Clinic. The same thing happens in the emergency room. One of my buddies out here—he had a fight with the resident one day to get a patient to come to this clinic. The patient had kidney stones. He said, 'I would like to see this patient in this clinic.' The resident said, 'Well, he has kidney stones, he belongs to the urology clinic.' My buddy said, 'There is no reason why we can't treat patients with kidney stones too.' He had to fight to get the patient to come to the General Medical Clinic."[3]

INTERVIEWS WITH GMC STAFF

The twelve members of the GMC staff (as of May 1956) were interviewed by a member of the research staff. The interviews were from one to two hours in length and were recorded; the records became anonymous.

Most of the staff felt that the students had received adequate medical training. However, all but two members agreed with the (by then) well-known complaints of the students that the GMC patients did not provide a wide enough variety of illnesses and specific pathological conditions. An excerpt from an interview with a GMC instructor who saw the problem in much the same way as the students did is presented below:

Q: What do you think about teaching "comprehensive care" to senior medical students?

A: I think it's very difficult. I'm not sure that the students are always as satisfied as if they were in a little different teaching situation. Perhaps a different plan, in which everyone is exposed to half and half [half clinics—half GMC] might be a reasonable compromise. The students might need both kinds of teaching. It seems to me that if we had enough time and enough of the right kind of patients to present to the student as much organic illness as represents an immediate challenge to his knowledge of specific problems there would be no gripe. But because many of the patients in this type of clinic represent a more custodial type of medical care, the students do not feel much challenge. They feel they are not seeing enough problems to determine whether or not they know how to solve them. It is a grave problem for a student who is very insecure. He wants to see everything, in case he should miss something he will need next week. He is afraid that next week he'll have a case of some exotic disease and he will not know how to handle it because he has never seen one. Perhaps this is a legitimate gripe on the student's part; perhaps it really represents only a manifestation of his own insecurity. He feels that if he sees everything in his medical school train-

[3] See Chapter 1 for a description of the role of the GMC in the hospital.

ing, he will be able to handle everything. The uncertainties of medicine are a lot more prominent in his thinking at this time. Actually, what happens is that he cannot see everything, because disease, like everything else, changes; and when the time comes that he is presented with a problem, he may have had no concrete example of this problem with which he has dealt previously. Pedagogically speaking, I am sure that really teaching people how to solve problems in general is the best principle. On the other hand, it is less satisfactory for the student's peace of mind than if he knows he has coped with a lot of different problems. Since the students feel that the GMC patients do not present a wide variety of organic illnesses, they feel they are not being taught as well as if they saw many different organic problems. Actually, it is probably much better to learn how to solve problems in general. But, as far as the students are concerned, they want to know they have handled specific things and have specific information, rather than general things and information. I think you could probably argue it both ways. If the time could be split so that the students were not exposed to GMC-type care and patients only, but saw both specialty clinic and GMC patients, that combination might ease the problem a little in their minds. I think next year the program will be better than it has been so far. I think the student should be dealing with both kinds of problems, but in a clinic such as this, you don't have any choice. We cannot throw the patient out because he doesn't have a specific organic illness; whereas, in a specialty clinic, only the patients with heart disease appear in the heart clinic, and when the student is exposed to heart clinic he sees people with heart disease.

Q: Do you think the student sees enough organic illness in GMC?

A: I can't answer that; the students say "no." This is a common gripe. I'm not at all sure that enough is not seen. I do not think there is ever enough to satisfy the student. He always wants to see more, always has a tremendous sense of insecurity, or, he reacts the other way and thinks he can handle everything, not realizing, in his own ignorance, his inadequacies. The common thing is to feel: "Well, I've handled this kind of a heart, but I don't know if I can handle that kind of a heart." The student feels inadequate. I think that in medical school, if possible, it would be better to turn out a student who felt more adequate, even though I'm not sure that is a primary function of medical education. I think it would be desirable if the students felt better prepared to face their work.

Q: You are not sure in your own mind, then, whether they do or do not see enough. . . .

A: No, I'm not sure. I am inclined to think that it would be desirable for them to see more. Yet, I'm also certain from the conversations I've had with those who have left the GMC and have gone into internship that there is apparently no significant difference [from conventionally trained fellow-interns] in their *ability* to handle problems, once they are exposed to the problems of internship.

To summarize, this section dealt with the answers to two questions: Why did the GMC students acquire as much medical knowledge as the control students, and why did the GMC students mistakenly believe they had not? Information obtained from various analyses strongly suggested that the GMC students learned as much about medicine as the control students because there was equal emphasis in both programs on teaching the organic aspects of medical care. The students to a large extent participated in highly similar activities, and, moreover, those activities specific to the GMC were unrelated to changes in scores on the test of medical knowledge. GMC students mistakenly believed they had not acquired as much medical knowledge as their peers primarily because they felt they had not seen as many patients who were acutely ill or as wide a variety of pathological conditions as the control students.

Individual Attributes Related to Medical Knowledge

The previous two sections dealt with the differences between *groups* and the reasons for these differences (or lack of them). This section concerns itself with the differences among *individuals* within these groups and how these individual differences were related both to initial (Pretest) scores and to changes in scores on the various measures. For example, was the acquisition of medical knowledge in the senior year related primarily to certain personality variables or primarily to academic ability? Was gain in medical knowledge a function of one personality trait in the GMC and of a different one in the control clerkship? Should it be found that one type of student profited most from the GMC and another type from the traditional medical clerkship, such information would be of considerable importance.

The order of presentation of findings concerning individual attributes is the same in all eight chapters of Part IV. First, the results concerning the relation between individual attributes and scores on the Pretest are reported for the entire class; second, findings concerning the relations between individual attributes and change from Pretest to Posttest I (first half of the year) and from Posttest I to Posttest II (second half of the year) are reported for the entire class. Next the relations between individual attributes and change from Pretest to Posttest I and from Posttest I to Posttest II are reported separately for each clerkship. Relations between individual attributes and Pretest scores are not reported for each clerkship group separately because these computations were not made. Although such information is always desirable, it was decided to expend resources in other directions. Thus, the sections on results pertaining to the GMC and results pertaining to the control group deal only with *change*, not with initial (Pretest) scores.

Results pertaining to the entire class. Medical Knowledge Pretest scores were correlated to some extent with virtually every other index of the students' academic ability at the Pretest administration in the classes of 1954 and 1955 (see Table 16.16). Students who had high scores on the MCAT, who obtained good grades in previous courses,

Table 16.16. Personal attributes correlated to a statistically significant degree ($p < .05$) with the Medical Knowledge Pretest (classes of 1954 and 1955)

Class of 1954 ($N = 79$)		Class of 1955 ($N = 70$)	
+.34	First-year grade average	+.35	Verbal Ability (MCAT)
+.52	Second-year grade average	+.29	Quantitative Ability (MCAT)
+.48	Cumulative grade average	+.30	Knowledge of Modern Society (MCAT)
+.36	Third-year grade average	+.34	Knowledge of Premedical Sciences (MCAT)
+.47	Competence as a physician (peer judgment)	+.35	Premedical grade average
+.36	Willingness and ability to work independently (peer judgment)	+.58	First-year grade average
+.59	Junior comprehensive examination	+.59	Second-year grade average
		+.44	Third-year grade average
		+.60	Cumulative grade average
		+.32	Grade in psychosomatics course
		+.29	Junior medical clerkship grade
		+.25	Junior pediatrics clerkship grade
		+.30	Junior OB-GYN clerkship grade
		+.34	Junior surgical clerkship grade
		—.28	Number of undergraduate credit hours in psychology
		+.30	Competence as a physician (peer judgment)
		+.41	Willingness and ability to work independently (peer judgment)
		+.27	Leadership (peer judgment)
		+.24	Sympathy to concept of comprehensive care (peer judgment)
		+.31	Aesthetic value

and who were well thought of by their peers were those who scored high on the Medical Knowledge test. Scores on this test, however, were not correlated with any of these indices at the Pretest administration in the class of 1956. No firm explanation of this difference can be made (but see Chapter 10 for further discussion of the class of 1956).

The fact that there were no relations of consequence between other measures (e.g., personality measures or attitude measures) and the Medical Knowledge test in any of the three classes studied was somewhat surprising.[4]

Because students were tested on medical knowledge at the beginning of the senior year (Pretest), at the end of the first half of the year (Posttest I), and at the end of the second half of the year (Posttest II), it was possible to study the relation of various personal attributes

[4] It is also of interest to note that the GMC staff's evaluations of students were related to measures of the students' academic ability only; they were not related to personality measures (see Chapter 24).

to gain in medical knowledge by comparing the differences in students' scores on each test administration and relating these differences to such measures as previous grade averages, peer judgments, etc.

There were no consistent relations between any of the measures of individual attributes used in this study and gain in medical knowledge in any of the three classes studied.

Results pertaining to the GMC. Peer judgments concerning medical knowledge were positively related to gain in medical knowledge from Posttest I to Posttest II in the 1956 GMC group. Although this finding, together with those data referring to peer judgments in Table 16.2, speak well for the keenness with which medical students evaluate one another, the authenticity of the evaluations they gave the research group, and the intrinsic value of students' evaluations of their peers, it does not shed much light on the type of student who acquired the most medical knowledge in the GMC.

Results pertaining to the control group. There were no consistent relations between measures of individual attributes and gain in medical knowledge from Posttest I to Posttest II in the 1956 control clerkship.

To summarize, Pretest scores on the Medical Knowledge test appeared to be entirely a function of previous academic performance. The measures of individual attributes employed in this study were, with only slight exception, unrelated to *gain* in medical knowledge during the senior year, regardless of whether the student participated in the GMC or the control clerkship. These findings indicate that the individual attributes studied in this project were unrelated to the acquisition of medical knowledge during the senior year.

Chapter 17

Medical Skill

Summary

In order to increase the student's skill in the application of knowledge (among other reasons) the GMC Program arranged for each student to see a patient for as many visits as the patient's problems required. To discover how well this effort succeeded, the research project developed a procedure for measuring a student's ability to integrate his knowledge of medicine with the facts about a patient and arrive at the correct answers about *that* patient's medical problems. The Medical Skill test required the student to use the information provided in the film and/or in the booklet of the Sound-Film Interview procedure, as well as his knowledge of medicine, to answer questions about the medical problems of the patient presented in the film.

Comparison of the GMC and control students with respect to the acquisition of medical skill revealed the same pattern of findings as the comparison with respect to the acquisition of medical knowledge. The experimental program neither impaired nor enhanced the students' acquisition of medical skill, although the students felt that participation in the GMC interfered with their efforts to acquire medical skill. And, as in the case of medical knowledge, it appeared that the GMC students acquired as much medical skill as the control students because equal emphasis was placed on this topic in both programs. Also, GMC students did not consider their patients valuable teaching material insofar as medical skill was concerned.

However, some of the special educational features of the GMC seemed to have important results. Greater participation in these special features, such as assuming more responsibility, led to greater appreciation of their importance.

That the GMC may have provided a different atmosphere from the control medical clerkship is indicated by the finding that the more docile, reticent student gained more medical skill in the GMC, while the more aggressive outgoing student made the greater gain in medical skill in the control clerkship.

The findings presented in this chapter must be treated with considerable caution because of the weaknesses of the test of medical skill.

Dependent Variables (Effects of the GMC)

There were two occasions (at the end of the first and second halves of 1956) on which it was possible to compare the effects of the GMC with the effects of the control medical clerkship and the surgery clerkship. On each occasion, the differences between the groups were such that they were attributable to random sampling.[1] Table 17.1 indicates the similarity of test results obtained by students in the GMC and control programs. Table 17.2 presents the results in more detail for all three clerkships.

In addition, the effect of the experimental program was evaluated in terms of the students' judgments of the helpfulness of their clerkships, of their own proficiency, and of the importance they attributed to two topics: applying the facts of organic medicine to clinical practice, and learning to organize diagnostic and therapeutic regimes. The students' responses to questions concerning their confidence in their ability to handle problems involving medical skill are also presented below.

The students' responses revealed a pattern similar to that found for medical knowledge. As can be seen in Tables 17.3 and 17.4, a smaller percentage of GMC than control students rated their clerkship as extremely or very helpful with respect both to applying the facts of organic medicine and to organizing diagnostic and therapeutic regimes. It is interesting in this connection to note that one surgery group followed the same pattern.

There were no significant differences between the GMC and control groups with respect to change in the percentage of students who rated as above average their own proficiency in applying their knowledge and in organizing diagnostic and therapeutic regimes (see Tables 17.5 and 17.6). Therefore, although the GMC students did not evaluate their clerkship as favorably as the control students evaluated theirs, it is important to note that, although they were not aware of it, the GMC students rated their own proficiency as high as the control students rated theirs.

[1] Comparisons of gain in medical skill were also made for the classes of 1954 and 1955. These data are not reported in detail because at that time the test of medical skill was not well enough developed to be useful.

Table 17.1. Change in medical skill from Pretest to Postest II (class of 1956)

	No. below median	No. above median	Total
GMC	17	17	34
Control	15	16	31
Total	32	33	65

Table 17.2. Difference between percentages of students expected and obtained in the high increase group: medical skill (class of 1956)

	Percentage expected	Percentage obtained	Difference
1956 I			
GMC ($N = 18$)	14	15	1
Control ($N = 13$)	10	9	—1
Surgery I ($N = 17$)	13	14	1
Surgery II ($N = 17$)	13	12	—1
1956 II			
GMC ($N = 16$)	12	15	3
Control ($N = 18$)	14	18	4
Surgery I ($N = 15$)	12	11	—1
Surgery II ($N = 16$)	12	6	—6

Because the form used in Table 17.2 for presenting the data will be used frequently in subsequent chapters, a brief explanation is offered here. There were 65 students in the class, of which 18 were in GMC. One half of the GMC students would, on the basis of chance, be expected to be in the group of students in the upper half of the score distribution (i.e., in the high increase group). One half of 18/65 equals .14, or 14% (see column 1). Actually, 15% of the GMC students were found to be in the upper half of the score distribution (see column 2). Thus, the discrepancy between the percentage expected on the basis of chance, and the percentage actually obtained in the high increase group was 1% (see column 3). The probability of obtaining a discrepancy of a given size by chance alone was calculated by means of the Chi-squared test. First- and second-half discrepancies were tested separately.

Table 17.3. Percentage of students rating their clerkship as extremely or very helpful in acquiring skill at applying the facts of organic medicine to clinical practice (1955 II, 1956 I and II)

	1955 II	1956 I	1956 II
GMC	41	61	31
Control	61	69	66
Surgery I	—	42	60
Surgery II	16	58	32

Table 17.4. Percentage of students rating their clerkship as extremely or very helpful in learning to organize diagnostic and therapeutic regimes (1955 II, 1956 I and II)

	1955 II	1956 I	1956 II
GMC	12	22	13
Control	39	15	33
Surgery I	—	6	13
Surgery II	5	47	6

Table 17.5. Change in percentage of students rating themselves above average in skill at applying the facts of organic medicine to clinical practice (1955 II, 1956 I and II)

	1955 II			1956 I			1956 II		
	Post I	Post II	Change	Pre	Post I	Change	Post I	Post II	Change
GMC	*	59	*	17	62	*45*	37	38	*1*
Control	*	45	*	8	61	*53*	33	44	*11*
Surgery I	*	—	*	6	24	*18*	73	53	*—20*
Surgery II	*	58	*	6	47	*41*	50	37	*—13*

* No data.

Table 17.6. Change in percentage of students rating themselves above average in knowing how to organize diagnostic and therapeutic regimes (1955 II, 1956 I and II)

	1955 II			1956 I			1956 II		
	Post I	Post II	Change	Pre	Post I	Change	Post I	Post II	Change
GMC	*	59	*	12	40	*28*	37	38	*1*
Control	*	61	*	16	61	*45*	33	33	*0*
Surgery I	*	—	*	6	35	*29*	46	67	*21*
Surgery II	*	52	*	0	35	*35*	50	31	*—19*

* No data.

Table 17.7. Change in percentage of students rating acquisition of skill at applying the facts of organic medicine to clinical practice as extremely or very important (1955 II, 1956 I and II)

	1955 II			1956 I			1956 II		
	Post I	Post II	Change	Pre	Post I	Change	Post I	Post II	Change
GMC	*	94	*	72	89	*17*	94	94	*0*
Control	*	78	*	77	69	*—8*	100	73	*—27*
Surgery I	*	—	*	95	95	*0*	80	87	*7*
Surgery II	*	79	*	82	100	*18*	81	82	*1*

* No data.

Table 17.8. Change in percentage of students rating learning to organize diagnostic and therapeutic regimes as extremely or very important (1955 II, 1956 I and II)

	1955 II			1956 I			1956 II		
	Post I	Post II	Change	Pre	Post I	Change	Post I	Post II	Change
GMC	*	88	*	88	83	*—5*	100	94	*—6*
Control	*	78	*	84	54	*—30*	94	78	*—16*
Surgery I	*	—	*	94	100	*6*	80	93	*13*
Surgery II	*	95	*	89	94	*5*	63	81	*18*

* No data.

More GMC students than control students continued to believe that acquiring skill at applying the facts of organic medicine to clinical practice was extremely or very important. As can be seen from Table 17.7, the percentage of GMC students rating this topic in this way increased or remained the same from pretest to posttest, whereas the percentage of control students so rating this topic decreased. The difference in change was statistically significant (at the .05 level of confidence) for the 1956 I and II students. The percentage of students rating learning to organize diagnostic and therapeutic regimes as extremely or very important decreased in both groups, but the decrease for the control clerkship was greater than that for the GMC—significantly so for the 1956 I students (see Table 17.8). In short, a larger proportion of GMC than control students evaluated medical skill highly.

There were no important or systematic differences between the GMC and control students in the amount of confidence they reported in their ability to deal with five problems involving medical skill.[2] Table 17.9 presents the change in the percentage of students who rated themselves as completely confident in their ability to handle these five problems.

To summarize, the GMC students in the class of 1956 performed as well as the control students on the objective test of medical skill. Also, their evaluations of themselves were as high as the control students', and they rated their confidence in their ability to deal with five problems involving medical skill as highly as did the control students. However, the GMC students did not evaluate the helpfulness of their clerkship in acquiring medical skill as highly as the control students evaluated theirs. This is the same pattern of results as that found in connection with medical knowledge and thereby strengthens the conclusion drawn from the former. Evidently, the experimental program neither impaired nor enhanced the acquisition of traditional medical knowledge and skill—although the students felt that the GMC had a deleterious effect.

Independent Variables (Reasons for the Effects of the GMC)

This section deals with the problems of why the GMC students acquired as much medical skill as the control students and why the students felt that GMC was less helpful in this respect than the control clerkship. These questions are similar to those discussed in relation to medical knowledge, and the same analyses were made in an attempt to answer them.

[2] One item, knowing what to do in an emergency, was an exception on one occasion (1955 II group).

Table 17.9. Change in percentage of students rating themselves as completely confident in their ability to deal with various problems (classes of 1955 and 1956)

	1955 I			1955 II			1956 I			1956 II		
	Pre	Post I	Change	Post I	Post II	Change	Pre	Post I	Change	Post I	Post II	Change
Knowing what to do in an emergency												
GMC	0	0	*0*	0	47	*47*	11	6	*—5*	0	6	*6*
Control	6	6	*0*	0	6	*6*	15	31	*16*	6	11	*5*
Being able to do a veni-puncture without difficulty												
GMC	60	55	*—5*	76	94	*18*	72	72	*0*	88	75	*—13*
Control	61	72	*11*	65	78	*13*	77	100	*23*	95	95	*0*
Having a doctor as a patient												
GMC	0	10	*10*	29	6	*—23*	17	11	*—6*	19	13	*—6*
Control	22	22	*0*	12	0	*—12*	8	23	*15*	17	17	*0*
Being able to make a diagnosis in a difficult case												
GMC	0	5	*5*	0	0	*0*	11	17	*6*	0	0	*0*
Control	6	0	*—6*	0	0	*0*	8	23	*15*	0	6	*6*
Deciding on appropriate medi-cation and dosage												
GMC	0	10	*10*	0	18	*18*	11	28	*17*	0	6	*6*
Control	6	28	*22*	6	17	*11*	15	23	*8*	17	22	*5*

ANALYSIS OF THE TEACHING CONFERENCES

The research psychologist's analysis of the teaching conferences revealed no differences in the teaching efforts in the two programs and no differences in the students' presentation of material to the staff.

The physician observer was able to rate almost every student's presentation (96% of 99 conferences in the GMC group, and 100% of 76 conferences in the control group) with respect to medical skill. As in the case of medical knowledge, the mean ratings of the two groups were virtually identical, and were at the mid-point of the seven-point rating scale (GMC = 4.0, control = 3.9).

The physician observer found that in virtually every conference in both programs the teacher devoted attention to the application of the facts of organic medicine to clinical practice. There was a very slight tendency for the GMC staff to go to the core of the problem less often than the control staff (see Table 17.10). There was, however, a slight tendency for the GMC staff to propose action related to the central aspect of patients' (organic) problems more frequently than the control staff, although the latter somewhat more often proposed action related to *both* central and peripheral aspects (see Table 17.11).

Both tables indicate, however, that there was little difference between the programs in the teaching of medical skill. Thus, the physician observer's ratings parallel the psychologist's analysis of the teaching conference. Apparently the application of medical knowledge was given equal emphasis by the instructors in each program.

STUDENTS' REPORTS OF ACTIVITIES ENGAGED IN

It will be recalled that both groups of students reported participating in highly similar activities, except for the fact that a smaller percentage of GMC students reported that they saw a wide variety of illnesses and specific organic illnesses (see Tables 16.10 and 16.11). One item, however, was not included in those lists because it so directly related to medical skill (see Table 17.12). Although a larger percentage of the 1956 I control students reported that they engaged in activities themselves, a smaller percentage of the 1956 II control students did so.

Table 17.10. Rating of staff with respect to their analysis of problems associated with application of the facts of organic medicine to clinical practice

	Percentage of conferences		
	Staff only recognized problem	Staff explored problem	Staff went to core of problem
GMC ($N = 91$)	42.8	46.2	11.0
Control ($N = 75$)	38.7	46.7	14.7

Table 17.11. Rating of staff with respect to relevance of action proposed by them to patients' medical (organic) problems

	Percentage of conferences			
	Not explicitly relevant	Related to peripheral aspects	Related to central aspects	Related to both aspects
GMC ($N = 90$)	5.6	16.7	60.0	17.8
Control ($N = 74$)	4.0	16.2	52.7	27.0

Table 17.12. Percentage of students indicating that engaging in activities rather than observing the staff was very frequently or always present in their clerkship (class of 1956)

	1956 I		1956 II	
	GMC	Control	GMC	Control
Engaging in activities yourself rather than observing the staff	45	77	63	55

Table 17.13. Percentage of students rating their staff as extremely or very helpful in acquiring medical skill (class of 1956)

	1956 I	1956 II
GMC	78	32
Control	77	61
Surgery I	30	86
Surgery II	64	44

Table 17.14. Percentage of students rating their staff as extremely or very proficient in medical skill (1955 II, 1956 I and II)

	1955 II	1956 I	1956 II
GMC	82	83	32
Control	72	69	78
Surgery I	—	47	87
Surgery II	58	59	63

Table 17.15. Percentage of students rating their patients as extremely or very helpful in acquiring medical skill (class of 1956)

	1956 I	1956 II
GMC	44	32
Control	85	72
Surgery I	42	87
Surgery II	82	82

Again, there seems to be little systematic difference between the GMC and control groups.

STUDENTS' REPORTS OF GENERAL CLERKSHIP EXPERIENCE

Both 1956 I groups rated their teachers almost identically, but in the 1956 II group a far smaller percentage of GMC students than control students believed their staff to be very or extremely helpful with respect to acquiring medical skill (see Table 17.13). And, as Table 17.14 indicates, a smaller percentage of GMC students in the 1956 II than in the 1956 I group had a high impression of the proficiency of the GMC staff. Moreover, a much smaller proportion of GMC than control students felt that the patients they saw were very or extremely helpful to them in acquiring medical skill (see Table 17.15).

It will be noted from Tables 17.13 and 17.14 that on one occasion only a small percentage of students rated the surgery staff and patients high on helpfulness, although a large proportion of students in the control clerkship rated their staff and patients as highly helpful on both occasions. This finding indicates that it cannot be assumed automatically that the reason for students' rating their clerkship low on helpfulness was the "comprehensive care" aspect of the GMC.

SPECIAL EDUCATIONAL TECHNIQUES OF THE GMC[3]

Several specific features of the GMC Program were found to be related to various aspects of medical skill. For example, those students in the 1956 I group who spent the greatest amount of time with their patients' families rated the GMC high on helpfulness with respect to acquiring skill in applying the facts of organic medicine to clinical practice. Those students who reported having a great deal of responsibility for the diagnosis and treatment of patients, and who reported that they had an opportunity to learn how to function as a member of a clinic team, were less anxious about ambiguous diagnostic problems after the GMC experience than before.

It is important to note that those GMC students with the smallest number of broken appointments, and those who reported having an opportunity to learn how to function as a member of a clinic team, reported that after their GMC experience they believed that having responsibility for patients was more important than they had believed it to be prior to entering the GMC. These results (all from the 1956 I group) indicate that fuller participation in the special features of the GMC Program was related to greater appreciation of the value of those features.

Conversely, those students in the 1956 II group who had the most broken appointments and who saw the most patients were the

[3] Only those results significant at the .05 level of confidence are reported here.

students who found the GMC to be of the greatest help in learning how to make diagnoses and treat patients. These results indicate that reduced participation in the GMC Program (as evidenced by seeing a large number of patients and as indirectly evidenced by having many patients break appointments) led to a higher evaluation of the GMC in terms of those objectives which were not peculiar to the GMC Program—a finding which complements the one mentioned in the previous paragraph.

Staff's evaluation of students

The information provided by this study indicates that because the GMC medical staff emphasized strongly the value of medical skill, the two groups did not differ with respect to their gains in Medical Skill scores. As pointed out in Chapter 16, the GMC medical staff evaluated the students solely on one dimension: the traditionally medical aspects of the students' performance. Consequently, it might be expected that, since both the experimental and control faculties evaluated students' performance on the same basis, both groups of students would be similar in acquisition of knowledge and skill.

Interviews with students and staff

The topic of acquisition of medical skill was not systematically explored by the interviewers, and few spontaneous remarks about it were made by either students or staff in the interviews. Consequently, the interviews contain little important information on this matter.

Analyses of the individual teaching conferences and of the staff's evaluation of students indicate that because equal emphasis was placed upon acquisition of medical skill in the experimental and control programs, the GMC students acquired as much skill in the application of medical knowledge as the control students.

GMC students very likely found their clerkship somewhat less helpful than the control students found theirs because the GMC students felt they failed to see enough patients with specific organic illnesses. Because of the rather close relation between medical knowledge and medical skill, it is not surprising to find quite similar results in connection with these two topics.

It is important to note that those students who participated most fully in the family care aspects of the GMC Program were those who found the GMC most helpful with respect to developing medical skill. Moreover, those students who assumed more responsibility for their patients and felt that they learned how to work as part of a clinic team reported that they became less anxious about ambiguous diagnostic problems. Finally, those students who participated most fully in the special features of the GMC were those who found these features to be of greater value than they had expected, while those students who did not participate fully in these activities found the GMC to be most helpful with respect to traditional objectives of a medical curriculum.

Individual Attributes Related to Medical Skill

In Chapter 16 it was shown that Pretest performance on the test of medical knowledge was entirely a function of previous academic performance. Moreover, *gain* in Medical Knowledge scores was also a function of previous academic performance as well as of learning which took place in the individual teaching conferences (see Chapter 14). Personality characteristics were found to be unrelated to either Pretest performance or change in performance on the test of medical knowledge.

The results obtained in connection with medical skill, however, were quite different. Personality characteristics, as well as measures of previous academic performance, were found to be related to scores on the test of medical skill.

Results pertaining to the entire class. Scores on the Pretest were clearly related to previous academic performance in the class of 1956. For example, the MCAT subtest, Knowledge of Premedical Sciences, and several grade averages (first-, second-, and third-year grade averages, cumulative grade average, and junior medical clerkship grade) were all positively related to Medical Skill test scores. Students' judgments of one another concerning amount of medical knowledge were also positively related to Medical Skill scores on the Pretest. These results are highly similar to those obtained in connection with the test of medical knowledge in the classes of 1954 and 1955.

It is interesting, however, to note that those students who reported more "fantasy about intellectual and professional accomplishments" scored higher on medical skill than those who reported less. Also students who had high scores on the Psychological-Mindedness scale of the California Psychological Inventory tended to have high Medical Skill scores on the Pretest.

MCAT scores and measures of previous academic performance were unrelated to gain in medical skill scores in the class of 1956. Certain personality characteristics were related to gain, however. Those students who made the greatest gain in medical skill had higher scores on Self-Acceptance (ACL), lower on Self-Criticality (ACL). They were persons likely to be seen by others as modest and shy rather than aggressive, determined, and energetic.[4] Moreover, those students who

[4] See H. G. Gough, *Reference Handbook for the Gough Adjective Check-List* (Berkeley: University of California Institute of Personality Assessment and Research, 1955).

gained more medical skill had high scores on Achievement via Conformance, indicating that they tended to be seen as capable, responsible, and cooperative rather than as easily disorganized under pressure to conform. The fact that students who gained also reported that they were not rewarded as adolescents for influencing others is congruent with the above indications of shyness and lack of aggressiveness.

Results pertaining to the GMC. Gain in medical skill seemed to be related to what might be called "docility." For example, GMC students in the class of 1956 who had low needs for exhibition (n Exhibition, EPPS), who did not have a tendency to be aggressive and outgoing (Dominance, CPI), who worried about their social adjustment to the behavior of others (Anxiety scale) were apt to gain more medical skill than students exhibiting the opposite pattern. Moreover, students who reported that they were not rewarded for scholastic success as adolescents also gained more medical skill.

Results pertaining to the control group. The students who gained medical skill in the 1956 control group tended to be quite the opposite from those who gained medical skill in the GMC. The students who gained in medical skill in the control clerkship were outgoing, apt to take the initiative in social affairs (Sociability, CPI), cooperative, capable, and confident in their work (Achievement via Conformance, CPI), and reported that they were rewarded as adolescents for influencing others.

A similar pattern appeared in the class of 1955. Students who might be characterized as insightful and assertive (Flexibility, CPI), aggressive, confident, outgoing (Dominance, CPI), and masculine (low scores on Femininity, CPI) gained medical skill in the control group.

Interest in the welfare of a patient's family was positively related to gain in medical skill in the control group. This is somewhat puzzling unless one assumes that students who were sociable, etc. (as described above) were simply interested in people. If this was the case, this finding confirms the above results.

Any conclusions must remain highly tentative because these results were obtained almost entirely from the class of 1956 only and also because of the imprecise nature of the Medical Skill test. However, there does seem to be some basis for inferring that whereas the more docile, reticent students gained more medical skill in the GMC, the more aggressive, outgoing students made the greater gain in medical skill in the control clerkship. This conclusion is offered mainly as a hypothesis for future exploration.

Chapter 18

Medical Attitudes

Summary

One of the more important purposes of the General Medical Clinic was to change students' attitudes. The staff of the GMC was particularly concerned about the medical student's attitudes toward the total care of the patient. Training the medical student in specialty clinics, it was argued, too often leads to "disease-centered" rather than "patient-centered" medical care. Consequently, the student treats only the present illness, and too often fails to develop a feeling of responsibility for the patient's total health problem. In an effort to inculcate "patient-centered" attitudes, the GMC provided various experiences not usually found in specialty clinics (e.g., continuous care of a patient, family visits, psychiatric and sociological consultation).

Experience in the GMC seemed to affect the students' attitudes toward comprehensive care. In a climate where the change in students' attitudes was mostly in the direction of increasing antipathy to the concept of comprehensive care, the GMC apparently reduced this antipathy. Furthermore, the GMC was successful to some extent in developing positive attitudes toward comprehensive care. This positive trend seemed to develop despite the personal disadvantages which the GMC student perceived in the actual practice of comprehensive care.

Apparently the most important factor affecting the GMC student's attitudes was the nature of his relation with his patient. Greater responsibility for the patient led to an increased sense of the importance of comprehensive care.

It was the better student as well as the one with healthy personality characteristics who was initially favorable to comprehensive care and who became more so. But changes in attitudes toward the supervision of patients' health seemed to require a strongly motivated student, as well as experience.

These conclusions appear to be firm ones.

Dependent Variables (Effects of the GMC)

ATTITUDES TOWARD COMPREHENSIVE CARE

Several attitudinal measures were employed in order to discover to what extent the GMC affected students' attitudes. The Medical Attitudes test provided measures of students' attitudes toward comprehensive care and toward health supervision (see Chapter 13).

Results presented in Table 18.1 indicate that there were no statistically significant differences among the clerkships in the 1956 class with respect to attitudes toward comprehensive care when the first or second halves are considered separately. However, when the scores at the beginning of the year are compared with the scores at the end of the year, the data indicate that the GMC students improved their attitudes relative to the control students. The difference between the expected and obtained percentages of GMC and control students in the high increase group was significant at the .05 level of confidence.

Tables 18.2, 18.3, and 18.4 present a somewhat more detailed comparison. Table 18.2 shows that approximately the same number of students in each clerkship developed more negative attitudes, remained unchanged, or developed more positive attitudes toward comprehensive care during the first half of the year (from Pretest to Posttest I). Table 18.3 indicates that approximately the same results occurred during the second half of the year (from Posttest I to Posttest II). However, Table 18.4 shows that when the comparison is made from the beginning (Pretest) to the end (Posttest II) of the senior year, the GMC apparently did affect students' attitudes toward comprehensive care—primarily by preventing the development of negative attitudes. Almost two thirds (19/31) of the control students developed negative attitudes, but the GMC students were divided almost equally among the negative change, no change, and positive change categories.

ATTITUDES TOWARD HEALTH SUPERVISION

There were no statistically significant differences among the clerkship groups with respect to change in attitudes toward health supervision (see Table 18.5). Table 18.6 indicates that there was a tendency for the GMC to have an effect during the first half of the year. Table 18.7 indicates almost identical results for the second half of the year. When the attitude change scores over the entire year are examined, it appears that the GMC had a slight negative effect on the students' attitudes toward health supervision (see Table 18.8).

The attitudes of the GMC and control students were also compared with respect to the students' total scores on the five subscales of the Medical Attitudes test: Attitudes toward Comprehensive Care, Health Supervision, Physician-Patient Relations, Behavior Disorders, and the

Table 18.1. Difference between percentages of students expected and obtained in the high increase group: attitudes toward comprehensive care (class of 1956)

	Percentage expected	Percentage obtained	Difference
1956 I			
GMC ($N = 18$)	13	11	—2
Control ($N = 13$)	10	8	—2
Surgery I ($N = 17$)	12	14	2
Surgery II ($N = 17$)	12	15	3
1956 II			
GMC ($N = 16$)	17	12	—5
Control ($N = 18$)	19	18	—1
Surgery I ($N = 15$)	16	17	1
Surgery II ($N = 16$)	17	22	5
1956 I and II			
GMC ($N = 34$)	27	34	7
Control ($N = 31$)	25	18	—7

Table 18.2. Change in attitudes toward comprehensive care from Pretest to Posttest I (1956 I)

	Negative change	No change	Positive change	Total
GMC	11	2	5	18
Control	8	3	2	13
Total	19	5	7	31

Table 18.3. Change in attitudes toward comprehensive care from Posttest I to Posttest II (1956 II)

	Negative change	No change	Positive change	Total
GMC	8	3	5	16
Control	6	7	5	18
Total	14	10	10	34

Table 18.4. Change in attitudes toward comprehensive care from Pretest to Posttest II (1956 I and II)

	Negative change	No change	Positive change	Total
GMC	12	10	12	34
Control	19	7	5	31
Total	31	17	17	65

Table 18.5. Difference between percentages of students expected and obtained in the high increase group: attitudes toward health supervision (class of 1956)

	Percentage expected	Percentage obtained	Difference
1956 I			
GMC ($N = 18$)	11	11	0
Control ($N = 13$)	8	5	—3
Surgery I ($N = 17$)	10	13	3
Surgery II ($N = 17$)	10	11	1
1956 II			
GMC ($N = 16$)	13	11	—2
Control ($N = 18$)	15	12	—3
Surgery I ($N = 15$)	12	12	0
Surgery II ($N = 16$)	13	18	5
1956 I and II			
GMC ($N = 34$)	30	28	—2
Control ($N = 31$)	27	29	2

Table 18.6. Change in attitudes toward health supervision from Pretest to Posttest I (1956 I)

	Negative change	No change	Positive change	Total
GMC	7	4	7	18
Control	8	2	3	13
Total	15	6	10	31

Table 18.7. Change in attitudes toward health supervision from Posttest I to Posttest II (1956 II)

	Negative change	No change	Positive change	Total
GMC	9	4	3	16
Control	10	4	4	18
Total	19	8	7	34

Table 18.8. Change in attitudes toward health supervision from Pretest to Posttest II (1956 I and II)

	Negative change	No change	Positive change	Total
GMC	16	9	9	34
Control	12	7	12	31
Total	28	16	21	65

Table 18.9. Difference between percentages of students expected and obtained in the high increase group: total score, Medical Attitudes test (class of 1956)

	Percentage expected	Percentage obtained	Difference
1956 I			
GMC ($N = 18$)	14	25	11
Control ($N = 13$)	10	6	—4
Surgery I ($N = 17$)	13	6	—7
Surgery II ($N = 17$)	13	14	1
1956 II			
GMC ($N = 16$)	15	12	—3
Control ($N = 18$)	17	15	—2
Surgery I ($N = 15$)	14	15	1
Surgery II ($N = 16$)	15	17	2
1956 I and II			
GMC ($N = 34$)	25	34	9
Control ($N = 31$)	23	14	—9

Team Concept. The scores on all these subscales were combined into a total score in order to measure "composite" attitude change. Results are presented in Table 18.9. In the 1956 I group the difference between the expected and obtained percentages of GMC and control students in the high increase group was statistically significant. In the 1956 II group the difference was not statistically significant, although the difference from Pretest to Posttest II (entire year comparison) was statistically significant.[1]

Apparently the GMC Program had a positive effect on the attitudes of students (as measured by the Medical Attitudes test). The fact that attitudes toward health supervision were not affected, although attitudes toward comprehensive care were, seems somewhat curious but can be partly accounted for by the nature of the items included in each of these tests. The items included in the Comprehensive Care scale concerned the *extensiveness* of medical care that should be given an individual (see Appendix 2), whereas the items in the Health Supervision scale concerned preventive medicine. Although there was definite variability in students' attitudes toward preventive medicine (health supervision), and although a fairly large percentage of students became more favorable in their attitudes toward preventive medicine, no relation between change and the GMC experience was found.

QUESTIONNAIRE RESPONSES

Further evidence that the GMC Program affected the attitudes of students (and that the effect was different on the first and second

[1] Note that this change was effected in the 1956 I but not the 1956 II GMC clerkship. This difference was noted in connection with medical knowledge and medical skill and is discussed in Chapter 25.

Table 18.10. Percentage of students rating their clerkship as extremely or very helpful in learning the principles of comprehensive care (1955 II, 1956 I and II)

	1955 II	1956 I	1956 II
GMC	65	72	44
Control	33	46	61
Surgery I	—	18	13
Surgery II	5	47	19

halves) comes from the students' questionnaire responses. It was expected that if the GMC succeeded in its attempt to instruct students in the practical application of the principles of comprehensive care, the GMC students would rate their clerkship as more helpful in this respect than the control students would rate their clerkship. The data presented in Table 18.10 show that in the 1955 II and 1956 I groups a significantly larger percentage of GMC students than control students rated their clerkship as extremely or very helpful with respect to learning about comprehensive care. However, in the 1956 II group the percentage of GMC students so rating their clerkship was smaller (to an almost statistically significant degree). These results agree quite well with those found in connection with the Medical Attitudes test.

There were no significant differences between the GMC and control groups with respect to change in the percentage of students who rated learning the practical application of the principles of comprehensive care as extremely or very important (see Table 18.11). However, when the results for the entire year are considered, the percentage of GMC students who thought this topic was extremely or very important remained the same from Pretest to Posttest II (63%), whereas the percentage of control students decreased significantly (.01) from 74% at the Pretest to 48% at Posttest II. This finding parallels the result mentioned earlier—the tendency for the GMC Program to hold attitudes toward comprehensive care constant during the time when the control students developed negative attitudes.

The students' attitudes toward participating in various educational activities were investigated by ascertaining the amount of im-

Table 18.11. Change in percentage of students rating learning practical application of the principles of comprehensive care as extremely or very important (1955 II, 1956 I and II)

	1955 II			1956 I			1956 II		
	Post I	Post II	Change	Pre	Post I	Change	Post I	Post II	Change
GMC	*	47	*	67	56	*—11*	75	63	*—12*
Control	*	33	*	69	46	*—23*	50	50	*0*
Surgery I	*	—	*	88	77	*—11*	60	54	*—6*
Surgery II	*	37	*	71	48	*—23*	44	57	*13*

* No data.

portance different students attributed to engaging in these activities. Table 18.12 presents the change in the percentage of students responding that it was extremely or very important to engage in certain activities or to have certain conditions present. There were very few, if any, consistent differences between the two groups in this respect. Although more GMC than control students changed during both halves with respect to the importance they attached to consultation with the medical specialties, other changes were either small or inconsistent.

If the GMC Program was effective in changing the students' attitudes in the direction of a broadened concept of medical practice, it might be expected that the GMC students would come to regard a greater variety of information about their patients as important for them to know. The students were therefore asked whether they thought the physician should have information about the patient's diet, occupation, marital status, and recreational activities[2] as part of his routine information about patients, or whether such information was to be obtained only when specifically indicated. There were no significant differences between the GMC and control groups with respect to change in the percentage of students who thought diet, occupation, and marital status should be routine information (see Table 18.13). However, for the 1955 I and 1956 I groups the percentage of GMC students who thought that the patient's recreational activities should be routine information increased significantly more than did the percentage of control students. There were no statistically significant differences for the 1955 II and 1956 II groups.

It should be pointed out that virtually all students thought that occupation and marital status should be routine information, and that a very large percentage of the students thought that diet should also be routine information.[3] Therefore, the only item in which change might be detected was the one dealing with recreational activities.

STUDENTS' CONCEPTIONS OF VARIOUS SPECIALISTS

A further effort to determine how the students changed their attitudes as a result of their experiences in the GMC was made by attempting to discover whether they changed their conceptions of themselves as persons. More specifically, the researchers tried to discover whether the student's self-concept changed so that he thought himself to be more like his conception of an internist, more like his conception of a surgeon, or more like his conception of a psychiatrist.

[2] Results concerning other types of information are reported in Chapters 21 and 23. For a complete list see Appendix 4.

[3] It should be pointed out that all students are expected to ask patients about their occupations, marital status, and diet.

Table 18.12. Change in percentage of students rating engaging in certain activities or having certain conditions present as extremely or very important (class of 1956)

	1956 I						1956 II					
	GMC			Control			GMC			Control		
	Pre	Post I	Change	Pre	Post I	Change	Post I	Post II	Change	Post I	Post II	Change
Following patients for several months	55	78	*23**	46	23	*—23**	44	31	*—13*	6	28	*22**
Having responsibility for diagnosis of patients	72	67	*—5*	84	85	*1*	76	82	*6*	67	78	*11*
Having responsibility for treatment of patients	78	66	*—12*	76	77	*1*	94	94	*0*	66	73	*7*
Engaging in activities yourself rather than observing the staff	100	78	*—22**	85	85	*0*	100	94	*—6*	67	77	*10*
Having opportunities for consultation with the medical specialties	72	94	*22**	77	61	*—16*	69	81	*12*	72	61	*—11*
Having staff supervision time readily available	88	83	*—5*	85	85	*0*	88	56	*—32**	78	67	*—11*
Having a high quality of staff supervision	94	100	*6*	77	93	*16*	100	94	*—6*	89	77	*—12*
Having specific staff suggestions for the interpretation of symptoms and treatment	83	72	*—11*	54	61	*7*	94	82	*—12*	94	66	*—28**
Learning the amount and dosage schedule for specific therapies	78	61	*—17*	54	53	*—1*	81	69	*—12*	50	39	*—11*
Learning the principles of therapy	99	95	*—4*	92	92	*0*	94	88	*—6*	89	77	*—12*
Developing physical examination skills	94	95	*1*	85	92	*7*	94	88	*—6*	95	67	*—28**
Developing skill in history taking	89	89	*0*	62	69	*7*	88	88	*0*	83	61	*—22**
Doing laboratory procedures	11	11	*0*	8	23	*15*	12	13	*1*	11	0	*—11*
Handling the medical problems of patients	89	100	*11*	84	85	*1*	88	88	*0*	78	89	*11*
Making rounds	78	61	*—17*	76	38	*—38**	63	50	*—13*	61	39	*—22**
Working with diagnostic problems	95	100	*5*	77	70	*—7*	75	62	*—13*	95	61	*—34**
Seeing a wide variety of illnesses	94	84	*—10*	85	77	*—8*	82	94	*12*	83	72	*—11*
Seeing unusual pathological conditions	39	50	*11*	15	46	*31**	38	69	*31**	50	55	*5*
Having patients with a definite pathology	39	56	*17*	39	62	*23**	44	50	*6*	39	44	*5*
Following the latest medical advances in books and journals	94	78	*—16*	77	54	*—23*	81	82	*1*	72	61	*—11*
Handling routine medical problems	67	67	*0*	77	69	*—8*	87	82	*—5*	45	67	*22**

* Significant change ($p < .05$).

Table 18.13. Change in percentage of students responding that a family physician should have various kinds of information as part of his routine information about patients (classes of 1955 and 1956)

	1955 I			1955 II			1956 I			1956 II		
	Pre	Post I	Change	Post I	Post II	Change	Pre	Post I	Change	Post I	Post II	Change
Diet												
GMC	80	90	*10*	76	59	*—17*	61	56	*—5*	69	69	*0*
Control	83	89	*6*	71	67	*—4*	85	77	*—8*	67	50	*—17*
Surgery I	71	76	*5*	89	74	*—15*	71	65	*—6*	47	73	*26*
Surgery II	56	71	*15*	89	89	*0*	47	71	*24*	81	63	*—18*
Occupation												
GMC	95	95	*0*	100	94	*—6*	89	89	*0*	100	94	*—6*
Control	100	95	*—5*	94	89	*—5*	100	92	*—8*	100	100	*0*
Surgery I	94	94	*0*	89	100	*11*	100	100	*0*	93	87	*—6*
Surgery II	95	100	*5*	100	100	*0*	94	100	*6*	88	100	*12*
Marital status												
GMC	90	90	*0*	100	100	*0*	78	95	*17*	100	88	*—12*
Control	100	95	*—5*	94	95	*1*	92	85	*—7*	89	89	*0*
Surgery I	100	100	*0*	84	95	*11*	94	88	*—6*	93	80	*—13*
Surgery II	95	94	*—1*	100	95	*—5*	88	100	*12*	88	94	*6*
Recreational activities												
GMC	40	70	*30**	53	53	*0*	11	50	*39**	38	38	*0*
Control	61	61	*0*	35	39	*4*	46	54	*8*	39	39	*0*
Surgery I	47	47	*0*	68	47	*—21*	41	24	*—17*	40	53	*13*
Surgery II	50	41	*—9*	63	42	*—21*	35	53	*18*	63	25	*—38**

* Significant change ($p > .05$).

Table 18.14. Adjectives checked significantly more often to describe one specialist than the other two (class of 1956)

Surgeon	Pre	Post II	Internist/ pediatrician	Pre	Post II	Psychiatrist	Pre	Post II
aggressive	x	x	sincere	x	x	defensive	x	x
egotistical	x	x	friendly	x	x	anxious	x	x
self-confident	x	x	conscientious	x	x	reflective	x	x
dominant	x	x	adaptable	x	x	complicated	x	x
opinionated	x	x	clear-thinking	x	x	idealistic	x	x
arrogant	x	x	fair-minded	x	x	preoccupied	x	x
determined	x	x	good-natured	x	x	insightful	x	x
assertive	x	x	pleasant	x	x	emotional	x	x
energetic	x	x	calm	x	x	changeable	x	x
alert		x	patient	x	x	unconventional	x	x
argumentative		x	gentle	x	x	unrealistic	x	x
masculine		x	appreciative	x	x	forgetful	x	
temperamental	x		helpful		x	leisurely	x	
organized	x		cheerful		x	restless	x	
sarcastic	x		conservative		x	sensitive	x	
aloof	x		easy going		x			
precise	x		kind		x			
impatient	x		dependable	x				
			tactful	x				
			logical	x				
			practical	x				
			understanding	x				
			thorough	x				

First, what were the students' conceptions of the "typical" internist (and pediatrician),[4] surgeon, and psychiatrist?

At the beginning (Pretest) and end (Posttest II) of the senior year students were asked to indicate on a checklist of 117 adjectives (see Appendix 3) those adjectives which they felt were descriptive of the typical internist (and pediatrician), the typical surgeon, and the typical psychiatrist. In Table 18.14 are presented those adjectives which were used significantly more often to describe one specialist than the other two. There was little change from beginning to end of the senior year in the adjectives checked for each specialist. The descriptions which emerge seem clear enough and seem to conform to the way laymen might well be expected to think of these specialists—the forbidding surgeon, the gentle internist, and the not-too-easily-understood psychiatrist.

In order to discover whether the student changed his conception of himself during the senior year and whether the change in self-conception resulted in the student's perceiving himself to be more like his conception of one of the three "typical" specialists, each student

[4] There may be some objection to the implication that internists and pediatricians have similar personalities. The objection is well taken; the two specialties were conjoined merely to reduce the number of test blanks to be filled out.

was also asked at the beginning and the end of the senior year to check those adjectives most descriptive of himself.

Thus, for each student there was obtained a Self-Surgeon Similarity score, a Self-Internist/Pediatrician Similarity score, and a Self-Psychiatrist Similarity score. The Self-Surgeon Similarity score, for example, was a ratio of the number of adjectives checked both for self and surgeon to the total number of adjectives checked on both the self-description and the surgeon description checklists. Changes from Pretest to Posttest II were computed for all three Self-Specialist Similarity scores, and the results are presented in Table 18.15. The only statistically significant difference in change was in connection with the Self-Surgeon Similarity scores—the GMC students apparently changing their self-conceptions in the direction of their conception of the surgeon. However, the GMC students did not change their self-descriptions to conform more closely with their concept of surgeons. An analysis of the components of the change scores revealed that the GMC students' Self-Surgeon Similarity scores were unchanged from Pretest to Posttest II. It was the control students who changed, and this change was a result of their having checked more unfavorable adjectives for the surgeon on Posttest II. Since all students tended not to check unfavorable adjectives as descriptive of themselves, the fact that the control students checked more unfavorable adjectives as descriptive of the surgeon resulted in a decrease in their Self-Surgeon Similarity scores. Since the GMC students were more favorable towards the surgeons to begin with, and became slightly more so, the difference between the two groups increased and became statistically significant.

Even though the results should not be interpreted to mean that the GMC students developed an increased sense of "identification" with surgeons, the fact remains that the control students did check more unfavorable adjectives for the surgeons at the end of the year than

Table 18.15. Difference between percentages of students expected and obtained in the high increase group: Self-Specialist Similarity scores (class of 1956)

	Percentage expected	Percentage obtained	Difference
Self-Surgeon Similarity			
GMC	52	65	13
Control	52	39	—13
Self-Internist/Pediatrician Similarity			
GMC	54	53	—1
Control	54	55	1
Self-Psychiatrist Similarity			
GMC	46	50	4
Control	46	42	—4

at the beginning, while the GMC students did not. Since it is often assumed, rightly or wrongly, that surgeons are unsympathetic to a broadened concept of medicine which includes and emphasizes psychological and social factors, it may seem strange that the GMC experience did not increase the students' tendency to describe the surgeon unfavorably while the control experience did. As the data in Table 18.15 indicate, however, all students, both at the Pretest and at Posttest II used an unflattering set of adjectives to decribe surgeons.

INTERVIEWS WITH STUDENTS

Interviews with the 20 GMC students and 17 control students of the 1955 I group indicated certain differences between these two groups of students in their attitudes toward comprehensive care. Although both groups defined the term comprehensive care in roughly the same way (i.e., used the same clichés such as "total care," and identified "comprehensive care" with "good medical care"), there was a difference between the groups with respect to their intentions to practice comprehensive care. Almost all students in both groups said they would try to practice comprehensive care, but GMC students, on the whole, qualified their answers by pointing out that such factors as time, number of patients, and type of practice would limit the extent to which they would practice comprehensive care. GMC students seemed to be much more aware of the implications of the term. More GMC students expressed some reservations when asked if all doctors should attempt to practice comprehensive care. Only 50% (10/20) of the GMC students said all doctors should attempt it, and 7 of the 10 qualified their answer by saying, in effect, "it all depends. . . . " In contrast, 85% (15/18) of the control students gave an unqualified "yes" to the question. Evidently the GMC students developed a much more realistic attitude toward comprehensive care.

GMC students in the class of 1954 also indicated that they had a more realistic conception of the practice of medicine. When asked if they had a better idea of practice as a result of their clerkship, almost all GMC students unhesitatingly answered "yes," whereas only about 50% of the control students answered "yes." GMC students also indicated that they anticipated being able to see fewer new patients, and have fewer revisits with patients, in a single day than did control students. In short, GMC students seemed much more aware of the fact that the practice of comprehensive medical care takes time.

To summarize, in the main, the GMC Program had a positive effect on students' attitudes. Fewer GMC students changed their attitudes toward comprehensive care in a negative direction than did control students, and more GMC students changed their attitudes in a positive direction (relative to the control students) on a total of five subscales of the Medical Attitudes test. More GMC than control students believed that the application of the principles of comprehensive care was important; more GMC students found their clerkship helpful with respect to learning these principles. There was some slight indication that GMC students were likely to consider a wider range of information about patients to be "routine."

No directly negative effects were observed, although there was a slight indication that more GMC students developed negative attitudes toward the supervision of patients' health. There were no important differences between the two groups with respect to the importance the students attached to various educational activities. Nor did the GMC experience seem to affect the students' self-conceptions. However, the combined experience of control medical clerkship and the surgery clerkship did have the effect of making students' already unflattering opinions of surgeons even more so. There was some evidence from interviews with students that GMC students had positive attitudes toward comprehensive care but were also much more aware of the implications of this term for the actual practice of medicine.

Independent Variables (Reasons for the Effects of the GMC)

The conclusion drawn in the immediately preceding discussion was that the GMC did affect students' attitudes toward comprehensive care. That is, the attitudes of students who participated in the GMC tended not to change, while the attitudes of those in the control clerkship changed in a negative direction. We now turn our attention to the problem of why this result occurred.

Analysis of the Teaching Conferences

There is some evidence to indicate that the teaching in the control medical clerkship was somewhat more conducive to positive attitude change than was the teaching in the GMC. Analysis of the Teaching Conference Records suggests that the teaching was somewhat more highly organized in the control clerkship. That is, the instructors in the control clerkship indicated more interrelations among the medical facts of the patients' problems than did the instructors in the GMC (see Table 18.16). (As pointed out in Chapter 14, there was a tendency for teaching of a more organized nature to be related to attitude change in the entire class.) There were no differences between the experimental and control groups, however, with respect to the manner in which students thought about their patients when presenting the patients' problems to their instructors.

The physician observer found that 86% of the records of the GMC teaching conferences and 76% of the records of the control conferences

Table 18.16. Rating of Teaching Conference Records with respect to maximum number of determinants in the matrix of each record (see Chapter 14)

	Number of conferences		
	Low no. of determinants	High no. of determinants	Total
GMC	10	9	19
Control	4	14	18
Total	14	23	37

contained sufficient information relevant to comprehensive care to enable him to rate the performance of student and staff on their willingness to apply the principles of comprehensive care. The two groups of students received different ratings—more GMC students than control students being rated high on willingness to apply the principles of comprehensive care (see Table 18.17).

The mean rating for the GMC students was 3.9 ($N = 19$), and for the control students 3.2 ($N = 16$). Since a seven-point rating scale was used, the average GMC rating was almost exactly at the center, and the control rating was somewhat lower. The physician observer found that the GMC staff members devoted attention to the application of the principles of comprehensive care in treating patients 28.3% ($N = 92$) of the time, and the control staff did so 28.4% ($N = 74$) of the time. The ratings of the staff's analyses of problems related to comprehensive care also indicated a high degree of similarity in the two teaching efforts (see Table 18.18). The two teaching staffs were rated differently, however, on the type of action they proposed with respect to comprehensive care (see Table 18.19).

The above results, although not entirely unequivocal, indicate that it is improbable that the change in GMC students' attitudes toward comprehensive care was due to their instructors' efforts in the individual teaching conferences.

Students' reports of activities engaged in

It is important to note that far more GMC than control students reported that they participated in continuity of patient care (see Table 18.20).

Students' reports of general clerkship experience

It will be recalled that, in the main, more GMC than control students reported that their clerkship was extremely or very helpful in increasing their ability to apply the principles of comprehensive care. In this connection, it is pertinent to note that fewer GMC than control students appraised their instructors as highly proficient in the application of the principles of comprehensive care (see Table 18.21). How-

Table 18.17. Rating of students with respect to their willingness to apply principles of comprehensive care to clinical practice

	No. below median	No. above median	Total
GMC	6	13	19
Control	12	4	16
Total	18	17	35

Table 18.18. Rating of staff with respect to their analysis of problems associated with comprehensive care

	Percentage of conferences		
	Staff only recognized problem	Staff explored problem	Staff went to core of problem
GMC ($N = 26$)	61.5	26.9	11.5
Control ($N = 21$)	66.7	23.8	9.5

Table 18.19. Rating of staff with respect to relevance of action proposed by them to principles of comprehensive care

	Percentage of conferences			
	Not explicitly relevant	Related to peripheral aspects	Related to central aspects	Related to both aspects
GMC ($N = 25$)	0.0	20.0	52.0	28.0
Control ($N = 22$)	22.7	22.7	31.8	22.7

Table 18.20. Percentage of students indicating that following patients for several months was very frequently or always present in their clerkship (class of 1956)

	1956 I		1956 II	
	GMC	Control	GMC	Control
Following patients for several months	78	15	63	23

Table 18.21. Percentage of students rating their staff as extremely or very proficient in applying the principles of comprehensive care (class of 1956)

	1956 I	1956 II
GMC	50	25
Control	62	56
Surgery I	18	33
Surgery II	59	32

Table 18.22. Percentage of students rating their staff as extremely or very helpful in acquiring proficiency in comprehensive care (class of 1956)

	1956 I	1956 II
GMC	67	19
Control	62	55
Surgery I	35	26
Surgery II	47	19

ever, more GMC than control students rated their instructors as helpful in contributing to the students' proficiency in applying the principles of comprehensive care (see Table 18.22); moreover, the GMC students found their patients helpful in this respect (see Table 18.23), although they did not find them helpful in acquiring medical knowledge and medical skill.

Although somewhat indirectly related to attitudes toward comprehensive care, the students' attitudes toward the patients' role in the students' education was investigated. Because patients in university hospitals not only receive treatment, but also serve as teaching aids, the students' reaction to the patients' dual role is indicative of their experience with patients. The students were asked to respond to the question: Do you look upon your contact with patients in medical school (1) primarily as an opportunity to learn medicine, (2) primarily as an opportunity to help patients, (3) as presenting equal opportunities to learn medicine and to help patients. As this question was one that survived the many revisions of the questionnaire, results (presented in Table 18.24) were available for all three classes. These results indicate that fewer GMC than control students considered their patient contacts to be primarily to learn medicine. (Practically all the remaining students responded that contacts were looked upon as presenting equal opportunities to learn medicine and to help patients; only a negligible number of students thought their patient contacts were primarily to help patients.) A larger percentage of GMC students changed their response to "equal opportunity" on four of the six occasions when comparisons were made. Thus, more GMC students looked upon their patient contacts as opportunities to help patients as well as to learn medicine—an attitude consistent with assuming more

Table 18.23. Percentage of students rating their patients as extremely or very helpful in acquiring proficiency in comprehensive care (class of 1956)

	1956 I	1956 II
GMC	72	62
Control	61	61
Surgery I	36	40
Surgery II	77	38

Table 18.24. Change in percentage of students responding that contact with patients was primarily to learn medicine (classes of 1954, 1955, and 1956)

	1954 I			1954 II			1955 I			1955 II			1956 I			1956 II		
	Pre	Post I	Change	Post I	Post II	Change	Pre	Post I	Change	Post I	Post II	Change	Pre	Post I	Change	Post I	Post II	Change
GMC	19	29	*10*	53	16	*—37*	35	25	*—10*	24	35	*11*	44	17	*—27*	50	19	*—31*
Control	30	28	*—2*	62	38	*—24*	33	56	*23*	59	50	*—9*	31	31	*0*	50	61	*11*
Surgery I	32	60	*28*	25	43	*18*	47	41	*—6*	32	42	*10*	53	35	*—18*	20	20	*0*
Surgery II	29	55	*26*	32	37	*5*	44	41	*—3*	47	32	*—15*	53	65	*12*	25	38	*13*

Table 18.25. Change in percentage of students responding that they had too little responsibility for diagnosis of patients (classes of 1954, 1955, and 1956)

	1954 I			1954 II			1955 I			1955 II			1956 I			1956 II		
	Pre	Post I	Change	Post I	Post II	Change	Pre	Post I	Change	Post I	Post II	Change	Pre	Post I	Change	Post I	Post II	Change
GMC	60	5	*—55*	74	5	*—69*	50	15	*—35*	76	24	*—52*	67	11	*—56*	63	19	*—44*
Control	70	72	*2*	62	19	*—43*	50	22	*—28*	35	17	*—18*	85	15	*—70*	56	28	*—28*
Surgery I	47	75	*28*	35	81	*46*	47	53	*6*	16	58	*42*	29	71	*42*	7	47	*40*
Surgery II	48	60	*12*	37	53	*16*	61	59	*—2*	21	63	*42*	35	47	*12*	19	63	*44*

responsibility for patients. This finding is particularly interesting in view of the fact that the patients were not considered by GMC students to be very helpful in acquiring medical knowledge or skill.

In addition to thinking of patient contacts as providing opportunities for helping patients as well as learning medicine, the GMC students felt they had more responsibility for diagnosis and treatment of patients than did other students. The percentage of students responding that they had too little responsibility for diagnosis of patients is presented in Table 18.25. At the end of their clerkship experience fewer GMC students responded that they had too little responsibility for diagnosis (this was found on all comparisons except for the 1955 II group). The differences between the GMC and control students were statistically significant for both the 1954 I and II groups. And in every case but one (1956 I) a larger percentage of GMC students than any other group changed their response from "too little responsibility" to "enough responsibility."

On all four comparisons presented in Table 18.26 fewer GMC students than other students responded that they had too little responsibility for treatment of patients at the end of their clerkship experience. The differences in percentages for the 1955 I and 1956 I groups were significant at the .05 level of confidence. On all four comparisons a larger percentage of GMC students changed their response to "enough responsibility."

Further substantiating the above findings concerning responsibility are the results presented in Table 18.27. On all six comparisons made, more GMC students came to think of themselves as doctors rather than as students in their contacts with patients.

In brief, the students' reports of their general clerkship experience indicate that the GMC students believed it was their experience with patients which contributed to their acquisition of proficiency in applying the principles of comprehensive care. Moreover, more GMC students felt that their clerkship provided equal opportunities to help patients and learn medicine. Finally, GMC students clearly felt more responsible for the diagnosis and treatment of their patients and more often thought of themselves as doctors than did the control students.

Special educational techniques of the GMC

As pointed out above, far more GMC than control students were able to follow patients for several months. Did participation in this activity have an effect on students' attitudes? Evidently it did not: there was no relation between change in attitude and the length of time a student took care of a patient. However, there was a negative relation between change in attitude and the extent to which the students judged

Table 18.26. Change in percentage of students responding that they had too little responsibility for treatment of patients (classes of 1955 and 1956)

	1955 I			1955 II			1956 I			1956 II		
	Pre	Post I	Change	Post I	Post II	Change	Pre	Post I	Change	Post I	Post II	Change
GMC	60	20	*—40*	82	29	*—53*	67	11	*—56*	69	31	*—38*
Control	44	56	*12*	65	44	*—21*	77	46	*—31*	50	33	*—17*
Surgery I	59	71	*12*	37	89	*52*	65	59	*—6*	20	67	*47*
Surgery II	61	76	*15*	37	63	*26*	53	59	*6*	31	63	*32*

Table 18.27. Change in percentage of students responding that they thought of themselves primarily as doctors rather than students in their contacts with patients (classes of 1954, 1955, and 1956)

	1954 I			1954 II			1955 I			1955 II			1956 I			1956 II		
	Pre	Post I	Change	Post I	Post II	Change	Pre	Post I	Change	Post I	Post II	Change	Pre	Post I	Change	Post I	Post II	Change
GMC	39	90	*61*	42	74	*32*	35	70	*35*	76	94	*18*	39	89	*50*	50	88	*38*
Control	25	44	*19*	29	43	*14*	39	61	*22*	47	61	*14*	54	62	*8*	61	61	*0*
Surgery I	21	20	*—1*	70	29	*—41*	47	76	*29*	58	32	*—26*	53	47	*—6*	87	73	*—14*
Surgery II	43	50	*7*	68	47	*—21*	72	47	*—25*	74	42	*—32*	53	65	*12*	69	81	*12*

this activity (following patients for several months) to be present. Table 18.28 indicates that those students who estimated that following patients for several months was an activity that was infrequently present were those who developed positive attitudes toward comprehensive care in the 1956 I group.

Of particular interest is the fact that those GMC students in the 1956 I group who reported having more responsibility for the treatment of patients not only changed their attitudes toward comprehensive care but, at the end of their GMC experience, believed the following activities to be more important than before entering the GMC: the opportunity to give psychotherapy, acquiring skill in managing patients' social problems, and seeing the families of patients. Incidentally, it was the nonauthoritarian students who accepted more responsibility for the treatment of patients.

It should be noted that these results were obtained for the 1956 I group, at which time the GMC was having an effect on students' attitudes, and at which time the GMC students reported having more responsibility for patients.

Staff's evaluation of students

Students' attitudes toward comprehensive care, insofar as they were known to the GMC staff, played no role in the staff's evaluation of the students, except with the first (1954 I) students to participate in the GMC. In that instance it was found that the staff did, in performance as well as plan, evaluate the students with respect both to medical knowledge and skill and to attitudes toward patient care. However, in the remaining five groups studied, all staff evaluations involved only the purely medical aspects of the students' relations with patients, in spite of intentions on the part of the staff to do otherwise.

Interviews with students

Fifteen of the eighteen students who had just completed six months in the GMC in the 1955 II group were interviewed by a member of the research staff. A report based on these interviews (written in 1955)

Table 18.28. Relation between frequency with which following patients for several months was reported to be present in the clerkship and change in attitudes toward comprehensive care from Pretest to Posttest I (1956 I)

	Infrequently present	Frequently present	
Positive attitude change	10	4	14
Negative attitude change	0	4	4
	10	8	18

is reproduced below. As may be seen, the report consists entirely of the interviewer's impressions of the students' attitudes:

There is no doubt whatsoever that the students' attitudes toward GMC as "an idea" (which represents the teaching of comprehensive care) are favorable. Every student but one expressed positive attitudes toward comprehensive care. Every student but one (the same one) was glad that he had been in the GMC, not only because he believed he received superior clinical (not ward) teaching, but also because he had an opportunity to participate in comprehensive care. Almost all the students complained about patient selection ("too many crocks") and the fact that they had not seen enough pathology; yet they preferred the GMC primarily because of the clinic teaching.

Almost all students mentioned that as a consequence of reports made to them about the clinic by the previous twenty students, their initial attitudes toward the GMC were poor, but these negative attitudes changed to definitely positive ones shortly after their experience in the clinic. The source of the negative attitudes seemed to lie mainly in reports made to them about personal relations with the GMC staff.

The "Tuesday afternoon conference" (family care conference) drew almost exactly the same response from all but one student—"boring." The reasons for this were expressed in much the same pattern by each student: "it's just common sense"; "they talked down to us"; "haven't gotten much out of these"; "repetitious"; "wasted effort"; "don't really learn"; "examples illustrate some point which is fairly obvious"; "poor planning"; "a waste of time"; "would know this anyway"; "left up in the air"; "worthless"; "say the same things about the same problem"; "monotonous." There seems no escape from the conclusion that the positive nature of the students' attitudes toward comprehensive care developed in spite of the family care conference.

The interview material does not throw much light on the problem of the reasons for the general positive attitude toward comprehensive care. Students felt that they received good medical teaching, but did not identify the source of their increased knowledge of psychological factors—if indeed they believed they had increased their knowledge here except by (increased?) common sense. Moreover, the conference designed to develop the role of both psychological and sociological factors in medical care was viewed with distinct disfavor, and the students denied having profited from it.

It may be that positive attitudes were developed through "general" contact with staff members. This explanation is dubious, however, because the students indicate that the staff is by no means of one mind concerning the matter of comprehensive care. Several students mentioned that the staff orientation toward comprehensive care was not uniform—that, in fact, the staff was divided on this matter, and one student mentioned that psychiatry was "undercut" in the Tuesday conference. The students themselves were divided on this issue, however; about as many said that the entire staff was favorable to comprehensive care as said that the staff was divided on this issue.

Students' diaries

Material from students' diaries also threw some light on the reasons for attitude change. For example, the following diary entry made by a senior medical student while in the surgery clerkship illustrates how responsibility for a patient may affect a student's behavior:

Well, today I found out one reason why I am a poor student. For days I have been lounging around on this clerkship, playing cards, etc., and doing as little as possible, even less than is absolutely necessary to get by. Why not, nothing I do on this clerkship means anything anyway! I am in no way responsible; I only get in the way of the busy men. But I don't think I realized what was wrong. Today, another student's patient was being discussed, and the need for his having skin grafting was mentioned. He was going to surgery tomorrow, but only to have his burns cleaned up (debrided), not to have grafts, because there was no skin. So, I found out which patients had died in the local hospitals during the past six hours, found a suitable dead person, arranged to get permission for the skin removal, and even drove out to Derby to get the permit signed. Coming back, I wondered why I had done more work in two hours for that old man than I did on this clerkship in a week. The reason is obvious—the skin is for a *patient*. All other activities on this clerkship are for practice, for play, unreal duties. I am unable to force myself to do needless things, even when I have much to lose by not doing them. Any teaching experience *must include* responsibility, or it is useless. The surgical clerkship gives the student *no* responsibility for the patient. I suspect that this situation is intentional, for obviously any student who knows any surgery is dangerous; he might do surgery when he gets out of school. Whether it is good or bad for nonspecialists to do surgery, it is a shame that one quarter of the medical curriculum must be sacrificed.

A diary entry made by a student while in the GMC also illustrates what responsibility for patients may signify to a senior medical student:

I'm getting a little tired of following somebody else's patient. My chief complaint is that I haven't yet had a single case in which I had the opportunity of doing the initial work-up on any phase of the patient's problem. All the patients I have seen have either had extensive diagnostic work done or have at least been worked up by somebody in this clinic already. Consequently, I do a full work-up in a half-hearted manner, because most of the stuff is already down in the chart with the exception of social, economic, and marital history, which is a little hard to take anyway. So it is hard to do a real whole-hog job of asking questions when the patient has already answered them two or three times before. Further, I am getting tired of hearing these folks compare their previous physicians in the GMC, with the implication that I had damn well better come up to these previous standards. Not that I have any serious paranoid feelings about this, it is just that this gets into the conversation with two thirds of my patients, and it seems that they are aware of this rapid shift and curious as to where I fit in. So, Dear Diary, my fondest wish tonight is to have some nice sick patient all my very own to come in with an empty folder and a tale of woe, that I can listen to, thump on the chest of, diagnose and cure, and discharge at long last, forever grateful.

INTERVIEWS WITH GMC STAFF

Although the staff were not unanimous in their statements about students' attitudes and the reasons why they might or might not change, one staff member did contrast the effect of the setting in which the students found themselves with the effect of the staff:

> I think the students' impression of overemphasis on comprehensive care has come primarily from the [group] conferences and not from work with individual patients. I think that [the extent to which comprehensive care is emphasized] in working with individual patients will be dependent upon our own staff. The staff has a setting in which comprehensive care can be emphasized; whether they do it or not depends on them.

Another faculty member noted that the group conferences did not leave the student with a feeling of achievement:

> A number of students think that there has been too much emphasis on social problems and too many conferences on the deplorable social situations and psychiatric [problems] too. But the way it is right now, there is only one meeting per week that deals with those problems exclusively, and I don't think that's too many. [We have] given up the family care conference where [the student] would have a whole afternoon of family and social problems. After going to a number of those, most of the students I talked to thought that was an excessive amount of time on that. It made quite a long afternoon out of it for what they were able to accomplish. . . .

Why did the experience in the GMC lead the GMC students to develop more positive attitudes toward comprehensive care? Apparently the most important factor was the "institutional demand" which the GMC placed on the students. The GMC, in fact as well as in plan, placed more of the responsibility for the patients' care on the shoulders of the students and thus created a situation which led to an appreciation of the importance of "total care." GMC students clearly felt more responsible for their patients, and those students who felt the greatest responsibility became more convinced of the value of providing comprehensive care. As might be expected, more GMC students felt that they were helping patients as well as learning medicine, more GMC students developed a willingness to apply the principles of comprehensive care to their patients, and more GMC students found their patients helped them to understand the value of comprehensive care. The principal cause of the change seems to have been the nature of the contact with the patient.

It seems doubtful that the direct effort of the staff had a large effect on the students. There is little to indicate that the GMC staff, either in individual student-staff conferences or in large group conferences, served to develop positive attitudes in the student. Neither do any of the specific educational features of the GMC (except the matter of responsibility mentioned above) seem to have been related to attitude change.

Individual Attributes Related to Medical Attitudes

Although the GMC apparently had an effect on students' attitudes toward comprehensive care, it did not, of course, change *every* student's attitude. Many students' attitudes did not change at all, and some changed for the worse. The following discussion deals with the problem of discovering which individual attributes were associated with attitude change.

ATTITUDES TOWARD COMPREHENSIVE CARE

Results pertaining to the entire class. Because the Medical Attitudes test was not used in this study until after the administration of the Pretest to the class of 1955, there were no data available concerning the relations between Pretest scores and attitudes toward comprehensive care for the class of 1955. However, the list of personality traits presented in Table 18.29 makes quite clear the type of student who had positive attitudes toward comprehensive care at Posttest I in the class of 1955. These students differed from those who had negative attitudes in terms of intellectual and interest modes, in terms of poise and self-assurance, and in terms of maturity and responsibility. Students who had positive attitudes were more efficient intellectually and more apt to seek achievement through their own independence and self-reliance. They had more poise and confidence, were more imaginative and spontaneous, and more effective in communication. Moreover, they were less conforming and more rebellious toward rules and restrictions—although responsibly so. They were also politically liberal and possessed nonauthoritarian attitudes.

There was only a slight tendency for these relations to occur at the Pretest in the class of 1956, however.

Table 18.29. Personal attributes correlated to a statistically significant degree ($p < .05$) with attitudes toward comprehensive care, Posttest I (class of 1955, $N = 53$)

—.45	F (Authoritarian) scale
+.35	Liberal Attitude scale
+.28	Tolerance (CPI)
+.36	Intellectual Efficiency (CPI)
+.41	Psychological-Mindedness (CPI)
+.43	Achievement via Independence (CPI)
+.40	Social Presence (CPI)
+.28	Capacity for Status (CPI)
+.35	Sociability (CPI)
+.34	Dominance (CPI)
+.32	Responsibility (CPI)

There was a definite positive relation between previous grades (as well as peer judgments of medical knowledge) and positive change in attitudes toward comprehensive care. Eight indices of previous academic performance were positively associated to a statistically significant degree ($p < .05$) with the development of more favorable attitudes toward comprehensive care. These indices included the following: first-year grade average, second-year grade average, third-year grade average, cumulative grade average, junior medical clerkship grade, junior surgery clerkship grade, psychopathology course grade, and peer judgments of medical knowledge. Clearly, it was the better students who developed more positive attitudes toward comprehensive care.

When the relation between personality characteristics and attitude change was examined, an interesting result appeared. It will be recalled that students who *initially* possessed positive attitudes were identified by the California Psychological Inventory as being intellectually efficient, socially poised, mature, and responsible. Students who *changed* in a positive direction were identified by their peers as sympathetic to comprehensive care, skillful in physician-patient relations, and responsible and mature. These students also reported being rewarded for responsibility in adolescence, but not rewarded for influencing others. They also reported, as might be expected, not being interested in major surgery as a specialty.

It seems quite clear that students with more desirable characteristics not only had positive attitudes toward comprehensive care at the Pretest, but changed their attitudes in a positive direction.

Results pertaining to the GMC and control groups separately. It is clear that the students with better academic records were the ones who changed positively their attitudes toward comprehensive care, whether they were in the control or experimental group. However, there was an interesting form of interaction between student characteristics and clerkship experience which throws further light on the effect of the GMC. Note the strong effect of the GMC on attitude change illustrated in Table 18.30. About two thirds (22/34) of the students in the GMC

Table 18.30. Change in attitudes toward comprehensive care from Pretest to Posttest II (class of 1956)

	Negative change	No change or positive change	Total
GMC	12	22	34
Control	19	12	31
Total	31	34	65

Table 18.31. Relation between academic record and change in attitudes toward comprehensive care from Pretest to Posttest II, GMC (class of 1956)

	Change in attitudes toward comprehensive care		
	Negative change	No change or positive change	
Upper half of class	4	13	17
Lower half of class	8	9	17
	12	22	34

either did not change their attitudes, or changed them in a positive direction; the remaining third (12/34) changed their attitudes in a negative direction.

Which students in the GMC group exhibited either no change or positive change—students with good academic records or students with poor academic records? Table 18.31 shows that it was the better students. Of the 17 students in the upper half of the class, 13 changed positively, whereas the lower half of the class was divided into two virtually equal groups of those who changed positively (or did not change) and those who changed negatively.

Refer once more to Table 18.30. Note that the control clerkship experience changed students' attitudes toward comprehensive care in a negative direction; about two thirds (19/31) of the control students became more negative in their attitudes toward comprehensive care. Which students in the control group changed negatively—students with good academic records or students with poor ones? As Table 18.32 indicates, it was clearly the poor students in the control clerkship who became negative toward comprehensive care. Moreover, the good student (as in the GMC) tended to change positively. Of the 19 students in the control clerkship who changed negatively, 15 were in the lower half of the class. Of the 12 who changed positively (or did

Table 18.32. Relation between academic record and change in attitudes toward comprehensive care from Pretest to Posttest II, control medical clerkship (class of 1956)

	Change in attitudes toward comprehensive care		
	Negative change	No change or positive change	
Upper half of class	4	10	14
Lower half of class	15	2	17
	19	12	34

Table 18.33. Relation between academic record, clerkship experience, and change in attitudes toward comprehensive care from Pretest to Posttest II (class of 1956)

	Change in attitudes toward comprehensive care: Negative change	Change in attitudes toward comprehensive care: No change or positive change	
GMC, upper half of class	4	13	17
Control, lower half of class	15	2	17
	19	15	34

not change), 10 were in the upper half of the class. Table 18.33 further illustrates this point.

These results may be summarized by pointing out that the GMC did not have a differential effect on good students in comparison with the control clerkship; the percentage of good students developing more positive attitudes toward comprehensive care was about the same (Tables 18.31 and 18.32). The GMC seems to have had its greatest effect on poor students, for in the control group almost all (15 out of 17) the poor students developed negative attitudes toward comprehensive care, while in the GMC as many poor students changed in a positive direction (or did not change) as changed in a negative direction. Perhaps the good students grasped the philosophy of comprehensive care independently of instruction, whereas the poor students had to be shown.[5]

Attitudes toward health supervision

Results pertaining to the entire class. In the class of 1955 students judged by their peers to be cooperative had positive attitudes toward health supervision on the Pretest. Students with strong social values also scored high on this attitude measure. Furthermore, mature, responsible students, whose drive for achievement was related to independence and self-reliance had positive attitudes toward health supervision, as in the case of attitudes toward comprehensive care

[5] There were 8 students (4 in the control clerkship and 4 in the GMC) in the upper half of the class of 1956 whose attitudes toward comprehensive care changed in a negative direction. An examination of their scores on the California Psychological Inventory and their rankings by their fellow students provided an interesting supplement to the above results. Of these 8 students, 5 were perceived by their fellow students as lacking responsibility and maturity, or achieved low scores on responsibility on the CPI. Two of the remaining 3 were high on authoritarianism. The third student made it quite clear that his sole interest was surgery and he was opposed to any expenditure of time and effort which interfered with this interest.

(see Table 18.34). Essentially the same results were obtained for the class of 1956. However, in this class, the students with positive attitudes at the Pretest also reported having an interest in the welfare of the patient's family and in administrative work.

It is of some interest to note that two MCAT subtests (Quantitative Ability and Knowledge of Premedical Sciences) were negatively related to scores on attitudes toward health supervision at the Pretest in the class of 1956.

The relations between individual attributes and change in attitudes toward health supervision did not present a coherent pattern of results. This may have been due to the positive relation between personality traits and change in attitude in the GMC group and the absence of such a relation in the control group (see below).

Results pertaining to the GMC. There were no relations between individual attributes and change in attitudes toward health supervision from Pretest to Posttest I in the class of 1956. However, in the same class the relations between individual attributes and change in attitudes toward health supervision from Posttest I to Posttest II formed a pattern consistent with results obtained regarding attitudes toward comprehensive care and Pretest scores on attitudes toward health supervision. Students who developed positive attitudes toward health supervision in the GMC were much like the students who developed positive attitudes toward comprehensive care, except that there was an "achievement" component present in connection with positive change toward health supervision which was lacking in connection with positive change toward comprehensive care. For example, students who became more positive toward health supervision had a need for achievement (n Achievement, EPPS); reported anxiety about accomplishment (Anxiety scale); were leaders among their peers (peer judgment); and scored low on the Femininity scale of the CPI. The drive for achievement, however, was apparently not of a competitive kind, for the attributes tolerance, communality, and psychological-mindedness from the California Psychological Inventory were also related to positive change

Table 18.34. Personal attributes correlated to a statistically significant degree ($p < .05$) with attitudes toward health supervision, Posttest I (class of 1955, $N = 53$)

+.33	Cooperation (peer judgment)
+.34	Social value (Allport-Vernon-Lindzey Study of Values)
+.28	Tolerance (CPI)
+.34	Achievement via Independence (CPI)
+.36	Social Responsibility (CPI)
+.34	Self-Acceptance (CPI)

in attitudes toward health supervision. High scores on these scales indicate maturity and responsibility, as well as a certain nonconformity.

Results pertaining to the control group. Students in the control group with high scores on the Tolerance scale of the CPI changed their attitudes in a positive direction. (Note that this personality trait was positively related to change in both experimental and control groups.) Students who reported not being rewarded for scholastic success as adolescents changed in a negative direction. This finding is confirmation of the "achievement" component noted for the GMC group.

To summarize, it appears rather clear that students who had achieved good academic standing and students with healthy personality characteristics were apt to be favorable to the concept of comprehensive care at the Pretest. Moreover, it was students with these characteristics who changed in a positive direction. The GMC had a positive effect on the better students and was not entirely unsuccessful with the poor ones. On the other hand, although the control clerkship had some positive effects on good students, it had a negative effect on the poor students.

Results concerning attitudes toward health supervision were not as clear. Evidently the GMC had little effect on this attitude, and although there was some indication that the better students developed positive attitudes toward health supervision while in the GMC, the result was not a firm one. The fact that there was a strong tendency for an achievement component to be related to changes in attitudes toward health supervision suggests that change in this respect occurred only with highly motivated students.

Chapter 19

Psychological Knowledge

Summary

As the preceding results show, the student in the GMC gained as much medical knowledge and skill as the control student and developed more positive attitudes toward comprehensive care. We turn now to the question of whether the GMC student increased his knowledge of the psychological components of medical care. A test of the student's knowledge of these psychological factors was included in the Sound-Film Interview (described in Chapter 13). Because this test was revised several times, however, results were available for the class of 1956 only.

Some evidence was found to suggest that the GMC student acquired more psychological knowledge than the control student. This result was certainly not firm, however, and it is by no means clear how to account for a difference between the two groups, if, indeed, there was a difference. The effect of the staff's teaching was not large, nor were the special educational features of the GMC discovered to have any important effect on the student. The most likely factor accounting for gain in psychological knowledge seems to have been an interrelation between general experience in the GMC, academic ability, and a willingness on the part of the student to forego social acceptability for the sake of achievement.

The tendency for the results from different sources to confirm one another indicates that these results are quite dependable.

Dependent Variables (*Effects of the GMC*)

The test data and the results obtained from the questionnaire and from interviews with students suggest that the GMC students gained more psychological knowledge than the control students. For example, although there were larger percentages of GMC than control students among those students who showed the greatest gain in psychological knowledge both from Pretest to Posttest I and from Posttest I to Posttest II, the difference between expected and obtained frequencies could have occurred by chance (see Table 19.1). However, when the comparison between the two groups is made over the entire year (from Pretest to Posttest II), it becomes apparent that the GMC increased the students' Psychological Knowledge scores to an almost statistically significant degree (see Table 19.2).

It should be pointed out that, although strict adherence to the usual significance levels would result in the conclusion that the GMC did not increase the students' knowledge of the psychological components of medical care, if the number of GMC students with scores above the median had been 21 instead of 20, the difference between the two groups would have been statistically significant ($p < .05$).

Evidence from the questionnaire suggests that the GMC students increased their knowledge in this area. For example, the GMC students rated their clerkship as more helpful in acquiring knowledge of the basic ideas of psychosomatic medicine and psychiatry than did the control students. As indicated in Table 19.3, a greater percentage of GMC students rated their clerkship as extremely or very helpful on three occasions, the differences between the GMC and control students being statistically significant (at the .05 level of confidence) for the 1955 II and 1956 II groups. And on three occasions more GMC students rated their own proficiency above average (see Table 19.4). The difference between the GMC and control students with respect to increase in self-ratings of proficiency was statistically significant for the 1956 I group, but fell short of significance for the 1956 II group. On the assumption that the groups in the class of 1955 did not differ in the initial percentage who rated their proficiency above average, the difference at Posttest II was statistically significant.

Interviews with students did not provide unequivocal data. For example, after interviewing fifteen students following their GMC experience in the 1955 II group, the interviewer made the following comment:

> The situation with respect to psychological knowledge is difficult to evaluate because the students do not seem sure of what they think. Most seem to believe that they learned *something* about physician-patient relations in the GMC, but many relegated this knowledge to "common sense" or "something I will pick up in practice." Only a small minority seemed to feel that they gained anything besides "greater awareness" of psychological and sociological factors—and there were few students who were certain about this.

But interviews with the 1955 I students provided data which supported the questionnaire results. For example, 63% of the 19 GMC

Table 19.1. Difference between percentages of students expected and obtained in the high increase group: psychological knowledge (class of 1956)

	Percentage expected	Percentage obtained	Difference
1956 I			
GMC ($N = 18$)	12	17	5
Control ($N = 13$)	9	8	—1
Surgery I ($N = 17$)	12	9	—3
Surgery II ($N = 17$)	12	11	—1
1956 II			
GMC ($N = 16$)	14	17	3
Control ($N = 18$)	16	14	—2
Surgery I ($N = 15$)	13	15	2
Surgery II ($N = 16$)	14	12	—2

Table 19.2. Change in psychological knowledge from Pretest to Posttest II (class of 1956)

	No. below median	No. above median	Total
GMC	14	20	34
Control	19	12	31
Total	33	32	65

$\chi^2 = 2.62; p = .11$

Table 19.3. Percentage of students rating their clerkship as extremely or very helpful in acquiring knowledge of the basic ideas of psychosomatic medicine and psychiatry (1955 II, 1956 I and II)

	1955 II	1956 I	1956 II
GMC	42	61	56
Control	0	46	28
Surgery I	—	0	0
Surgery II	11	12	6

Table 19.4. Change in percentage of students rating themselves above average in knowledge of the basic ideas of psychosomatic medicine and psychiatry (1955 II, 1956 I and II)

	1955 II			1956 I			1956 II		
	Post I	Post II	Change	Pre	Post I	Change	Post I	Post II	Change
GMC	*	58	*	11	73	*62*	25	44	*19*
Control	*	17	*	16	31	*15*	23	23	*0*
Surgery I	*	—	*	18	24	*6*	67†	59	*—8*
Surgery II	*	43	*	12	24	*12*	44	50	*6*

* No data.

† The reason for the rather large percentage of students rating themselves above the average prior to their surgery clerkship is that one half of the students in each surgery group had been in the GMC.

students said they learned a great deal about rapport and handling patients in their clerkship, whereas only 12% of the 17 control students said this.

Interviews with the 1954 II students were not directed to this point and therefore yielded no information concerning psychological knowledge. Interviews with the first students to participate in the GMC (the 1954 I group) led the interview analyst to draw one interesting conclusion:

> The impression given in the interviews is that the students believe that formal training in interpersonal relations would not be successful and that much can be learned from watching doctors at work. Apparently, skill in interpersonal relations is illustrated, rather than explained.

To summarize, it seems likely that the GMC students acquired more psychological knowledge than the control students. The analysis of the objective test data indicated a definite trend in favor of the GMC. Also, more GMC than control students definitely felt that their clerkship was helpful, and more GMC students felt that they were above average with respect to proficiency in the psychological aspects of medical care. Although the data from the interviews with students were not unequivocal, the safest conclusion would appear to be that there was a definite tendency for the GMC students to acquire more knowledge about the psychological components of medical care. The following discussion concerns the problem of what caused this result.

Independent Variables (Reasons for the Effects of the GMC)

Analysis of the teaching conferences

No differences in the manner in which students were taught or in the manner in which they thought about their patients were discernible from the analysis of the Post-Conference Interviews or the Teaching Conference Records. That is, there were no differences in the number of psycho-social facts which student and teacher discussed about a given patient or in the extent to which these facts were interrelated. The physician observer found that 56% of the GMC conferences and 60% of the control conferences contained sufficient information to make a rating of the students' psychological knowledge. The average ratings (on a seven-point scale) are given in Table 19.5. These ratings con-

Table 19.5. Mean ratings of students on psychological knowledge (class of 1956)

	1956 I	1956 II	1956 I and II
GMC ($N = 18$)	4.1	4.3	4.2
Control ($N = 17$)	4.1	4.0	4.0

firm the test results: there was a slight tendency for GMC students to be higher on psychological knowledge.

It appears that the GMC staff members devoted attention to knowledge of the basic ideas of psychosomatic medicine somewhat less frequently than did control clerkship staff members (see Table 19.6). On the other hand, the GMC staff apparently were more thorough in their analysis of the psychological problems of patients (see Table 19.7).

The general complaint voiced by most GMC students (and staff) about the disheartening nature of the GMC patients seems also to have been noted by the physician observer. For example, there was a tendency for the GMC patients to be rated as somewhat less stimulating than the control patients (see Table 19.8). But the conferences in both clerkships received approximately the same ratings with respect to their helpfulness to the students (see Table 19.9).

Although the psychologist's analyses of the teaching conferences by means of Teaching Conference Records and Post-Conference Interviews indicated no differences between the two groups, the physician observer's ratings showed some slight differences. It seems possible, though somewhat unlikely, that the tendency for GMC students to acquire more psychological knowledge can be attributed directly to the teaching which the students received in the individual teaching conferences.

Students' reports of activities engaged in

Some clues to the reason for the slight difference between the GMC and control groups in the acquisition of psychological knowledge may be found in the students' reports of activities in which they participated during their respective clerkships. For example, the data in Table 19.10 illustrate that particularly in the 1956 II group more GMC than control students engaged in activities likely to increase knowledge of the psychological components of medical care. More GMC than control students reported that they had opportunity for psychiatric consultation, had opportunity to give psychotherapy, had opportunity to handle emotional problems of patients, spent time exploring social and emotional factors when taking a history, and advised patients on their personal problems. However, about the same percentage of both groups found that the staff gave direct instruction in physician-patient relations. The data in Table 19.10 support the hypothesis mentioned in the chapter on medical attitudes: that the GMC provided a situation in which the student had an opportunity to assume more responsibility for the patient's total health problem. (It should be pointed out, however, that the differences between the two 1956 I groups were small and were occasionally in the control clerkship's favor.)

Table 19.6. Percentage of conferences in which the staff member devoted attention to knowledge of the basic ideas of psychosomatic medicine

GMC ($N = 92$)	37.0
Control ($N = 75$)	45.3

Table 19.7. Rating of staff with respect to their analysis of problems associated with knowledge of the basic ideas of psychosomatic medicine

	Percentage of conferences		
	Staff only recognized problem	Staff explored problem	Staff went to core of problem
GMC ($N = 34$)	61.8	32.4	5.9
Control ($N = 34$)	82.4	14.7	2.9

Table 19.8. Rating of teaching conferences with respect to degree to which patients' psychological problems were potentially stimulating to students

	Percentage of conferences						
	Negative effect on stimulation	Not stimulating	Slightly	Somewhat	Moderately	Very	Extremely
GMC ($N = 99$)	3.0	58.6	22.2	7.1	7.1	2.0	0.0
Control ($N = 76$)	6.6	48.7	17.1	11.8	13.2	2.6	0.0

Table 19.9. Rating of teaching conferences with respect to their helpfulness to students' learning about psychosomatic medicine

	Percentage of conferences						
	A hindrance	Not helpful	Slightly	Somewhat	Moderately	Very	Extremely
GMC ($N = 99$)	5.1	61.6	18.2	6.1	6.1	2.0	1.0
Control ($N = 76$)	9.2	56.6	15.8	10.5	5.3	2.6	0.0

Table 19.10. Percentage of students indicating that certain activities were very frequently or always present in their clerkships (class of 1956)

	1956 I		1956 II	
	GMC	Control	GMC	Control
Having opportunities for psychiatric consultation for your patients	61	54	75	23
Having opportunities to give psychotherapy	28	46	56	17
Handling the emotional problems of patients	44	46	56	34
Spending a lot of time exploring social and emotional factors when taking a history	17	15	50	11
Advising patients on their personal problems	33	30	56	11
Having the staff give direct instruction in physician-patient relations	12	23	25	22

Table 19.11. Percentage of students reporting very little or no reading about psychosomatic medicine and psychiatry (class of 1956)

	1956 I	1956 II
GMC	45	50
Control	92	78
Surgery I	82	93
Surgery II	94	100

GMC students reported doing more reading about psychosomatic medicine and psychiatry than did the other students (see Table 19.11). In both the 1956 I and II groups fewer GMC students reported very little or no reading in the area of psychosomatic medicine and psychiatry (statistically significant difference, $p < .05$).[1]

STUDENTS' REPORTS OF GENERAL CLERKSHIP EXPERIENCE

More GMC students found their teachers to be helpful with respect to acquiring psychological knowledge than did the control students (see Table 19.12). (This response confirms the observation made by the physician who rated the teaching conferences, see Table 19.7.) Somewhat more GMC than control students found their teachers to be highly proficient as well, although the differences were very small in the class of 1956 (see Table 19.13). However, more GMC than control students clearly thought their patients were helpful in enabling them to acquire psychological knowledge (see Table 19.14).

These results contrast with those obtained in connection with medical knowledge and skill. In those areas GMC students thought the GMC to be unsatisfactory (unhelpful) because the patients were not good teaching material (did not present enough variety or enough specific organic illness). But, in the main, the students believed that their teachers were proficient and helpful with respect to traditional medical knowledge. When psychological knowledge is considered, however, the reverse was true. GMC students thought the GMC clerkship as a whole was very helpful (and more students felt above average with respect to their proficiency in psychological knowledge than with respect to their proficiency in medical knowledge). Moreover,

[1] Of interest, aside from the difference between the GMC and control students' responses to this question, is the surprisingly large percentage of students who reported very little or no reading about psychosomatic medicine and psychiatry. When the responses of all students were combined, 77% of the 1956 I group and 80% of the 1956 II group reported that they had done very little or no reading about psychosomatic medicine and psychiatry. While it is true that significantly more GMC students reported reading than other students, it is interesting to note that even in a program emphasizing the importance of the emotional problems of patients, approximately half the students reported doing very little if any reading about psychosomatic medicine and psychiatry.

Table 19.12. Percentage of students rating their staff as extremely or very helpful in acquiring psychological knowledge (class of 1956)

	1956 I	1956 II
GMC	61	44
Control	46	17
Surgery I	0	0
Surgery II	12	0

more GMC students thought their patients were helpful with respect to the acquisition of psychological knowledge than believed the staff were helpful, and fewer thought the staff proficient in psychological knowledge than thought them proficient in medical knowledge.

Special educational techniques of the GMC

None of the special techniques employed by the GMC were related to gain in Psychological Knowledge test scores. This is an interesting finding in view of the fact that GMC students reported participating in more activities assumed to be conducive to the acquisition of this type of knowledge.

Staff's evaluation of students

The GMC staff's evaluations of six groups of approximately twenty students each were carefully studied (see Chapter 24). There was no indication that the staff's evaluations included consideration of the students' knowledge of the psychological aspects of medical practice. In each case, the medical staff (with the possible exception of the psychiatrist) evaluated the students with respect to their knowledge of medicine alone.

Interviews with students

Viewpoints of some of the students in the class of 1954 just prior to graduation are interesting. Most of the students (from both groups) felt that the subject of interpersonal relations in general, although important, could not be satisfactorily included in the curriculum either

Table 19.13. Percentage of students rating their staff as extremely or very proficient in psychological knowledge (1955 II, 1956 I and II)

	1955 II	1956 I	1956 II
GMC	42	33	26
Control	17	30	17
Surgery I	—	0	0
Surgery II	5	18	0

Table 19.14. Percentage of students rating their patients as extremely or very helpful in acquiring psychological knowledge (class of 1956)

	1956 I	1956 II
GMC	83	75
Control	46	34
Surgery I	0	26
Surgery II	24	0

because it would involve personal problems or because personalities already developed could not be changed. The general feeling was that either a doctor was "good with patients" or he was not, and there was not much to be done about it except to cultivate a friendly approach to patients. This attitude was also expressed in a discussion about patients with emotional problems: common sense was considered an important attribute, and any kind of training in handling patients was often seen as neither useful nor possible.

This impression was supported by the fact that when students were asked to describe the behavior of a doctor who was "good with patients" they found this almost impossible to do, giving vague answers like "he's kind," "he seems interested in them," or "he's a gentleman." Only their descriptions were vague, however; they seemed quick to recognize a good or bad relation between doctor and patient and were ready to imitate the good and condemn the bad. This, of course, suggests (among other things) that the behavior of the staff is an important factor in determining students' attitudes toward physician-patient relations.

A sizeable percentage of students in the 1955 I group were critical of the GMC staff's efforts in the field of psychosomatic medicine and psychiatry. Sixty per cent (12/20) of the students felt that some members of the GMC staff belittled the practice of psychosomatic medicine and psychiatry and that some would not cooperate with students (or other instructors) in considering these problems of patients. As one student put it: "I think many of them inflict their anxieties on the students, that they try to scare out some of the new students from further inquiry (in the area of psychological problems), telling them that it is time consuming and that they'll never get anywhere anyway."

An excerpt from an interview with a GMC student in the class of 1956 illustrates the point that at least some GMC staff members did not encourage students to study the psychological aspects of patients' problems:

Q: Did the staff—not the psychiatrist, but the internists and pediatricians—did they help you diagnose psychological problems?

A: It seemed to me at least that the staff did not make any attempt to investigate the psychological problems of the patient. When we—at least this is my own experience—gave them the history and told them what the physical findings were, I then mentioned to them that I thought a lot of complaints were on a psychogenic level, and all they did was nod their heads, they didn't try to investigate by talking to the patients themselves and showing me how many of the problems were actually psychogenic. It seem to me the internists let that problem go and put it in the hands of the psychiatrist. They told me, yes, they recognized that this sounded like a psychogenic problem, and probably it would be a good idea next time to have the psychiatrist or someone go in and perhaps talk with the patient. But they themselves made no effort—at least to my mind. I don't want to speak unkindly of them, because I thought they did a good job. They were busy, but I don't think they went any too deeply into the psychogenic problems themselves.

Q: Did you learn anything about therapy—giving therapy to patients with psychological problems?

A: Not as such; now I don't know if this is psychotherapy—let's put it this way. One of the articles I read not so long ago stressed the fact that you should give superficial psychotherapy to hypertensive patients. Well, I think that this was the kind of psychotherapy I was giving to some of my patients—superficial psychotherapy. I was trying to talk to them, talk their problems over with them; but actually I did not learn to go too deeply into anybody's emotional problems. It was just a superficial situation in which I tried to put the patient at ease as we talked together. If this is called psychotherapy—and probably it has an element of psychotherapeutics in it—then I did do that.

Some GMC students (20%) said that a few of the staff tended to overemphasize the psychosomatic aspects of treatment. Fifty per cent (9/18) of the control students said that there was little instruction in this field; 11% (2/18) remarked that the control staff belittled psychosomatic medicine and psychiatry. Some (28%) of the control students criticized members of the staff for the manner in which they handled patients, although more (40%) of the GMC students made this criticism too.

The interviews with the 1955 II group were less detailed and did not provide further information in this area.

INTERVIEWS WITH GMC STAFF

The twelve GMC staff physicians were asked about the kinds of psychological concepts they used in discussing the psychological problems of patients with students. The parts of two interviews which include typical replies are presented below:

Q: I'm going to ask you about a specific case in which you felt that you did a good job of pointing out the value of comprehensive care to the student. Can you think of an example where a student presented a patient to you, and the student was pretty much oblivious to some of the psychological and sociological factors, and in which you pointed them out to the student, and the student then developed a better grasp of the case?

A: This usually, I think, comes up most frequently in areas of chronic disease. The child with acute tonsillitis doesn't as a rule present these problems unless something else turns up in the history. I can think specifically of a case of rheumatic fever one of the students picked up on discharge from the hospital. The patient had a lot of personality changes related, I'm sure, to her long period of hospitalization as well as to withdrawal which she developed because of a very insecure home situation to begin with. Associated with this were the other aspects of care of a child with inactive rheumatic fever in the home. I think first of all from the standpoint of her psychological problem the student did see better that this at the present time was actually her major disease; the rheumatic fever was no longer active and didn't present a real problem in itself. Most of his time was then spent in dealing with the end result of the emotional problem which she had developed on the ward. When the patient was readmitted, unfortunately with a different student, with a new attack of rheumatic fever, we tried to think in terms of what we could do for this hospital admission to prevent the sort of reaction she had developed previously from having been removed from her home and her normal environment. Although it was a different student, one might like to believe that had it been the same one, he could have foreseen the difficulty himself and tried to use preventive measures at that time. From the standpoint of the other areas in the care of rheumatic fever which go more into the sociological aspects of the problem, I think he came to see that he had to know specifically how many rooms were in the house, how many beds, how many floors, whether there were stairs, how far she lived from the school, so that we could outline a specific program, which could really not be done until we knew how many times she had to go up and down stairs in school, what arrangements could be made for her to get some rest at recess and lunch time. We evaluated these things with the help of the public health nurse, and actually in this case the student took it upon himself to go out to the home and out to the school to see at first hand exactly what the situation would be. He was then able to outline a program of increasing physical activity for her until we got her back to full physical activity. I think this is the sort of thing that unless one has a conscious awareness of these related social problems, if you want to call them that, one is apt to tell the child that he can do so much in terms of physical activity, but leave the child and the family in a state of utter confusion as to what it really is they should or should not do.

Q: Returning for a moment to the psychological problem of withdrawal in this particular case, I'd like to get an idea about the level at which the conversation took place with the student in this particular case. For example, the sociological problem was a fairly concrete matter with respect to exercise and so on; however, with respect to the psychological problem, would you tell me what kind of explanatory concepts you used with the student when you talked about withdrawal?

A: I'm sure that the approach most of the internists and pediatricians in the clinic take is a fairly superficial one because we have not had specific training in psychiatry ourselves, but at the same time I think in many cases it's one we can work with ourselves. In this particular case we did have the assistance of our pediatric psychiatrist and for several sessions sat down with her so that a good bit of the discussion of the more fundamental aspects of the problem was brought up by the pediatric psychiatrist, but I think still on a fairly superficial level. I know therapy was certainly on an extremely superficial level. There was no effort at retrogressive psychotherapy, and it was simply a matter of deciding whether this child had had a more severe emotional reaction to her hospitalization than another child from a different environment. It seemed fairly apparent that she had, in that she was completely uncommunicative with any of the medical personnel both during and after her hospitalization. We discussed first of all the role of the hospitalization itself in terms of the fears that the child might have had. The student suggested the fear of needles and unpleasant things that were happening to her physically. He did not, I recall very clearly, bring up the matter of separation from her home and her mother—the thing that both the psychiatrist and I felt was probably the primary factor. I think the student did come to see that this probably was the primary factor. We found out that after discharge and in her own home environment she was quite a different child from the one that we had seen in the clinic, although still by no means a normal child. I think he came to see that separation was one of the most important aspects. This child had originally been very acutely ill, had been given last rites several times, and pulled through. At that time there had been no discussion with her by ward personnel, physician, or even her parents, as far as we knew, as to why this was being done, to perhaps make the situation a little easier. There was some discussion as to why this particular child should have felt more insecure in the hospital than another child; the fact that she was unable to carry with her a feeling of love and security developed in the home was brought out. I think this is probably about as far as we went into the mechanics of the problem. As far as therapy went, it was a matter of trying to get her to express some of the things that she did fear. In this particular situation we decided that there was very little that could be done to make her home situation any more secure. The mother did not speak English, had to talk to us through an interpreter; there were eight children in the family; this girl was in the middle. This was one area in which we had to pretty much draw the line, feeling that we couldn't do all that even a student might do by working with the mother, getting the mother perhaps to see areas in which she could make the child feel more secure. We tried to have the student discuss with the child some of her fears and give her a better understanding of her illness and what it meant to her both at the present time and in the future.

Following is the interview with the second GMC faculty member:

Q: Now I'd like you to think of an instance in which you taught a student something about comprehensive care, an instance in which you made your point clearly. Could you think of a good example and tell me about it, preferably a case which the student discussed with you and didn't see some of the psychological implications, and in which you pointed them out to him.

A: Hmmm. You won't think I've done a very good job. I can't think right off hand.

Q: I'm wondering about the level of the explanatory concepts you used when you talked to the students about these problems. For example, at one end of the scale you could be talking about the patient's "id" and at the other end of the scale you could be talking about how well the patient "gets along" with people. I am just wondering whereabouts in between there you work with the students?

A: Well, I work with them pretty far up the scale, I think. That is, if you want to call the "id" pretty far up the scale. I don't go clear up to the top, because I'm afraid that I'm not really able to go clear to the top, but I go as far up as possible because I think that's important.

Q: It's fairly complicated?

A: No, I don't think I use fairly complicated concepts or even abstract types of things, but on the other hand I don't go clear down the scale and just use very superficial terms such as any lay person might. I try to go into a little bit more detail and try to interpret some little things that the patient might be experiencing to the student in terms of the patient's own psyche and mental mechanisms, and so forth.

Q: What sort of terms did you use to discuss the patient's problem?

A: In one case we talked in terms of repressed hostility for the father. In this particular case the patient (a young girl) actually decided she didn't want to go out and didn't relate well to the opposite sex. It turned out that her father had left her at an early age and left the mother in charge of the brood—it was quite a brood, as a matter of fact—and we talked a little bit about hostility to the father, and father figures, and went on down the line. Actually she was not able to express her hostility for him, which caused guilt association.

Q: I'm just curious about how you gained this kind of knowledge yourself; in what part of your training did you pick up this kind of knowledge? As a student? Through experience? Through association with psychiatrists? From your reading?

A: First of all, is this uncommon knowledge? I think it's very important for people who deal in internal medicine to know these things. I think everyone who graduated from this university is probably very well versed in psychiatry. I have spent a lot of time in large institutions . . . and actually spent three months on the psychiatric ward at a hospital doing nothing but psychiatry. But I think a great deal of it actually comes from working with psychiatrists down here and having these things pointed out time and again, then applying it as you see situations come up. Seems to work fairly well.

The interviewer also made an attempt to discover to what extent GMC staff members thought formal preparation in the fields of psychology and sociology might be necessary in order successfully to instruct senior medical students in these aspects of medical care. Virtually all staff members felt that formal instruction would be unnecessary; the majority seemed to feel that one learned a sufficient amount from contact with psychiatrists and sociologists. Excerpts from two interviews are presented below:

Q: Would you suggest any kind of special preparation for someone who was going to teach in a comprehensive care clinic? That is, if you were talking to someone who said to you, "I'm going to be an instructor in a clinic where they teach comprehensive care," would you suggest that that person take any specific steps to prepare himself for that kind of teaching?

A: I'm not sure just what one would recommend to a person who had completed most of his training, if this is the sort of person that you're talking about. I don't know of any specific courses at the present time on a postgraduate level that would prepare him specifically for this. But certainly there are some that could help one in performing this role a little better in a setting such as the General Medical Clinic. I think that experience in private practice is of value; I think it's of value to anyone in academic medicine, but not at all essential. I think that most people might be a little better in this particular setting by virtue of that experience. Perhaps some people in whom it would be a disadvantage.

Q: Private practice might be a disadvantage?

A: Yes. It might make them a little less idealistic. I think from my own standpoint that had I had courses in sociology and psychology, at some point, I would have been better prepared for this.

Q: Would you recommend such courses or would you consider this as sort of a luxury item—if you have it, so much the better, but it isn't going to hold you back any if you don't?

A: I think from my standpoint, having a sociologist available to the clinic, participating in our programs, taught me a great deal about exactly what we were doing, and I'm sure I have developed a much better understanding of the reasons why patients and staff react in the ways they do.

Q: Have you taken any specific steps to prepare for teaching in the comprehensive care clinic, aside, say, from talking to the sociologist?

A: No, I think the only thing I've done is a little more reading in sociology, particularly in this area.

Q: Could you mention the kind of things you've read?

A: *The Health of Regionville* has been the one book that, I think, stands out as being of primary help to me. I haven't gone back into any basic study of sociology. I'm not sure that's necessary in itself.

Q: Have you attended any seminars or lectures in sociology or psychology or psychiatry?

A: No, I don't think I have attended seminars or lectures or read about any other area specifically in leading to this.

Q: Do you read any journals outside the what might be called traditional medical sphere?

A: I think perhaps the only other thing that I probably would not have done had I not gotten specifically interested in medical education is to read the *Journal of Medical Education*. And, of course, I've had the opportunity here, without going elsewhere, to talk with a lot of people who have other programs, and I think this has been of some value.

Q: How about the *American Journal of Psychiatry*? Have you read that?

A: I read isolated articles, specifically around a particular patient, perhaps, often, I'm sure, stimulated by our over-all comprehensive care program. Before we had a psychosomatic conference, for instance, I sat down for myself, having to participate in that conference, and tried to read a little more on psychosomatic medicine than I probably would have done otherwise.

Following is the interview with a second GMC faculty member:

Q: What kind of preparation would you suggest for someone who was going to teach in a comprehensive care clinic? That is, suppose you knew someone who told you that he was going to be an instructor in a clinic like the General Medical Clinic. Could you suggest anything to him; would you recommend to him that he do anything to prepare himself?

A: Well, I'm sure he'd need more than the general knowledge and ability to teach internal medicine, or pediatrics, as the case may be. Yes, I think it would be an excellent idea for him to talk to our sociologist, for instance, about the social and economic problems of the patients, their religious background, and their religious teaching; talk with social service and see exactly what is offered by various community agencies; and actually look in on the agencies and learn a little bit about their roles, and so forth. Actually, I think any good citizen should do it. No one has time to do this, but I certainly think that if you are going to teach good comprehensive medical care you should have an idea of all these things, actually even going out into the areas where these people live and seeing about the housing conditions and the family set-ups, etc. I think that would be not only fascinating from your own personal standpoint, but instructive to you as far as good citizenship in the community is concerned, and invaluable in teaching good comprehensive medical care.

Q: Is there anything in the way of formal preparation you would suggest?

A: Could you elaborate on that?

Q: Like any courses, or seminars, or meetings—to take an extreme example, you might urge the new doctor to take a residency in psychiatry.

A: Oh, I don't think a formal course would really be required. I think a good outline of things that you could do and should do, acquainting yourself with all the matters which you would need to know for comprehensive medical care would be enough. I suppose if they offered a brief didactic refresher course on all aspects of the thing it might actually become boring. I feel that it might. I don't think you need to know any more psychiatry than you have to know in the general practice of medicine anyway. And you certainly need to know your medicine and be able to teach it, that goes without saying.

Q: So that you feel that, say, the average internist has sufficient knowledge to be able to cope with most of the emotional problems, say, or social problems that patients. . . .

A: I don't think you can generalize that. I don't believe that you can. I think that—on the other hand, I don't know how you would pick your staff.

Q: The medical staff?

A: Yes, I don't know how you'd decide which internists have had this training. I mean some people are not cut out for it. But I think some people make it their business to do good comprehensive medical care in their offices, and, on the other hand, I think some probably are content with diagnosing and prescribing on purely organic grounds or perhaps engage in very superficial psychotherapy. What separates one from the other, and how you would find out about it, I'm not sure, but I don't think those who treat patients in a cold, rather distant, manner are going to teach good comprehensive medical care, although they may be brilliant internists and very fine doctors, and probably would be excellent in their own situation.

Q: You think it's probably more a function of the personality, say, his way of doing things, rather than a matter of acquisition of formal knowledge?

A: Yes, I think so. I think most internists could certainly do it. I think, however, that some of them are neither interested in it nor want to do it.

Q: In your own work, have you done anything different from what you would have done if you'd been teaching, say, in the control medical clerkship, the specialty clinics? That is, do you find that you have read anything different, attended any seminars?

A: You mean as far as comprehensive care is concerned?

Q: Yes.

A: Well, I read Lyle Saunders' book.[2] I've talked with social service on specific problems and talked with the sociologist about specific problems, and I certainly would not have done this in a specialty clinic. There I probably would have done what was indicated medically, and then if the patient was having a difficult time because of that, just refer him on to one of the social agencies. I think I have done a little bit more than I would have ordinarily along those lines.

Q: Do you find that you've read anything, say, in the field of psychiatry or psychology that you wouldn't have otherwise?

A: Not that I wouldn't have otherwise. I mean, I just don't think that you can ever separate one from the other and I think that you should try to keep up a little bit on all aspects of it. By virtue of having a mixed group of specialists in one organization, for instance a psychiatrist and a pediatrician along with me, it's been fascinating to discuss a problem, for instance, and have the psychiatrist suggest, well, do you think this could be a manifestation of thus and so, or here is an excellent article on this type of situation, and of course out of interest I read these articles, and I'm sure I wouldn't have either known about the articles or had much inclination to read them otherwise. So from that standpoint I guess I have.

Assuming that participation in the GMC did in fact lead to an increase in psychological knowledge, what factors might have produced this effect? The evidence presented above by no means leads to a definite answer. However, the results of the psychologist's analysis of the Teaching Conference Records and the Post-Conference Interviews, the ratings of the teaching conferences made by the physician observer, the staff's evaluation of students, and interviews with students and staff, all suggest that the effect of the staff's teaching was not large.

The students' reports of activities engaged in and their reports of their clerkship experience suggest that the general nature of the clinic was such that more experience with patients was gained, and more activities assumed to lead to more knowledge about patients were engaged in. But no actual relation was found between these experiences and activities and gain in psychological knowledge.

In short, the tendency for the students in the GMC Program to acquire more psychological knowledge was not readily explainable in terms of either the staff's teaching or the students' general experience in the clinic.

Individual Attributes Related to Psychological Knowledge

The results reported below indicate that acquisition of psychological knowledge was more highly related to individual characteristics of students than to educational programs in the senior year.

Results pertaining to the entire class. Students who obtained high

[2] *Cultural Difference and Medical Care: The Case of the Spanish-Speaking People of the Southwest* (New York: Russell Sage Foundation, 1954).

Pretest scores on the Psychological Knowledge test had already shown some predilection for this topic (see Table 19.15 for a complete list of correlations for the class of 1956). Not only were they good students, according to their peers, but they were interested in the inner experiences of others, according to their scores on the Psychological-Mindedness scale of the CPI. It is noteworthy that in the previous class peer judgments of likeability, cooperation, and skill in developing good relations with patients were all positively correlated with scores on the Psychological Knowledge Pretest. Scores on the Psychological-Mindedness scale were also correlated with Psychological Knowledge Pretest scores in 1955.

The results reported above present rather a consistent pattern. Students who were seen as good students by their peers had high

Table 19.15. Personal attributes correlated to a statistically significant degree ($p < .05$) with Psychological Knowledge test (class of 1956)

Pretest ($N = 65$)	Posttest I ($N = 65$)	Posttest II ($N = 65$)
+ Amount of medical knowledge (peer judgment)	+ Verbal Ability (MCAT)	+ Verbal Ability (MCAT)
+ General Anxiety scale	+ Knowledge of Modern Society (MCAT)	+ Quantitative Ability (MCAT)
+ Psychological-Mindedness (CPI)	+ Knowledge of Premedical Sciences (MCAT)	+ Knowledge of Modern Society (MCAT)
+ Achievement via Independence (CPI)	+ First-year grade average	+ Knowledge of Premedical Sciences (MCAT)
+ Flexibility (CPI)	+ Third-year grade average	+ Third-year grade average
	+ Cumulative grade average	+ Cumulative grade average
	+ Junior surgical clerkship grade	+ Junior medical clerkship grade
	+ Competence as a physician (peer judgment)	+ Amount of medical knowledge (peer judgment)
	+ Amount of medical knowledge (peer judgment)	+ Liberal Attitude scale
	+ Frequency of fantasy about intellectual and professional accomplishments (self-rating)	+ Frequency of fantasy about intellectual and professional accomplishments (self-rating)
	+ Psychological-Mindedness (CPI)	— Interest in minor surgery (self-rating)
	+ Achievement via Independence (CPI)	— Amount of reward for ability to get along with others as an adolescent (self-rating)
		+ Achievement via Independence (CPI)
		— Self-Control (CPI)
		+ Need Aggression

Pretest scores on the Psychological Knowledge test. Moreover, on at least one occasion they were seen by their fellow students as likeable, cooperative, and as being skillful in establishing good relations with patients. In two different classes they were interested in the inner experiences of others (as measured by the Psychological-Mindedness scale of the CPI). Also, a strong interest in achievement coupled with a tendency toward nonconformity were related to high Pretest scores on the Psychological Knowledge test.

Students who had performed well in the judgment of both instructors and fellow students throughout the first three years of medical school gained more psychological knowledge than did students with less commendable records, whether or not they participated in a program which stressed such material. Students who were in the upper half of the class of 1956, and who were judged by their fellow students to be competent, gained in psychological knowledge from Pretest to Posttest I. There is evidence that the same students gained from Pretest to Posttest II as well.

Results pertaining to the GMC and control groups separately. Gain in psychological knowledge was not completely a function of academic ability, however, for although the GMC students did not make statistically significant gains over the control students, a definite Pretest–Posttest II trend was apparent (see Table 19.2). In short there seems to have been a joint effect, or interaction, between academic ability and GMC experience, so that the GMC had its effect on the better students. Tables 19.16 and 19.17 illustrate the nature of this joint effect in the class of 1956.

Note that the GMC had a positive effect on good students and that the control clerkship had a negative effect on poor students. Note also that the GMC had about the same effect on poor students as the control clerkship had on good students. In short, good students in the GMC Program were likely to gain more psychological knowledge; poor students in the GMC were about as likely to gain psychological knowl-

Table 19.16. Relation between peer judgments of competence as a physician and change in psychological knowledge from Pretest to Posttest II, GMC (class of 1956)

		Change in psychological knowledge		
		Below median	Above median	
Competence as a physician	High	3	10	13
Competence as a physician	Low	11	10	21
		14	20	34

Table 19.17. Relation between peer judgments of competence as a physician and change in psychological knowledge from Pretest to Posttest II, control medical clerkship (class of 1956)

		Change in psychological knowledge		
		Below median	Above median	
Competence as a physician	High	9	10	19
Competence as a physician	Low	10	2	12
		19	12	31

edge as good students in the control program; and poor students in the control program were likely to gain less. It is of considerable interest to note that somewhat similar results occurred in connection with change in attitudes toward comprehensive care (see Chapter 18).

Personality characteristics associated with gain in psychological knowledge in the GMC differed from those associated with gain in the control program. In the GMC more psychological knowledge was acquired by students who were oriented toward independent achievement, i.e., had strong needs for achievement (n Achievement); who were not much affected by needs to be accepted by others (low scores on n Affiliation); and who scored high on need for aggression (n Aggression). These students seem to be those who were willing to "buck the tide"—and were capable of doing it.

But in the control clerkship the students who worried about their ability to solve ambiguous diagnostic problems; who had strong values for utility, i.e., strong economic values (Allport-Vernon-Lindzey Study of Values); and who indicated that during adolescence they were rewarded for influencing others were the students who acquired more psychological knowledge.

These results should be compared with the results presented in connection with change in medical attitudes and psychological skill. It is significant that much the same pattern of personality characteristics was associated with differential change in these variables.

Chapter 20

Psychological Skill

Summary

The previous chapter was concerned with the question of whether the General Medical Clinic student acquired more psychological knowledge than the control student. This chapter deals with the question of whether the GMC student acquired more skill than the control student in the *application* of psychological knowledge, for one of the aims of the GMC was to increase the student's skill in the application of knowledge of the psychological components of medical care. This objective had two aspects: increasing the student's skill in applying the basic ideas of psychosomatic medicine and psychiatry, and increasing his skill in establishing and maintaining good physician-patient relations. Each aspect is discussed separately below.

There were no important differences between the experimental and control groups with respect to the various measures of psychological skill employed in this project, although the GMC students estimated their psychological skill to be higher than the control students estimated theirs to be.

Although no differences were found between the psychologist's analyses of the individual teaching conferences, the physician observer's ratings indicate that the GMC staff gave more attention to application of psychological knowledge than the staff of the control clinic. Very likely it is this difference which resulted in more GMC students' reporting that they believed their staff was helpful with respect to learning how to establish good relations with patients. Another reason for the difference between the two groups' estimations of their psychological skill seems to be related to the differences in types of patients and the nature of the relations between student and patient. The GMC student had more opportunity to perceive, and become involved in, the psychological problems of patients. Larger experience with this type of problem apparently led the students to feel that they were developing greater skill, for those GMC students who participated most fully in the special features of the GMC believed it to be very helpful with respect to developing skills in working with patients.

It must be pointed out, however, that these differences in experiences were unrelated to the acquisition of psychological skill as measured by tests. This lack of difference might well be attributed to the inaccuracy of the tests were it not for the fact that individual attributes *were* related to gain in psychological skill as measured by these tests.

Individual attributes of students, in fact, seem to have been more important than educational experiences in relation to the acquisition of psychological skill. The more academically successful student, who was also relatively disinterested in social acceptance, was clearly more likely to be psychologically skillful than the student exhibiting opposite characteristics. It must be pointed out, however, that this type of student developed a type of skill indicated by ability to answer questions about a particular patient's problem. That is, the "independent achiever" developed a skill which might be described as an intellectual, or *cognitive,* skill. But the ability to *perceive intuitively* the characteristics of a patient was a function of a different set of attributes. This skill was developed by the student who was concerned about his social status and who was successful in actually achieving good relations with others. The GMC seems to have increased this type of student's ability to perceive accurately patients' characteristics.

It is difficult to say how dependable these results are. There have been virtually no previous attempts to measure psychological skill, and the procedures used in this study leave much to be desired.

The manner in which teaching, the students' study of the patient, and the students' personality characteristics interact to increase this skill remains an open question. The results of this study suggest that the latter is more important than the former two. Equally important, however, is the fact that these results also raise questions about the nature of psychological skill itself.

Dependent Variables (Effects of the GMC)

SKILL AT APPLYING THE BASIC IDEAS OF PSYCHOSOMATIC MEDICINE AND PSYCHIATRY TO CLINICAL PRACTICE

Students were asked questions about each patient's psychological characteristics as these were displayed during the six-minute sound-films administered as part of the Sound-Film Interview. Correct answers to these questions depended upon the students' skill in interpreting the cues presented in the films (see Chapter 13). This test was used first with

Table 20.1. Means and standard deviations for increase in Psychological Skill scores (1956 II)

	Mean increase	Standard deviation
GMC ($N = 8$)*	23.4	17.5
Control ($N = 9$)*	24.7	12.1
Surgery I ($N = 19$)	24.4	11.3
Surgery II ($N = 19$)	29.2	14.3

* Data available for only half the group because of test revisions.

the 1955 II group. On that occasion the GMC students improved less than the control students, but the differences in mean change scores were not statistically significant (see Table 20.1). The results for the class of 1956 were similar to those for the 1955 II students—only chance differences existed among the groups (see Table 20.2). The results obtained with this test, then, indicate that the GMC did not increase the students' skill in applying their knowledge of psychology.

The data from the questionnaire, however, indicate that the students felt the GMC had a positive effect on their psychological skill. For example, the GMC students rated their clerkship as more helpful in this respect, and they evaluated their own proficiency higher, than did control students.

Results concerning the students' responses about the helpfulness of their clerkships are presented in Table 20.3. For the 1955 II and 1956 II groups, a higher percentage (statistically significant) of GMC than control students rated their clerkship as extremely or very helpful. The difference between the GMC and control percentages for the 1956 I group was not statistically significant. On two of three occasions, then, more GMC than other students rated their clerkship as extremely or very helpful.

Table 20.2. Difference between percentages of students expected and obtained in the high increase group: psychological skill (class of 1956)

	Percentage expected	Percentage obtained	Difference
1956 I			
GMC ($N = 18$)	13	12	−1
Control ($N = 13$)	10	6	−4
Surgery I ($N = 17$)	12	11	−1
Surgery II ($N = 17$)	12	18	6
1956 II			
GMC ($N = 16$)	12	15	3
Control ($N = 18$)	14	14	0
Surgery I ($N = 15$)	12	8	−4
Surgery II ($N = 16$)	12	14	2

Table 20.3. Percentage of students rating their clerkship as extremely or very helpful in acquiring skill at applying the basic ideas of psychosomatic medicine and psychiatry to clinical practice (1955 II, 1956 I and II)

	1955 II	1956 I	1956 II
GMC	47*	61	50*
Control	11	77	22
Surgery I	—	0	0
Surgery II	5	12	6

* Difference between GMC and other groups statistically significant ($p < .05$).

The results presented in Table 20.4 definitely indicate that the GMC students felt more proficient than did other students. Statistically significantly more GMC than control students rated their own proficiency above average. It will be noted that a high percentage of surgery clerkship students rated their proficiency above average in the 1956 II group. Apparently this relatively high percentage was effected by the previous clerkship. A high percentage of 1956 II students rated themselves above average upon entering surgery, and the change in percentage of students so rating themselves was small.

To summarize, the objective test results indicate only chance differences between the GMC and control groups in the acquisition of skill in applying the basic ideas of psychosomatic medicine and psychiatry to clinical practice. The questionnaire results, however, reveal that the GMC students rated their clerkship as more helpful. GMC students also rated their own proficiency higher than control students rated their proficiency.

Skill in establishing and maintaining good physician-patient relations

The development of the test of this type of skill is explained in detail in Chapter 13. The rationale of this test might be summarized in the

Table 20.4. Change in percentage of students rating themselves above average in skill at applying the basic ideas of psychosomatic medicine and psychiatry to clinical practice (1955 II, 1956 I and II)

	1955 II			1956 I			1956 II		
	Post I	Post II	Change	Pre	Post I	Change	Post I	Post II	Change
GMC	*	53	*	23	66	*43*†	25	50	*25*†
Control	*	17	*	39	23	*—16*	22	17	*—5*
Surgery I	*	—	*	6	24	*18*	60	67	*7*
Surgery II	*	42	*	12	24	*12*	38	50	*12*

* No data.
† Difference between GMC and control groups statistically significant ($p < .05$).

following way. If a physician is to be skillful in establishing and maintaining good relations with patients, he must be effective in communicating with them, and his effective communication depends on his accurate perception of them. To communicate effectively, the physician must accurately perceive (among other things) the patient's intelligence, his vocabulary level, and his personality characteristics. Mistaken judgments about any of these are likely to prevent effective communication and thus prevent the development of rapport. Consequently, the students were asked to make judgments about these (and other) aspects of the patients they saw in the Sound-Film Interview.

The accuracy of the students' perceptions of patients was compared before and after participation in the various clerkships. The results indicate that the control students improved more in the accuracy of their estimation of patients' characteristics than did the GMC students. (It is interesting to note that the failure of the GMC students to improve as much as the control students appears to be due to their increased responsiveness to the individual differences among patients. This point is developed in detail in Chapter 21.)

Estimating age. The students were asked to estimate the age of each patient filmed. (This task was used because it is a very simple one; it was used only with the class of 1956.) The accuracy of these estimations was computed by the Random Comparison Method described in Chapter 13. The results indicate that there were no differences between the 1956 I groups, but that the 1956 II control students improved over the GMC students to a statistically significant degree (see Table 20.5).

Estimating intelligence. The students were also asked to estimate the intelligence of the patients in the films. There were no statistically significant differences among the groups (see Table 20.6).

Table 20.5. Difference between percentages of students expected and obtained in the high increase group: accuracy in estimating age (class of 1956)

	Percentage expected	Percentage obtained	Difference
1956 I			
GMC ($N = 18$)	12	8	—4
Control ($N = 13$)	12	12	0
Surgery I ($N = 17$)	9	9	0
Surgery II ($N = 17$)	13	17	4
1956 II			
GMC ($N = 16$)	10	8	—2
Control ($N = 18$)	12	18	6
Surgery I ($N = 15$)	10	6	—4
Surgery II ($N = 16$)	10	9	—1

Table 20.6. Difference between percentages of students expected and obtained in the high increase group: accuracy in estimating intelligence (class of 1956)

	Percentage expected	Percentage obtained	Difference
1956 I			
GMC ($N = 18$)	13	14	1
Control ($N = 13$)	13	15	2
Surgery I ($N = 17$)	10	9	—1
Surgery II ($N = 17$)	14	12	—2
1956 II			
GMC ($N = 16$)	13	12	—1
Control ($N = 18$)	14	11	—3
Surgery I ($N = 15$)	12	14	2
Surgery II ($N = 16$)	13	15	2

Estimating vocabulary level. It was felt that one of the advantages to be gained from experience in the GMC would be an increased awareness of the need for the doctor to use an appropriate vocabulary when communicating with the patient. In order for the doctor to do so, he must make an accurate estimation of the patient's vocabulary level. It seemed likely that the GMC students' increased contact with a given patient would not only emphasize this need, but improve the students' ability in this respect as well. For this reason GMC students were expected to improve in the accuracy of their estimations of patients' vocabulary level more than the control students.

As explained in Chapter 13, each patient was given the vocabulary test from the Wechsler-Bellevue Intelligence Scale. The students were to estimate the first word the patient defined incorrectly (task A) and the first three consecutive words the patient defined inaccurately (task B). These estimations, made on the basis of the students' observations of the patient during the Sound-Film Interview, were compared with the patient's actual performance on the vocabulary test in order to discover how accurate the students' estimations were.

Group differences in Accuracy scores for task A—estimating the first word missed—for the class of 1954 are presented in Table 20.7. This table shows the means, variances, and ranks of the means for the various groups. In the Pretest–Posttest I comparison, the control group was superior to the other groups, the difference from the class mean being significant at the .05 level of confidence. The differences obtained in the Posttest I—Posttest II comparison were not significant. An examination of the trend of these data in the ranks of the groups fails to reveal a discernible pattern. The significant superiority of the control group in the first-half comparison was not supported by the second-half comparison in which the control students improved less than the GMC students.

Table 20.7. Means, variances, and ranks for Accuracy scores: estimating vocabulary level, task A (class of 1954)

	Pretest		Posttest I		Pre–Post I		Rank of mean
1954 I							
	Mean	Variance	Mean	Variance	Mean	Variance	
GMC	74.74	214.4	58.57	184.2	—16.68	303.9	3
Control	60.00	577.7	57.95	349.3	—3.39	513.6	1
Surgery I	67.89	374.5	50.05	236.0	—18.58	391.9	4
Surgery II	67.50	258.7	59.53	286.6	−8.89	351.9	2
1954 II							
	Posttest I		Posttest II		Post I–Post II		Rank of mean
	Mean	Variance	Mean	Variance	Mean	Variance	
GMC	53.74	294.2	50.79	189.2	—2.95	182.4	3
Control	55.55	270.9	50.71	333.1	—4.80	327.5	4
Surgery I	57.67	277.3	59.57	280.1	1.90	290.4	2
Surgery II	58.95	245.7	61.50	255.0	2.83	464.5	1

Group differences in Accuracy scores for task B—estimating the first three words missed consecutively—are presented in Table 20.8. None of the comparisons was statistically significant.

Analysis of the accuracy of the estimations made by the students in the class of 1955 indicated that for both first- and second-half comparisons, the differences on both tasks A and B among the groups were due to chance (see Tables 20.9 and 20.10). Although the data from the class of 1956 were analyzed in a somewhat different fashion, similar

Table 20.8. Means, variances, and ranks for Accuracy scores: estimating vocabulary level, task B (class of 1954)

	Pretest		Posttest I		Pre–Post I		Rank of mean
1954 I							
	Mean	Variance	Mean	Variance	Mean	Variance	
GMC	72.63	187.8	72.90	229.8	0.26	595.8	2
Control	75.00	258.3	68.16	231.5	—7.61	727.5	4
Surgery I	72.10	185.0	71.10	335.7	—1.10	646.7	3
Surgery II	70.00	231.5	70.53	261.6	0.89	529.2	1
1954 II							
	Posttest I		Posttest II		Post I–Post II		Rank of mean
	Mean	Variance	Mean	Variance	Mean	Variance	
GMC	70.00	308.5	59.32	212.8	—10.68	287.5	4
Control	71.60	290.1	62.33	203.6	—9.50	285.1	3
Surgery I	71.19	258.2	65.57	225.4	—5.62	256.8	1
Surgery II	70.05	211.2	61.50	186.4	—7.39	243.2	2

Table 20.9. Means, variances, and ranks for Accuracy scores: estimating vocabulary level, task A (class of 1955)

1955 I	Pretest		Posttest I		Pre–Post I		Rank of mean
	Mean	Variance	Mean	Variance	Mean	Variance	
GMC	74.50	204.7	59.65	340.9	—14.85	572.5	4
Control	66.11	290.4	60.17	340.1	—5.94	617.0	2
Surgery I	73.33	266.6	69.33	198.2	—4.00	249.4	1
Surgery II	74.70	224.9	64.88	167.7	—9.82	371.5	3

1955 II	Posttest I		Posttest II		Post I–Post II		Rank of mean
	Mean	Variance	Mean	Variance	Mean	Variance	
GMC	69.94	128.7	61.18	198.6	—9.12	189.8	4
Control	64.24	234.7	54.44	191.3	—8.94	311.5	3
Surgery I	65.16	305.3	58.95	262.0	—6.21	233.4	2
Surgery II	54.63	320.4	56.84	347.9	2.21	570.6	1

results were obtained; no statistically significant differences between the groups on task A or task B appeared for either first- or second-half comparisons (see Tables 20.11 and 20.12).

Estimating personality characteristics. Perhaps an even more important skill than the correct appraisal of a patient's intelligence and vocabulary level, is the correct (and swift) appraisal of a patient's personality. The development and maintenance of good relations with patients demands that the physician respond in an appropriate

Table 20.10. Means, variances, and ranks for Accuracy scores: estimating vocabulary level, task B (class of 1955)

1955 I	Pretest		Posttest I		Pre–Post I		Rank of mean
	Mean	Variance	Mean	Variance	Mean	Variance	
GMC	72.50	108.7	70.15	252.1	—2.35	401.6	3
Control	73.33	25.5	60.72	208.5	—12.61	445.5	4
Surgery I	70.56	149.6	72.89	267.0	2.82	481.5	1
Surgery II	65.88	165.3	65.35	221.2	—0.53	504.9	2

1955 II	Posttest I		Posttest II		Post I–Post II		Rank of mean
	Mean	Variance	Mean	Variance	Mean	Variance	
GMC	72.89	258.0	63.53	58.1	—9.88	275.2	4
Control	65.35	230.8	59.44	160.8	—5.94	304.6	3
Surgery I	67.58	216.6	64.21	203.3	—3.37	277.4	2
Surgery II	63.79	283.4	64.21	98.0	0.42	351.2	1

Table 20.11. Difference between percentages of students expected and obtained in the high increase group: accuracy in estimating vocabulary level, task A (class of 1956)

	Percentage expected	Percentage obtained	Difference
1956 I			
GMC ($N = 18$)	12	12	0
Control ($N = 13$)	9	9	0
Surgery I ($N = 17$)	12	15	3
Surgery II ($N = 17$)	12	8	—4
1956 II			
GMC ($N = 16$)	10	11	1
Control ($N = 18$)	11	14	3
Surgery I ($N = 15$)	9	11	2
Surgery II ($N = 16$)	10	5	—5

way to the individuality of his patients. This can be done only if the physician can accurately estimate what sort of person his patient is—and this requires that he accurately estimate the patient's personality characteristics. To discover whether the GMC had an effect on the students' skill in making such estimations, a test of this skill was developed in connection with the Sound-Film Interview.

The students made estimations about seven aspects of the patient's personality. Since these seven estimations were made for both the overt and covert aspects of the patient's personality, a total of fourteen estimations were made by each student for each patient.

Results of the comparisons of the four groups for the classes of 1954 and 1955 are presented in Table 20.13. The data in this table refer to increase in accuracy of estimations from pretest to posttest. The number of times each group obtained the rank of first *or* second in increased

Table 20.12. Difference between percentages of students expected and obtained in the high increase group: accuracy in estimating vocabulary level, task B (class of 1956)

	Percentage expected	Percentage obtained	Difference
1956 I			
GMC ($N = 18$)	14	14	0
Control ($N = 13$)	10	9	—1
Surgery I ($N = 17$)	13	15	2
Surgery II ($N = 17$)	13	11	—2
1956 II			
GMC ($N = 16$)	16	12	—4
Control ($N = 18$)	17	23	6
Surgery I ($N = 15$)	15	12	—3
Surgery II ($N = 16$)	16	15	—1

Table 20.13. Number of times each group was first or second with respect to increase in accuracy of estimations of personality characteristics (classes of 1954 and 1955)*

	1954 I	1954 II	1955 I	1955 II
GMC	8	3	1	4
Control	5	5	11	5
Surgery I	7	10	10	11
Surgery II	8	10	6	8

* Expected number = 7.

accuracy is indicated in each column. Thus, because there are fourteen scales, there were fourteen opportunities for a group to be listed as first or second in gain in accuracy. The chance expectancy of being listed as being first or second versus being listed as third or fourth is 14/2, or seven. The deviations from this number were tested by Chi-squared (with three degrees of freedom). This statistical test indicated that the GMC students were first or second in gain in accuracy less frequently than one would expect on the basis of chance in three of the four GMC-control comparisons.[1] The GMC experience, then, did not increase the students' accuracy in judging patients' personality characteristics. In fact, participation in the GMC definitely hampered the students in this respect.

The results for the class of 1956 were analyzed in a somewhat more detailed fashion. The four groups were compared with respect to their gain in accuracy in estimating the overt aspects of personality separately from their gain in accuracy in estimating the covert aspects of personality. No significant differences among the groups were obtained in connection with either task (see Tables 20.14 and 20.15).

To summarize, GMC students rated their own proficiency in applying their knowledge of psychology higher than the control students rated their proficiency. However, there were no statistically significant differences between the two groups on the multiple-choice test. Differences which did appear on the interpersonal perception test of skill generally favored the control students. There was no evidence to support the GMC students' impressions that they possessed greater proficiency in this area.

Independent Variables (Reasons for the Effects of the GMC)

The previous discussion suggests that there was little evidence to indicate that the GMC increased the students' skill in coping with the psychological problems of patients. The following discussion is concerned with the question of why this result occurred.

[1] Note that this test favors acceptance of the null hypothesis.

Table 20.14. Difference between percentages of students expected and obtained in the high increase group: accuracy in estimating overt personality characteristics (class of 1956)

	Percentage expected	Percentage obtained	Difference
1956 I			
GMC ($N = 18$)	14	12	—2
Control ($N = 13$)	10	8	—2
Surgery I ($N = 17$)	13	17	4
Surgery II ($N = 17$)	13	12	—1
1956 II			
GMC ($N = 16$)	12	11	—1
Control ($N = 18$)	14	14	0
Surgery I ($N = 15$)	12	12	0
Surgery II ($N = 16$)	13	15	2

Analysis of the teaching conferences

The psychologist's analysis of the Teaching Conference Records and the Post-Conference Interviews revealed no differences between the GMC and control groups with respect to the manner in which students were taught or the manner in which they presented their patients to the staff.

The physician observer found that ratings of the students on psychological skill could be made in 60% of the GMC records and 59% of the control records. The mean rating for GMC students ($N = 18$) was 4.1, and the mean rating for control students ($N = 17$) was 4.0 (on a seven-point scale). The physician observer found GMC staff members devoted attention to the application of the basic ideas of psychosomatic medicine and psychiatry in 34% of their conferences, while the control staff devoted attention to this topic in 48% of their con-

Table 20.15. Difference between percentages of students expected and obtained in the high increase group: accuracy in estimating covert personality characteristics (class of 1956)

	Percentage expected	Percentage obtained	Difference
1956 I			
GMC ($N = 18$)	14	12	—2
Control ($N = 13$)	10	8	—2
Surgery I ($N = 17$)	13	17	4
Surgery II ($N = 17$)	13	12	—1
1956 II			
GMC ($N = 16$)	13	11	—2
Control ($N = 18$)	14	14	0
Surgery I ($N = 15$)	12	12	0
Surgery II ($N = 16$)	13	15	2

Table 20.16. Rating of staff with respect to their analysis of problems associated with the application of psychological knowledge to clinical practice

	Percentage of conferences		
	Staff only recognized problem	Staff explored problem	Staff went to core of problem
GMC ($N = 32$)	62.5	34.4	3.1
Control ($N = 36$)	66.7	25.0	8.3

ferences. The control staff and the GMC staff received almost identical ratings on their analyses of problems associated with the application of psychological knowledge to clinical practice (see Table 20.16). However, the GMC staff more frequently proposed action which was related to the central aspects of the patient's psychological problems than did the control staff (see Table 20.17). Although 21% of the conferences in both clerkships included discussion of physician-patient relations, the GMC staff apparently went much further in analysis of problems associated with these relations (see Table 20.18). Also, the action proposed by the GMC staff was more often related to central aspects of the patient's problem than was the action proposed by the control staff (see Table 20.19).

In short, although the psychologist's analyses of the teaching conferences indicated slight differences between the two clerkships, the ratings of the physician observer indicated that some differences did exist. The physician observer noted that the GMC staff proposed more relevant action and dealt more thoroughly with the matter of physician-patient relations than did the control staff.

Students' reports of activities engaged in

The data presented in Table 20.20 indicate that the two 1956 I clerkships differed very little, but the 1956 II clerkships differed greatly; far more 1956 II GMC students than control students reported that they had opportunities to participate in activities relating to developing skill in interpersonal relations.

Students' reports of general clerkship experience

More GMC students found their teachers helpful with respect to acquiring skill in applying the basic ideas of psychosomatic medicine and psychiatry than did students in other clerkships (see Table 20.21). But in the class of 1956 more control students than GMC students rated their teachers as extremely or very proficient in this respect (see Table 20.22). This was not true for the 1955 II group.

Table 20.17. Rating of staff with respect to relevance of the action proposed by them to patients' psychological problems

	Percentage of conferences			
	Not explicitly relevant	Related to peripheral aspects	Related to central aspects	Related to both aspects
GMC ($N = 32$)	6.2	25.0	50.0	18.8
Control ($N = 38$)	23.7	26.3	34.2	15.8

Table 20.18. Rating of staff with respect to their analysis of problems associated with establishing good physician-patient relations

	Percentage of conferences		
	Staff only recognized problem	Staff explored problem	Staff went to core of problem
GMC ($N = 20$)	60.0	30.0	10.0
Control ($N = 16$)	81.2	18.8	0.0

Table 20.19. Rating of staff with respect to relevance of action proposed by them to problems of physician-patient relations

	Percentage of conferences			
	Not explicitly relevant	Related to peripheral aspects	Related to central aspects	Related to both aspects
GMC ($N = 20$)	10.0	25.0	45.0	20.0
Control ($N = 16$)	18.8	31.2	37.5	12.5

Table 20.20. Percentage of students indicating that certain activities were very frequently or always present in their clerkship (class of 1956)

	1956 I		1956 II	
	GMC	Control	GMC	Control
Having opportunities to explain to patients their prognosis, limitations, etc.	66	76	82	39
Having opportunities to give psychotherapy	28	46	56	17
Handling the emotional problems of patients	44	46	56	34

Table 20.21. Percentage of students rating their staff as extremely or very helpful in acquiring skill at applying the basic ideas of psychosomatic medicine and psychiatry to clinical practice (class of 1956)

	1956 I	1956 II
GMC	50	51
Control	38	11
Surgery I	0	0
Surgery II	6	0

Table 20.22. Percentage of students rating their staff as extremely or very proficient in applying the basic ideas of psychosomatic medicine and psychiatry to clinical practice (1955 II, 1956 I and II)

	1955 II	1956 I	1956 II
GMC	24	28	19
Control	6	39	28
Surgery I	—	0	13
Surgery II	11	12	6

Definitely more GMC than other students found their patients helpful with respect to acquiring skill in applying the basic ideas of psychosomatic medicine and psychiatry to clinical practice (see Table 20.23). In fact, the utility of the patients *in this respect* seems to be the one aspect of the GMC about which its students were in high agreement.

In brief, more GMC students than control students found their clerkship helpful in acquiring skill in psychological aspects of medical practice. However, the students felt that the nature of the patients contributed more to this difference than the proficiency of the staff.

Special educational techniques of the GMC

In the 1956 II group those GMC students who had the fewest contacts with the families of their patients, and those who had the fewest conferences with the social workers and the public health nurse gained the most in Psychological Skill test scores. No other relations between special techniques of the GMC and Psychological Skill scores were found.

However, in the 1956 I group those students who had the largest number of ward contacts with the families of their patients increased the importance they attached to treating the emotional problems of patients. And in the same group those students who reported frequently having responsibility for patients also increased the importance they attached to having opportunities to give psychotherapy.

Students in the 1956 I group who found the GMC to be very helpful with respect to increasing their skill in physician-patient relations were those who reported having responsibility for the diagnosis

Table 20.23. Percentage of students rating their patients as extremely or very helpful in acquiring skill at applying the basic ideas of psychosomatic medicine and psychiatry to clinical practice (class of 1956)

	1956 I	1956 II
GMC	89	69
Control	46	28
Surgery I	12	34
Surgery II	18	0

and treatment of their patients, reported thinking of themselves more as doctors than as students, reported that they found the GMC more helpful than they had expected with respect to acquiring more of the basic facts of clinical medicine, reported that they found the GMC more helpful than they expected with respect to learning the practical application of the principles of comprehensive care, and reported that they had expected (prior to entering the GMC) that the GMC would be helpful with respect to learning to organize diagnostic and therapeutic regimes. And those GMC students in the 1955 I group who saw the fewest patients found the GMC to be of the most help in establishing and maintaining good physician-patient relations.

In short, those students who more often saw patients' families and accepted responsibility for patients perceived the importance of psychological factors; those students who accepted responsibility, thought of themselves as doctors, and felt that they had learned more in the GMC than they had expected, reported the GMC a good place in which to increase their skill in physician-patient relations.

Staff's evaluation of students

As indicated previously, the GMC staff evaluated the students almost wholly in terms of their medical knowledge and skill. They distinguished this type of performance from students' ability to develop good relations with patients only for the 1954 I group.

Interviews with students

Little material in the interviews with the classes of 1954 and 1955 was directly related to skill in working with patients. However, after the 1955 Posttest I both GMC and control students did discuss this topic, albeit somewhat briefly, with the interviewer. Of the GMC students, 40% (8/20) reported that the staff helped them establish good physician-patient relations by suggesting ways in which they could achieve better rapport with patients. Only 17% (3/18) of the control students mentioned that their teachers had helped them in this way.

A few GMC students (20%, 4/20) and a similar percentage of control students felt that the staff were helpful because they had provided a good example. Approximately an equal percentage in both groups, however, asserted that formal training could not be given in this area because, they said, such skills can be acquired only through experience. Some (28%) of the control students mentioned that the staff tended to behave tactlessly toward patients. The response of most (44%) of the control students, however, was that they were given little or no training in this area.

In the 1955 I group, then, the GMC students reported more instruction in establishing good physician-patient relations than did the control students.

To summarize, evidently the GMC did provide an environment which was likely to enhance the acquisition of psychological skill. Although no differences were found between the psychologist's analyses of the teaching conferences, some differences were found in the ratings made by the physician observer. Although many GMC students were unimpressed with the proficiency of their teachers in connection with psychological skill, the students did believe the staff was helpful, and the patients particularly helpful, in this regard. Moreover, those students who participated most in the special features of the GMC reported the GMC to be a good place in which to develop skill in physician-patient relations.

Individual Attributes Related to Psychological Skill

The results reported below suggest that, as in connection with psychological knowledge, the acquisition of psychological skill was more a function of individual attributes than of participation in either clerkship. The nature of the relations between individual attributes and psychological skill provides an interesting comparison with those between individual attributes and psychological knowledge. It appears that students who had already acquired knowledge about psychological factors, and who continued to do so, were successful academically. They were "independent achievers." These independent achievers also obtained high Pretest scores in psychological skill, and they acquired more psychological skill *as measured by objective tests.*

However, when psychological skill was measured in terms of *ability to perceive accurately the characteristics of patients,* quite a different set of attributes was involved. Students who had high Pretest scores (and who gained in skill) were not only concerned about their social status, but were successful in achieving good relations with others. On the other hand, they were not very successful in their academic work.

Measurement by objective test

Results pertaining to the entire class. There were no relations of consequence between measures of previous academic performance and Pretest scores on the Psychological Skill test.

Personality characteristics, however, were related to Pretest scores on the Psychological Skill test. (These personality characteristics were similar to those related to Pretest scores on the Psychological Knowledge test, as well as to Pretest scores on attitudes toward comprehen-

Table 20.24. Relation between cumulative grade average and change in psychological skill from Posttest I to Posttest II, all groups (1956 II)

		Change in psychological skill		
		Below median	Above median	
Cumulative grade average	Above median	11	20	31
Cumulative grade average	Below median	21	13	34
$\chi^2 = 4.48; p < .05$		32	33	65

sive care.) Results from the California Psychological Inventory indicated that such personality characteristics as an interest in achievement through independence and self-reliance (Achievement via Independence, CPI), frequent fantasy about intellectual and professional accomplishments, a tendency to think of oneself in positive terms (Self-Acceptance, ACL) and to be tolerant and nonjudgmental (Tolerance, CPI) identify the student who had a high Pretest score on the objective test of psychological skill.

Although this section is primarily concerned with Pretest scores, the individual attributes associated with Psychological Skill scores on Posttest II were so striking that they should be mentioned here. First-, second-, and third-year grade averages, the junior medical clerkship grade, and the cumulative grade average were all positively associated with Psychological Skill scores. Amount of medical knowledge as judged by fellow students was also positively associated with these scores. The following self-ratings were associated with Psychological Skill scores on Posttest II: frequency of fantasy about intellectual and professional accomplishments, importance attached to intellectual and professional accomplishments, anxiety concerning responsibilities for patients when practicing medicine, and worry about peer acceptance as a friend. Confirming the finding from the California Psychological Inventory (and the self-ratings) was the fact that the Edwards Personal Preference Schedule Need for Achievement scale was also positively associated with Psychological Skill scores on Posttest II.

When all 1956 II clerkships were considered, third-year grade averages, premedical grade averages, and cumulative grade averages were positively associated with gain in Psychological Skill scores from Posttest I to Posttest II (see Table 20.24). This same relation was apparent when the control and GMC clerkships only were compared (see Table 20.25).

Students who were uneasy about their social relations, i.e., those students who reported worrying about their social adjustment and

Table 20.25. Relation between cumulative grade average and change in psychological skill from Posttest I to Posttest II, GMC and control groups (1956 II)

		Change in psychological skill		
		Below median	Above median	
Cumulative grade average	Above median	4	13	17
Cumulative grade average	Below median	11	6	17
$\chi^2 = 4.29; p < .05$		15	19	34

about their acceptance by their peers, also gained in psychological skill. Students who reported that they had not been rewarded for responsibility as adolescents gained in psychological skill from Posttest I to Posttest II.

When the period from Pretest to Posttest II is considered, the students who gained in psychological skill reported worrying about acceptance by peers (see above), but somewhat surprisingly reported little interest in the welfare of patients' families and reported not being rewarded for responsibility as adolescents. There may well be some reason for these students to "worry" about acceptance by others. It will be noted that these students did not receive favorable ratings by their peers on leadership, likeability, etc., although their academic accomplishments were recognized, i.e., they received high ratings by fellow students on medical knowledge.

Results pertaining to the GMC. In the GMC group the better students (as indicated by cumulative grade average) gained in psychological skill from Posttest I to Posttest II (see Table 20.26). The relations between personality characteristics and gain in psychological skill in the GMC group were similar to those found in the entire class. For example, students who liked to be on their own (n Autonomy) and who were unconcerned about relations with others in connection with

Table 20.26. Relation between cumulative grade average and change in psychological skill from Posttest I to Posttest II, GMC (1956 II)

		Change in psychological skill		
		Below median	Above median	
Cumulative grade average	Above median	1	8	9
Cumulative grade average	Below median	5	2	7
$p < .05$		6	10	16

achievement (scored low on Achievement via Conformance, Good Impression, and n Exhibition) acquired more psychological skill in the GMC.

This descriptive pattern from two personality tests (CPI and EPPS) is confirmed by data from students' self-reports. Students who acquired psychological skill in the GMC also reported that they had little interest in the welfare of a patient's family, were not rewarded for influencing others as adolescents, were not rewarded for scholastic success as adolescents, and were not rewarded for responsibility as adolescents.

Results pertaining to the control group. The results obtained in connection with the control group indicated that much the same sort of students who profited in the GMC gained psychological skill from Posttest I to Posttest II in the control program.

To summarize, it seems quite clear that students who acquired psychological skill as measured by multiple-choice, objective test items were likely to be academically successful, but socially independent. Moreover, they seemed to recognize that their independence separated them from their fellows, i.e., they indicated worrying about relations with others. It should be pointed out that the data supporting this finding came from five different sources: the California Psychological Inventory, the Edwards Personal Preference Schedule, students' judgments of one another, students' reports about themselves, and grade averages.

Measurement by ability to estimate personality characteristics

Because a detailed examination of the relations of each psychological test to each interpersonal perception task (estimation of age, intelligence, vocabulary level, and personality characteristics) categorized by class and group would result in a proliferation of data and tables, only the general results emerging from the study of these relations will be presented.

Results pertaining to the entire class. High scores on the Quantitative Ability subtest of the MCAT were negatively related to accurate perceptions of patients' characteristics on three of the four interpersonal perception tasks at the Pretest administration.

Certain individual attributes were related to accuracy. Students who reported that they worried about their social adjustment and their social acceptance, who were authoritarian and generally anxious, and who were not psychologically-minded were the more accurate perceivers.

There was a fairly definite tendency for certain peer ratings to be associated with the accurate perception of personality characteristics.

Those students whose peers thought them likeable, sympathetic to comprehensive care, responsible and mature, willing and able to work independently, and leaders were the more accurate perceivers.

All these results point in one direction—students who were concerned about social relations and successful in achieving high status among their peers were accurate perceivers of the personality characteristics of patients at the Pretest.

There was a tendency for the same traits that characterized students who were initially accurate perceivers to characterize also those students who increased most in accuracy. For example, those students who reported worrying about peer acceptance increased their accuracy more than those who did not report this worry. And students with strong feelings about their social relations (high n Affiliation, EPPS; high score on the Sociability scale, CPI) increased their accuracy scores the most.

Results pertaining to the GMC. There was some indication that the same personality traits related to increased perceptual accuracy in the entire class were also related to increased perceptual accuracy in the GMC. Students who were concerned with their social relations (high score on Sociability scale, CPI; high n Affiliation, EPPS), increased their accuracy in two of the tasks. And GMC students who were socially responsible (high score on Social Responsibility, CPI), tolerant (high score on Tolerance, CPI), and who rated themselves high on "fear of failure" increased their accuracy from Pretest to Posttest II.

Results pertaining to the control group. There were no discernible trends in relations between individual attributes and change in accuracy of the perception of patients' personality characteristics in the control group.

To summarize, the results concerning relations between individual attributes and the acquisition of psychological skill present a consistent picture and lead to a definite conclusion. Students who were independent achievers acquired more psychological skill when this was measured by objective test items. These students were more likely to improve in psychological skill if they were in the GMC than if they were in the control clerkship.

Students who were interested in social acceptance and who were successful in their efforts to achieve it acquired more psychological skill when this was measured in terms of ability to perceive accurately the personality characteristics of patients.

Chapter 21

Psychological Attitudes

Summary

One of the more important aims of the GMC was to promote positive attitudes toward the psychological aspects of medical care. Therefore, an effort was made to develop several tests of students' attitudes toward psychosomatic medicine and psychiatry, physician-patient relations, and other psychological aspects of medicine. Some of these tests were of the direct "question and answer" variety, and some were less direct and less obvious to the student (see Chapter 13).

Experience in the GMC apparently affected the students who participated in it by changing their attitudes toward emotional problems (as well as in other ways). GMC students seemed somewhat more aware of and more convinced of the importance of psychological factors. But the GMC did not much affect the students' attitudes toward physician-patient relations or toward patients.

These results seemed to stem from the same causes—high similarity of teaching experiences in both groups, and dissimilarity of patient material in the groups. That is, although GMC students became more aware of, and sympathetic to, psychological problems, they were not more inclined to want to cope with them or even to develop more fully their relations with patients. These negative results apparently occurred because GMC patients involved students in a large number of psychological problems, most of which were not related to the students' central desire—acquisition of medical knowledge.

Some students did change their attitudes toward physician-patient relations as well as toward psychological factors. These students tended to be more intelligent as well as more mature and responsible. Students who tended to increase their perceptions of individual differences among patients were relatively more anxious, authoritarian, and highly concerned with, although not successful in, their relations with others.

Dependent Variables (Effects of the GMC)

ATTITUDES TOWARD BEHAVIOR DISORDERS

The subscale Attitude toward Behavior Disorders of the Medical Attitudes test was used to measure changes in students' attitudes. In the 1956 I group the increase in the percentage of GMC students who developed more favorable attitudes (in contrast to the percentage expected on a chance basis) was sufficiently great to warrant accepting the conclusion that the GMC had a positive effect on students' attitudes (see Table 21.1). In the 1956 II group, however, there were only chance differences among the four groups. Thus, with respect to the problem of *relative* change among the four groups, the GMC was found to have a statistically significant effect on one occasion, but not on the other.

When the GMC and control clerkships are compared with respect to *absolute* change, it is also apparent that the GMC had its effect on the 1956 I but not the 1956 II group (see Table 21.2).

Of 18 GMC students in the 1956 I group, 13 (or approximately two thirds) changed in a positive direction, while of 13 control students, 8 (or approximately two thirds) changed in a negative direction. However, because roughly half the GMC students changed in a negative direction in the 1956 II group, the over-all effect of GMC does not quite achieve statistical significance, although a trend is clearly present (see Table 21.3).

Thus, although almost twice as many GMC students as control students changed in a positive direction, the large number (13) of GMC students who changed in a negative direction prevents a definite confirmation of the hypothesis that the GMC would affect students' attitudes toward behavior disorders. (It should be pointed out that during the senior year more of the total group of students changed their attitudes in a negative direction than in a positive direction—31 compared with 20.)

To summarize, the GMC had a perceptible but not a marked effect on students' attitudes toward psychosomatic medicine and psychiatry, as measured by the Behavior Disorders subscale of the Medical Attitudes test.

ATTITUDES TOWARD THE PHYSICIAN-PATIENT RELATION

The Physician-Patient Relations subscale of the Medical Attitudes test was used to compare changes in students' attitudes toward physician-patient relations. The relative change among the four clerkships is presented in Table 21.4. The data indicate that the differences among the clerkships could have arisen by chance in both the 1956 I and II groups;

Table 21.1. Difference between percentages of students expected and obtained in the high increase group: attitudes toward behavior disorders (class of 1956)

	Percentage expected	Percentage obtained	Difference
1956 I			
GMC ($N = 18$)	14	23	9
Control ($N = 13$)	10	8	—2
Surgery I ($N = 17$)	13	9	—4
Surgery II ($N = 17$)	13	11	—2
1956 II			
GMC ($N = 16$)	14	11	—3
Control ($N = 18$)	16	18	2
Surgery I ($N = 15$)	13	14	1
Surgery II ($N = 16$)	14	15	1

Table 21.2. Change in attitudes toward behavior disorders from Pretest to Posttest I (1956 I) and from Posttest I to Posttest II (1956 II)

	Negative change	No change	Positive change	Total
1956 I				
GMC	3	2	13	18
Control	8	2	3	13
Total	11	4	16	31
1956 II				
GMC	9	2	5	16
Control	6	5	7	18
Total	15	7	12	34

Table 21.3. Change in attitudes toward behavior disorders from Pretest to Posttest II (1956 I and II)

	Negative change	No change	Positive change	Total
GMC	13	8	13	34
Control	18	6	7	31
Total	31	14	20	65
$\chi^2 = 2.72; p > .05$				

Table 21.4. Difference between percentages of students expected and obtained in the high increase group: attitudes toward physician-patient relations (class of 1956)

	Percentage expected	Percentage obtained	Difference
1956 I			
GMC ($N = 18$)	13	18	5
Control ($N = 13$)	10	8	—2
Surgery I ($N = 17$)	12	9	—3
Surgery II ($N = 17$)	12	12	0
1956 II			
GMC ($N = 16$)	16	15	—1
Control ($N = 18$)	18	22	4
Surgery I ($N = 15$)	15	11	—4
Surgery II ($N = 16$)	16	17	1

Table 21.5. Change in attitudes toward physician-patient relations from Pretest to Posttest I (1956 I)

	Negative change	No change	Positive change	Total
GMC	6	5	7	18
Control	8	4	1	13
Total	14	9	8	31

that is, the GMC apparently did not succeed in developing more favorable attitudes toward physician-patient relations than did the control medical clerkship or the surgery clerkship, although the trend of results in the 1956 I group slightly favors GMC.

This trend in the 1956 I group also appears when GMC students are compared with control students on an absolute rather than a relative basis (see Table 21.5). As in the case of attitudes toward psychosomatic medicine and psychiatry, however, the GMC's advantage was lost on the 1956 II group (see Table 21.6). When the period from the beginning of the senior year (Pretest) to the end of the senior year (Posttest II) is considered, there appears to have been no difference between the GMC and control students' change in attitudes toward physician-patient relations (see Table 21.7).

There is, in short, little evidence to suggest that the GMC affected students' attitudes toward the physician-patient relation, as measured by the Medical Attitudes test. (Again it is of some importance to note that approximately half (35/65) the class became less favorable in its attitudes toward the physician-patient relation during the senior year.)

Differential memory

The two procedures discussed above were direct tests of students' attitudes. That is, inasmuch as students were asked to indicate agreement or disagreement with a particular statement, the meaning of which was fairly obvious, the students were aware of the implications of their answers. To measure students' attitudes in a somewhat less direct fashion, an attempt was made to discover the amount of personal

Table 21.6. Change in attitudes toward physician-patient relations from Posttest I to Posttest II (1956 II)

	Negative change	No change	Positive change	Total
GMC	6	5	5	16
Control	4	9	5	18
Total	10	14	10	34

Table 21.7. Change in attitudes toward physician-patient relations from Pretest to Posttest II (1956 I and II)

	Negative change	No change	Positive change	Total
GMC	17	11	6	34
Control	18	9	4	31
Total	35	20	10	65

and social information they remembered in contrast to medical information. The students were asked a series of multiple-choice questions about each patient seen in the Sound-Film Interview; roughly half the questions concerned personal and social facts about the patient, and half concerned medical facts. All the information had been given by the patient during the interview; a period of about twenty minutes intervened between the showing of the film and the memory test. Two scores were computed—a Memory for Medical Facts score and a Memory for Personal and Social Facts score. It was assumed that students' attitudes would determine the kind of information they remembered. That is, if students were primarily oriented toward the medical problems of patients, they would remember medical facts about patients to the exclusion of personal and social facts, and vice versa.

Tables 21.8, 21.9, and 21.10 present the results for the classes of 1954, 1955, and 1956, respectively. Each table shows the mean increase in the Memory for Medical Facts score from Pretest to Posttest I and from Posttest I to Posttest II for each year. In both the 1954 I and II groups GMC students' scores increased by *smaller* amounts than those of the other clerkship students. The same result occurred in the 1956 II groups. In these three instances the results were statistically significant ($p < .05$). Although the differences among the groups on the

Table 21.8. Means and standard deviations for increase in Memory for Medical Facts scores (class of 1954)

	Mean increase	Standard deviation
1954 I		
GMC ($N = 18$)	0.90	5.93
Control ($N = 17$)	4.72	5.87
Surgery I ($N = 17$)	4.33	5.76
Surgery II ($N = 17$)	6.79	6.62
1954 II		
GMC ($N = 16$)	0.50	8.13
Control ($N = 18$)	6.80	7.16
Surgery I ($N = 15$)	2.00	5.21
Surgery II ($N = 16$)	2.62	8.43

Table 21.9. Means and standard deviations for increase in Memory for Medical Facts scores (class of 1955)

	Mean increase	Standard deviation
1955 I		
GMC ($N = 18$)	0.80	8.83
Control ($N = 13$)	0.00	6.32
Surgery I ($N = 17$)	—	—
Surgery II ($N = 17$)	2.50	8.71
1955 II		
GMC ($N = 16$)	5.89	12.9
Control ($N = 18$)	6.25	13.1
Surgery I ($N = 15$)	6.63	13.2
Surgery II ($N = 16$)	5.68	11.1

remaining three occasions were not statistically significant, it seems likely that on the basis of the results mentioned above the GMC increased students' Memory for Medical Facts scores less than the other clerkships did.

As Tables 21.11, 21.12, and 21.13 indicate, however, the GMC did not facilitate students' memory for personal and social material—at least as measured by the Memory for Personal and Social Facts test. There were no statistically significant differences among the clerkships (except in the 1954 II group, and this did not favor the GMC and was due entirely to the large gain made by a surgery group). Yet when change in Memory for Personal and Social Facts scores from Pretest to Posttest II were compared for GMC and control students in the class of 1956 there appeared to be a trend in favor of the GMC (see Table 21.14).

However, the surprising fact that GMC students were found to be somewhat poorer on both memory measures in 1954 and 1955 led to the re-examination of the content of the Memory for Personal and Social

Table 21.10. Difference between percentages of students expected and obtained in the high increase group: memory for medical facts (class of 1956)

	Percentage expected	Percentage obtained	Difference
1956 I			
GMC ($N = 18$)	14	14	0
Control ($N = 13$)	10	6	—4
Surgery I ($N = 17$)	13	20	7
Surgery II ($N = 17$)	13	11	—2
1956 II			
GMC ($N = 16$)	12	8	—4
Control ($N = 18$)	13	14	1
Surgery I ($N = 15$)	11	8	—3
Surgery II ($N = 16$)	12	18	6

Table 21.11. Means and standard deviations for increase in Memory for Personal and Social Facts scores (class of 1954)

	Mean increase	Standard deviation
1954 I		
GMC ($N = 18$)	0.11	4.97
Control ($N = 17$)	3.06	4.88
Surgery I ($N = 17$)	1.44	5.21
Surgery II ($N = 17$)	1.58	4.42
1954 II		
GMC ($N = 16$)	0.89	4.42
Control ($N = 18$)	1.10	4.62
Surgery I ($N = 15$)	1.14	7.51
Surgery II ($N = 16$)	4.88	5.29

Table 21.12. Means and standard deviations for increase in Memory for Personal and Social Facts scores (class of 1955)

	Mean increase	Standard deviation
1955 I		
GMC ($N = 18$)	0.15	6.41
Control ($N = 13$)	0.61	9.07
Surgery I ($N = 17$)	—	—
Surgery II ($N = 17$)	3.68	5.76
1955 II		
GMC ($N = 16$)	0.44	8.66
Control ($N = 18$)	1.50	11.28
Surgery I ($N = 15$)	0.37	8.86
Surgery II ($N = 16$)	2.74	8.42

Table 21.13. Difference between the percentages of students expected and obtained in the high increase group: memory for personal and social facts (class of 1956)

	Percentage expected	Percentage obtained	Difference
1956 I			
GMC ($N = 18$)	14	12	—2
Control ($N = 13$)	10	8	—2
Surgery I ($N = 17$)	13	18	5
Surgery II ($N = 17$)	13	12	—1
1956 II			
GMC ($N = 16$)	12	12	0
Control ($N = 18$)	14	9	—5
Surgery I ($N = 15$)	12	12	0
Surgery II ($N = 16$)	12	17	5

Table 21.14. Change in memory for personal and social facts from Pretest to Posttest II (1956 I and II)

	No. below median	No. above median	Total
GMC	14	20	34
Control	18	13	31
Total	32	33	65
$\chi^2 = 1.85; p = .20$			

Facts test. Re-examination of the test items led to the conclusion that they frequently involved highly specific, often superficial, details of the patient's life which were not highly pertinent to his personal or social problems. Because it seemed likely that students might focus upon the personal or social problem of a patient and still forget the superficial details involved in the test items, a different procedure was evolved and administered to the class of 1956 (in addition to the procedure just described).

The new test (called Memory for Latent Material) was intended to measure the students' memory for the personal and social characteristics of the patient, rather than mere personal and social details mentioned in the filmed interview. Although it proved to be impossible to refine the new procedure sufficiently to be useful for the 1956 administration, this test did permit students to make as many inferences about the patient as they cared to make. Thus it was possible to compare the GMC and control students with respect to their willingness to make inferences about the patients' personal and social behavior. It was hypothesized that GMC students would be more willing to make inferences about the personality characteristics of the patients seen in the films because they would attach greater importance to these features. No differences were found among the groups, however (see Table 21.15).

Table 21.15. Difference between percentages of students expected and obtained in the high increase group: memory for latent material (class of 1956)

	Percentage expected	Percentage obtained	Difference
1956 I			
GMC ($N = 18$)	13	12	—1
Control ($N = 13$)	10	6	—4
Surgery I ($N = 17$)	12	12	0
Surgery II ($N = 17$)	12	17	5
1956 II			
GMC ($N = 16$)	11	12	1
Control ($N = 18$)	13	12	—1
Surgery I ($N = 15$)	11	8	—3
Surgery II ($N = 16$)	11	14	3

In summary, the GMC program apparently had little effect on the students' memory for personal and social information compared with memory for medical information, nor did it affect the students' willingness to make inferences about patients' personality characteristics.

Attitudes toward patients

A further attempt was made to measure students' attitudes toward patients in a manner which would not appear obvious to the students. Equally, if not more, important was the fact that it was thought necessary to discover whether any subtle attitude changes took place—changes which the students might not be aware of. For these purposes, the students' estimations (made during the Sound-Film Interview) of patient's characteristics were studied. As pointed out in Chapter 20, there is reason to believe that the GMC students improved somewhat less than the control students in ability to make accurate estimations of patients' characteristics—particularly of their personality characteristics. However, it was possible to study not only students' accuracy but the extent to which they tended to perceive individual differences among patients (see them as individuals). If, for example, the students perceived the filmed patients as unique individuals, each differing from the others, their estimates of the patients' characteristics would vary widely. On the other hand, should the students perceive all the patients as very much alike ("stereotype" them), their estimations of the patients' characteristics would tend to be the same for all patients. In short, the variability in the students' estimates of the patients' characteristics provided an index of their tendency to individualize patients, and thus provided a measure of their attitudes toward patients. The following sections deal with each estimation task separately.

Perception of individual differences in age. Table 21.16 indicates

Table 21.16. Difference between percentages of students expected and obtained in the high increase group: perception of individual differences in age (class of 1956)

	Percentage expected	Percentage obtained	Difference
1956 I			
GMC ($N = 18$)	14	9	—5
Control ($N = 13$)	10	9	—1
Surgery I ($N = 17$)	13	17	4
Surgery II ($N = 17$)	13	15	2
1956 II			
GMC ($N = 16$)	12	15	3
Control ($N = 18$)	14	11	—3
Surgery I ($N = 15$)	12	11	—1
Surgery II ($N = 16$)	12	14	2

Table 21.17. Difference between percentages of students expected and obtained in the high increase group: perception of individual differences in intelligence (class of 1956)

	Percentage expected	Percentage obtained	Difference
1956 I			
GMC ($N = 18$)	14	14	0
Control ($N = 13$)	10	11	1
Surgery I ($N = 17$)	13	14	1
Surgery II ($N = 17$)	13	12	—1
1956 II			
GMC ($N = 16$)	12	12	0
Control ($N = 18$)	14	22	8
Surgery I ($N = 15$)	12	11	—1
Surgery II ($N = 16$)	12	6	—6

that there were no statistically significant differences among the clerkship groups with respect to change in perception of individual differences in age.

Perception of individual differences in intelligence. The results shown in Table 21.17, however, indicate that in the 1956 II group the control students changed more than the GMC students, for the former perceived larger differences among patients. Furthermore, when the performance of the GMC and control students is compared from Pretest to Posttest II, the control students clearly increased their perception of individual differences among patients with respect to intelligence more than did GMC students (see Table 21.18).

Perception of individual differences in vocabulary level. There were no statistically significant differences among the clerkship groups in the class of 1955 with respect to change in the variability in estimates of either the first word missed in the vocabulary test (task A, see Table 21.19) or the first three words missed consecutively (task B, see Table 21.20).

There were statistically significant differences in the 1956 I group with respect to change in the variability in the students' estimates of

Table 21.18. Change in perception of individual differences in intelligence from Pretest to Posttest II (1956 I and II)

	No. below median	No. above median	Total
GMC	22	12	34
Control	10	21	31
Total	32	33	65
$\chi^2 = 6.83$; $p = .01$			

Table 21.19. Difference between percentages of students expected and obtained in the high increase group: perception of individual differences in vocabulary level, task A (class of 1955)

	Percentage expected	Percentage obtained	Difference
1955 I			
GMC ($N = 18$)	14	17	3
Control ($N = 13$)	13	14	1
Surgery I ($N = 17$)	12	13	1
Surgery II ($N = 17$)	12	7	—5
1955 II			
GMC ($N = 16$)	12	8	—4
Control ($N = 18$)	12	11	—1
Surgery I ($N = 15$)	13	13	0
Surgery II ($N = 16$)	13	18	5

the first word missed in the vocabulary test—one surgery group increasing its variability the most (see Table 21.21). There were no differences among the clerkships with respect to variability in estimates of the first three words missed consecutively when each half of the year is considered separately (see Table 21.22). However, when the comparison is made over the entire year, it can be seen that the control students made a statistically significant gain over the GMC students (see Table 21.23).

Perception of individual differences in personality characteristics. There was some indication that the GMC students became more sensitized to personality differences among patients. It will be recalled that the students were required to estimate how the patient had rated himself on eight personality traits as well as where the patient "really

Table 21.20. Difference between percentages of students expected and obtained in the high increase group: perception of individual differences in vocabulary level, task B (class of 1955)

	Percentage expected	Percentage obtained	Difference
1955 I			
GMC ($N = 18$)	14	18	4
Control ($N = 13$)	13	13	0
Surgery I ($N = 17$)	12	7	—5
Surgery II ($N = 17$)	12	13	1
1955 II			
GMC ($N = 16$)	12	14	2
Control ($N = 18$)	12	11	—1
Surgery I ($N = 15$)	13	13	0
Surgery II ($N = 16$)	13	13	0

Table 21.21. Difference between percentages of students expected and obtained in the high increase group: perception of individual differences in vocabulary level, task A (class of 1956)

	Percentage expected	Percentage obtained	Difference
1956 I			
GMC ($N = 18$)	14	12	—2
Control ($N = 13$)	10	12	2
Surgery I ($N = 17$)	13	6	—7
Surgery II ($N = 17$)	13	20	7
1956 II			
GMC ($N = 16$)	12	14	2
Control ($N = 18$)	14	14	0
Surgery I ($N = 15$)	12	11	—1
Surgery II ($N = 16$)	12	12	0

Table 21.22. Difference between percentages of students expected and obtained in the high increase group: perception of individual differences in vocabulary level, task B (class of 1956)

	Percentage expected	Percentage obtained	Difference
1956 I			
GMC ($N = 18$)	14	11	—3
Control ($N = 13$)	10	14	4
Surgery I ($N = 17$)	13	8	—5
Surgery II ($N = 17$)	13	17	4
1956 II			
GMC ($N = 16$)	12	14	2
Control ($N = 18$)	14	14	0
Surgery I ($N = 15$)	12	9	—3
Surgery II ($N = 16$)	12	14	2

Table 21.23. Change in perception of individual differences in vocabulary level (task A and task B) from Pretest to Posttest II (1956 I and II)

	No. below median	No. above median	Total
GMC	21	13	34
Control	11	20	31
Total	32	33	65

$\chi^2 = 4.48; p = .05$

Table 21.24. Number of times each group was first or second with respect to increase in variability in estimations of personality characteristics (class of 1955)*

	1955 I	1955 II
GMC	15	13
Control	4	9
Surgery I	0	5
Surgery II	14	5

* Expected number = 8.

Table 21.25. Difference between percentages of students expected and obtained in the high increase group: perception of individual differences in patients' self-ratings (class of 1956)

	Percentage expected	Percentage obtained	Difference
1956 I			
GMC ($N = 18$)	14	17	3
Control ($N = 13$)	10	5	—5
Surgery I ($N = 17$)	13	15	2
Surgery II ($N = 17$)	13	12	—1
1956 II			
GMC ($N = 16$)	12	17	5
Control ($N = 18$)	14	12	—2
Surgery I ($N = 15$)	12	12	0
Surgery II ($N = 16$)	12	9	—3

was" on these same eight traits.[1] Table 21.24 indicates the number of times each clerkship group was first or second in order of increase in the perceived differences among patients on all sixteen trait scales. The results shown in both columns of Table 21.24 differ from chance expectancy and indicate that GMC students tended to individualize the filmed patients more than did other students.

The data for the class of 1956 were analyzed in a more detailed fashion. The changes in perceived differences among patients were studied in terms of each type of estimate (students' estimations of patients' self-ratings and students' estimations of patients' "real score"). The variability in estimates of patients' self-ratings on all eight traits was averaged and pretest-posttest difference scores were computed for each student. This distribution of differences was divided at the median and the number of students expected (by chance) in the upper half of the distribution was computed. Differences between the number of students expected by chance and the number actually occurring in the upper half of the distribution were evaluated by the Chi-squared method. The data presented in Table 21.25 (in terms of percentages) indicate that the differences among the groups were due to chance, although there was a tendency for GMC students to increase their perception of individual differences more than control students.

The change in variability in students' estimates of the patients' "real scores" on the eight personality traits was studied in the same way. The results shown in Table 21.26 indicate that there were no statistically significant differences among the groups in this respect. Thus, the results for the class of 1956 did not confirm those obtained for the class of 1955.

[1] Eight scales were used in the computation of variability and seven in the computation of accuracy because it was difficult to obtain a criterion of accuracy for one scale.

Table 21.26. Difference between percentages of students expected and obtained in the high increase group: perception of individual differences in patients' real scores on personality scales (class of 1956)

	Percentage expected	Percentage obtained	Difference
1956 I			
GMC ($N = 18$)	14	12	—2
Control ($N = 13$)	10	11	1
Surgery I ($N = 17$)	13	15	2
Surgery II ($N = 17$)	13	12	—1
1956 II			
GMC ($N = 16$)	12	12	0
Control ($N = 18$)	14	15	1
Surgery I ($N = 15$)	12	12	0
Surgery II ($N = 16$)	12	11	—1

Perception of differences between overt and covert personality characteristics. The students were asked to estimate how each patient rated (described) himself on eight personality traits. In effect, the patient said, "This is the sort of person I am"; the students' task was to estimate what sort of person the patient said he was. The patient's description of himself might be termed the overt aspect of personality. The students were also asked to estimate the patient's "real score" on the same eight personality traits. The students were, in effect, asked to guess what sort of person the patient really was—to describe the covert aspects of the patient's personality. The differences between the two estimates made by the students provided a measure of the extent to which the students perceived differences between the overt and covert aspects of personality.

The results presented in Table 21.27 indicate that the GMC students in the class of 1955 clearly increased their perceptions of the difference between the overt and covert aspects of personality more than the control students did. (Both 1955 I and II results are statistically sig-

Table 21.27. Difference between percentages of students expected and obtained in the high increase group: difference between estimations of overt and covert personality characteristics (class of 1955)

	Percentage expected	Percentage obtained	Difference
1955 I			
GMC ($N = 20$)	14	22	8
Control ($N = 18$)	12	11	—1
Surgery I ($N = 17$)	11	4	—7
Surgery II ($N = 17$)	11	11	0
1955 II			
GMC ($N = 17$)	12	18	6
Control ($N = 17$)	12	14	2
Surgery I ($N = 19$)	13	8	—5
Surgery II ($N = 19$)	13	10	—3

nificant.) However, this result was not confirmed by the data from the class of 1956 (see Table 21.28).

To summarize, in an effort to measure the students' attitudes toward patients in a manner which would not be obvious to the students, the students' estimations of the characteristics of the patients in the films were studied. The results indicate that the GMC had no differential effect on the students' attitudes toward patients in the class of 1956, but that the GMC may well have caused the students in the class of 1955 to increase their perception of individual differences among patients and to become more alert to difference between the overt and covert aspects of personality.

Questionnaire responses

The comparison of the 1956 II students' ratings of the helpfulness of their clerkships with respect to improving their ability to establish and maintain good physician-patient relations indicates that there was an important (and statistically significant) difference between the GMC and the control clerkship (see Table 21.29), more GMC students reporting that their clerkship was extremely or very helpful.

Table 21.30 presents the percentage of students rating themselves above average in ability to establish and maintain good physician-patient relations. Although the percentage of students rating themselves above average increased in all 1956 I groups, the increase among GMC students was significantly greater than among control students. (Note the large percentage of students who rated themselves above average in this respect.) Interestingly enough, there was a decline in the percentage of students in all groups (except one) who felt that it was extremely or very important to maintain good physician-patient relations, the decline being larger in the 1956 II GMC group than in any other group (see Table 21.31).[2]

The students were also asked how important they thought it was to have various activities or conditions present. This question was asked on three occasions: just prior to commencing the senior year (Pretest), after participation in various clerkships in the first half of the year (Posttest I), and again after participation in various clerkships in the second half of the year (Posttest II). The results are presented in Table 21.32. Apparently quite large percentages of students felt that

[2] The tendency for students to find those aspects of medical care in which they felt most proficient to be the least important is discussed in detail in Chapter 25. This finding is particularly important since the students generally had a high opinion of their knowledge and skill in interpersonal relations. Note also the parallel between this result and the finding reported above that a large percentage of students developed negative attitudes toward various aspects of comprehensive care in the senior year.

Table 21.28. Difference between percentages of students expected and obtained in the high increase group: difference between estimations of overt and covert personality characteristics (class of 1956)

	Percentage expected	Percentage obtained	Difference
1956 I			
GMC ($N = 18$)	14	14	0
Control ($N = 13$)	10	9	—1
Surgery I ($N = 17$)	14	14	0
Surgery II ($N = 17$)	14	15	1
1956 II			
GMC ($N = 16$)	12	14	2
Control ($N = 18$)	14	12	—2
Surgery I ($N = 15$)	11	11	0
Surgery II ($N = 16$)	12	12	0

Table 21.29. Percentage of students rating their clerkship as extremely or very helpful in improving ability to establish and maintain good physician-patient relations (1955 II, 1956 I and II)

	1955 II	1956 I	1956 II
GMC	59	78	63
Control	55	77	39
Surgery I	—	47	27
Surgery II	16	65	12

Table 21.30. Change in percentage of students rating themselves above average in ability to establish and maintain good physician-patient relations (1955 II, 1956 I and II)

	1955 II			1956 I			1956 II		
	Post I	Post II	Change	Pre	Post I	Change	Post I	Post II	Change
GMC	*	89	*	34	94	*60*	69	69	*0*
Control	*	79	*	54	77	*23*	61	44	*—17*
Surgery I	*	—	*	36	71	*35*	100	80	*—20*
Surgery II	*	63	*	18	59	*41*	76	88	*12*

* No data.

Table 21.31. Change in percentage of students rating improving ability to establish and maintain good physician-patient relations as extremely or very important (1955 II, 1956 I and II)

	1955 II			1956 I			1956 II		
	Post I	Post II	Change	Pre	Post I	Change	Post I	Post II	Change
GMC	*	53	*	89	61	*—28*	82	56	*—26*
Control	*	61	*	62	30	*—32*	50	61	*11*
Surgery I	*	—	*	70	59	*—11*	60	60	*0*
Surgery II	*	74	*	88	70	*—18*	38	44	*6*

* No data.

Table 21.32. Change in percentage of students rating engaging in certain activities or having certain conditions present as extremely or very important (class of 1956)

	1956 I						1956 II					
	GMC			Control			GMC			Control		
	Pre	Post I	Change	Pre	Post I	Change	Post I	Post II	Change	Post I	Post II	Change
A. Having opportunities to explain to patients their prognoses, limitations, etc.	83	77	*—6*	85	69	*—16*	69	88	*19*	55	67	*12*
B. Having opportunities for psychiatric consultation for your patients	28	50	*22**	31	31	*0*	32	25	*—7*	17	50	*33**
Having opportunities to give psychotherapy	33	39	*6*	15	23	*8*	25	38	*13*	11	28	*17**
Handling the emotional problems of patients	39	66	*27**	46	38	*—8*	50	31	*—19*	17	28	*11*
C. Having the staff give direct instruction in physician-patient relationships	23	17	*—6*	15	15	*0*	13	6	*—7*	6	33	*27**
Spending a lot of time exploring social and emotional factors when taking a history	0	17	*17**	0	0	*0*	0	6	*6*	11	0	*—11*
Advising patients on their personal problems	11	22	*11*	8	16	*8*	19	6	*—13*	17	6	*—11*

* Significant change ($p < .05$)

it was important to be able to explain to patients their prognosis, limitations, etc., and there was not much change with respect to this item. Only about one third of the students, however, felt that it was very or extremely important to have opportunities for experience with the psychiatric problems of patients. It should be noted that of the four statistically significant changes in group B activities (Table 21.32), three (the largest) took place in the GMC group. Apparently the GMC experience led students to believe these conditions to be more important than they had believed before. It is quite clear from Table 21.32 that few students believed Group C activities to be very important, and there was essentially no change in regard to these activities.

The GMC apparently did affect the students' attitudes toward the importance of acquiring skill at applying the basic ideas of psychosomatic medicine and psychiatry to clinical practice (see Table 21.33), although this effect was quite small in the 1956 II group.

The GMC apparently did not differ from the control clerkship in its effects upon students' attitudes toward the type of information that should be routinely gathered (see Table 21.34). Nor were there any consistent differences among the groups with respect to students' confidence in their ability to handle a series of interpersonal relations problems (see Table 21.35).

In short, the data from the questionnaire indicate that experience in the GMC definitely increased the importance which students attached to learning to apply their knowledge of the psychological aspects of medical care. However, as the data from the Attitude toward Physician-Patient Relations scale also suggest, the GMC students did not develop a greater appreciation of the importance of physician-patient relations.

Interviews with students

Students in the class of 1954 who participated in the GMC were not enthusiastic about treating patients with "psychogenic" illnesses. Of

Table 21.33. Change in percentage of students rating acquisition of skill at applying the basic ideas of psychosomatic medicine and psychiatry to clinical practice as extremely or very important (1955 II, 1956 I and II)

	1955 II			1956 I			1956 II		
	Post I	Post II	Change	Pre	Post I	Change	Post I	Post II	Change
GMC	*	59	*	34	66	*32*	25	38	*13*
Control	*	22	*	61	38	*—23*	28	33	*5*
Surgery I	*	—	*	36	24	*—12*	67	27	*—40*
Surgery II	*	58	*	53	30	*—23*	44	31	*—13*

* No data.

Table 21.34. Change in percentage of students responding that a family physician should have various kinds of information as part of his routine information about patients (classes of 1955 and 1956)

	1955 I			1955 II			1956 I			1956 II		
	Pre	Post I	Change	Post I	Post II	Change	Pre	Post I	Change	Post I	Post II	Change
Relations with friends, relatives, and associates												
GMC	40	20	*—20*	29	35	*6*	28	50	*22*	44	31	*—13*
Control	17	33	*16*	12	17	*5*	31	62	*31*	22	33	*11*
Surgery I	29	29	*0*	26	37	*11*	41	35	*—6*	53	27	*—26*
Surgery II	22	12	*—10*	26	32	*6*	24	29	*5*	56	25	*—31*
Religion												
GMC	65	65	*0*	47	59	*12*	44	50	*6*	31	44	*13*
Control	33	44	*11*	35	44	*9*	46	46	*0*	39	11	*—28*
Surgery I	59	53	*—6*	53	26	*—27*	29	12	*—17*	33	27	*—6*
Surgery II	28	29	*1*	58	47	*—11*	35	59	*24*	63	19	*—44*
Aspirations and goals in life												
GMC	50	30	*—20*	29	24	*—5*	17	33	*16*	25	31	*6*
Control	22	44	*22*	29	33	*4*	0	46	*46*	22	28	*6*
Surgery I	29	47	*18*	42	42	*0*	35	18	*—17*	33	47	*14*
Surgery II	22	12	*—10*	32	26	*—6*	12	29	*17*	44	25	*—19*
Fears, worries, and problems												
GMC	80	95	*15*	71	82	*11*	56	78	*22*	81	69	*—12*
Control	95	100	*5*	59	78	*19*	69	77	*8*	72	72	*0*
Surgery I	88	65	*—23*	95	89	*—6*	100	71	*—29*	87	80	*—7*
Surgery II	72	65	*—7*	100	84	*—16*	82	82	*0*	69	69	*0*

Table 21.35. Change in percentage of students responding that they felt completely confident in their ability to deal with various problems (classes of 1955 and 1956)

	1955 I			1955 II			1956 I			1956 II		
	Pre	Post I	Change	Post I	Post II	Change	Pre	Post I	Change	Post I	Post II	Change
When a patient has an emotional outburst of crying, swearing, or something like that												
GMC	20	15	*—5*	18	24	*6*	28	28	*0*	6	13	*7*
Control	22	28	*6*	12	17	*5*	15	62	*47*	28	22	*—6*
Surgery I	12	6	*—6*	26	21	*—5*	24	18	*—6*	47	53	*6*
Surgery II	11	24	*13*	16	21	*5*	12	18	*6*	38	25	*—13*
Preventing a patient from becoming embarrassed during a pelvic examination												
GMC	30	45	*15*	53	53	*0*	50	61	*11*	50	50	*0*
Control	44	67	*23*	29	50	*21*	54	69	*15*	33	33	*0*
Surgery I	29	47	*18*	58	42	*—16*	47	35	*—12*	67	80	*13*
Surgery II	50	35	*—15*	53	63	*10*	24	47	*23*	63	38	*—25*
Talking with the family of a patient who has just died												
GMC	0	10	*10*	12	18	*6*	17	33	*16*	6	19	*13*
Control	17	17	*0*	18	17	*—1*	23	54	*31*	17	22	*5*
Surgery I	12	12	*0*	11	21	*10*	12	6	*—6*	40	53	*13*
Surgery II	17	18	*1*	16	11	*—5*	6	18	*12*	44	19	*—25*

Table 21.35. (continued)

	1955 I			1955 II			1956 I			1956 II		
	Pre	Post I	Change	Post I	Post II	Change	Pre	Post I	Change	Post I	Post II	Change
Having to tell a patient that the tests performed on him do not reveal the cause of his problems												
GMC	40	60	*20*	53	65	*12*	33	61	*28*	38	44	*6*
Control	61	61	*0*	29	39	*10*	54	85	*31*	61	56	*—5*
Surgery I	24	47	*23*	58	47	*—11*	47	47	*0*	80	67	*—13*
Surgery II	44	35	*—9*	63	37	*—26*	59	53	*—6*	63	69	*6*
Deciding what to tell a patient who has a serious and irremediable illness												
GMC	5	5	*0*	0	26	*26*	11	22	*11*	13	19	*6*
Control	6	17	*11*	0	11	*11*	8	46	*38*	22	28	*6*
Surgery I	6	0	*—6*	5	35	*30*	18	24	*6*	33	40	*7*
Surgery II	11	0	*—11*	16	11	*—5*	6	12	*6*	31	44	*13*

the GMC students 53% (18/34) expressed dislike of treating such patients, whereas only 29% (10/35) of the control students expressed dislike of this type of problem. Moreover, although 23% (8/34) of the GMC students felt they would enjoy working with patients with psychogenic problems because they presented a challenge, 29% (10/35) of the control students were willing to treat these patients because of the challenge they presented.

When asked about their ideas on handling such patients, however, both groups of students gave very vague answers, mostly based on the assumption that "there's not much you can do, except talk to them, and listen to them," apparently for the purpose of encouraging the patient to understand his own problems. Some answers directly reflected the students' recent experiences. For example, one GMC student said:

> I think one thing that has been brought out very vividly in my experience in the GMC is that the doctor plays the role of the person the patient can become dependent upon. I had several patients down there whose life was completely empty—so far as having some one to lean on. They needed some one to draw their strength from, and I think the doctor was the one person they had. I think that's a big point in psychotherapy as far as the general practitioner is concerned.

Because of the scheduling arrangement (see Chapter 10), 10 of the 18 students in the spring surgery clerkship had previously been in the GMC, and 8 had been in the control medical clerkship. If the GMC experience had indeed had an effect on students different from that of the control medical clerkship, it seemed that this effect might be evidenced by a differential response to the surgery clerkship. Consequently, these students were interviewed about their surgery experience. Although virtually all students were of one mind (9/10 of the GMC students, 6/8 of the control students) concerning the fact that on the surgery clerkship little or no attention was given to the psychological or social aspects of illness, the effects of this experience were difficult to assess, mainly because the surgery experience seemed to have opposite effects on different GMC students. For example, one GMC student who said that he had learned from the surgery staff how *not* to handle patients, stated:

> Of course I was impressed by GMC—we were constantly impressed down there by the value of this [psychological factors in illness]; and to suddenly come from that extreme to this extreme, where you see it apparently forgotten that a patient is a human being, irritates me tremendously. . . . I've heard it stated too often that we won't bother about [psychological factors] because they're not important. . . . It really hurts the surgeons to call in a psychiatrist . . . and even interns are somewhat like that. . . . They've caught the disease. . . .

But another GMC student said:

Well, I notice in myself—I just figured this out the other day—that during the last few weeks I've come to regard the patient less as a person and more as a disease condition since I've been on surgery. I think that has been imparted to me by the general attitude of the surgery staff. . . .

Apparently, then, a negative reaction to surgery could reinforce an effect of the GMC, but surgery might reverse the influence of the GMC as well.

Interviews with the class of 1955 did not provide further information.

To summarize, two pieces of evidence suggest that the GMC had a positive effect on students' attitudes toward psychosomatic medicine and psychiatry. First, on one occasion the GMC students made a statistically significant gain over the control students on the Behavior Disorders subscale of the Medical Attitudes test. Second, the increase in the percentage of GMC students who thought it was important to have psychiatric consultation available for their patients was greater to a statistically significant degree than the increase in the percentage of control students who felt that way.

It seems doubtful, however, that the GMC had an important effect on students' attitudes toward physician-patient relations. First, there was no difference between the two groups with respect to change on the Physician-Patient Relations subscale of the Medical Attitudes test. Second, the percentage of GMC students who felt that this was an important topic decreased as much as (and on one occasion more than) the percentage of control students who felt this way.

Attempts to measure students' attitudes in less direct ways suggest that although the GMC induced its students to individualize patients more (and thus stereotype them less) than the control students, this effect was small and inconsistent. GMC students did not change very much or differ from the control students with respect to the kind of information about patients they considered to be routine. The same was true with respect to the confidence GMC students had concerning their ability to deal with certain emotional problems.

In short, the evidence suggests that the GMC increased the students' sense of the importance of psychological problems, but did not, in the main, deepen the students' concern over physician-patient relations.

Independent Variables (Reasons for the Effects of the GMC)

This section deals with the question of why the experimental and control groups differed so little with respect to attitudes toward behavior disorders and physician-patient relations.

Table 21.36. Mean ratings of students with respect to attitudes toward emotional problems (class of 1956)

	1956 I	1956 II	1956 I and II
GMC ($N = 19$)	3.9	3.9	3.9
Control ($N = 15$)	3.9	3.3	3.5

Analysis of the teaching conferences

The ratings of the students' attitudes and the instructors' attitudes by the physician observer indicate that there was little difference with respect to the teaching conferences between the experimental and control groups. The physician observer found that 60% of the Teaching Conference Records in the GMC, and 59% of the records in the control group contained sufficient information to enable him to rate on a seven-point scale the students' attitudes toward emotional problems. There was only a slight difference in favor of the GMC students in these ratings (see Table 21.36).

Sixty-one per cent of the conferences in the GMC and 59% of the conferences in the control clerkship contained sufficient information to enable the physician observer to rate the staff's attitudes toward emotional problems. There seems to have been little difference between the GMC staff and the control medical clerkship staff in this respect (see Table 21.37).

Somewhat different results were obtained, however, in connection with the physician observer's rating of students' and staff's attitudes toward patients. Ratings could be made of students' attitudes toward patients in 90% of the GMC records and 89% of the control records. The ratings were virtually identical for both groups—the mean rating of 19 GMC students being 3.9, and that of 18 control students 3.8. The instructors in both clinics revealed their attitudes toward patients somewhat less frequently than did the students; ratings could be made of only 65% of the GMC records and only 58% of the control records. The GMC staff apparently expressed favorable attitudes toward patients somewhat less frequently than did the control medical clerkship staff (see Table 21.38).

Table 21.37. Rating of staff with respect to their attitudes toward emotional problems in illness

	Percentage of conferences						
	Low						High
GMC ($N = 56$)	1.8	19.6	28.6	10.7	28.6	10.7	0.0
Control ($N = 45$)	2.2	13.3	26.7	20.0	31.1	6.7	0.0

Table 21.38. Rating of staff with respect to their attitudes toward patients

	Percentage of conferences						
	Low						High
GMC ($N = 60$)	0.0	13.3	23.3	40.0	21.7	1.7	0.0
Control ($N = 44$)	0.0	2.3	22.7	40.1	34.1	0.0	0.0

The above analysis of the teaching conferences suggests that one reason the GMC had little if any effect on students' attitudes toward physician-patient relations was that the instructors in the two groups differed little in their attitudes.

STUDENTS' REPORTS OF GENERAL CLERKSHIP EXPERIENCE

As Table 21.39 indicates, in the 1956 II group there was a sharp drop in the percentage of GMC students who felt that their instructors were extremely, very, or moderately helpful in improving their ability to establish and maintain good physician-patient relations. The GMC students apparently believed that in this respect their patients were more helpful than their instructors (see Table 21.40). Note that except for the 1956 II control group the comparisons in Tables 21.39 and 21.40 indicate that the students found their patients more helpful than their instructors. A large drop in the 1956 II group was also noted in connection with the GMC students' appraisal of their staff's ability to develop good relations with patients (see Table 21.41).

However, on five of six occasions more GMC than control students reported deriving a great deal of satisfaction from their relations with patients (see Table 21.42). And on all six occasions more GMC than control students reported that patients had been discussed with them as individual persons rather than as disease entities (see Table 21.43).

In brief, it appears that a substantial percentage of GMC students felt that they had learned something about physician-patient relations from their patients, and more GMC than control students felt this way. Apparently the largest, most consistent effect on the students came from the patients and the situation in which the students found them-

Table 21.39. Percentage of students rating their staff as extremely, very, or moderately helpful in improving ability to establish and maintain good physician-patient relations (class of 1956)

	1956 I	1956 II
GMC	61	19
Control	69	67
Surgery I	24	26
Surgery II	30	31

Table 21.40. Percentage of students rating their patients as extremely or very helpful in improving ability to establish and maintain good physician-patient relations (class of 1956)

	1956 I	1956 II
GMC	67	57
Control	77	62
Surgery I	36	53
Surgery II	71	38

Table 21.41. Percentage of students rating their staff as extremely or very proficient in establishing and maintaining good physician-patient relations (1955 II, 1956 I and II)

	1955 II	1956 I	1956 II
GMC	53	39	12
Control	56	54	39
Surgery I	—	18	27
Surgery II	16	53	31

Table 21.42. Percentage of students responding that they derived a great deal of satisfaction from their physician-patient relations (classes of 1954, 1955, and 1956)

	1954 I	1954 II	1955 I	1955 II	1956 I	1956 II
GMC	81	68	65	76	83	56
Control	56	71	39	50	62	33
Surgery I	25	38	59	26	41	27
Surgery II	55	42	35	47	35	25

Table 21.43. Percentage of students responding that patients had been discussed as individual persons in their clerkship (classes of 1954, 1955, and 1956)

	1954 I	1954 II	1955 I	1955 II	1956 I	1956 II
GMC	67	84	70	76	83	56
Control	32	50	61	44	69	56
Surgery I	15	20	12	21	0	27
Surgery II	10	11	6	42	29	31

Table 21.44. Relation between change in students' estimations of the helpfulness of the GMC with respect to learning the basic facts of clinical medicine and change in attitudes toward behavior disorders from Posttest I to Posttest II (1956 II)

		Change in attitudes toward behavior disorders		
		Below median	Above median	
Change in estimation	Above median	3	8	11
Change in estimation	Below median	6	0	6
$p = .04$		9	8	17

selves, rather than from the staff (see also Chapters 18 and 20). But the fact that GMC students did not develop positive attitudes toward physician-patient relations indicates that greater experience does not necessarily lead to more positive attitudes.

Special educational techniques of the GMC

Those students in the 1956 II group who reported the GMC to be more helpful than they had expected with respect to learning the basic facts of clinical medicine (excluding psychosomatic medicine) were those who tended to improve their attitudes toward behavior disorders (see Table 21.44). Moreover, those students in the 1956 II group who found the GMC more helpful with respect to traditional medicine than they had expected also came to regard psychosomatic medicine and psychiatry as more important than they had regarded them prior to participating in the GMC ($p < .05$). These results suggest that when students felt they were receiving adequate training in the traditional areas of medicine, they were more likely to accept the importance of psychological factors in medical care.

On the other hand, those students who reported frequent visits to their patients' homes found this activity less important after the GMC than before ($p < .05$ for 1956 I group).

Students in the 1956 II group who reported that the staff frequently gave them direct instruction in physician-patient relations tended to change their attitudes in a positive direction (see Table 21.45). Moreover, those GMC students who felt that the staff frequently gave them direct instruction in physician-patient relations decided that psychosomatic medicine and psychiatry were more important topics after they had participated in the GMC than they had previously believed them to be ($p < .05$ for 1956 II group).

Apparently students who felt they were receiving adequate training in the traditional aspects of medical care were more apt to develop a higher regard for psychosomatic medicine and psychiatry. Di-

Table 21.45. Relation between frequency of direct instruction in physician-patient relations and change in attitudes toward physician-patient relations from Posttest I to Posttest II (1956 II)

		Change in attitudes toward physician-patient relations		
		Below median	Above median	
Frequency of direct instruction	Above median	1	9	10
Frequency of direct instruction	Below median	5	2	7
$p = .01$		6	11	17

rect instruction in physician-patient relations also seemed to have an effect on students' attitudes.

Interviews with students

Students' responses in interviews demonstrated clearly that experience in the GMC resulted in different attitudes toward the psychological aspects of medical care. For example:

Q: I wonder how well you think the GMC accomplished these aims?
A: Pretty well. They converted a lot of us. I had a lot of satisfying patient relations in the clinic. I made a lot of friends with the patients, and I got to know some very nice people, and I learned a lot of medicine. I saw a lot of organic pathology, and I had a lot of people who knew a lot more than I did tell me about what I was finding. I don't see how you could find a better set-up with that many students.

Q: Do you feel that your training has equipped you to handle the patient with psychological problems?
A: Yes, I think so. I think they stress it a little too much down at GMC. I don't think it takes that much. I think that if you are going to try and treat them with psychotherapy, you have got to have a lot more training than you are going to get in medical school. If you are going to try to do so-called superficial psychotherapy, or just relieve their anxiety, I think just common sense will take care of it pretty well on most of their patients. I don't think it is something that has to be stressed too much. Maybe I'm wrong.

Q: The statement is frequently made that about 50% of the patients that a GP will see in practice are suffering primarily from a psychogenic illness; do you feel that this is correct?
A: So many people have told me that, that I'm inclined to believe it. Actually my own experience with people, not necessarily patients, makes me think it might even be more than that.
Q: Did you ever make an estimate of what it might be?
A: In general practice, maybe 70% or 80%. It is more now than it has ever been.
Q: Do you think your training in school will help you handle these patients?
A: It supposedly helps you recognize these problems, and that is the important thing. If you recognize them you have conquered more than half of the problems. I think most of the cases that you get can be treated by just plain common sense for one thing. Secondly, . . . if you understand your own problems and your own self and your own philosophy of life, etc., I feel you can transfer this . . . and you can see where the patient's faults lie and what his problems are. I think it depends on the individual's ability and imagination how to bring this point up with patients. I know the psychiatrists tell us to just let the patient talk, and this starts the therapy, and you probably will help a tremendous amount by that method alone. I think that it is only the psychotic ones that you will have to take to the hospital. The rest I think you can help, but this depends on the doctor himself and his willingness to handle the patient's problems.
Q: Have you had any training in medical school in handling psychological problems (other than common sense)?

A: Oh, yes, they told us to let the patient talk and you listen. I think one of the hardest things to do is listen, and let the patient talk on and on about his problems. I think that is probably the most important thing they have emphasized to us. Secondly, gain the patient's confidence in your ability to handle his problems, medical, surgical or mental, and get the patient to elaborate fully what is really bothering him. I think once that is done then you have gone over the biggest part, and by a superior follow-up you have done much to take care of the better part of his trouble.

. . . I want to keep on good terms with this patient so that she will continue to tell me when things are bothering her. She must have many problems at her advanced age (eighty-six), for the world has become very complicated and sort of moved on by her. If she will tell me about these problems, I can help her with them, and she won't have to rile her ulcer so much.

GMC students in the 1955 I group pointed out that the staff's attitudes were not always conducive to changing students' attitudes in a positive direction. For example, some (60%) of the students indicated that certain members of the GMC staff deliberately disparaged the practice of psychosomatic medicine and would not cooperate in the efforts of students or other staff men to take all the problems of the patients into consideration. One student made this comment:

. . . Poor [psychiatrist], I feel sorry for him. In the conferences they would ask him, "Well, now, what's the psychiatry department's offer for this alcoholic? . . . I'm sure you could treat this with the psychiatric approach." This was belittling what the poor guy was trying to do. . . . This belittled it to us too, because we listen to these things, you know. . . . I think it was a shame they would belittle his stand.

INTERVIEWS WITH THE GMC STAFF

Parts of interviews with certain GMC staff members are reproduced below to convey some indication of the staff's attitudes toward the psychological problems of patients.

Q: Would you be able to give me a good example of how you've gotten some of the ideas of comprehensive care across to the student?

A: Yes, there's one that would be a good example: a man came in . . . he was blind. To my recollection the student considered him an insoluble custodial problem. The man's blindness was due to an injury, and it wasn't going to change. This is what the student characterized as a "crock." Actually, it turned out that the man did not expect anything to be done about the blindness; he was there because he wanted attention. Of course, the first thing that a physician frequently gives a patient with an insoluble problem is hostility. I don't know why this happens. It seems to be a characteristic response—that you don't like patients for whom you can't do something. In any event, the student became less hostile toward the patient's insoluble problem when he perceived that this man wanted someone who was interested in him; and first with supervision and later with some assistance from the staff and perhaps from the psychiatrist—I don't remember the details—he [the student] was able to help this man get along better in his situation. It seems to me that the social worker was able to get the man some aids for the blind, something that both the man and the student had been unaware of; or it was funds, or God knows what. I don't know that we solved the blind man's problem; he still cannot see. But, somebody listened to his story and sympathized with him; I think we even gave him some pills that helped cheer him up at one time. All sorts of services were rendered this man, which made life a little better for him. And this all started out with a "crock." I think the man felt he had benefited in some way from medical attention; this was a multifaceted approach, perhaps, to his problem—I think we also changed his convalescent home. We manipulated environment, helped with economic things, etc., etc., all of which were more necessary for him than trying to put a new eyeball in his head, which couldn't be done. I think this goes for almost all problems.

Q: How did this help the student?

A: Until the student actually works with such a patient's problem, his immediate response is hostility, something like, "Well, let's get rid of him; there's nothing I can do for him." But through this type of experience the student begins to understand that if he looks beneath the surface, there are other things that will help to satisfy the patient's needs. The patient knows he can't get new eyes; if he comes to you and says, "I'm blind, I have trouble," the first thought is to take him at face value—that he wants new eyes. He doesn't really want new eyes; he wants other things to be done for him. Unless you can think of him as an entire organism—how this happens, what his blindness means to him in many facets, and what can possibly be useful to him—and unless you understand those things you are not carrying out your potentialities as a physician. You just send him back to remain blind. The student should at least have an idea that many things can be done to help patients with problems, because the problems are not simple but complex. That is what comprehensive care is about.

Q: I wonder whether you could give me an idea of the kind of explanatory concepts you use when you talk to the students about these patients' psychological problems?

A: I'm not sure exactly what you want here.

Q: Let me just give you an example. You could say to the student on a very superficial level, "This happened because his wife nagged at him." On a very complicated level, you could talk about the patient's ego structure. . . .

A: I think that I, personally, not being well versed in the technical aspects and patois of fields other than internal medicine, am more likely to bring it down to practical, specific terminology, like "nagging." There are certain situations, however, where I would be very apt to make simple explanations of things that a psychiatrist would discuss in terms such as you used. For instance, I would point out the type of personality that might be associated with a hypertensive patient. But I would not be able to phrase it in terms of whether the difficulty was at the anal level or the oral level, or whatever. I would be apt to say, "A hypertensive patient has difficulty handling his drives and satisfactions; and an ulcer patient might be characterized as someone needing satisfactions that are oral." I use oral in that sense, because it fits the ulcer pattern. Sometimes it gets more complicated; but generally I would not use technical terms because I would not know about them. I might use simple concepts, like the "organ language" of Weiss and English, I think. I don't think that I could formulate these concepts in the terms of psychiatrists, for two reasons: first of all, I don't understand them well myself, and secondly, students do not take to that kind of description very well.

A psychiatrist who participated in the General Medical Clinic had this to say about the staff's attitudes:

In my opinion, the clinic had an enthusiastic beginning with a great deal of staff interaction which should have led to increased interest, awareness, and endeavor toward overcoming some of the problems of teaching comprehensive medicine to senior medical students. However, during the third, or definitive, year (1956) there seems to have been a letdown, with decreased enthusiasm and regression to older and more familiar methods of teaching, primarily centered around the disease process rather than the patient as an individual. There are probably several reasons for this, including a distinct difference between the students seen in the last year (1956) and those seen in the previous years. In general, the students were less interested and more resistant to this [comprehensive] method of teaching. The increase in resistance of the students is a field for intensive study in itself.

In addition, the lack of conference time at which the total staff was present, resulting in a lessened interaction and communication between staff members, seemed responsible for some of the change in attitudes toward teaching in the clinic. A third factor is the basic resistance of people, including physicians, to awareness of underlying psychological and unconscious problems.

In my opinion, some of these problems could have been obviated by maintaining conferences and additional total staff interaction as well as by more consideration of the background and training of the teachers on the staff.

Because of increased awareness of emotional problems as related to all forms of illness, I think the time has come to face the fact that physicians need adequate training in psychology and psychiatry so that they can understand and work with the emotional problems of their patients. If this is true for physicians in general, then teachers of medical students will require excellent training in the understanding of such problems.

I do not think that the questions of how this training should be conducted or how much training is necessary can be answered without further study of training processes, as well as of the basic personality factors and motivations which are present in physicians, both practicing and teaching.

To summarize, experience in the GMC apparently could impress students with the importance of psychological factors in medicine. But the evidence presented above indicates that the students were more likely to have been affected by their experiences with patients than by their teaching conferences with the staff. It appears that experiences with patients also account for the fact that more positive attitudes toward physician-patient relations were not developed. In short, although GMC students increased their sense of the importance of psychological problems, their enthusiasm for close relations with patients diminished rather than increased. Both these results seem to have occurred because of the type of patient the GMC students worked with.

Individual Attributes Related to Psychological Attitudes

The results reported below indicate that change in attitudes is largely a function of personality characteristics.

ATTITUDES TOWARD BEHAVIOR DISORDERS

Results pertaining to the entire class. There were no statistically significant relations between any individual attributes and Pretest scores on the Behavior Disorders subscale of the Medical Attitudes test, although there was a definite *tendency* for three CPI measures (Achievement via Independence, Tolerance, and Intellectual Efficiency) to be positively related to scores on the Behavior Disorders subscale on all three test administrations in the class of 1956.

There was some indication that the more intelligent, responsible, and self-accepting students were those who developed more positive attitudes toward behavior problems. The Verbal Ability subtest of the MCAT, cumulative grade averages, and the Intellectual Efficiency scale of the CPI were positively (and statistically significantly) associated with change in attitudes. The CPI scales Social Responsibility and Self-Acceptance were also related to attitude change (see, for example, Table 21.46).

Results pertaining to the GMC and control groups separately. Results obtained for the GMC and control students tended to be similar to those obtained for the class as a whole. Thus, change in attitudes toward behavior disorders seems to have been a function of intelligence and certain personality variables.

It is important to note that essentially the same individual attributes were associated with change in attitudes toward behavior disorders and gain in psychological knowledge and skill.

Table 21.46. Relation between self-acceptance and change in attitudes toward behavior disorders from Pretest to Posttest II (class of 1956)

		Change in attitudes toward behavior disorders			
		Negative change	No change	Positive change	
Self-acceptance	Above median	12	6	14	32
Self-acceptance	Below median	19	8	6	33
$\chi^2 = 5.04; p = .08$		31	14	20	65

Table 21.47. Relation between psychopathology course grade and change in attitudes toward behavior disorders from Pretest to Posttest II (class of 1956)

		Change in attitudes toward physician-patient relations		
		Below median	Above median	
Psychopathology course grade	Above median	13	19	32
Psychopathology course grade	Below median	22	11	33
$\chi^2 = 4.43; p = .05$		35	30	65

ATTITUDES TOWARD PHYSICIAN-PATIENT RELATIONS

Results pertaining to the entire class. Two personality traits were the only individual attributes associated with attitudes toward physician-patient relations at the Pretest; these were the CPI scales Good Impression and Sense of Well-Being. Both relations fell just short of statistical significance, however. Both these scales were positively associated with this attitude measure on all three test administrations in the class of 1956.

Two interpretations might be made of this result. First, since subjects who score high on the Good Impression scale have been found to be those whose test scores are likely to be invalid because they are attempting to create a good impression,[3] it might be inferred that the medical students who scored high on this measure were giving specious responses. On the other hand, subjects scoring high on this scale have also been found to be more cooperative, adaptable, and outgoing, and, as might be expected, concerned about the impression they make on others. It may be that these qualities are characteristic of students who value physician-patient relations highly.

Because the test sheets were anonymous, the research was carried on by an "outside" group, and the student (and faculty) atmosphere provided support for students who did not have strong positive attitudes toward physician-patient relations, it seems likely that the Good Impression scale of the CPI accurately describes the characteristics of students who value physician-patient relations.

In the class of 1956 students with better grades in the psychopathology course tended to be those who developed more positive attitudes toward physician-patient relations (see Table 21.47). Students in the class of 1955 who received high grades in the course in psychosomatic medicine were generally the ones who subsequently developed positive attitudes toward physician-patient relations. Also those students

[3] See H. G. Gough, *Manual for the California Psychological Inventory* (Palo Alto: Consulting Psychologists Press, 1957).

whose competence as a physician was ranked high by their peers, and those students who indicated they were not interested in research, tended to change their attitudes positively.

Results pertaining to the GMC. Among the students who participated in the GMC, course grades in psychopathology were positively related to change in attitudes toward physician-patient relations from Pretest to Posttest II. Those students who were judged by their peers to be responsible and mature, and those who reported not being interested in major surgery, were those who developed more positive attitudes toward physician-patient relations from Pretest to Posttest I.

Results pertaining to the control group. Scores on the Good Impression scale were positively related to change in attitudes toward physician-patient relations in the control group.

In summary, two conclusions seem apparent. Initial positive attitudes toward physician-patient relations were a function of personality traits—principally the tendency to be adaptable and make a good impression on others. The development of increasingly positive attitudes toward physician-patient relations seems to have been related both to a prior interest in psychological matters (as indicated by grades in previous courses concerned with psychopathology) and to personality characteristics.

Perception of individual differences among patients

The tendency to perceive differences among patients in the Sound-Film Interview rather than to see patients as "all alike" was studied rather carefully. The individual attributes of students were studied in relation to both Pretest scores and change from Pretest to Posttest I and from Posttest I to Posttest II. Rather than enumerate separately the individual attributes related to change in perception of individual differences among patients with respect to their intelligence, vocabulary level, and personality characteristics, a general summary is presented below.

Results pertaining to the entire class. There were no consistent, statistically significant relations between any of the individual attributes studied and the perception of individual differences. However, there were persistent *tendencies* for two personality traits (flexibility and leadership) to be related to perception of certain individual differences. The CPI subscale Flexibility was positively related to the Pretest perception of individual differences among patients with respect to their intelligence and vocabulary level (see Table 21.48).

Analysis of the relations between individual attributes of students

Table 21.48. Relation between flexibility and perception of individual differences among patients (class of 1956)

Flexibility score	Perception of individual differences in intelligence			Perception of individual differences in vocabulary level: First word missed (task A)			Perception of individual differences in vocabulary level: First three words missed (task B)		
	Below median	Above median		Below median	Above median		Below median	Above median	
Pretest									
Above median	15	19	34	13	21	34	15	19	34
Below median	19	12	31	19	12	31	17	14	31
	34	31	65	32	33	65	32	33	65
	$p > .05$			$p > .05$			$p > .05$		
Posttest I									
Above median	15	19	34	15	19	34	12	22	34
Below median	19	12	31	17	14	31	20	11	31
	34	31	65	32	33	65	32	33	65
	$p > .05$			$p > .05$			$p = .05$		
Posttest II									
Above median	15	19	34	13	21	34	12	22	34
Below median	17	14	31	19	12	31	20	11	31
	32	33	65	32	33	65	32	33	65
	$p > .05$			$p > .05$			$p = .05$		

and increases in their perception of individual differences among patients revealed interesting but somewhat unexpected findings.[4]

Students who increased their perception of individual differences among patients tended to be anxious, authoritarian persons. Anxiety test scores were positively related to increased perception of individual differences in the classes of 1955 and 1956. And students scoring high on the F (Authoritarian) scale, and low on the CPI subtests Flexibility, Tolerance, and Achievement via Independence, were those (in the class of 1956) who increased their perception of individual differences, as did those students who reported that they worried about their social adjustment. Students who increased their perception of individual differences apparently were not well accepted by their peers. Peer judgments of likeability and of ability and willingness to work independently were negatively related to increase in the perception of individual differences in both the classes of 1955 and 1956. Peer judgments of leadership and of skill in physician-patient relations (class of 1955) and peer judgments of competence as a physician (class of 1956) were also negatively related to increased perception of individual differences.

It will be recalled that increased accuracy in perceiving characteristics of patients was associated with anxiety, authoritarianism, and concern over social relations. Note, however, that successful social relations were found to be positively related to increased accuracy (see Chapter 20). Increase in the perception of individual differences among patients was also associated with anxiety, authoritarianism, and concern over social relations; but in this case, unsuccessful social relations were associated with the increased perception of differences among patients.

Results pertaining to the GMC. There was a tendency for certain indices of academic performance to be negatively related to change in the perception of individual differences when the entire class was considered. These tendencies became more pronounced when the results from the GMC group alone were studied. For example, second-year grade average (classes of 1955 and 1956) and first- and third-year grade averages (class of 1956) were negatively related to change in the GMC group. Peer judgments of skill in physician-patient relations (class of 1955) and peer judgments of competence as a physician (class of 1956) were also negatively related to the increased perception of individual differences in the GMC group.

[4] All the relations reported in this section were statistically significant at the .05 level of confidence. Statistical tests were made by means of the Chi-squared test, with four-fold tables, median breaks, and *N*'s approximating 70 (change from Pretest to Posttest II) and approximating 35 (change from Pretest to Posttest I or from Posttest I to Posttest II).

It is of considerable interest that (in the class of 1955) those students who received higher grades in the psychosomatic medicine course and the course in psychiatry were those students *in the GMC* who increased their perception of individual differences.

Results pertaining to the control group. A pattern similar to the one described for the GMC group was found in the control clerkship, although it was not as pronounced. As in the "entire class" results reported above, peer judgments of likeability, of skill in physician-patient relations, and of responsibility and maturity were negatively related to change in the control group.

Perception of differences between overt and covert personality characteristics

Results pertaining to the entire class. Students in the class of 1956 who were rated highly by their peers on leadership and on ability and willingness to work independently increased their perception of the differences between overt and covert aspects of patients' personalities, as did students who obtained high scores on the Social Responsibility subscale of the CPI.

Results pertaining to the GMC and control groups separately. There was some indication that the more anxious students were more apt to perceive differences between overt and covert aspects of patients' personalities. This result was obtained with one group of GMC students and with another group of control students.

To summarize, intelligent, responsible, self-accepting students developed more positive attitudes toward behavior disorders. There was a tendency for students with somewhat similar characteristics to develop more positive attitudes toward physician-patient relations.

Anxious, authoritarian students who were concerned about social relations and who were unsuccessful in establishing good relationships with others were apt to increase their perception of individual differences among patients. Comparison of this result with an earlier one (that anxious, authoritarian students who were successful in their relations with others increased the accuracy with which they perceived the characteristics of patients) indicates the following relation: anxious, authoritarian students who fail to develop good relations overreact to the individuality of others, misjudge them, act inappropriately, and worsen their relations with others; but anxious, authoritarian students who succeed in developing good relations with others accurately perceive the characteristics of others, judge them correctly, act appropriately, and improve their relations with others.

Although the above interpretation should be treated with caution because of the scarcity of research in this area, it should be pointed out that most of the results discussed above were obtained with a fairly large number of subjects ($N = 65$), and most were found in connection with two different tasks and in two different classes. The above results, therefore, should be considered hypotheses worthy of further research.

Furthermore, it should be pointed out that intelligence and academic ability seem to be positively related to the intellectual or cognitive type of attitude change indicated by objective tests, while personality characteristics and relations with others seem to be related to changes in intuitive perceptions of others.

Chapter 22

Sociological Knowledge and Skill

Summary

In previous chapters medical knowledge was treated separately from medical skill, and psychological knowledge was treated separately from psychological skill. Sociological knowledge and skill, however, are included in one chapter because in the development of the tests it became apparent that a distinction between sociological knowledge and sociological skill was not practicable. GMC students learned about relations between sociological factors and medical care by the case method alone, not by studying basic sociology and then applying the knowledge thus acquired (as, of course, was the case with respect to medical knowledge). Thus, GMC students did not study sociology in its broad sense, but learned about those aspects of sociology which were directly applicable to a particular patient's problem. In short, knowledge and skill were developed simultaneously.

GMC students found their clerkship more helpful with respect to acquiring sociological knowledge and skill, and believed themselves to be more proficient, than the control students did, although the test data indicated no differences between the two groups.

The lack of difference in test results is readily explainable in terms of the staff's teaching: there were only slight differences in the manner in which the students were taught by their medical instructors. On the other hand, GMC students reported considerable experience with the social problems of their patients, far more opportunities to work with social workers and the public health nurse, and believed this experience to be more useful to them than the control students did. But this type of experience was found to be unrelated to gain in sociological knowledge as measured by objective tests (at least in the class of 1956). As might be expected, GMC students did not improve their sociological knowledge and skill over the control students.

Table 22.1. Means and standard deviations for increase in sociological knowledge and skill (1955 II)

	Mean increase	Standard deviation
GMC ($N = 9$)*	20.44	7.54
Control ($N = 8$)*	0.25	12.68
Surgery I ($N = 19$)	4.16	14.62
Surgery II ($N = 19$)	5.26	14.19

* Data available for only half the group because of test revisions.

As noted in connection with psychological knowledge, students with greater potential for achievement were those who had higher scores on the test of sociological knowledge and skill at the beginning of the senior year (Pretest).

Because the results from various sources corroborate one another, these results seem to be dependable ones.

Dependent Variables (Effects of the GMC)

Students were asked questions in the Sound-Film Interview about the social aspects of each patient's problems. Because this test was revised following its trial administrations, the first results available were those for the 1955 II group.

The results, presented in Table 22.1, indicate that the 1955 II GMC students clearly acquired more sociological knowledge and skill than the control students. Each of the differences between the mean increase for the GMC students and the mean increases for the other three clerkship groups was statistically significant ($p < .01$). The analysis of change was also made in another fashion. The 55 subjects were divided into two groups—those whose "gain scores" were above the median of the distribution of gain scores, and those whose "gain scores" were below the median. All 9 GMC students were in the group whose "gain scores" were above the median.

Table 22.2. Difference between percentages of students expected and obtained in the high increase group: sociological knowledge and skill (class of 1956)

	Percentage expected	Percentage obtained	Difference
1956 I			
GMC ($N = 18$)	14	15	1
Control ($N = 13$)	10	11	1
Surgery I ($N = 17$)	13	9	—4
Surgery II ($N = 17$)	13	15	2
1956 II			
GMC ($N = 16$)	11	14	3
Control ($N = 18$)	13	18	5
Surgery I ($N = 15$)	11	8	—3
Surgery II ($N = 16$)	11	6	—5

Table 22.3. Change in sociological knowledge and skill from Pretest to Posttest II (class of 1956)

	No. below median	No. above median	Total
GMC	18	16	34
Control	16	15	31
Total	34	31	65

Results for the class of 1956 are presented in Table 22.2. With respect to the 1956 I group, the differences between the number of students expected and obtained in the high increase group could easily have occurred by chance. It is interesting to note that in the 1956 II group the GMC and control students differed to a statistically significant degree ($p < .05$) from students in the two surgery clerkships, but the GMC students did not significantly differ from the control students. As might be expected, the experience in surgery was less helpful with respect to acquiring sociological knowledge and skill than was the experience in the two medical clerkships.

Apparently the GMC experience had a strong effect on the 1955 II students' acquisition of sociological knowledge and skill, but this effect was not repeated in either the 1956 I or II groups (see Table 22.3).

The GMC students' responses to the questionnaire, however, clearly indicated that they found the GMC helpful with respect to acquiring skill in recognizing and managing social problems (see Table 22.4). Moreover, as Table 22.5 suggests, the 1955 II GMC students very likely increased their feelings of proficiency in this regard more than the control students.[1] This result also occurred in the 1956 I group, but there were small and inconsistent differences in change among the 1956 II groups.

The high percentage of students in the 1956 II surgery groups who rated themselves above average at Posttest I is due to the fact that one half of these students had been in GMC (see Chapter 10).

In short, data from the objective tests indicate that there was no difference between the two 1956 groups, although the GMC students thought they had increased their skill in managing social problems.

Independent Variables (Reasons for the Effects of the GMC)

Were there any factors related to the teaching methods in the two clinics to account for the fact that the GMC students believed their clerkship more helpful, and believed themselves more proficient in

[1] This conclusion cannot be a definite one because Pretest data are not available.

Table 22.4. Percentage of students rating their clerkship as extremely or very helpful in acquiring skill at recognizing and managing social problems in clinical practice (1955 II, 1956 I and II)

	1955 II	1956 I	1956 II
GMC	59	78	56
Control	22	30	28
Surgery I	—	0	0
Surgery II	5	24	0

managing social problems, although the objective test data indicated that there was no difference between the two groups?

ANALYSIS OF THE TEACHING CONFERENCES

The psychologist's analyses revealed no pertinent differences between the teaching conferences in the GMC and those in the control clerkship during 1956.

The ratings made by the physician observer also indicated little difference between the two clinics' teaching conferences, although there was some evidence that the GMC staff pursued sociological matters somewhat further than did the control staff. The physician observer found that 95% of the GMC teaching conferences and 88% of the control clerkship conferences contained sufficient information to permit rating. The mean ratings of students on sociological skill in each group were virtually identical—3.7 in the GMC and 3.6 in the control medical clerkship (on a seven-point scale). The percentage of conferences in which the staff member devoted attention to skill in handling social problems in clinical practice was identical in both groups (24%). There was some indication, however, that more GMC staff members dealt more thoroughly with social problems (see Table 22.6). Moreover, there was a definite tendency for the action proposed by the GMC staff members to be more relevant to the patients' problems (see Table 22.7). There was little difference between the two groups with respect to the extent to which the teaching conferences were helpful

Table 22.5. Change in percentage of students rating themselves above average in skill at recognizing and managing social problems in clinical practice (1955 II, 1956 I and II)

	1955 II			1956 I			1956 II		
	Post I	Post II	Change	Pre	Post I	Change	Post I	Post II	Change
GMC	*	65	*	17	77	*60*	31	38	*7*
Control	*	33	*	31	31	*0*	29	18	*—11*
Surgery I	*	—	*	6	24	*18*	60	74	*14*
Surgery II	*	47	*	6	36	*30*	56	44	*—12*

* No data.

Table 22.6. Rating of staff with respect to their analysis of problems associated with skill at handling social problems in clinical practice

	Percentage of conferences		
	Staff only recognized problem	Staff explored problem	Staff went to core of problem
GMC ($N = 22$)	59.1	22.7	18.2
Control ($N = 18$)	66.7	22.2	11.1

to the students' acquisition of sociological knowledge (see Table 22.8). Nor was there much difference between the two groups concerning the extent to which the patients' sociological problems seemed potentially stimulating to the medical students (see Table 22.9).

There were, in short, no large differences between the two groups' teaching conferences with respect to social factors. However, the physician observer's ratings indicated that the GMC staff did consider social factors more thoroughly and somewhat more frequently than did the control staff.

STUDENTS' REPORTS OF ACTIVITIES ENGAGED IN

Table 22.10 illustrates rather clear differences between the activities engaged in by GMC students and those engaged in by the students in the control medical clerkship in 1956. The GMC students had much greater opportunities than the control students to work with social workers and the public health nurse, as well as to see families of patients and to take complete social histories.

STUDENTS' REPORTS OF GENERAL CLERKSHIP EXPERIENCE

In the 1956 I group virtually all GMC students reported that they found the patients' personal and social histories had frequently or almost always been useful to them, although only about one third of the control students made similar reports. This difference became very small in the 1956 II group, however (see Table 22.11).

Table 22.7. Rating of staff with respect to relevance of action proposed by them to patients' social problems

	Percentage of conferences			
	Not explicitly relevant	Related to peripheral aspects	Related to central aspects	Related to both aspects
GMC ($N = 23$)	26.1	17.4	39.1	17.4
Control ($N = 18$)	33.3	22.2	38.9	5.6

Table 22.8. Rating of teaching conferences with respect to their helpfulness to students' learning about social problems in clinical practice

	Percentage of conferences						
	Hindrance	Not helpful	Slightly	Somewhat	Moderately	Very	Extremely
GMC ($N = 98$)	2.0	64.3	20.4	9.2	2.0	2.0	0.0
Control ($N = 76$)	7.9	67.1	14.5	9.2	1.3	0.0	0.0

Table 22.9. Rating of teaching conferences with respect to degree to which patients' problems were potentially stimulating to students

	Percentage of conferences						
	Negative effect on stimulation	Not stimulating	Slightly	Somewhat	Moderately	Very	Extremely
GMC ($N = 99$)	3.0	53.5	31.3	7.1	3.0	1.0	1.0
Control ($N = 76$)	4.0	60.5	26.3	4.0	5.3	0.0	0.0

Table 22.10. Percentage of students indicating that certain activities were very frequently or always present in their clerkships (class of 1956)

	1956 I		1956 II	
	GMC	Control	GMC	Control
A. Having opportunities to consult with the ancillary services (social worker and public health nurse)	89	54	76	39
Using ancillary services in patient care	50	31	50	39
Learning the skills that the social worker has, and when to utilize them	39	8	32	17
B. Handling the social problems of patients	39	31	44	23
Seeing the families of patients	22	8	25	12
Taking complete social histories	33	23	57	11
Learning how to function as a member of a clinic team	39	30	44	28
Making home visits	6	0	13	11

Table 22.11. Percentage of students responding that patients' personal and social histories had almost always or frequently been of use (class of 1956)

	1956 I	1956 II
GMC	89	31
Control	31	22
Surgery I	6	33
Surgery II	30	31

Table 22.12. Percentage of students rating their patients as extremely or very helpful in acquiring skill at recognizing and managing social problems in clinical practice (class of 1956)

	1956 I	1956 II
GMC	72	50
Control	61	45
Surgery I	6	26
Surgery II	30	6

GMC students apparently found their work with patients useful in acquiring knowledge about social factors related to medicine (see Table 22.12). However, control students believed their patients to be almost equally helpful in this respect. (Note, however, the large differences between the medical clerkships and the surgical clerkships.) On the other hand, there were smaller differences among these four groups with respect to their evaluations of their staff's helpfulness (see Table 22.13). It should be noted that far fewer students believed their teachers were helpful in acquiring sociological knowledge and skill than believed their patients were helpful in this respect (see Chapters 16, 18, 19, 20, and 21). The students' perceptions of the staff's helpfulness were very likely directly related to their feeling that the staff was not very proficient in these matters (see Table 22.14). In the 1955 II group there was a statistically significant difference ($p < .05$) between GMC students' ratings of staff proficiency and the ratings made by other groups.[2]

The students reported reading very little about social phenomena relating to medicine. In fact, the data presented in Table 22.15 show that a large percentage of students in every group reported that they had read nothing pertaining to this area. (Somewhat similar results were obtained in connection with psychological knowledge.) Note, however, that the 1956 I GMC students were exceptional in this respect.

Special educational techniques of the GMC

The results presented below suggest a pattern that has been observed in connection with findings presented earlier (Chapters 16, 17, 19, and 20). That is, there was a tendency for participation in the special educational features of the GMC to be unrelated to gain in tests of *knowledge*, although such participation was positively related to change in *attitudes* toward the topics under consideration, as well as toward the GMC itself.

For example, in the 1956 I group those students who felt that the

[2] It should be pointed out that this was the GMC group which clearly improved over the other groups on the test of sociological knowledge and skill.

Table 22.13. Percentage of students rating their staff as extremely or very helpful in acquiring skill at recognizing and managing social problems in clinical practice (class of 1956)

	1956 I	1956 II
GMC	28	6
Control	38	22
Surgery I	0	0
Surgery II	18	6

staff often gave them direct instruction in physician-patient relations made the least gain on the test of sociological knowledge and skill. The same held true for the students who reported making a large number of home visits. But it is significant that those 1956 I students who actually made the larger number of home contacts with families were also those who reported the GMC to be most helpful with respect to acquiring skill at managing social problems of patients.

However, more participation in the GMC led to the development of more positive attitudes toward the value of the GMC itself with respect to sociological knowledge and skill. In the 1956 II group those students who felt that the GMC was helpful with respect to acquiring skill at managing the social problems of patients were those who reported the following conditions to be present (for them) in the GMC: following patients for several months and finding the GMC more helpful than they had expected with respect to learning how to organize diagnostic and therapeutic regimes.

In the 1956 I group those students who found the GMC helpful in acquiring knowledge and skill in utilizing the ancillary services were those who reported that they had made a large number of home visits, actually did have a large number of home visits, and found the GMC more helpful than they had expected.

It should be remembered, however, that greater participation did not lead to increased knowledge about the social components of medical care.

Interviews with students

The GMC students of the class of 1954 clearly had more contacts with the social workers than the control students, although approxi-

Table 22.14. Percentage of students rating their staff as extremely or very proficient in sociological knowledge and skill (1955 II, 1956 I and II)

	1955 II	1956 I	1956 II
GMC	47	28	12
Control	22	38	28
Surgery I	—	12	0
Surgery II	5	35	6

Table 22.15. Percentage of students reporting no reading at all about social aspects of medicine (class of 1956)

	1956 I	1956 II
GMC	39	75
Control	69	50
Surgery I	88	73
Surgery II	88	81

mately equal percentages of each group had favorable attitudes toward social workers. Of the GMC students, 56% said they had a great deal of contact with social workers; only 16% of the control students said this. When asked if the social workers were helpful, 83% of the GMC students said yes, and 79% of the control medical clerkship students indicated that they had a favorable attitude toward social workers.

The answers of the GMC students showed, too, that they were grateful to the social workers for taking work off their shoulders and saving them time:

> I think they save an invaluable amount of time, and the more I go along the more I realize that time is your enemy perhaps; you have to cut down and weed out those things that can be handled by a social worker and use that social worker, rather than trying to spread your work out so that you can handle it all. . . .

Most GMC students also seemed to feel that although the social worker's role was a valuable one in the hospital, they could not expect to use such agencies in private practice, either because their patients would not need this kind of help or because the machinery for it simply would not exist:

> I don't think I will be overloaded (in practice) with problems that I can refer to a social worker. I don't think there are very many social workers out in practice themselves; I think they are usually associated with a hospital. . . .

> . . . We are not going to have a social worker that we can push the neurotics on in practice. . . .

The type of help given by social workers was seen by the GMC students as largely financial (67%), finding out about and taking care of the patient's family (62%), and counselling (38%). The control students' ideas of the social workers' function emphasized care of the family (91%), fewer (43%) mentioning financial details, and even fewer (26%) citing counselling.

Students in the 1955 I group ($N = 20$) were asked what they had learned in the past six months about the function of the social worker, the sociologist, and the public health nurse. As might be expected from their closer contact, GMC students felt they had learned more about each than did control students.

Most of the GMC students (55%) said they had learned a great deal about the function of the social workers. A majority (59%) said they had had a great deal of contact with social workers, and the rest (41%) said they had had "some" contact. Of these contacts, 50% were mainly consultations, and 39% were both consultations and referrals; there were no contacts which were only referrals. Time was ample for these contacts, according to most of the students.

Treatment of patients was made easier by the help of the social workers, said 74% of the GMC students; the rest said their help was sometimes valuable and sometimes not. Fewer control students reported that they gained knowledge of the social service and its work: only 18% had learned a great deal, 41% had learned a little, and 24% had learned merely that they were available to help; 89% reported very little contact, and only one student a great deal.

Aside from greater contact with social service, more GMC than control students reported contacts with the medical sociologist. Students in both groups seemed to have had about equal contact with the public health nurse.

There seems to be little doubt that the GMC students had more experience with social service than the control students.

Students' diaries

One GMC student's diary entry indicates how he felt he was helped by direct instruction about how to overcome cultural barriers:

> Nothing but praise for the staff man in this regard [physician-patient relations] this day. . . . This was a difficult patient to relate to, but I learned all sorts of things about getting along with Spanish-Americans from the staff man today. Particularly the importance of trying to get only a very few things across to them and getting these few points firmly implanted so that the whole family could repeat them back to us in English and Spanish both. This was probably the most valuable help of the week if not of the entire service. This has always been a problem to me, and I feel quite confident that I can do a lot better in this field from now on. . . .

Another quotation from the diary of the same student illustrates the conflict between the desire to acquire "basic physiological knowledge" and the desire to learn "diagnosis and management":

> I picked up a wonderful little book at the library tonight called *Pulmonary Edema*. The subject of this monograph was not only the diagnosis and treatment of acute pulmonary edema, but also the results of many significant studies on the etiology and pathogenesis of this condition. Although this is a very common symptom, there seems to be very little actually known about just what causes it. The common clinical explanation has seemed to be grossly inadequate, and though fairly good for working principles, completely overlooks important physiologic findings in animal

experiments. I was particularly pleased with this book because it seems that in this clinic [GMC] a lot of emphasis on basic physiology is overlooked in the interest of diagnosis and management. It has always appealed to me that before any of these end results can be realized, a basic understanding of physiology and pathology must be achieved. I find myself woefully lacking in many fields in regard to this basic physiological knowledge. This book allowed me to fill in one small gap at any rate.

Individual Attributes Related to Sociological Knowledge and Skill

Results pertaining to the entire class. In the class of 1956 four measures of individual attributes were not only positively related to Pretest scores on the Sociological Knowledge and Skill test, but were closely related to Posttest I and II scores on this test. These measures were the MCAT subtest Knowledge of Modern Society, the CPI subtest Achievement via Independence, the CPI subtest Intellectual Efficiency, and fantasy about professional and intellectual accomplishments (see Table 22.16). (It should be pointed out that these measures were

Table 22.16. Relations between various individual attributes and sociological knowledge and skill (class of 1956)

	Sociological Knowledge and Skill scores								
	Pretest			Posttest I			Posttest II		
	Low	High		Low	High		Low	High	
Knowledge of Modern Society									
High*	12	17	29	10	19	29	11	18	29
Low	27	9	36	20	16	36	21	15	36
	39	26	65	30	35	65	32	33	65
Achievement via Independence									
High	17	18	35	10	25	35	16	19	35
Low	22	8	30	20	10	30	16	14	30
	39	26	65	30	35	65	32	33	65
Intellectual Efficiency									
High	21	17	38	10	28	38	17	21	38
Low	18	9	27	20	7	27	15	12	27
	39	26	65	30	35	65	32	33	65
Fantasy about intellectual and professional accomplishments									
High	15	14	29	11	22	33	10	23	33
Low	24	12	36	19	13	32	22	10	32
	39	26	65	30	35	65	32	33	65

* Splits were made as close to the median as possible.

also related to Pretest scores on the Psychological Knowledge test, see Table 19.15.) These results suggest that those students with greater achievement potential were those who obtained higher Pretest scores on the Sociological Knowledge and Skill test.

Because of the relatively large amount of statistical regression of the Pretest on the Posttests, studies of individual differences in change were not meaningful.

Chapter 23

Sociological Attitudes

Summary

One of the important goals of the GMC was to develop among the students positive attitudes toward the social aspects of medical care. The GMC staff believed that because medical students often fail to appreciate the importance of these factors, and fail to recognize the value of the services performed by the social work staff and other ancillary services, the students therefore fail to utilize effectively these services. One of the tasks of the research project, then, was to discover whether participation in the GMC led to more positive attitudes toward the ancillary services and the social components of medical care.

The GMC had a positive effect on students' attitudes during the first half of 1956, but not during the second; consequently its net effect relative to the control medical clerkship was small. Although more GMC than control students felt they were proficient in utilizing the ancillary services, the two groups did not differ with respect to the importance they attached to the ancillary services. Few students in either group found much significance in working with the ancillary services. It is noteworthy, however, that those students who participated most fully in the special educational features of the GMC developed positive attitudes toward the importance of the ancillary services and social factors in medicine. Lack of participation led to the opposite result. There was a tendency for brighter students to develop more positive attitudes toward the ancillary services.

Dependent Variables (Effects of the GMC)

Attitudes toward the social aspects of medicine were measured by the Team Concept subscale of the Medical Attitudes test (see Chapter 13). The results presented in Table 23.1 illustrate a pattern similar to that found earlier—a definite, statistically significant increase in posi-

Table 23.1. Difference between percentages of students expected and obtained in the high increase group: attitudes toward the team concept (class of 1956)

	Percentage expected	Percentage obtained	Difference
1956 I			
GMC ($N = 18$)	13	23	10
Control ($N = 13$)	10	5	—5
Surgery I ($N = 17$)	12	8	—4
Surgery II ($N = 17$)	12	12	0
1956 II			
GMC ($N = 16$)	15	12	—3
Control ($N = 18$)	17	20	3
Surgery I ($N = 15$)	14	12	—2
Surgery II ($N = 16$)	15	17	2

tive attitudes on the part of GMC students (relative to the control students) in the first half of the year; but no difference between the groups in the second half of the year.

Table 23.2 compares the GMC and the control students on an absolute basis.

The effect of the GMC is particularly striking in the 1956 I group, but equally noticeable is the similarity of the two clerkships in the 1956 II groups.[1] Students in the two clerkships did not differ with respect to change from Pretest to Posttest II, that is, from the beginning to the end of the senior year, although there was a definite trend in favor of the GMC.[2]

In the 1955 II, 1956 I, and 1956 II groups GMC students rated their clerkship higher than control students rated theirs (see Table 23.3).

GMC students clearly believed themselves proficient in utilizing the ancillary services, and equally clearly the control medical clerkship students did not believe themselves proficient in this respect (see Table 23.4). But assignment to the GMC did not result in students' attaching greater importance to acquiring skill in utilizing these services (see Table 23.5). Nor did GMC students attach greater importance to skill at recognizing and managing social problems in clinical practice (see Table 23.6).[3]

Students in both groups were asked how important it was to have certain activities or conditions present in their training. Table 23.7

[1] Explanations of the consistent differences between first- and second-half results are presented in Chapter 25.

[2] Note that roughly one half of the entire class developed less positive attitudes toward the team concept.

[3] The inverse relation between students' estimations of the importance of a skill and their proficiency in it is developed at greater length in Chapter 25.

Table 23.2. Change in attitudes toward the team concept from Pretest to Posttest I (1956 I), from Posttest I to Posttest II (1956 II), and from Pretest to Posttest II (1956 I and II)

	Negative change	No change	Positive change	Total
1956 I				
GMC	3	5	10	18
Control	10	2	1	13
Total	13	7	11	31
1956 II				
GMC	8	3	5	16
Control	5	9	4	18
Total	13	12	9	34
*1956 I and II**				
GMC	16	5	13	34
Control	20	7	4	31
Total	36	12	17	65

* $\chi^2 = 5.42$; $.05 < p < .10$

Table 23.3. Percentage of students rating their clerkship as extremely or very helpful in learning to utilize ancillary services (1955 II, 1956 I and II)

	1955 II	1956 I	1956 II
GMC	53	89	57
Control	11	54	39
Surgery I	—	0	0
Surgery II	0	6	0

Table 23.4. Change in the percentage of students rating themselves above average in knowing how to utilize ancillary services (1955 II, 1956 I and II)

	1955 II			1956 I			1956 II		
	Post I	Post II	Change	Pre	Post I	Change	Post I	Post II	Change
GMC	*	59	*	12	73	*61*	6	38	*32*
Control	*	6	*	0	23	*23*	11	12	*1*
Surgery I	*	—	*	6	6	*0*	4	67	*20*
Surgery II	*	32	*	0	12	*12*	56	12	*—44*

* No data.

Table 23.5. Change in the percentage of students rating acquisition of knowledge and skill at utilizing ancillary services as extremely or very important (1955 II, 1956 I and II)

	1955 II			1956 I			1956 II		
	Post I	Post II	Change	Pre	Post I	Change	Post I	Post II	Change
GMC	*	30	*	28	28	*0*	26	32	*6*
Control	*	17	*	31	23	*—8*	17	11	*—6*
Surgery I	*	—	*	42	24	*—18*	27	20	*—7*
Surgery II	*	26	*	35	18	*—17*	25	6	*—19*

* No data.

Table 23.6. Change in the percentage of students rating acquisition of skill at recognizing and managing social problems in clinical practice as extremely or very important (1955 II, 1956 I and II)

	1955 II			1956 I			1956 II		
	Post I	Post II	Change	Pre	Post I	Change	Post I	Post II	Change
GMC	*	35	*	34	28	*—6*	37	26	*—11*
Control	*	28	*	15	15	*0*	23	33	*10*
Surgery I	*	—	*	35	18	*—17*	14	27	*13*
Surgery II	*	27	*	47	41	*—6*	31	13	*—18*

* No data.

indicates the responses of GMC and control students to various activities or conditions related to social factors in medical care. Although there are statistically significant differences scattered throughout Table 23.7, these differences do not consistently favor one program or the other.[4]

GMC students did not differ in any marked way from control students with respect to the kind of information they considered routine. There was, however, a statistically significant increase on two occasions in the percentage of GMC students who indicated that information about a patient's physical environment should be considered routine (see Table 23.8).

Almost every student felt that it was the doctor's responsibility to investigate social and environmental factors which might be affecting the health of the patients (see Table 23.8), though very few students felt that the doctor should actually carry out the investigation himself (see Table 23.9).

Interviews with students at the end of the first half of 1955 confirmed the results found by means of the questionnaire. About three fourths of the students in each group indicated that it was important to have social workers on the staff, but about one half of these qualified this by referring specifically to charity hospitals.

Approximately 50% of the students in each group indicated that it was important to discuss social factors in relation to medical care, although slightly more control students (56%) than GMC students (32%) reported they were fairly interested in social factors.

To summarize, it was evidently possible for the GMC to affect students' attitudes toward the team concept, for the GMC did change students' attitudes in a positive direction in the 1956 I group. However, because the GMC was unsuccessful in this respect in the 1956 II group,

[4] Note that, in the main, a smaller percentage of students found the activities listed in Table 23.7 to be important at the end of the senior year than at the beginning of the senior year.

Table 23.7. Change in percentage of students rating engaging in certain activities or having certain conditions present in the clerkship as extremely or very important (class of 1956)

	1956 I						1956 II					
	GMC			Control			GMC			Control		
	Pre	Post I	Change	Pre	Post I	Change	Post I	Post II	Change	Post I	Post II	Change
Making home visits	17	17	*0*	16	23	*7*	19	0	*—19**	0	6	*6*
Having opportunities to consult with the ancillary services (social worker, public health nurse)	33	45	*12*	31	23	*—8*	32	19	*—13*	6	22	*16**
Using ancillary services in patient care	44	39	*—5*	38	31	*—7*	25	19	*—6*	0	11	*11*
Learning the skills that the social worker has and when to utilize them	39	28	*—11*	15	8	*—7*	37	12	*—25**	11	11	*0*
Learning the philosophy and point of view of social work	23	33	*10*	23	23	*0*	19	0	*—19**	11	17	*6*
Handling the social problems of patients	11	39	*28**	16	15	*—1*	25	19	*—6*	12	11	*—1*
Seeing the families of patients	34	28	*—6*	23	8	*—15*	38	12	*—26**	17	6	*—11*
Taking complete social histories	0	11	*11*	0	0	*0*	13	25	*12*	6	6	*0*
Learning how to function as a member of a clinic team	67	50	*—17*	84	39	*—45**	63	51	*—12*	44	34	*—10*

* Significant change.

Table 23.8. Change in percentage of students responding that a family physician should have various kinds of information as part of his routine information about patients (classes of 1955 and 1956)

	1955 I			1955 II			1956 I			1956 II		
	Pre	Post I	Change	Post I	Post II	Change	Pre	Post I	Change	Post I	Post II	Change
Income												
GMC	65	80	*15*	77	76	*—1*	50	72	*22*	69	63	*—6*
Control	67	83	*16*	59	61	*2*	62	69	*7*	56	72	*16*
Surgery I	65	65	*0*	68	58	*—10*	53	65	*12*	67	33	*—34*
Surgery II	61	71	*10*	95	58	*—37*	76	59	*—17*	75	63	*—12*
Physical environment												
GMC	80	80	*0*	65	82	*17**	72	89	*17**	63	50	*—13*
Control	67	78	*11*	59	50	*—9*	92	77	*—15*	72	67	*—5*
Surgery I	76	59	*—17*	79	63	*—16*	65	65	*0*	80	67	*—13*
Surgery II	61	65	*4*	79	63	*—16*	76	71	*—5*	88	69	*—19*
Social standing												
GMC	15	5	*—10*	24	18	*—6*	11	33	*22*	6	25	*19*
Control	11	11	*0*	6	11	*5*	8	31	*23*	17	0	*—17*
Surgery I	6	24	*18*	5	16	*11*	0	0	*0*	33	0	*—33*
Surgery II	11	6	*—5*	11	5	*—6*	12	24	*12*	31	6	*—25*
Nationality or ethnic background												
GMC	70	90	*20*	59	76	*17*	61	83	*22*	44	44	*0*
Control	44	67	*23*	47	78	*31*	54	77	*23*	56	61	*5*
Surgery I	65	65	*0*	79	53	*—26*	53	41	*—12*	80	67	*—13*
Surgery II	56	41	*—15*	79	63	*—16*	53	59	*6*	81	81	*0*
Education												
GMC	60	60	*0*	88	71	*—17*	44	78	*34*	44	50	*6*
Control	44	61	*17*	59	39	*—20*	62	77	*15*	61	50	*—11*
Surgery I	71	76	*5*	58	63	*5*	47	53	*6*	80	47	*—33*
Surgery II	72	71	*—1*	63	53	*—10*	65	53	*—12*	75	50	*—25*
Political affiliation												
GMC	5	5	*0*	0	0	*0*	0	0	*0*	0	6	*6*
Control	0	0	*0*	0	0	*0*	0	8	*8*	0	0	*0*
Surgery I	0	0	*0*	0	0	*0*	0	0	*0*	0	0	*0*
Surgery II	0	0	*0*	5	5	*0*	0	0	*0*	6	6	*0*

* Significant change.

Table 23.9. Change in percentage of students responding that doctor should take primary responsibility for investigating social and environmental factors which may be affecting the health of a patient (classes of 1955 and 1956)

	1955 I			1955 II			1956 I			1956 II		
	Pre	Post I	Change	Post I	Post II	Change	Pre	Post I	Change	Post I	Post II	Change
Seeing to it that investigation is made												
GMC	95	90	*—5*	94	88	*—6*	78	95	*17*	100	88	*—12*
Control	83	89	*6*	94	89	*—5*	77	85	*8*	83	89	*6*
Surgery I	100	88	*—12*	89	95	*6*	82	88	*6*	93	80	*—13*
Surgery II	78	100	*22*	89	79	*—10*	76	94	*18*	88	94	*6*
Actually carrying out the investigation												
GMC	20	30	*10*	12	29	*17*	6	6	*0*	6	6	*0*
Control	6	0	*—6*	6	17	*11*	8	0	*—8*	11	17	*6*
Surgery I	18	12	*—6*	11	11	*0*	18	0	*—18*	7	7	*0*
Surgery II	11	6	*—5*	21	16	*—5*	12	18	*6*	0	0	*0*

the net effect of the GMC over the entire year was small. GMC students found their clerkship to be more helpful and judged their own proficiency in utilizing the ancillary services higher than the control students judged theirs.

There was no effect, however, upon the students' views about the importance of learning to utilize the ancillary services. Nor were there differences between the GMC and control students' judgments of the importance of engaging in activities relevant to learning about the social problems of patients. There were also no differences in the students' attitudes toward the importance of gathering information about patients' social problems.

Independent Variables (Reasons for the Effects of the GMC)

The GMC seems to have changed students' attitudes so that they became more favorable toward the team concept in medicine—on one occasion, at least. Yet, in the main, the GMC had little effect on the importance which GMC students attached to the ancillary services. Why did these results occur?

Analysis of the teaching conferences

The results of the psychologist's analyses of the teaching conferences, as well as the ratings made by the physician observer, indicate little, if any, difference between the two groups. The psychologist's analyses suggest that the student-staff conferences in the two programs included roughly the same number of psycho-social facts and involved an approximately equal number of interrelations among those facts.

The physician observer found that 78% of the conferences in the GMC and 70% of the conferences in the control clerkship contained sufficient information to permit rating the students' attitudes toward social problems. The mean rating for the GMC students was 3.7; the mean rating for the control students was 3.6 (on a seven-point scale).

Sixty-five percent of the GMC conferences permitted a rating of the GMC staff, and 77% of the control conferences permitted a rating of the staff. Table 23.10 presents a comparison of the two groups.

Table 23.10. Rating of staff with respect to their attitudes toward social problems in illness

	Percentage of conferences						
	Low						High
GMC ($N = 59$)	1.7	15.2	28.8	20.3	27.1	6.8	0.0
Control ($N = 58$)	0.0	3.4	48.3	15.5	29.3	1.7	1.7

Table 23.11. Percentage of students rating their staff's attitudes toward social service as very positive (class of 1956)

	1956 I	1956 II
GMC	72	31
Control	38	39
Surgery I	6	20
Surgery II	12	13

There were, then, virtually no differences between the two groups with respect to the teaching in the student-staff conferences.

STUDENTS' REPORTS OF GENERAL CLERKSHIP EXPERIENCE

A large majority of the 1956 I GMC students believed the GMC staff to have very positive attitudes toward social service;[5] however, this finding was not repeated with the 1956 II group (see Table 23.11). Fewer GMC students found their teachers helpful in learning to utilize the ancillary services (see Table 23.12), although on the whole more GMC students than control students thought their teachers were proficient in this respect (see Table 23.13). And, as noted in connection with psychological knowledge, skill, and attitudes (Chapters 19, 20, and 21), far more GMC students than control students found their patients helpful in learning to utilize the ancillary services (see Table 23.14).

SPECIAL EDUCATIONAL TECHNIQUES OF THE GMC

Students in the 1956 I group who had the largest number of home contacts with families, and students in the 1956 II group who felt they had the most responsibility for their patients, were those who developed positive attitudes toward the team concept in medicine (as measured by the Medical Attitudes test).

Students in the 1956 I group who felt they had the most responsibility for their patients, and students in the 1956 II group who found the GMC more helpful than they had expected it to be with respect to learning how to establish and maintain good physician-patient relations were those who came to attach greater importance to seeing the families of patients. Also, those students in the 1956 II group who reported making the largest number of home visits were those who came to attach greater importance to following patients for several months.

Attitude change among GMC students, then, was a function of the extent to which a student participated in the special features of the

[5] Note that this was the period during which GMC students definitely developed positive attitudes toward the team concept.

Table 23.12. Percentage of students rating their staff as extremely or very helpful in learning to utilize ancillary services (class of 1956)

	1956 I	1956 II
GMC	39	25
Control	54	23
Surgery I	0	0
Surgery II	6	0

GMC. More responsibility, more experience with patients' families, more home visits, and more experience in learning how to maintain good relations with patients, led to increased appreciation of the importance of social factors in medicine.

The students who came to attach increased importance to acquiring skill at managing patients' social problems were those who reported having more responsibility for their patients (1956 I), who found the GMC more helpful than they had expected with respect to acquiring knowledge about psychosomatic medicine and psychiatry (1956 I), and had a larger number of visits per patient (1956 II). Moreover, in the 1956 I group a positive relation was found between change in the importance students attached to the acquisition of knowledge and skill at utilizing the ancillary services and the degree to which students thought of themselves as doctors rather than students.

In both 1956 I and II groups increased estimations of the importance of learning the skills and usefulness of the social worker were positively related to the extent to which the GMC was found to be more helpful than expected with respect to learning psychosomatic medicine and psychiatry, and in the 1956 II group were positively related also to the extent to which the GMC was found to be helpful with respect to learning clinical medicine.

Evidently those students who indicated that they did not participate extensively in the special programs of the GMC were those who became less convinced that it was important to learn how to function as a member of a clinic team. For example, in the 1956 II group those students who made the fewest home visits, had the greatest number

Table 23.13. Percentage of students rating their staff as extremely or very proficient in utilizing ancillary services (1955 II, 1956 I and II)

	1955 II	1956 I	1956 II
GMC	65	50	31
Control	28	39	34
Surgery I	—	6	13
Surgery II	11	35	12

Table 23.14. Percentage of students rating their patients as extremely or very helpful in learning to utilize ancillary services (class of 1956)

	1956 I	1956 II
GMC	83	44
Control	31	34
Surgery I	12	20
Surgery II	24	0

of broken appointments, saw the fewest patients in the GMC, and thought of themselves more as students than doctors were those who thought it less important, after participating in the GMC, to learn how to function as a member of a clinic team. Those students with the opposite experience and attitudes found it more important to learn this skill. The above data give rather clear support to the hypothesis that participation in the educational features of the GMC led to positive changes in attitudes toward the importance of the ancillary services and social factors in medicine.

Interviews with students

GMC students apparently had greater opportunities for contact with the social worker and public health nurse. Data from the interviews with the students in the class of 1955 concerning this point are presented in Table 23.15.

Seventy-four per cent of the GMC students said that treatment of patients was made easier by social workers; the remainder (26%) said their help was sometimes useful, sometimes not.

A few more GMC than control students reported that they had learned a great deal about the function of the public health nurse, but nearly all students in both groups said they learned something about this—and almost all students agreed that treatment of patients was made easier by the public health nurse.

Table 23.15. Percentage of students reporting various degrees of learning about function of social workers and of contact with social service (class of 1955)

	A great deal	Little	Nothing	Coder could not classify
Learning about function of social workers				
GMC	55	20	5	20
Control	18	41	24	17
Contact with social service				
GMC	59	41	0	0
Control	6	89	0	6

It seems quite evident, then, that GMC students did, in fact, have much greater contact with the ancillary services than did control students.

Further interview material is presented in detail below to indicate the conflict between learning to recognize and cope with pathology and to deal with other types of patients' problems:

Q: How did you feel about being assigned to the GMC?

A: I was glad that I had been. When I was a sophomore I lived in the basement of the house in which a senior lived who was on GMC. He liked it very much, so I was glad that I had been assigned to the GMC.

Q: What did you think you would like about it?

A: Well, I thought that I'd like having more responsibility for the care of the patient and more direct contact with them as their doctor.

Q: Was there anything that you thought you might not like about it? Were all your feelings positive, or were some of them negative?

A: Well, I'd heard some bad things before I came, too. I was on surgery, and I'd been down here some during my junior year in the emergency room and I had seen many times where the intern would return to the doctor's room and say "I've got a crock out here, what shall we do with him?" and everyone would say in a chorus, "Send him to GMC," so I had already heard that lots of the crocks showed up within GMC. I anticipated this.

Q: Did that bother you particularly?

A: Well, yes. Nobody likes crocks.

Q: Why not?

A: They're a nuisance. There is nothing ever wrong with them and they are even so peculiar they never have diseases other people do. But they've got five to ten times more complaints; they're more demanding, they're never satisfied, they're never cured. These are all the satisfactions of medicine—to make a diagnosis, to treat the person, and to cure him. None of these things are successful with a crock. That's where I suppose the name stems from. It's not that they aren't sick in the sense that they feel sick, it's just that they are crocks that don't ever get well.

Q: Has your attitude changed since then? Are you more positive about GMC than you were when you came in, or less?

A: Well, I'm less so. I feel that I haven't gotten as much in my senior year as I should have in terms of medical education. I may be able to deal with patients in the sense that they frequently point out to us here; that this sort of thing is going to make up the greater part of your practice, and you have to learn to deal with these people. It seems to me that the advantage they are pointing out to us is in terms of financial gain. I feel I haven't seen as much pathology in my senior year as I did in my junior year because of the GMC, and therefore I don't feel I've gotten all I could have in my senior year in terms of seeing pathology and learning to diagnose it, or learning to treat it. In that respect I feel I am even more fortunate than some of the other students on GMC because I have had perhaps half dozen patients that were very interesting, and have had some disease, but I know some other people say they have had less than that.

Q: You don't consider that lack of pathology, for example, was offset by gaining insight into patients? It isn't worth it, as far as you can see?

A: Well, I think that people who require insight into their problems aren't apt to die because of a mis-diagnosis. They will keep complaining (as I said in my definition of what I thought was a crock)—they keep complaining in spite of what you do. What I'm most interested in is that when I go out into practice I won't miss some organic problem that I didn't have an opportunity to see while I was in medical school, because I spent my time in GMC. The emphasis in this program is how to have a continued patient-doctor relation regardless of what the patient's illness is. The patients aren't selected as they are in other clinics. When you go to attend a clinic you may see thirty diabetics in one clinic in one afternoon and then thirty orthopedics in another one, and a dermatology clinic and so on. But if nobody else knows what to do with them and they are a pain in the neck they wind up in GMC—if they are really interesting problems they don't show up here. I can illustrate that. One day I had a young boy with rheumatic fever, and he had multiple cardiac lesions as a result of this, and it turned out that he belonged to the rheumatic fever clinic and we couldn't do anything to him; we couldn't keep him in this clinic. In fact, they were very irate that he had come to this hospital.

That would probably have been an interesting patient. At least it illustrated to me that patients with pathology are guarded pretty jealously in other clinics. It would have been a good student case, but we didn't get to keep him, nevertheless.

Q: Do you get anything out of your continued patient contact? Are you learning from this?

A: Yes, I am. I have a better ability now to continue relations with a patient that has a chronic disease, one that I don't expect to benefit a great deal with medication, and that will progress probably until his death—or a patient that I won't change except merely to be able to relieve his symptoms. I've learned somewhat how to talk to these people, how to explain their diseases to them, and how to keep their spirits up, which in a sense is about all I can do as their physician. I have learned that, yes. Much of it is just common sense, understanding, and a desire to be helpful to these people. But it also takes some practice which I have had an opportunity to do here at the clinic—probably more practice than I would have had in other types of clinics which are designed so that you don't necessarily see the same patient again. I've made some mistakes which would probably not have been too well accepted in a private practice. If I hadn't made them here I might have made them after I had started in practice. And there are things which at first didn't seem too important to me, or didn't seem unusual to me. After I made the mistake I realized that if I had another such patient I wouldn't do it quite that way, and by that time I had thought of some other way I would do it.

Q: Was the staff helpful with respect to learning how to deal with patients?

A: No, I don't think in our usual presentations to the staff that we ever discussed much about their emotional needs, unless we were talking to psychiatrists.

Q: Why was that?

A: Well, I think (and it is my impression that the medical staff feels this way too) that while we are medical students we need to learn about diseases as well as recognize the whole patient. This clinic is light in that sense, in the amount of pathology we see, and I'm sure I've seen more healthy normal patients than I have sick patients since I've been in this clinic. That doesn't seem right to me. That may be exactly what I'll see in practice, but while I'm here in the factory, so to speak, where all the pathology is presented, it seems to me that I've missed an opportunity to see pathology while I'm a student. There are certain specialty clinics that I haven't been able to attend that I wish I could have, and the other people in the other programs have. I've never had any training of any kind in dermatology and yet I believe from what I've read that about 20% of a person's practice is concerned with dermatology. I've had no training in my medical school in that particular field. Now as for the total care of the patient—which I believe in, subscribe to heartily—I have had a better chance to practice it than the people in the other clinics. This is the largest part of your practice, people who are not really sick but simply need some support, and I have had a better chance to practice that than other people. But the point I resent is this: I've devoted too much of my time to that kind of patient while I'm in the learning stage. This is fine when I'm out in practice and it's a question of keeping a patient or discharging him from a financial point of view as well as concern for the patient. But I wonder how many dermatological lesions I won't recognize or won't be able to treat successfully because I haven't attended any of those clinics. This seems to me just as important in the long run as knowing how to talk to a patient that doesn't have any organic disease.

Students' diaries

The following material is quoted from the diary of an exceptionally good student who did not participate in the GMC. This student was primarily interested in medical knowledge for its own sake and had little interest in comprehensive care. The material is presented here because it illustrates so clearly the complexity of one student's attitudes toward patients. The diary entries also illustrate a type of material which this research did not attempt to deal with. (The pseudonym Appeley is used for the diarist.)

Patient A: "This family was referred by a private doctor . . . for a definitive workup, and they are 'paying patients.' It is always a source of amazement to me that these people are always more patient and understanding of time delays and more willing to receive 'the full treatment,' and more pleased for getting it, than are our charity cases. Mother was very pleased at receiving a 'medical center workup' of the case."

Patient B: "This patient is uncooperative, disinterested, and stupid, and at the present time represents a classical therapeutic failure." On a revisit of the same patient, Appeley stated: "I am unable to manage this patient. Hence, I will prescribe insulin that he asks for and let him merrily kill himself. . . . Patient cannot be managed. Will watch him go to hell. In practice, one would refuse to treat this case."

Patient C: Although the patient being described here was considered valuable to Appeley because she had a "very interesting disease," and therefore served to focus his attention on "an important group of diseases," the following comments indicate his attitude toward the patient: "This patient is a bum who also is an Oriental . . . has abandoned four children to the state home . . . husband is also a bum. . . . Their existence is at an animal level—rehabilitation would be a greater waste of money than their support."

Doctor-patient relations were considered to have no function: "This is essentially veterinary medicine." After a revisit by this same patient, Appeley stated: "Patient has become conscious, friendly, and cooperative—but is frightfully stupid."

But Appeley showed an entirely different attitude toward other patients.

Patient D: "This patient eventually signed out of the hospital. I believe that this would not have occurred if my routine duties had permitted me more time with her. On the day of her initial interview, I saw seven patients in the OB Clinic, did five CBC's, eight routine urines, three deliveries. In the following days similar duties prevented further interviews. I feel that a good relation would, of itself, have been of immeasurable psychotherapeutic benefit to this patient. With some airing of her dependency needs and conflicts, the true organic nature of her illness would, I believe, be more clear—that is, without subjective distortion of symptoms."

In discussing the therapy of this patient, Appeley stated: "I believe that adequate psychotherapy here might well have been the major benefit to this patient. Certainly organic therapy would have little effect unless some attempt was made to deal with problems in the psychiatric sphere."

Appeley had the following to say when discussing the satisfactions derived from his work with the above patient: "This was a most frustrating patient. The problems that she presented were interesting, but the diagnoses were never made. As previously mentioned, I believe that with adequate time to form a good patient-physician relation, I could have prevented her premature departure from the hospital. Work with this patient today was fearfully inadequate. It was not fair to the patient, to the institution, or to the student. It was a half-done, botched job that chagrins me to write about and galls me to accept as an educational experience. All that was needed to fulfill not only my goals, but those of the patient and the institution as well, was time for an adequate workup. This commodity was not obtained today, or in the patient's subsequent hospital course. Results? A failure for all concerned."

The following comments come from different parts of one day's entry in the diary: "The patient's maternal grandmother accompanied her and her mother, and was obviously the controlling functionary in the family group. She constantly interrupted the mother during the taking of the history, corrected the child, and answered questions directed at the mother. The mother had to consult with her before answering even the simplest questions relating to the development of her child. The grandmother was quite critical of the child—i.e., 'She was always the slowest of my grandchildren,' etc. . . . Feel that there is probably a division of authority between the mother and grandmother, which is giving rise to an appreciable sense of insecurity in this child. . . . Management must be carried on through the mother alone, in an effort to shift responsibility and authority to the proper individual without the intervening grandmother-mother figure. . . . Any person who could subject a child to an enema two or three times a week for years has inherent a streak of sadism, unforgivable stupidity, or a psychotic aberration, and I fear that my strong feeling on this matter may have shown through as strong disapproval to this mother. Disapproval, indeed, of an act which may symbolically represent her idea of motherhood. . . . Likewise, I feel perhaps that modern medical advice was meeting ears prepared by a century of folk medicine, and that the mother not only did not believe what I told her, but will not follow the advice given to the further psychiatric and possibly organic detriment of her child.

"In some way rapport was not achieved with this mother to my satisfaction—I am not confident of this most necessary relation—this is obvious from rereading my last two paragraphs, but as I try to pin down the objective reasons for this feeling, I cannot. . . . Perhaps in my efforts to contact the mother, I in some way offended or trod upon her own relation with patient's grandmother. . . . I am afraid that this patient will not return for her next appointment because of this failure."

Future research will have to cope with problems of the sort suggested by the above material. The fact that the same student can be so harshly disapproving and indifferent that he is willing to let one patient "merrily kill himself," yet exhibit the sympathetic understanding of the behavior of the last mentioned family while regretting his own ineptitude, suggests a research problem of considerable magnitude and difficulty.

Individual Attributes Related to Sociological Attitudes

Results pertaining to the entire class. In the class of 1955 there was a persistent tendency for the better students to develop more positive attitudes toward the team concept from Posttest I to Posttest II. In the

Table 23.16. Relation between verbal ability, clerkship experience, and change in attitudes toward the team concept from Pretest to Posttest II (class of 1956)

		Change in attitudes toward team concept		
		Negative change	No change or positive change	
GMC				
Verbal ability	High	3	10	13
Verbal ability	Low	13	8	21
Control				
Verbal ability	High	12	7	19
Verbal ability	Low	8	4	12
		36	29	65

class of 1956, however, there were no definite and consistent findings in this respect, possibly because the GMC and control clerkships affected similar kinds of students differently (see below).

Results pertaining to the GMC and control groups separately. There was some indication (as noted in connection with change in attitudes toward comprehensive care) that the GMC had its greatest positive effect on the brighter students, when "brightness" is measured by the Verbal Ability subtest of the MCAT.

The Verbal Ability subtest is very likely a good indicator of students' intelligence, since most studies of intelligence show verbal ability to be an integral component of intelligence as it is commonly measured. Assuming that the Verbal Ability subtest does indicate intelligence, data presented in Table 23.16 suggest that the GMC was more likely to develop positive attitudes toward the team concept among brighter students than among less intelligent ones.

Part V

SPECIAL STUDIES

Introduction to Part V

Three special studies were undertaken in connection with the general research concerning the evaluation of the General Medical Clinic. The first of these, discussed in Chapter 24, is a detailed study of individual differences in student performance in the GMC. The second, discussed in Chapter 25, concerns a special problem which emerged during the course of the research—the Scheduling Effect. This problem was not anticipated, but it was studied carefully and is reported on separately because of its great importance in the present study and its serious implications for medical education in general. Chapter 26 describes the relations between the various measures of individual attributes employed in this study and grade averages on the assumption that such results are of general interest.

Chapter 24

Students' Performance in the GMC

One of the aims of the Individual Differences Section of the research project was to ascertain what, if any, individual attributes were correlated with performance in the General Medical Clinic and to examine these attributes to discover what type of student would be likely to perform well in this type of clinical setting. (The term individual attributes includes aptitude test scores, previous academic performance, and certain peer-judged attributes, as well as personality characteristics.)

The basic procedure was simply to compute correlations between ratings of performance and all the available measures of individual attributes. As was expected, a serious difficulty occurred in connection with obtaining suitable measures of the various components of performance in the clinic. This problem and the steps taken to solve it, which are discussed in detail below, led to some valuable findings about the nature of the clinic: in the course of investigating this problem, it became apparent that each member of the GMC staff was rating students almost wholly in terms of his own idiosyncratic concept of what constituted a good medical student, rather than differentiating among the various components of performance, as it had been hoped he would.

Ratings of Performance

Obtaining satisfactory measures of performance proved the chief problem in the study of students' performance in the GMC. In view of the difficulties that arose from the use of staff ratings for this purpose, one might question the wisdom of using them in the first place. The answer is that staff ratings were the only practicable and meaningful measures of students' performance. A possible alternative to staff ratings would have been ratings by independent observers in the clinic.

However, aside from the cumbersome nature of this procedure and the practical impossibility of getting competent persons to act as observers, the ratings thus produced would have been open to the objection that they did not accurately represent performance. That is, each student's performance in the clinic was, by definition, the degree to which he achieved appropriate knowledge, skill, and attitudes *from the point of view of the group attempting to inculcate these abilities and attitudes*—the GMC staff. Any other person's judgment would be colored by other values possibly inconsistent with, and undoubtedly not identical with, those of the GMC staff. For this reason, and also because the staff members were thoroughly familiar with the students' performance (they "checked" the students more than fifteen times during a twenty-two-week clerkship and saw them frequently on other occasions), staff ratings seemed the only logical choice as measures of performance.

The actual ratings and the methods of using them varied somewhat from group to group. The changes in rating procedures are discussed in detail in the second section of this chapter. It is sufficient here to state that the members of the staff of the GMC were asked to rate the students on their knowledge, skill, and attitudes in the areas of medicine, psychology, and sociology.

Procedures of Analysis

The basic procedure was to compute correlations between the measures of individual attributes and the various ratings. The index used was the product-moment correlation coefficient (r). This basic procedure and the analysis of the criterion problem were supplemented by two additional studies. The first of these was a further analysis of selected ratings, which was aimed at determining which individual attributes were considered by the raters in making their judgments. The second was an analysis of individual attributes associated with unexpected performance in the GMC, in which an attempt was made to ascertain what personality traits characterized students who performed markedly better or markedly worse in the GMC than their previous work in medical school would have indicated likely.

THE CRITERION PROBLEM

Before proceeding to the presentation and analysis of results, it is necessary to discuss in detail the problems of obtaining adequate measures of performance. As explained above, the only available and practicable measures were the ratings made by the members of the GMC staff; these ratings were intended to reflect various elements of the students' performance, corresponding to the objectives of the GMC: acquisition of medical, psychological, and sociological knowledge, skill, and attitudes. However, after mildly encouraging results with the first group of students (1954 I), it became apparent that the staff's ratings were inadequate in two respects: *intra*-rater correlations were much too high—that is, individual raters were not discriminating sufficiently among the various components of a student's performance; and *inter*-rater reliabilities were somewhat lower than had been desired—that is, there was not sufficient agreement among different raters of the same student. These two problems were separate, and separate steps were taken to reduce each one; yet they were related in the sense that they both occurred because each rater actually evaluated the student's performance wholly in terms of a single component (or at most two components), and in each case the component was unique to the staff member in question. If the raters individually had been able to distinguish among the various elements of performance, the intra-rater correlations would have been much lower; if all staff members had rated in terms of a single common component, the inter-rater reliabilities would have been much higher. To explain this dual problem more fully, it is necessary to describe in some detail the manner in which it emerged as the data from the various groups were analyzed.

Emergence of the Problem

1954 I group. Ratings on a list of nineteen components of performance were obtained for the first student group ($N = 21$). Nine of these were factor analyzed. Table 24.1 presents the results of these procedures. The factor structure shows that seven ratings were highly correlated with one or the other of two (rotated) factors, termed interpersonal relations and medical knowledge and skill. In other words, the raters were apparently distinguishing only two components instead of the many they had been expected to distinguish. This, however, was not at the time regarded as an especially discouraging result. The two components revealed in the factor analysis indicated that the raters were making some distinctions; there was also the possibility that there were only two components of the students' performance.

The inter-rater reliability coefficients,[1] also presented in Table 24.1, were regarded as somewhat lower than they should have been: the range of reliabilities for eleven ratings was from .36 to .73; the median reliability was .57. (The usual minimum reliability for this sort of material is .70.)

1954 II group. Ratings on a list of twenty-one components were

[1] Reliabilities were computed by correlating the mean of the ratings of students made by one half of the raters with the mean of the ratings made by the other half. The two groups of raters were randomly selected.

Table 24.1. Factor structure and inter-rater reliability coefficients of staff ratings, 1954 I students ($N = 21$)

	Interpersonal relations component	Medical knowledge and skill component	Reliability
Concern for patient	.83	.02	*
Skill in physician-patient relations	.83	.24	*
Attitudes toward physician-patient relations	.79	.28	*
Case presentation	.33	.90	.67
Judgment	.38	.87	.66
Physical examination	.33	.87	.46
Medical knowledge	.16	.84	.73
Independence of work	.03	.66	*
Personal adjustment	.15	.41	*

* Pooled ratings.

obtained for the 1954 II student group ($N = 18$). Again, selected ratings were factor analyzed. Reliabilities were computed (in the same manner as before) for all twenty-one ratings. The results appear in Table 24.2. All ratings but one, preference for working independently, were highly correlated with a single factor. This was regarded as a rather disturbing result. However, as may be seen from Table 24.2, the reliability coefficients for these ratings were considerably better than those for the 1954 I group: the range of reliabilities for all twenty-one ratings was from .51 to .91; the median reliability was .80.

1955 I group. Essentially the same procedure was followed for the 1955 I group ($N = 20$). Table 24.3 presents the inter-rater reliabilities and intra-rater correlations for selected ratings. As had been the case

Table 24.2. Factor structure and inter-rater reliability coefficients of staff ratings, 1954 II students ($N = 18$)

	Single rating component	Reliability
Concern for patient	.86	.88
Skill in physician-patient relations	.86	.86
Attitudes toward physician-patient relations	.91	.85
Case presentation	.85	.76
Judgment	.90	.80
Physical examination	.95	.77
Medical knowledge	.91	.87
Independence of work	.32	.71
Personal adjustment	.84	.89
Likeability	.88	.87

Table 24.3. Intra-rater correlation coefficients and inter-rater reliability coefficients of staff ratings, 1955 I students ($N = 20$)

	2	3	4	5	6	7	8	9	10	11	Relia-bility
1. Medical knowledge	.95	.91	.88	.83	.81	.82	.82	—.57	.68	.95	.97
2. Medical skill		.97	.95	.92	.91	.93	.89	—.56	.78	.99	.96
3. Attitudes toward medicine			.98	.93	.95	.96	.95	—.60	.84	.96	.73
4. Knowledge of physician-patient relations				.96	.95	.95	.93	—.58	.83	.94	.91
5. Skill in physician-patient relations					.91	.90	.87	—.69	.89	.91	.89
6. Attitudes toward patients						.98	.95	—.47	.81	.90	.78
7. Attitudes toward emotional problems							.95	—.48	.81	.93	.89
8. Attitudes toward ancillary services								—.59	.82	.89	—
9. Anxiety about uncertainties									—.82	—.57	—
10. Personal adjustment										.78	—
11. Over-all rating											.88

with the 1954 II group, the reliabilities were reasonably good, but the ratings were very highly intercorrelated.

At this point it was clear that a serious criterion problem existed. On two of three separate occasions only one component had appeared in the GMC staff's ratings of the students' performance. The staff had been expected to discriminate among students' knowledge, skill, and attitudes in the areas of traditional medicine, the psychological aspects of medicine, and the social aspects of medicine (see Chapters 10 and 11). However, the results to this point indicated that the staff, in the main, was evaluating students in terms of a single component, or at most, two components. Also, on one of three occasions, the interrater reliabilities were somewhat low, although on the other two occasions these seemed satisfactory.

Naturally the question then arose of the accuracy of the staff's evaluations. Possibly there was only one component (or at most two) of students' performance. Evidence from research in personality assessment made this possibility seem doubtful; current opinion about medical students made it extremely doubtful that the student who was interested and competent in the field of organic medicine was also the student who would be competent and interested in the psychological and social aspects of patient care. Two other kinds of information, from other parts of the research project, also strongly militated against the hypothesis that students' performance really contained only one or two components: these were the students' ratings of one another and the objective test data.

Students had been asked to rate one another on the same components of performance as the staff. Correlations among the students' ratings were found to be approximately .4 or .5. No correlation was as high as .8, the typical value found in correlations among staff ratings. Moreover, objective test measurements of some of the same components produced still lower correlations (approximately .2 or .3) than those among student ratings. In short, peers discriminated more sharply among the components of performance in the GMC than did clinic instructors, and objective tests discriminated even more sharply than did peers. Since these results were found in three separate groups of students, it seems clear that differences might well have existed which should have enabled the instructors to make valid discriminations.

Preliminary Attempts to Solve the Problem

The most obvious first step toward solving the criterion problem seemed to be to improve the methods of collecting the ratings. Therefore, three changes in the rating procedure were introduced: first, the definitions of the components of performance in terms of which students were to be rated were made more specific; second, the number of components to be rated by a GMC staff member was reduced; and third, the rating task was simplified.

From time to time, staff members had raised questions about the definitions of the areas of performance on which they were to rate the students. Therefore, an attempt was made to clarify the meaning of each area. Each staff member was interviewed, and his definition of each component was obtained. The specific question asked was: Which actions of a student do you think of when making this rating? From the replies to this question, a preliminary list of behavioral descriptions for each component was drawn up. Tentative rating forms, which included behavioral referents, were then made. These forms were discussed with staff members, and final revisions were made in the light of staff suggestions. This discussion also helped the staff to familiarize themselves with the new forms prior to using them.

The second change in the data collection procedure was reduction of the number of ratings a GMC staff member was asked to make. Staff members were asked which areas of performance they preferred to rate. On the basis of this expression of preference, and after a conference with the director of the GMC, four groups of raters were established: group 1 consisted of staff physicians with more than five years' experience; group 2 consisted of staff physicians with less than five years' experience; group 3 was made up of the psychiatrically oriented members of the GMC staff;[2] and group 4 consisted of ancillary staff members (social workers and public health nurses). Table 24.4 shows that although group 1 rated on all components, group 2 did not rate on psychological components, group 3 did not rate on medical components, and group 4 did not rate on either medical or psychological components. A student's score was the median rating he received on each component.

The third change was to simplify the rating procedure. It was felt that one reason for the inadequacy of the ratings might be that the raters, finding the rating task irksome and time consuming, tended to make their judgments in a hasty and perfunctory manner. Therefore, instead of requiring each rater to rate each student individually on a five-point scale for each component, each rater was now asked to sort cards (each containing a student's name) into six piles for each rating, the piles denoting varying degrees of excellence. (The use of a six-category scale was a change from the five-category scale previously

[2] Actually this group varied in makeup from one rating situation to another. It consisted of a single psychiatrist plus one other staff member, usually an internist.

Table 24.4. Components of performance rated (by preference) by various groups of staff members

	Group 1 (more experienced physicians)	Group 2 (less experienced physicians)	Group 3 (psychiatrically oriented physicians)	Group 4 (ancillary staff members)
Medical knowledge	x	x		
Medical skill	x	x		
Initiative in learning medicine	x	x		
Psychological knowledge	x		x	
Psychological skill	x		x	
Attitudes toward emotional problems	x		x	
Skill in physician-patient relations	x	x	x	x
Attitudes toward patients	x	x	x	x
Sociological skill	x	x	x	x
Attitudes toward social problems	x	x	x	x
Attitudes toward comprehensive care	x	x	x	x
Number of ratings	11	8	8	5

employed.) Each sort was recorded by a member of the research group while the rater studied the description of the next component on which the students were to be rated. Then any questions the rater might have were answered, the cards were reshuffled, and the next sort was made. In this way, the demands upon the staff member's time were reduced to thirty to forty-five minutes, and since the ratings were made in the presence of a member of the research staff, some potential confusions and misunderstandings were undoubtedly eliminated.

These three revisions were incorporated into the rating procedure, and the staff used the new rating forms to evaluate the members of the 1955 II group. Despite these changes the median correlation among ratings for the 1955 II student group ($N = 17$) was .87 (see Table 24.5). The lowest correlation was .67. The improvements in data collection procedure had not reduced to any appreciable extent the degree of relation among ratings of this group of students. Again, it was possible to represent the structure of the correlation matrix in terms of a single component, very likely medical knowledge.

Study of the GMC Staff as Raters

At this point the performance of the individual raters came under closer scrutiny. In contrast to the previous procedure of intercorrelating *mean* ratings of students, *all* the ratings made by *each* rater were intercorrelated. Similarly, instead of randomly dividing the raters into two

Table 24.5. Intra-rater correlation coefficients of staff ratings, 1955 II students ($N = 17$)

	2	3	4	5	6	7	8	9	10	11
1. Medical knowledge	.93	.88	.86	.80	.72	.91	.67	.80	.82	.77
2. Medical skill		.89	.92	.88	.78	.93	.75	.89	.88	.83
3. Initiative in learning medicine			.91	.93	.84	.90	.74	.84	.87	.84
4. Psychological knowledge				.93	.77	.89	.75	.86	.88	.83
5. Psychological skill					.91	.92	.86	.92	.92	.92
6. Attitudes toward emotional problems						.87	.86	.88	.84	.92
7. Skill in physician-patient relations							.82	.90	.85	.89
8. Attitudes toward patients								.87	.89	.95
9. Sociological skill									.95	.92
10. Attitudes toward social problems										.94
11. Attitudes toward comprehensive care										

groups and computing reliabilities, all ratings on each component (and there were as many ratings on a component as there were raters) were intercorrelated. The data for the 1955 II, 1956 I, and 1956 II students were all analyzed in this way. The results of applying this procedure to the data obtained from the 1955 II group are summarized in Table 24.6.

Intra-rater correlations

In the upper part of Table 24.6 the correlations among ratings made by each member of the GMC staff are summarized. The high median intra-rater correlation (.81) is particularly significant. (Replication of this study on the next two groups of students yielded over-all median intra-rater correlations of .68 and .75, respectively.) Thus, with one or two possible exceptions, each staff member of the experimental medical clinic was evaluating students' performance in terms of a single

Table 24.6. Intra-rater and inter-rater correlation coefficients of staff ratings, 1955 II students ($N = 17$)

	No. of ratings	No. of correlations	Range	Median r
Intra-rater correlations				
A. (More experienced physician)	11	55	.42 – .98	.81
B. " " "	11	55	.54 – .95	.76
C. " " "	11	55	.53 – .94	.79
D. " " "	11	55	—.06 – .91	.68
E. (Less experienced physician)	8	28	.40 – .93	.80
F. " " "	8	28	.48 – .88	.71
G. " " "	8	28	.73 – .93	.83
H. " " "	8	28	.68 – .92	.83
I. (Psychiatrist)	8	28	.71 – .95	.86
J. (Social worker)	5	10	.81 – .94	.89
K. " "	5	10	.76 – .95	.89
L. (Public health nurse)	5	10	.56 – .92	.77
Over-all median				.81
Range of medians				.68 – .89
Inter-rater correlations				
Medical knowledge	7	21	.14 – .67	.38
Medical skill	7	21	.02 – .79	.45
Initiative in learning medicine	7	21	.04 – .72	.31
Psychological knowledge	6	15	.01 – .74	.39
Psychological skill	6	15	.19 – .61	.37
Attitudes toward emotional problems	6	15	—.11 – .61	.32
Skill in physician-patient relations	12	66	.11 – .75	.43
Attitudes toward patients	12	66	—.04 – .79	.41
Sociological skill	12	66	—.13 – .78	.33
Attitudes toward social problems	12	66	—.20 – .77	.31
Attitudes toward comprehensive care	12	66	—.16 – .85	.36
Over-all median				.37
Range of medians				.31 – .45

component. Despite the efforts to spell out the several elements of performance in the new clinic, the staff members were not making distinctions among students' medical, psychological, and sociological knowledge, skill, and attitudes. It will be recalled that the students and the objective tests were making these distinctions.

Inter-rater correlations

The correlations among all raters for each rating were also computed; the results of this procedure are indicated in the lower part of Table 24.6. It is significant that the median inter-rater correlations were much lower than the intra-rater correlations. There were also more negative correlations among raters than among ratings by one rater. The over-all median inter-rater correlation was .37. (Replication of this study on two subsequent groups of students yielded an over-all median inter-rater correlation of .30 for each group.) Thus it appears that, although only one component appeared in the ratings of each rater, each rater rated on a different component. Staff members differed widely among themselves concerning which students were performing well and which were performing poorly.

In short, the improvement of the rating procedure did not solve the problem of single, unique rating components; analysis of the individual raters confirmed the fact of single, unique components.

Independent observations

These results raised questions of whether the aims of the experimental clinic were being carried out in the GMC teaching. If each instructor was evaluating students in terms of a single component, unique to the instructor, was it not possible that in his teaching he was likewise focusing on that same single component—which other teachers were not emphasizing? Data obtained from the student-staff conferences raised similar questions. The following is an excerpt from a report by a physician (not a member of the GMC staff and totally unaware of the rating problem) who analyzed recordings of the student-staff conferences:

> The way the student-staff conference proceeded after the student's initial presentation was almost always very much like all the other student-staff conferences *of a particular staff man.* Some staff men were interested in the student's knowledge of all laboratory procedures relevant to the case, others were interested in the pathology that might be found, and some focused on the social problems of the patients. Some inexorably stuck to organic diseases, while others discounted the organic and handled patients as psycho-social problems. . . . Some worked hard only if the student did so first; others insisted that the student cerebrate whether he liked it or not.

Two points about these comments are especially noteworthy. First, the physician observer remarked that each staff man "almost always" proceeded in the same way. This behavior is what might be expected if the staff were evaluating students in terms of a single component. Second, the physician observer remarked that each staff physician proceeded in a unique way. Independent observations of the teaching situation, then, confirmed the conclusions drawn from the analysis of GMC staff's ratings of students.

This result, supported as it is by the independent conclusions of a medically trained observer, constitutes a most important finding: it indicates that staff ratings are probably a highly inadequate device for evaluating medical students. Accurate and effective evaluation is hardly likely to occur when each evaluator bases his judgment on a single-dimensioned concept of what constitutes a good medical student, and when each evaluator's concept is different from that of every other evaluator. Yet this is precisely what this part of the study indicates. Moreover, it is improbable that the amount of disagreement among raters is generally suspected: for the raters in the present study differed only in what they *did* when they evaluated actual students; they substantially agreed in what they *said* they considered to be desirable characteristics in medical students. It should also be noted that the present results were obtained under conditions less likely to produce halo effects and individual rater idiosyncracies than would be the case in the usual medical situation, in which there would be less pressure to differentiate among different kinds of performance.

Solutions to the Problem

Low inter-rater reliabilities

The problem of low inter-rater reliability was attacked first. The solution was found in a statistical technique for estimating errors in ratings.[3] By means of this (analysis of variance) technique it was

[3] See J. P. Guilford, *Psychometric Methods* (New York: McGraw-Hill, 1954). The rationale for this procedure is represented in terms of conventional test theory. The basic formula in test theory, "raw score equals true score plus error score," is modified by this procedure to read, "raw score equals true score plus several error component scores." The errors are assumed to be additive and unrelated to each other. The component suspected of contributing the most error to the data was the *relative* halo or "rater-ratee interaction error." The halo component is described as relative because it represents the degree of over-valuation or under-valuation of a student by a rater relative to the over- or under-valuation of the same student by the other raters. As expected, an analysis of variance study of several sets of data showed that halo effect, or rater-ratee interaction, was important. In every one of nine analyses made, rater-ratee interaction variance proved to be significant beyond the .01 level. On the other hand, the contributions of leniency error and reaction error to the ratings were seldom significant.

possible to calculate the contributions of three kinds of *constant error* (rater-ratee interaction error, leniency error, reaction error) to ratings.

The error scores were subtracted from the original ratings to provide "corrected" or "adjusted" ratings. Table 24.7 presents an example of the inter-rater reliability coefficients before and after the ratings have been adjusted. The differences are striking. Some reliabilities increased as much as .40; the smallest increase in reliability was .15. In subsequent analyses *de*creases in reliability value were obtained on occasion, but in general the later results were similar to those presented here. (The decreases in agreement are mentioned here primarily to demonstrate the fact that increases were not mere statistical artifacts, but functions of the data obtained.)

Thus, removal of three kinds of errors increased the amount of agreement among raters to a considerable degree, and one of the two inadequacies of the staff ratings was thereby eliminated.

High intra-rater correlations

Attention now shifted to the problem of high correlations among ratings. Removal of relative halo and the other errors from ratings was expected to result in lower intra-rater correlations; however, it did not do so. The median correlation among adjusted ratings of the 1955 II student group was .86, compared with a median of .87 prior to adjustment of the ratings. Clearly, although relative halo error was causing low agreement among staff members, it was not causing the high correlations among ratings.

A fresh approach was therefore made to the problem of high intrarater correlation. It will be recalled that considerable evidence, including the independent observations of a medically trained witness, had appeared, which suggested that in their teaching, the internists, pediatricians, and other medical specialists were concentrating largely on their own specialties; the psychiatrists were concentrating on the psy-

Table 24.7. Inter-rater reliability coefficients of original ratings and adjusted ratings by staff members A, B, and C

	Original ratings			Adjusted ratings		
	*r*AB	*r*AC	*r*BC	*r*AB	*r*AC	*r*BC
Medical knowledge	.57	.67	.29	.80	.90	.81
Psychological knowledge	.43	.59	.41	.87	.79	.84
Attitudes toward patients	.33	.42	.30	.73	.63	.45
Sociological skill	.35	.17	.16	.56	.57	.62
Attitudes toward comprehensive care	.34	.40	.01	.79	.76	.60
Median *r*	.35	.42	.29	.79	.76	.62
Over-all median *r*		.35			.76	

chological aspects of medical care; and the members of the ancillary staff on social problems in medicine. If this was true, each group of raters would have little knowledge of the students' competence outside its own area of competence; there might be a tendency among medically trained raters, for example, to base all their ratings of a given student upon his medical competence alone. Likewise, the psychiatrists might tend to base all ratings on the student's psychological competence. This might then be the source of the high intra-rater correlations, since (as shown in Table 24.4) several groups of raters were rating students on components of performance that were outside their (the raters') special fields of competence.

On the above hypothesis, the number of ratings used was further restricted, as shown in Table 24.8. From the ratings made by the medically trained raters, four were selected (medical knowledge, medical skill, initiative in learning medicine, and attitudes toward comprehensive care); from the ratings made by the psychiatric group five were selected (psychological knowledge, psychological skill, attitudes toward emotional problems, skill in physician-patient relations, and attitudes toward patients); and from the ratings made by the ancillary staff three were selected (sociological skill, ability to work with ancillary services, and attitudes toward social problems). The other ratings were disregarded.

Table 24.8. Components of performance rated (by restriction procedure) by various groups of staff members

	Group 1 (more experienced physicians)	Group 2 (less experienced physicians)	Group 3 (psychiatrically oriented physicians)	Group 4 (ancillary staff members)
Medical knowledge	x	x		
Medical skill	x	x		
Initiative in learning medicine	x	x		
Psychological knowledge			x	
Psychological skill			x	
Attitudes toward emotional problems			x	
Skill in physician-patient relations			x	
Attitudes toward patients			x	
Sociological skill				x
Attitudes toward social problems				x
Ability to work with ancillary services				x
Number of ratings	3	3	5	3

Although intra-rater correlations remained high, it now became possible to distinguish four components, based on the means of ratings by each of the four rater groups. The first of these (based on ratings made by group 2, less experienced physicians) was designated medical knowledge. The second (based on ratings by group 1, more experienced physicians) was designated medical skill.[4] The third component (based on ratings made by group 3, psychiatrically oriented members of the medical staff) was designated psychological knowledge. The fourth component (based on ratings made by group 4, members of the ancillary staff) was designated attitudes toward patients' social problems. It should be borne in mind that these are somewhat arbitrary designations, and that when these terms are used below *they really refer to ratings made by the various groups of raters.*

RESULTS OF ADJUSTMENTS

On the basis of the two procedures outlined above, ratings for the 1955 II students were adjusted, and correlations were computed. The correlations among the four groups of raters, and thus the correlations among the four components of performance, were noticeably lower than those based on unrestricted ratings. To illustrate these results, one rating has been selected from those made by each of the four rater groups. Table 24.9 shows the intra-rater correlations based on the original ratings; Table 24.10 shows these correlations based on adjusted ratings. Table 24.11 shows the median inter-rater reliabilities based on the adjusted ratings. The results were encouraging, and to test further the value of the adjustment procedure, it was applied to the ratings of the 1955 I, 1956 I, and 1956 II student groups.

The ratings of the 1955 I group were adjusted in a manner similar to that described above. Table 24.12 shows that the intra-rater correlations were lower than they had been, and the median inter-rater reliabilities were sufficiently high.

The 1956 I and II student groups' ratings were also adjusted. The correlations and reliabilities of the adjusted ratings for each of these groups are presented in Tables 24.13 and 24.14. The results were somewhat better than those achieved with the 1955 I group.

Summary

To summarize, ratings of students by the GMC staff members were found to be inadequate because students were not being evaluated in

[4] These two designations were based on the hypothesis that the more experienced physicians would be better able to recognize medical skill as distinguished from medical knowledge, and on the fact that the ratings by the less experienced physicians were more highly correlated with previous academic performance, a measure presumably reflecting medical knowledge.

Table 24.9. Intra-rater correlation coefficients of original staff ratings, 1955 II students ($N = 17$)

		1	2	3
1	Medical skill			
2	Medical knowledge	.93		
3	Psychological knowledge	.92	.86	
4	Attitudes toward social problems	.88	.82	.88

Table 24.10. Intra-rater correlation coefficients of adjusted and restricted staff ratings, 1955 II students ($N = 17$)

		1	2	3
1	Medical skill			
2	Medical knowledge	.68		
3	Psychological knowledge	.55	.43	
4	Attitudes toward social problems	.60	.59	.50

Table 24.11. Median inter-rater reliability coefficients of original and of adjusted and restricted staff ratings, 1955 II students ($N = 17$)

	Original	Adjusted and restricted
Medical skill	.47	.81
Medical knowledge	.24	.57
Psychological knowledge	.74*	.74
Attitudes toward social problems	.41	.90

* No adjustment of ratings was possible because only two raters were in the group.

Table 24.12. Intra-rater correlation coefficients and median inter-rater reliability coefficients of adjusted and restricted staff ratings, 1955 I students ($N = 20$)

		1	2	3
Intra-rater correlations				
1	Medical skill			
2	Medical knowledge	.90		
3	Psychological knowledge	.83	.73	
4	Attitudes toward social problems	.72	.47	.79
Median inter-rater reliabilities				
	Medical skill		.59*	
	Medical knowledge		.79*	
	Psychological knowledge		.69*	
	Attitudes toward social problems		.83	

* No adjustment of ratings was possible because only two raters were in the group.

Table 24.13. Intra-rater correlation coefficients and median inter-rater reliability coefficients of adjusted and restricted staff ratings, 1956 I students ($N = 18$)

	1	2	3
Intra-rater correlations			
1 Medical skill			
2 Medical knowledge	.90		
3 Psychological knowledge	.48	.43	
4 Attitudes toward social problems	.33	.45	.28
Median inter-rater reliabilities			
Medical skill		.74	
Medical knowledge		.81	
Psychological knowledge		—*	
Attitudes toward social problems		.72	

* Only the psychiatrist rated all students. Each of four internists worked closely with one quarter of the student group and the psychiatrist. Each of the four internists rated the students he worked with.

terms of the several components of performance in the clinic, but in terms of each staff member's single-dimensioned, unique concept of good performance. That is, if a student was rated high on one component of his performance, he was rated high on all—knowledge, skill, and attitudes. From the standpoint of student evaluation, it is only a slight exaggeration to say that there were almost as many General Medical Clinics as there were staff members—and each one was different from all the others.

Several steps of a trial-and-error nature were taken in an effort to solve this problem. First, the rating procedures were changed and improved. This did not help. Second, statistical manipulation of the ratings made by the staff was undertaken so as to eliminate halo effects, or "rater-ratee" interaction. This step improved the amount of agree-

Table 24.14. Intra-rater correlation coefficients and median inter-rater reliability coefficients of adjusted and restricted staff ratings, 1956 II students ($N = 17$)

	1	2	3
Intra-rater correlations			
1 Medical skill			
2 Medical knowledge	.72		
3 Psychological knowledge	.57	.23	
4 Attitudes toward social problems	.37	.19	.37
Median inter-rater reliabilities			
Medical skill		.56	
Medical knowledge		.61	
Psychological knowledge		.20*	
Attitudes toward social problems		.79†	

* The psychiatrist rated all students. One internist was judged to have more knowledge of students' psychological knowledge than other staff members. The mean of the two ratings was the criterion score.

† No adjustment of ratings was possible because only two raters were in the group.

ment among raters, but separate components, corresponding to the objectives of the clinic, did not appear. These (relatively) separate components did appear, however, when the ratings made by a staff member on components outside his discipline were ignored.

The final establishment of measures for evaluating the performance of GMC students rested on the above steps. Although the final result was not altogether satisfactory, it provided a reasonably useful technique. Further refinements were precluded by the fact that the research project was scheduled to terminate with the study of the class of 1956.

RELATIONS BETWEEN INDIVIDUAL ATTRIBUTES AND STAFF RATINGS

The discussion of the relations between individual attributes and staff ratings is divided into two parts. The first reports a preliminary study concerning the first two GMC groups of students (1954 I and II). The second part reports the relations between individual attributes and staff ratings (as adjusted by the two procedures explained above) in the 1955 I, 1955 II, 1956 I, and 1956 II groups. Reliability data for the measures of individual attributes are presented in Chapter 15.

Preliminary Study Based on Original Staff Ratings

The studies of the 1954 I and II groups involved correlating all the 38 measures of individual attributes with all the components of performance rated by the staff (19 and 21, respectively). Then, because many (but not all) of the ratings were highly intercorrelated, two factor analyses of selected ratings and attributes were carried out, one on each set of data. These factor analyses made possible the definitions of independent (uncorrelated) components[5] in the ratings and the ascertainment of the degree of correlation between attribute measures and the rating components.[6] It is these correlations which will be presented in the report of the results of the preliminary study.

1954 I GROUP

Two components were found in the staff's ratings of the 1954 I group. These were medical skill and knowledge and interpersonal relations.

The medical skill and knowledge component was so named because

[5] Actually it would be more accurate to say *nearly uncorrelated*; the rotations of factors was oblique, not orthogonal, which led to small correlations between factors.

[6] The results of the preliminary study are reported in full in John R. Davis, "Predicting Students' Performance in a General Medical Clinic" (unpublished doctoral dissertation, University of Colorado, 1955). Only the data germane to our purpose are presented in this section.

Table 24.15. Correlation coefficients between individual attributes and the medical skill and knowledge component of staff ratings, 1954 I students ($N = 21$)

MCAT	
Verbal Ability	.06
Quantitative Ability	—.36
Knowledge of Premedical Sciences	.21
Premedical grade average	.51*
First-year grade average	.41*
Second-year grade average	.67*
Peer-judged competence as a physician	.50*
Peer-judged leadership	.63*
Peer-judged likeability	.09
F (Authoritarian) scale	—.45*
Liberal Attitude scale	.50*
Study of Values scale	
Theoretical	.11
Aesthetic	.21
Religious	—.45*

* $p < .05$.

four aspects of performance—ability to perform a physical examination, ability to present a case to the staff, judgment, and medical knowledge—were almost perfectly correlated with this component. Correlations between the individual attributes included in the factor analysis and this component are shown in Table 24.15.

Both staff and peer judgments of competence made before the students' senior year were related to the medical skill and knowledge component of performance in the GMC. All three grade averages were positively and highly correlated with this component, as were students' evaluations of one another's competence as a physician. Peer-judged leadership and liberal attitudes were positively correlated with this component; authoritarianism (as measured on the F scale) and religious values were negatively correlated with it to a statistically significant degree.

The second component in staff ratings of the 1954 I GMC group was termed interpersonal relations. Three aspects of performance—concern for patients as individuals, ability to develop good physician-patient relations, and grasp of the value of physician-patient relations—defined this second component. Table 24.16 shows that few individual attributes were significantly correlated with this component. Peer-judged competence as a physician, which had been positively correlated with the medical skill and knowledge component, was negatively correlated with interpersonal relations. Liberal attitudes and theoretical values (concern for the discovery of truth) were positively correlated with the interpersonal relations component. The measures of previous academic performance were negatively correlated with this component, though not to a very high degree.

Table 24.16. Correlation coefficients between individual attributes and the interpersonal relations component of staff ratings, 1954 I students ($N = 21$)

MCAT	
Verbal Ability	—.01
Quantitative Ability	—.11
Knowledge of Premedical Sciences	—.08
Premedical grade average	—.31
First-year grade average	—.19
Second-year grade average	—.21
Peer-judged competence as a physician	—.67*
Peer-judged leadership	—.34
Peer-judged likeability	—.11
F (Authoritarian) scale	—.06
Liberal Attitude scale	.52*
Study of Values scale	
Theoretical	.58*
Aesthetic	.00
Religious	—.19

* $p < .05$.

1954 II GROUP

The elements of the staff's evaluation of the 1954 II group's performance in the GMC were found to be very highly intercorrelated. That is, only one component could be defined by the several aspects of performance on which ratings were made. Few attributes were associated with this component to a significant degree (see Table 24.17). The only positive correlations of significant degree were between peer-judged leadership and staff ratings, and peer-judged likeability and staff ratings. Verbal ability was negatively correlated with high staff ratings among 1954 II students.

Table 24.17. Correlation coefficients between individual attributes and the single component of staff ratings, 1954 II ($N = 18$)

MCAT	
Verbal Ability	—.38*
Quantitative Ability	—.07
Knowledge of Premedical Sciences	—.19
Premedical grade average	—.20
First-year grade average	.13
Second-year grade average	.09
Peer-judged competence as a physician	—.15
Peer-judged leadership	.48*
Peer-judged likeability	.58*
F (Authoritarian) scale	.09
Liberal Attitude scale	—.07
Study of Values scale	
Theoretical	—.14
Aesthetic	—.22
Religious	.09

* $p < .05$.

In summary, two findings of importance had emerged thus far. First, only one individual attribute, peer-judged leadership, was positively correlated to a statistically significant degree with performance in *both* GMC groups of students. Second, although previous academic performance was positively and highly correlated with one component of performance in the 1954 I group, this correlation was considerably lower in the 1954 II group; in fact, it almost disappeared. A detailed investigation of this and similar phenomena is reported later.

Study Based on Adjusted Staff Ratings

Students who participated in the GMC during the 1954–55 and 1955–56 years were rated on approximately seventeen components of performance. The adjustments of these ratings, which were necessary in order to provide more reliable and less interrelated scores, have been described. An additional rating, general improvement, was obtained for the 1956 I and II groups. The ratings of the few staff members most familiar with each student's work were averaged to obtain ratings on this component. These ratings were not correlated to any appreciable degree (highest $r = -.23$) with ratings on other components in the 1956 I group. The same was true of the 1956 II group, except that the general improvement ratings were rather highly correlated with attitudes toward social problems ($r = .51$).

The following sections discuss correlations between the various measures of individual attributes and the five components of performance in the following order: correlations between individual attributes and medical knowledge (ratings by less experienced physicians); correlations between individual attributes and medical skill (ratings by more experienced physicians); correlations between individual attributes and psychological knowledge (ratings by psychiatrists); correlations between individual attributes and attitudes toward patients' social problems (ratings by members of the ancillary staff); and correlations between individual attributes and ratings of general improvement. Results for four student groups—1955 I, 1955 II, 1956 I, and 1956 II—are considered.

Medical knowledge

The medical knowledge component represented the mean of adjusted ratings made by the less experienced staff physicians. The relations between ratings on this component and the seven categories of individual attributes are discussed separately.

Correlations between aptitude for medical education and medical knowledge. The correlation coefficients between aptitude measures

Table 24.18. Correlation coefficients between scores on Medical College Admission subtests and adjusted staff ratings on medical knowledge (classes of 1955 and 1956)

	1955 I (N = 20)	1955 II (N = 17)	1956 I (N = 17)	1956 II (N = 15)
Verbal Ability	.42	—.13	.17	—.19
Quantitative Ability	.52*	.28	.39	—.03
Knowledge of Modern Society	.41	.05	.08	—.15
Knowledge of Premedical Sciences	.54*	.32	.24	—.30

* $p < .05$.

(the four subtests of the Medical College Admission Test) and ratings on medical knowledge for the four GMC groups are presented in Table 24.18.

Since Verbal Ability scores are likely to be highly associated with general intelligence, it was expected that students with more verbal ability would be rated more highly on medical knowledge than those with less of this ability. This expectation was borne out in the 1955 I group ($r = .42$) but not in any other group. Knowledge of premedical sciences was more consistently related positively to this component of performance than was any other aptitude measure (see Table 24.18). However, a correlation of —.30 was found in the last group studied—the 1956 II group.

In general, it would seem that the aptitude measures are of negligible value in identifying GMC students likely to be rated as possessing superior knowledge of medicine.

Correlations between previous academic performance and medical knowledge. Correlations between previous academic performance and the medical knowledge component of performance for the four GMC groups are presented in Table 24.19. It will be remembered that the indices of academic performance were more highly correlated with first-

Table 24.19. Correlation coefficients between previous academic performance indices and adjusted staff ratings on medical knowledge (classes of 1955 and 1956)

	1955 I (N = 20)	1955 II (N = 17)	1956 I (N = 17)	1956 II (N = 15)
Premedical grade average	.47*	—.04	—.03	—.53*
First-year grade average	.61†	.27	.13	.34
Second-year grade average	.76†	.37	.13	.34
Third-year grade average	.85†	.29	.56*	.21
Cumulative grade average	.82†	.38	.41	.35
Junior medical clerkship grade	.74†	.45	.52*	.09

* $p < .05$.
† $p < .01$.

half ratings than with second-half ratings in the class of 1954 (see Tables 24.15 and 24.17). This fluctuation appeared again in the data for the class of 1955, and to a lesser extent in those for the class of 1956.

The indices of academic performance most consistently related to ratings on medical knowledge were the cumulative grade average, the third-year grade average (an index of the student's performance immediately prior to the GMC), and the junior medical clerkship grade (an index of the student's performance in a clerkship which most nearly resembles the GMC). These correlations averaged approximately .50. First- and second-year grade averages also were consistently correlated in a positive direction with ratings, but the degree of relation was much lower than with the other three indices of previous academic performance. Thus, previous academic performance in medical school seemed to be a good predictor of students' performance in the GMC. This was especially true when the measures pertained to previous academic performance that was close in time to the GMC experience and when the measures reflected performance in a clerkship that closely resembled the GMC.

Correlations between peer-judged attributes and medical knowledge. The correlations between peer-judged attributes and medical knowledge ratings for the four GMC groups are shown in Table 24.20. The most notable finding here was that peer-judged competence as a physician was highly and consistently correlated in a positive direction with ratings on medical knowledge.

Perhaps somewhat less expected was the finding that the students'

Table 24.20. Correlation coefficients between peer-judged attributes and adjusted staff ratings on medical knowledge (classes of 1955 and 1956)

	1955 I ($N = 20$)	1955 II ($N = 17$)	1956 I ($N = 17$)	1956 II ($N = 15$)
Competence as a physician (nomination)	.38	.56*	.53*	.68†
Willingness and ability to work independently	.58†	.56*	.47	.09
Leadership				
ranking	.48*		.56*	.20
nomination		.35		
Likeability				
ranking	—.07		.27	—.04
nomination		.36		
Skill in developing good physician-patient relations	.20	.36	.65†	—.01
Sympathy to the concept of comprehensive care	.23	.42	.43	—.12

* $p < .05$.
† $p < .01$.

Table 24.21. Correlation coefficients between attitude measures and adjusted staff ratings on medical knowledge (classes of 1955 and 1956)

	1955 I ($N = 20$)	1955 II ($N = 17$)	1956 I ($N = 17$)	1956 II ($N = 15$)
F (Authoritarian) scale	—.01	.11	—.00	—.51*
General Anxiety scale	—.18	—.31	—.21	—.02
ACL Self-Acceptance scale	.14	—.12	.04	.11
ACL Self-Criticality scale	—.38	.08	.16	—.44

* $p < .05$.

estimations of their peers' willingness and ability to work independently was highly correlated with the medical knowledge rating in the first three of the four groups ($r = .58$, .56, and .47, respectively). However, this correlation fell off sharply in the fourth group ($r = .09$). Peer-judged leadership, the only individual attribute consistently related to performance ratings in the 1954 class, was also substantially correlated with the medical knowledge rating in the 1955 and 1956 classes. The pattern of correlation between likeability and medical knowledge in the two 1955 groups ($r = -.07$ and .36, respectively) resembled the pattern found in the previously reported data for the 1954 class ($r = .09$ and .58, respectively). However, in the 1956 class, the pattern was not quite the same. The "pattern" phenomenon will be taken up again later.

Peer-judged skill in developing physician-patient relations, and sympathy to the concept of comprehensive care, were positively correlated with medical knowledge in three of the four groups in 1955 and 1956.

Correlations between attitudes and medical knowledge. The correlations between medical knowledge ratings and the various attitude measures are shown in Table 24.21. (The four attitude measures used here were not all of the same order; that is, the F-scale involved the highly generalized attitude of authoritarianism, whereas the General Anxiety scale, and the Self-Acceptance and Self-Criticality scales involved attitudes toward oneself.)

In general, it can be stated that the attitudes measured were only occasionally correlated with medical knowledge ratings. The only consistent relation discovered involved general anxiety, which was negatively related to medical knowledge in all four groups. However, the degree of relation was too small to support an interpretation.

Correlations between values and medical knowledge. Correlations between values (as measured by the Study of Values scale) and medical knowledge ratings are shown in Table 24.22. In general, no consistent relations appeared between these individual values and medical knowledge. In the 1955 II group highly rated students tended to

Table 24.22. Correlation coefficients between scores on Study of Values scales and adjusted staff ratings on medical knowledge (classes of 1955 and 1956)

	1955 I (N =20)	1955 II (N = 17)	1956 I (N = 17)	1956 II (N = 15)
Theoretical value	—.28	—.47	.16	.15
Aesthetic value	.02	—.48*	.15	.06
Social value	.11	.20	—.39	—.36
Religious value	—.05	.18	—.03	—.45
Economic value	—.02	.22	—.07	.36
Political value	.29	.20	.05	.40

* $p < .05$.

have weaker theoretical and aesthetic values. And in the 1956 II group more highly rated students tended to have stronger politico-economic values and weaker socio-religious values. However, it would be unsafe to draw any conclusions from these data.

Correlations between CPI data and medical knowledge. Correlations between personality traits as measured by the California Psychological Inventory and medical knowledge ratings are shown in Table 24.23. These correlations appeared to be fairly high, but strikingly inconsistent from group to group. It would be more accurate, however, to say that they *alternate* in value from group to group. The fluctuations in the correlations involving the personality trait tolerance illustrate this alternating pattern. In the 1955 I group this correlation was .04, but in the 1955 II group it was .43; in the 1956 I group it was −.56, but in the 1956 II group it was .39. The other five personality traits show the same alternating pattern. Were these mere random fluctuations, totally unrelated to ratings of medical students? Or did these fluctuations represent a persistent phenomenon reflected in the interaction of student and staff? These questions were investigated and the results are presented later in this chapter. It is sufficient to point out here that, as in the case of the attitude and value measures used

Table 24.23. Correlation coefficients between scores on California Psychological Inventory scales and adjusted staff ratings on medical knowledge (classes of 1955 and 1956)

	1955 I (N = 20)	1955 II (N = 17)	1956 I (N = 17)	1956 II (N = 15)
Tolerance	.04	.43	—.56*	.39
Social Presence	—.04	.41	—.45	.57*
Flexibility	—.16	.40	—.17	—.22
Sociability	.18	.43	—.50*	.27
Dominance	.46*	.25	—.45	.31
Responsibility	.23	.42	—.35	.09

* $p < .05$.
Magnitude of correlations involving other CPI scales was not noteworthy.

in this study, personality traits were not consistently associated with ratings on medical knowledge.

Correlations between needs and medical knowledge. The correlations between the data produced by the Edwards Personal Preference Schedule and medical knowledge ratings are shown in Table 24.24. (The Edwards Schedule was administered only to the two 1956 groups.) It appeared that students' needs for achievement were positively correlated with medical knowledge in the 1956 II group, although needs for autonomy and change were negatively related to medical knowledge. These results suggest that the student whose medical knowledge was considered to be superior apparently was strongly concerned with doing his best, did not strongly feel the need to be independent of others, and was not continually seeking new activities and diversions.

To summarize, the principal finding was that the earlier evaluations made by the medical school faculty (previous academic performance) were the best predictors of the medical knowledge evaluations of the GMC students, made by the less experienced staff physicians. A related finding was that previous grades were better predictors when the previous course closely resembled the GMC and was close in time to the GMC experience. Evaluations made by fellow students were also fairly good predictors of ratings on medical knowledge, especially when the dimension which the peer judgment purported to measure was similar to the component of performance rated by the staff.

Measures of attitudes, values, and personality characteristics fluctuated widely in their relations to ratings on medical knowledge.

Finally, most of the foregoing summary statements must be qualified by the fact that the results varied widely from group to group.

Medical skill

Evaluation of students' performance in terms of medical skill was made by the more experienced staff members of the GMC. The correlations

Table 24.24. Correlation coefficients between scores on Edwards Personal Preference Schedule scales and adjusted staff ratings on medical knowledge (class of 1956)

	1956 I ($N = 17$)	1956 II ($N = 15$)
n Achievement	.08	.53*
n Autonomy	—.08	—.64†
n Change	—.07	—.62*
n Abasement	.31	.02
n Nurturance	—.31	—.18
n Exhibition	—.31	.08

* $p < .05$.
† $p < .01$.
Magnitude of correlations involving other EPPS scales was not noteworthy.

Table 24.25. Correlation coefficients between scores on Medical College Admission subtests and adjusted staff ratings on medical skill (classes of 1955 and 1956)

	1955 I ($N = 20$)	1955 II ($N = 17$)	1956 I ($N = 17$)	1956 II ($N = 15$)
Verbal Ability	.44*	.14	.26	—.07
Quantitative Ability	.38	.22	.18	—.36
Knowledge of Modern Society	.38	.20	.10	.20
Knowledge of Premedical Sciences	.43	.32	.16	—.42

* $p < .05$.

between individual attributes and medical skill ratings are discussed according to the seven categories of individual attributes.

Correlations between aptitude for medical education and medical skill. The correlations between aptitude for medical education (as revealed in the four subtests of the Medical College Admission Test) and the medical skill ratings are shown in Table 24.25. Except for the 1956 II group there was a generally positive relation between the subtest scores and ratings on medical skill in the GMC. As in the case of the ratings on medical knowledge, however, there was a general lessening of the relation from the 1955 I to the 1956 II group, at which time there was a definite tendency for the relations to be reversed. Correlations between Quantitative Ability scores and medical skill ratings, for example, occurred in the following order: .38, .22, .18, —.36. Correlations between scores on Knowledge of Premedical Sciences and medical skill ratings occurred in the following order: .43, .32, .16, —.42.

Correlations between previous academic performance and medical skill. The correlations between the various measures of previous academic performance and medical skill ratings are shown in Table 24.26. As with the medical knowledge ratings, grade averages were correlated highly with medical skill in the 1955 I, 1955 II, and 1956 I groups, but not in the 1956 II group. This pattern was especially characteristic of three indices: junior medical clerkship grade ($r = .68$, .60, .74, and

Table 24.26. Correlation coefficients between previous academic performance indices and adjusted staff ratings on medical skill (classes of 1955 and 1956)

	1955 I ($N = 20$)	1955 II ($N = 17$)	1956 I ($N = 17$)	1956 II ($N = 15$)
Premedical grade average	.27	—.12	.13	—.40
First-year grade average	.40	.05	.26	—.04
Second-year grade average	.57†	.38	.27	.16
Third-year grade average	.77†	.39	.76†	.10
Cumulative grade average	.64†	.30	.59*	.00
Junior medical clerkship grade	.68†	.60*	.74†	—.16

* $p < .05$.
† $p < .01$.

—.16, in order); third-year grade average ($r = .77$, .39, .76, and .10, in order); and cumulative grade average ($r = .64$, .30, .59, and .00, in order).

The correlations were especially high for the 1955 I group. It is important to note that two correlations—that between the third-year grade average and medical skill, and that between the junior medical clerkship grade and medical skill—were also very high in the 1956 I group ($r = .76$ and .74, respectively). Thus, the pattern of fluctuation in the value of the correlation coefficients mentioned above in connection with the medical knowledge ratings, made by the less experienced physicians, also appeared in the data involving the medical skill ratings, made by the more experienced physicians. That is, previous academic performance was more closely related to staff evaluations for students in the first-half groups than for students in the second-half groups. This result occurred with the two different groups of raters for two classes (1955 and 1956).

Correlations between peer-judged attributes and medical skill. The correlations between the various peer-judged attributes and the medical skill ratings are shown in Table 24.27. Peer-judged competence as a physician was the attribute most consistently (positively) correlated with medical skill, correlations for the two 1956 groups being particularly high. Again, the results obtained with the ratings by more experienced physicians paralleled the results obtained with the ratings by less experienced physicians. The correlations involving willingness to work independently and leadership exhibited the previously mentioned pattern, i.e., they were high in the first-half group and low

Table 24.27. Correlation coefficients between peer-judged attributes and adjusted staff ratings on medical skill (classes of 1955 and 1956)

	1955 I ($N = 20$)	1955 II ($N = 17$)	1956 I ($N = 17$)	1956 II ($N = 15$)
Competence as a physician (nomination)	.33	.30	.60*	.59*
Willingness and ability to work independently	.44*	.10	.42	.14
Leadership				
ranking	.46*		.47	.27
nomination		.08		
Likeability				
ranking	.11		.14	.14
nomination		.26		
Skill in developing good physician-patient relations	.34	.52*	.53*	.04
Sympathy to the concept of comprehensive care	.38	.48*	.47	—.02

* $p < .05$.

in the second-half group for each year. In general, the correlations between peer-judged attributes and medical skill ratings were not very different from correlations between peer-judged attributes and medical knowledge ratings.

Correlations between attitudes and medical skill. Correlations between the various measures of attitudes and the medical skill ratings are shown in Table 24.28. Although no attitude measure was highly correlated with this component, it is worth noting that both the F (Authoritarian) and General Anxiety scales were negatively related to this rating in every group studied; and the negative correlation between F-scale measures of authoritarianism and the medical skill ratings in the 1956 II group was rather high ($r = -.49$). The only other correlation that seems to merit attention here is that, in the 1956 II group particularly, self-acceptance tended to be *positively* correlated with ratings on medical skill, and self-criticality to be *negatively* correlated with it ($r =$ .37 and −.42, respectively).

Correlations between values and medical skill. Correlations between measures of values and the medical skill ratings are shown in Table 24.29. No systematic pattern of relations appeared here, nor were any correlations high enough to seem meaningful.

Correlations between CPI data and medical skill. Correlations between scores on the various California Psychological Inventory scales and the medical skill ratings are shown in Table 24.30. As with the medical knowledge ratings, made by the less experienced staff members, correlations between the CPI data and ratings on medical skill, made by the more experienced staff members, were found to alternate markedly from fairly high in the positive direction to fairly high in the negative direction.

Correlations between needs and medical skill. The correlations between needs (as revealed by the Edwards Personal Preference Schedule) and the medical skill ratings are shown in Table 24.31. Two needs, for change and for autonomy, were very highly correlated with medical skill in the 1956 II group ($r = -.83$ and −.80, respectively). Need for achievement was positively correlated with this rating to a near-significant degree ($r = .42$) in the 1956 II group. Thus, students with need structures like those of students rated high on medical knowledge were also rated high on medical skill in the 1956 II group (see Table 24.24).

To summarize, the kinds of personal attributes found to be related to evaluations of students' medical skill (ratings by more experienced faculty members) were almost identical with those found to be related to evaluations of medical knowledge (ratings made by less experienced

Table 24.28. Correlation coefficients between attitude measures and adjusted staff ratings on medical skill (classes of 1955 and 1956)

	1955 I ($N = 20$)	1955 II ($N = 17$)	1956 I ($N = 17$)	1956 II ($N = 15$)
F (Authoritarian) scale	—.24	—.21	—.09	—.49
General Anxiety scale	—.20	—.21	—.38	—.06
ACL Self-Acceptance scale	.18	—.08	—.03	.37
ACL Self-Criticality scale	—.36	.10	.17	—.42

Table 24.29. Correlation coefficients between scores on Study of Values scales and adjusted staff ratings on medical skill (classes of 1955 and 1956)

	1955 I ($N = 20$)	1955 II ($N = 17$)	1956 I ($N = 17$)	1956 II ($N = 15$)
Theoretical value	—.09	—.34	—.04	—.05
Aesthetic value	.05	—.33	.21	.00
Social value	.28	.32	—.32	—.30
Religious value	—.05	.29	.09	—.01
Economic value	—.17	—.02	—.23	.27
Political value	.11	.00	.04	.09

Table 24.30. Correlation coefficients between scores on California Psychological Inventory scales and adjusted staff ratings on medical skill (classes of 1955 and 1956)

	1955 I ($N = 20$)	1955 II ($N = 17$)	1956 I ($N = 17$)	1956 II ($N = 15$)
Tolerance	.12	.35	—.25	.50
Intellectual Efficiency	.28	.34	—.11	.43
Social Presence	.04	.35	—.30	.47
Flexibility	.01	.48*	—.23	—.19
Capacity for Status	.42	.32	—.32	.21
Sociability	.22	.22	—.42	.42
Dominance	.48*	.18	—.42	.47

* $p < .05$.
Magnitude of correlations involving other CPI scales was not noteworthy.

Table 24.31. Correlation coefficients between scores on Edwards Personal Preference Schedule scales and adjusted staff ratings on medical skill (class of 1956)

	1956 I ($N = 17$)	1956 II ($N = 15$)
n Change	—.07	—.83*
n Autonomy	.14	—.80*
n Dominance	—.23	.46
n Achievement	.19	.42

* $p < .01$.
Magnitude of correlations involving other EPPS scales was not noteworthy.

faculty members). Because of the rather high correlation between the ratings of the more experienced and less experienced members of the faculty, this result was to be expected. Previous academic performance as seen by faculty and present competence as seen by student peers were the attributes most highly related to staff ratings on medical skill. Measures of attitudes, values, and personality characteristics varied widely in their relations to ratings on medical skill, a finding which also parallels the finding in the case of ratings on medical knowledge.

Psychological knowledge

The relations between individual attributes and the psychological knowledge ratings made by the psychiatrically oriented staff members of the GMC are discussed below.

Correlations between aptitude for medical education and psychological knowledge. Correlations between the measures of aptitude for medical education and the psychological knowledge ratings are shown in Table 24.32. Apparently the conventional measures of aptitude for medical education do not predict students' performance with respect to learning about the psychological aspects of patient care, for the aptitude measures were not positively correlated with the psychological knowledge ratings to any appreciable degree. Indeed, Knowledge of Premedical Sciences was correlated —.45 with this rating in the 1956 I group.

Correlations between previous academic performance and psychological knowledge. Correlations between measures of previous academic performance and the psychological knowledge ratings are shown in Table 24.33. Except for significant positive correlations between both second- and third-year grade averages and this rating in the 1955 I group ($r = .44$ and .59, respectively), grade averages were not highly related to ratings on psychological knowledge. Grades in two single courses (psychopathology and psychosomatics) were positively correlated with psychological knowledge, but the strength of these relations varied considerably.

Table 24.32. Correlation coefficients between scores on Medical College Admission subtests and staff ratings on psychological knowledge (classes of 1955 and 1956)

	1955 I ($N = 20$)	1955 II ($N = 17$)	1956 I ($N = 17$)	1956 II ($N = 15$)
Verbal Ability	.06	—.33	.14	—.14
Quantitative Ability	.07	—.04	—.30	—.35
Knowledge of Modern Society	.08	—.05	—.14	.18
Knowledge of Premedical Sciences	.07	.17	—.45	—.26

Table 24.33. Correlation coefficients between previous academic performance indices and staff ratings on psychological knowledge (classes of 1955 and 1956)

	1955 I ($N = 20$)	1955 II ($N = 17$)	1956 I ($N = 17$)	1956 II ($N = 15$)
Premedical grade average	.14	—.18	—.37	.09
First-year grade average	.18	—.14	—.12	—.19
Second-year grade average	.44*	—.06	—.15	.13
Third-year grade average	.59†	—.18	.13	.31
Cumulative grade average	.41	—.12	.02	.00
Psychopathology course grade	.35	.22	.12	.43
Psychosomatics course grade	.45*	.21	—	—
Junior medical clerkship grade	.53*	.42	.29	.04

* $p < .05$.
† $p < .01$.
— Grades not available for these students.

The junior medical clerkship grade was also positively related to this rating ($r = .53$, .42, .29, and .04, respectively). It will be noted, however, that the strength of these relations was less than the strength of the relations between this grade and the medical knowledge and medical skill ratings.

Correlations between peer-judged attributes and psychological knowledge. Correlations between peer-judged attributes and the psychological knowledge ratings are shown in Table 24.34. The most interesting feature here is the positive direction of all of the correlations. No one measure was more consistently related to the rating than any other measure. In other words, general acceptability to peers seems to be correlated positively, though not to a high degree, with high ratings on psychological knowledge.

Table 24.34. Correlation coefficients between peer-judged attributes and staff ratings on psychological knowledge (classes of 1955 and 1956)

	1955 I ($N = 20$)	1955 II ($N = 17$)	1956 I ($N = 17$)	1956 II ($N = 15$)
Competence as a physician (nomination)	.15	.05	.30	.38
Willingness and ability to work independently	.33	.16	.19	.34
Leadership				
ranking	.48*		.37	.34
nomination		.19		
Likeability				
ranking	.27		.20	.31
nomination		.25		
Skill in developing good physician-patient relations	.38	.20	.28	.29
Sympathy to the concept of comprehensive care	.37	.23	.29	.35

* $p < .05$.

Table 24.35. Correlation coefficients between attitude measures and staff ratings on psychological knowledge (classes of 1955 and 1956)

	1955 I ($N = 20$)	1955 II ($N = 17$)	1956 I ($N = 17$)	1956 II ($N = 15$)
F (Authoritarian) scale	—.38	—.20	—.16	—.58*
General Anxiety scale	—.13	—.14	—.18	—.29
Liberal Attitude scale	.32	—.01	.40	—.11
ACL Self-Acceptance scale	.32	—.16	.15	.56*
ACL Self-Criticality scale	—.34	.08	—.04	—.52*

* $p < .05$.

Correlations between attitudes and psychological knowledge. Correlations between the various attitude measures and the psychological knowledge ratings appear in Table 24.35. Authoritarian attitudes (which would result in a tendency to perceive emotionally ill patients as "weak") were, as expected, negatively correlated with the psychological knowledge ratings ($r = -.38$, $-.20$, $-.16$, and $-.58$, respectively).

Scores on the General Anxiety scale were also negatively correlated with these ratings in every group. But the correlation values were lower than those obtained for the F scale ($r = -.13$, $-.14$, $-.18$, and $-.29$, respectively).

In the 1956 II group self-acceptance was positively correlated with psychological knowledge to a significant degree ($r = .56$), and self-criticality was negatively correlated to a significant degree ($r = -.52$).

The above findings support rather well the general notion that students who are relatively permissive, accepting of themselves and others, and less anxious than most, are more likely to develop good relations with patients.

Correlations between values and psychological knowledge. Correlations between scores on the Study of Values scale and the psychological knowledge ratings are shown in Table 24.36. No important correla-

Table 24.36. Correlation coefficients between scores on Study of Values scales and staff ratings on psychological knowledge (classes of 1955 and 1956)

	1955 I ($N = 20$)	1955 II ($N = 17$)	1956 I ($N = 17$)	1956 II ($N = 15$)
Theoretical value	—.13	—.14	.01	—.16
Aesthetic value	—.11	—.32	.27	.20
Social value	.33	.26	.12	.02
Religious value	—.29	.22	—.17	.17
Economic value	.11	.00	—.21	—.24
Political value	.18	—.05	—.13	—.06

Table 24.37. Correlation coefficients between scores on California Psychological Inventory scales and staff ratings on psychological knowledge (classes of 1955 and 1956)

	1955 I ($N = 20$)	1955 II ($N = 17$)	1956 I ($N = 17$)	1956 II ($N = 15$)
Tolerance	.32	.49*	—.20	.50
Intellectual Efficiency	.14	.22	—.17	.51*
Psychological-Mindedness	.15	.06	—.40	.40
Achievement via Independence	.48*	.14	—.04	.35
Dominance	.34	.37	.05	.40
Achievement via Conformance	.47*	.28	—.21	.70†
Responsibility	.40	.61†	—.34	.29
Good Impression	.48*	.50*	—.13	.46
Sense of Well-Being	—.04	.37	—.28	.43
Self-Control	.41	.25	—.27	.31
Socialization	.04	—.30	—.44	.49

* $p < .05$.
† $p < .01$.
Magnitude of correlations involving other CPI scales was not noteworthy.

tions were found between the Study of Values scores and psychological knowledge.

Correlations between CPI data and psychological knowledge. Correlations between the California Psychological Inventory scales and the psychological knowledge ratings are shown in Table 24.37. As with ratings on medical knowledge and medical skill, correlations between these personality traits and the ratings on psychological knowledge fluctuated considerably. More important is the fact that the fluctuations followed a pattern of alternations identical to that found between these personality traits and ratings on medical knowledge and medical skill.

It should be noted here that the direction of the correlations in three of four groups was such that it provides empirical support (as do the correlations between attitudes and psychological knowledge) for the hypothesis that the student with more desirable personality characteristics is likely to be more effective in the area of interpersonal relations.

Correlations between needs and psychological knowledge. Correlations between needs (as indicated by the Edwards Personal Preference Schedule) and the psychological knowledge ratings are shown in Table 24.38. In the two 1956 groups the more highly rated students seemed to have stronger needs for exhibition and weaker needs for aggression and autonomy than lower rated students. Two other needs—for change and for heterosexuality—were related to this rating rather strongly, but not in the same direction in both groups.

Table 24.38. Correlation coefficients between scores on Edwards Personal Preference Schedule scales and staff ratings on psychological knowledge (class of 1956)

	1956 I ($N = 17$)	1956 II ($N = 15$)
n Exhibition	.50*	.32
n Aggression	—.42	—.39
n Autonomy	—.31	—.42
n Change	—.03	—.49
n Heterosexuality	.40	—.39

* $p < .05$.
Magnitude of correlations involving other EPPS scales was not noteworthy.

It will be recalled that the two performance ratings previously discussed, medical knowledge and medical skill, tended to be highly and fairly consistently associated in a positive direction with previous grades in medical school. This was not true of the psychological knowledge ratings, which included proficiency in the areas of psychiatry, psychosomatic medicine, doctor-patient relations, etc. Psychological knowledge tended instead to be associated with attitudes and personality characteristics—attributes which had not been correlated with ratings on medical knowledge and medical skill.

Medical College Admission Test scores were not correlated with psychological knowledge. This was not surprising, since there is no MCAT subtest concerned with psychological knowledge.

Peer-judged attributes were generally related to this rating in a positive direction, although not strongly so; they were definitely less strongly related to psychological knowledge than they were to medical knowledge and to medical skill.

Attitudes and personality characteristics, however, were definitely associated with ratings on psychological knowledge. The nature of the relation supports the hypothesis that the student most likely to be highly evaluated by the psychiatrically oriented members of the staff was the nonauthoritarian, permissive, well-adjusted, responsible, tolerant student, who was also interested in achievement. It must be emphasized, however, that a definite exception to this hypothesis was found: in the 1956 I group exactly the reverse was true. This exception is in accord with the alternation in results which was also found for the medical knowledge and medical skill ratings.

Attitudes toward patients' social problems

The mean of the adjusted ratings on attitudes toward patients' social problems, made by the social workers and public health nurse, was the fourth component of performance used in the study of GMC students. These ratings were correlated with eight categories of individual at-

Table 24.39. Correlation coefficients between scores on Medical College Admission subtests and adjusted staff ratings on attitudes toward patients' social problems (classes of 1955 and 1956)

	1955 I ($N = 20$)	1955 II ($N = 17$)	1956 I ($N = 17$)	1956 II ($N = 15$)
Verbal Ability	.10	.10	—.10	.08
Quantitative Ability	—.06	.19	.04	—.59*
Knowledge of Modern Society	.06	.28	—.23	.58*
Knowledge of Premedical Sciences	—.10	.55*	—.24	—.44

* $p < .05$.

tributes, the seven used in the preceding sections plus a group of self-ratings.

Correlations between aptitude for medical education and attitudes toward patients' social problems. Correlations between the four measures of aptitude for medical education and attitudes toward patients' social problems are shown in Table 24.39. Although, as can be seen from the table, some fairly high correlations appeared in individual groups, no correlations appeared with any appreciable degree of consistency among the various groups. For example, knowledge of premedical sciences was highly correlated with this rating in the 1955 II group ($r = .55$), but this relation was sharply reversed in the 1956 II group ($r = -.44$). In the 1956 II group quantitative ability was negatively correlated with this rating to a high degree ($r = -.59$) and knowledge of modern society was positively correlated with this rating to a similarly high degree ($r = .58$). Since these relations do not appear for any of the other groups, these data are highly inconsistent.

Correlations between previous academic performance and attitudes toward patients' social problems. Correlations between this rating and previous academic performance are shown in Table 24.40. These correlations were similar to those discussed in the preceding para-

Table 24.40. Correlation coefficients between previous academic performance indices and adjusted staff ratings on attitudes toward patients' social problems (classes of 1955 and 1956)

	1955 I ($N = 20$)	1955 II ($N = 17$)	1956 I ($N = 17$)	1956 II ($N = 15$)
Premedical grade average	—.08	—.36	.25	.16
First-year grade average	—.08	—.12	—.19	.03
Second-year grade average	.26	.23	—.34	—.02
Third-year grade average	.50*	—.12	.04	—.01
Cumulative grade average	.20	—.03	—.18	—.04
Public health course grade	.14	.02	.15	—.15
Junior medical clerkship grade	.44*	.12	.21	—.33

* $p < .05$.

graph. That is, no consistent relations appeared, although there were some rather high correlations in individual groups, for example, those between the rating and both third-year grade average and junior medical clerkship grade for the 1955 I group ($r = .50$ and .44, respectively). It is interesting to note that the grade received in the public health course was unrelated to attitudes toward social problems.

Correlations between peer-judged attributes and attitudes toward patients' social problems. Correlations between peer-judged attributes and this rating appear in Table 24.41. Although only four strong relations were found (all in the 1955 I group), these results are interesting because most correlations were positive. This finding parallels the finding with respect to psychological knowledge ratings. However, a more striking feature of these data is the appearance of a pattern similar to the one noted in the correlations between previous academic performance and ratings on both medical knowledge and medical skill. That is, for all peer judgments except competence and willingness to work independently and competence as a physician, correlations with attitudes toward social problems in the first-half group of each class were higher than correlations in the second-half group. Thus, it appears that physicians differentiated students in the first-half groups in both classes on components of performance correlated with previous academic performance, and the ancillary service staff differentiated the same students on components highly correlated with peer-judged skill in developing physician-patient relations, peer-judged sympathy to the comprehensive care concept, peer-judged likeability, and peer-judged leadership. However, these relations were weaker in the second-half groups.

Correlations between self-ratings and attitudes toward patients' social problems. Correlations between four self-ratings and ratings on attitudes toward social problems for three groups are shown in Table 24.42.[7] There is some indication that those students who reported they had been rewarded for good interpersonal relations as adolescents, that they had become confident with respect to interpersonal relations early in life, and that they were interested in the welfare of patients' families were likely to be rated high on attitudes toward patients' social problems.

Correlations between objective measures of attitudes and ratings on attitudes toward patients' social problems. Correlations between students' attitudes (as measured by the F-scale and the General Anxiety scale) and students' attitudes toward patients' social problems (as rated by the ancillary staff) are shown in Table 24.43. These relations were

[7] The self-ratings in Table 24.42 were not obtained from the 1955 I group.

Table 24.41. Correlation coefficients between peer-judged attributes and adjusted staff ratings on attitudes toward patients' social problems (classes of 1955 and 1956)

	1955 I ($N = 20$)	1955 II ($N = 17$)	1956 I ($N = 17$)	1956 II ($N = 15$)
Competence as a physician (nomination)	.34	.26	.21	.48
Willingness and ability to work independently	.42	.21	—.07	.13
Leadership				
ranking	.55*		.40	.09
nomination		.08		
Likeability				
ranking	.46*		.40	.21
nomination		—.03		
Skill in developing good physician-patient relations	.59†	.20	.42	.06
Sympathy to the concept of comprehensive care	.57†	.10	.31	—.07

* $p < .05$.
† $p < .01$.

Table 24.42. Correlation coefficients between self-ratings and adjusted staff ratings on attitudes toward patients' social problems (1955 II, 1956 I and II)

	1955 II ($N = 17$)	1956 I ($N = 17$)	1956 II ($N = 15$)
Amount of reward for ability to get along with others as an adolescent	.41	.23	.34
Age at which confident in ability to develop satisfying interpersonal relations (high score = early age)	—.32	.71†	.52*
Interest in welfare of patient's family	.04	.21	.43
Anxiety concerning ambiguous diagnostic problems	—	.09	.74†

* $p < .05$.
† $p < .01$.
– Test not administered to 1955 class.
Magnitude of correlations involving other self-ratings was not noteworthy.

Table 24.43. Correlation coefficients between attitude measures and adjusted staff ratings on attitudes toward patients' social problems (classes of 1955 and 1956)

	1955 I ($N = 20$)	1955 II ($N = 17$)	1956 I ($N = 17$)	1956 II ($N = 15$)
F (Authoritarian) scale	—.37	.06	—.21	—.09
General Anxiety scale	—.24	—.12	—.02	—.04

Table 24.44. Correlation coefficients between scores on Study of Values scales and adjusted staff ratings on attitudes toward patients' social problems (classes of 1955 and 1956)

	1955 I ($N = 20$)	1955 II ($N = 17$)	1956 I ($N = 17$)	1956 II ($N = 15$)
Theoretical value	.17	—.18	—.01	.02
Aesthetic value	.06	—.30	—.29	—.32
Social value	.31	.03	.30	.24
Religious value	—.17	.31	.33	.36
Economic value	—.16	.11	—.11	.05
Political value	—.11	—.14	—.11	—.53*

* $p < .05$.

all very weak. There was evidently a tendency for authoritarianism and anxiety to be negatively correlated with high staff ratings (a tendency consistent with the same findings in connection with psychological knowledge ratings); but this tendency was not strong enough to warrant any definite inferences.

Correlations between values and attitudes toward patients' social problems. Correlations between values (as revealed by the Study of Values scale) and the adjusted ratings of attitudes toward patients' social problems are shown in Table 24.44. The most noteworthy characteristic of these data was the generally positive direction of correlations between social values and staff ratings on attitudes toward social problems ($r = .31$, .03, .30, and .24, respectively). Except for the 1955 I group, the same can be said for religious values ($r = -.17$, .31, .33, and .36, respectively). The finding with respect to social values was not surprising, since a value for helping others might be presumed to make a person more sensitive to and considerate of the problems of others.

Correlations between CPI data and attitudes toward patients' social problems. The correlations between individual attributes (as measured by the CPI) and the ratings on attitudes toward social problems are shown in Table 24.45. These relations were similar to those obtained in connection with psychological knowledge (see Table 24.37). That is, the correlations were generally (in three of four groups) positive, a finding which suggests that those persons who possess personality characteristics ordinarily meeting with approval (tolerance, responsibility, interest in achievement) were likely to be rated high by the ancillary staff on attitudes toward social problems.

The correlations between personality characteristics and attitudes toward patients' social problems showed fluctuations similar to those noted in Tables 24.23, 24.30, and 24.37.

Correlations between needs and attitudes toward patients' social problems. Correlations between needs (as revealed by the Edwards

Table 24.45. Correlation coefficients between scores on California Psychological Inventory scales and adjusted staff ratings on attitudes toward patients' social problems (classes of 1955 and 1956)

	1955 I ($N = 20$)	1955 II ($N = 17$)	1956 I ($N = 17$)	1956 II ($N = 15$)
Tolerance	.43	.35	—.31	.46
Good Impression	.48*	.11	—.20	.45
Achievement via Conformance	.46*	.18	—.18	.34
Dominance	.41	—.30	—.14	.19
Psychological-Mindedness	.46*	.09	—.39	—.11
Intellectual Efficiency	.14	.41	—.54*	.47
Social Presence	.37	—.00	—.48*	—.10
Socialization	—.26	—.06	—.25	.52*

* $p < .05$.
Magnitude of correlations involving other CPI scales was not noteworthy.

Personal Preference Schedule) and this rating for the two 1956 groups are shown in Table 24.46. (The Edwards Schedule was not administered to the class of 1955.) Only two of these correlations require comment here. Need for affiliation (for companionship with and acceptance by others) was fairly highly related to attitudes toward social problems in both 1956 groups ($r = .36$ and .31). Need for affiliation is the motivational aspect of the interpersonal relations component of personality. Skill in developing physician-patient relations (one of the components of performance in the GMC) represents the ability aspect of the same personality component. Thus, more evidence is adduced for the influence of the students' facility in interpersonal relations on the ratings made by ancillary service staff. The high negative correlation between need for heterosexuality and this rating for the 1956 II group ($r = -.62$) is a curious finding for which no explanation is offered.

To summarize, Medical College Admission Test scores and previous academic performance were found to be essentially unrelated to ratings by the ancillary staff on attitudes toward social problems. Both these findings paralleled those regarding psychological knowledge. In

Table 24.46. Correlation coefficients between scores on Edwards Personal Preference Schedule scales and adjusted staff ratings on attitudes toward patients' social problems (class of 1956)

	1956 I ($N = 17$)	1956 II ($N = 15$)
n Affiliation	.36	.31
n Heterosexuality	.23	—.62*

* $p < .05$.
Magnitude of correlations involving other EPPS scales was not noteworthy.

Table 24.47. Correlation coefficients between scores on Medical College Admission subtests and staff ratings on general improvement (class of 1956)

	1956 I ($N = 17$)	1956 II ($N = 15$)
Verbal Ability	—.09	—.05
Quantitative Ability	.41	—.51*
Knowledge of Modern Society	—.19	.31
Knowledge of Premedical Sciences	—.19	—.38

* $p < .05$.

contrast, however, to the psychological knowledge results, is the fact that the ratings made by the ancillary staff on attitudes toward patients' social problems were in the main unrelated to attitude and value measures.

Those correlations which consistently appeared between this rating and such indications of personality as certain peer-judged attributes, self-ratings, and personality measures obtained with the CPI, indicated that facility in interpersonal relations characterized students with high ratings on attitudes toward social problems.

General improvement

The two GMC groups of the 1956 class were rated by all staff members on amount of change toward the ideal GMC student. The mean of the ratings made by those staff members who had most often checked a student in the clinic constituted a student's general improvement rating. Correlations between this rating and the various measures of individual attributes are reported below.

Correlations between aptitude for medical education and general improvement. Correlations between the four measures of aptitude for medical education and the general improvement ratings are shown in Table 24.47. No correlations appearing here were both statistically significant and consistent. Quantitative ability was negatively correlated with general improvement to a significant degree in the 1956 II group, but positively correlated to a near-significant degree in the 1956 I group ($r = -.51$ and $.41$, respectively). Knowledge of premedical sciences was negatively correlated with the ratings in both groups ($r = -.19$ and $-.38$, respectively), but the degree of correlation was too low to warrant any definite inference.

Correlations between previous academic performance and general improvement. Correlations between measures of previous academic performance and the general improvement ratings are shown in Table 24.48. Those indices which were positively correlated to a high degree with the medical knowledge and medical skill ratings (junior medical

Table 24.48. Correlation coefficients between previous academic performance indices and staff ratings on general improvement (class of 1956)

	1956 I ($N = 17$)	1956 II ($N = 15$)
Premedical grade average	.21	.37
First-year grade average	.04	—.08
Second-year grade average	—.10	.20
Third-year grade average	—.48*	—.32
Cumulative grade average	—.12	—.16
Junior medical clerkship grade	—.50*	—.37

* $p < .05$.

clerkship grade, cumulative grade average, and third-year grade average) were negatively correlated with the general improvement ratings. Such a reversal of direction in relations is usual when measures of *improvement* in qualities are compared with measures of qualities themselves. The students with the most opportunity for improvement are those nearer the bottom than the top of the scale. Nevertheless, one of the grade averages, the premedical grade average, was positively related to the improvement rating in both student groups.

Correlations between peer-judged attributes and general improvement. Correlations between peer-judged attributes and the general improvement ratings appear in Table 24.49. None of these correlations was high enough to attain significance; moreover, only one was consistent in direction for both groups. All but likeability were negative in the 1956 I group and positive in the 1956 II group. Likeability was positively correlated with this rating in both groups, but the correlation values were too small to be noteworthy.

Correlations between self-ratings and general improvement. Correlations between self-ratings of several kinds and ratings on general im-

Table 24.49. Correlation coefficients between peer-judged attributes and staff ratings on general improvement (class of 1956)

	1956 I ($N = 17$)	1956 II ($N = 15$)
Competence as a physician (nomination)	—.38	.24
Willingness and ability to work independently	—.10	.17
Leadership (ranking)	—.08	.06
Likeability (ranking)	.26	.19
Skill in developing good physician-patient relations	—.08	.20
Sympathy to the concept of comprehensive care	—.23	.20

provement for the 1956 groups appear in Table 24.50. Worry about adequacy of knowledge of differential diagnosis was rather highly correlated with general improvement ($r = .52$).

Correlations between attitudes and general improvement. Correlations between a number of attitude measures and the general improvement ratings are shown in Table 24.51. The one correlation of apparent significance here was that between the Self-Acceptance scale (adjective check-list) and the general improvement rating in the 1956 II group ($r = .58$). However, this correlation was not consistent; it was negative in the 1956 I group ($r = -.35$). The relations between other attitude measures and ratings on general improvement were both weak and inconsistent.

Correlations between values and general improvement. Correlations between scores on the Study of Values scale and the general improvement ratings are shown in Table 24.52. No strong relations appeared.

Correlations between CPI data and general improvement. Correlations between scores on the CPI scales and the general improvement ratings are shown in Table 24.53. It is interesting to note the nature of five personality measures which were positively correlated to a high degree with this rating in the 1956 II group. These five personality characteristics (ability to create a good impression, responsibility, self-control, sense of well-being, and socialization) all represent various components of the tendency to present oneself in a favorable light.

Correlations between needs and general improvement. Correlations between needs (as revealed in the Edwards Personal Preference Schedule) and the general improvement ratings are shown in Table 24.54. In both groups needs for intraception were fairly highly correlated with

Table 24.50. Correlation coefficients between self-ratings and staff ratings on general improvement (class of 1956)

	1956 I ($N = 17$)	1956 II ($N = 15$)
Amount of reward for ability to get along with others as an adolescent	.04	.46
Age at which confident in ability to develop satisfying interpersonal relations (high score = early age)	—.33	.49
Worry about adequacy of knowledge of differential diagnosis	—.06	.52*

* $p < .05$.
Magnitude of correlations involving other self-ratings was not noteworthy.

Table 24.51. Correlation coefficients between attitude measures and staff ratings on general improvement (class of 1956)

	1956 I ($N = 17$)	1956 II ($N = 15$)
F (Authoritarian) scale	.24	—.30
General Anxiety scale	.17	—.20
Liberal Attitude scale	—.35	.16
ACL Self-Acceptance scale	—.35	.58*
ACL Self-Criticality scale	.12	—.33

* $p < .05$.

Table 24.52. Correlation coefficients between scores on Study of Values scales and staff ratings on general improvement (class of 1956)

	1956 I ($N = 17$)	1956 II ($N = 15$)
Theoretical value	—.24	—.07
Aesthetic value	—.08	.13
Social value	.07	—.03
Religious value	.19	.04
Economic value	.25	.08
Political value	—.20	—.22

Table 24.53. Correlation coefficients between scores on California Psychological Inventory scales and staff ratings on general improvement (class of 1956)

	1956 I ($N = 17$)	1956 II ($N = 15$)
Self-Acceptance	—.47	—.34
Good Impression	—.28	.77†
Responsibility	.04	.70†
Self-Control	—.01	.70†
Sense of Well-Being	.09	.65†
Socialization	.10	.61*
Achievement via Conformance	—.26	.47
Tolerance	.00	.40

* $p < .05$.
† $p < .01$.
Magnitude of correlations involving other CPI scales was not noteworthy.

Table 24.54. Correlation coefficients between scores on Edwards Personal Preference Schedule scales and staff ratings on general improvement (class of 1956)

	1956 I ($N = 17$)	1956 II ($N = 15$)
n Exhibition	—.45	—.50
n Heterosexuality	—.29	—.42
n Intraception	.31	.43
n Aggression	.20	—.64*
n Endurance	—.08	.42

* $p < .01$.
Magnitude of correlations involving other EPPS scales was not noteworthy.

general improvement ratings ($r = .31$ and .43, respectively); that is, the students who improved more felt a need to examine and understand themselves. These findings were not surprising, for a student who reviews his own performance is likely to change, and hence improve.

These results, moreover, were quite consistent with the findings for the CPI Self-Acceptance scale. Students who did not accept their shortcomings were perceived as having improved more during their GMC clerkship than did other students. Thus, a willingness to find but not condone faults in oneself can be expected to be related to improvement in performance. A result similar to this was found in the study of change in students' medical knowledge. Students who were relatively anxious about the inadequacy of their knowledge of differential diagnosis gained relatively more medical knowledge from Pretest to Posttest I and from Posttest I to Posttest II. All these findings could mean that concern about a recognized shortcoming motivated these students to improve themselves to a greater extent than students not so motivated.

Two needs were negatively correlated with general improvement in both groups: need for exhibition and need for heterosexuality ($r =$ −.45 and −.50; −.29 and −.42, respectively). Finally, need for aggression was strongly correlated in a negative direction with general improvement for the 1956 II group ($r = -.64$).

To summarize, indices of previous performance, which were positively related to ratings on medical knowledge and skill, were negatively related to ratings on general improvement in the GMC. This finding was to be expected, for it indicates that those students with the most apparent room for improvement were the ones who were perceived as having improved most. It must be pointed out, however, that although the poorer students improved the most, still the better students received the highest absolute ratings by the GMC staff.

Ratings on improvement were correlated with several scales of the California Psychological Inventory. These correlations suggest that the students who improved could be described as methodical, given to self-criticism, cooperative, warm, calm, patient, persistent, conscientious, and valuing work and effort for its own sake. An independent confirmation of these findings is the fact that students indicating high needs for aggression were rated low on general improvement by the GMC staff.

Summary

The broad finding of this study of students' performance in the GMC was that the traditional medical components of performance (medical knowledge and medical skill) tended to be correlated with previous grades in medical school and similar measures, but to be unrelated to other individual attributes; whereas the psychological and sociological components of performance tended to be correlated with attitudes and personality characteristics rather than with measures of previous academic performance. In general, students whose previous academic performance was relatively low were seen as having improved the most.

The study of the first two groups that participated in the GMC (the 1954 I and II students) led to three important findings: only one or two components appeared in the staff's ratings of the students' performance; the direction of most of the relations between individual attributes and ratings reversed from the first-half to the second-half groups; and only one individual attribute (peer-judged leadership) was consistently related to ratings.

As a result of these findings, questions were raised about the adequacy of the GMC staff ratings, and steps were taken to remove certain inadequacies. Four components of performance were isolated from the staff ratings of the classes of 1955 and 1956: medical knowledge, medical skill, psychological knowledge, and attitudes toward patients' social problems. For two student groups a fifth component was available: general improvement.

The medical knowledge ratings, which were made by the less experienced staff members, were definitely related to previous academic performance in medical school. The students with good grades in previous clinics and courses were rated high on medical knowledge in the GMC. Also those students who were judged by their peers as competent physicians, capable of independent work, leaders, skillful in doctor-patient relations, and sympathetic to the concept of comprehensive care, were rated high on medical knowledge. Almost exactly the same correlations were found between individual attributes and the medical skill ratings made by the more experienced members of the GMC staff as were found between individual attributes and the medical knowledge ratings.

Somewhat different results were obtained in connection with ratings of students in the area of psychiatry, psychosomatic medicine, doctor-patient relations, etc. Previous grade averages were not closely associated with ratings on psychological knowledge, and peer ratings were noticeably less highly correlated with psychological knowledge than with the ratings on medical knowledge and skill. On the other hand, although there were exceptions, students' attitudes and personality characteristics were associated with ratings on psychological knowledge. The students who received high ratings could be characterized as less authoritarian (permissive in their relations with others) and less anxious than those who received low ratings. Moreover, highly rated students were likely to appear as informal, having poise and self-assurance, being mature and responsible, having a certain amount of achievement drive and intellectual efficiency, as well as being interested in and responsive to the inner needs and experiences of others. The highly rated students did not have strong needs for aggression, for autonomy, or for change. All the evidence from measures of personality (and to a certain extent from the judgments of students by their peers) indicated that persons rated high on psychological knowledge exhibited many more desirable personality characteristics—from the current viewpoint of mental hygiene—than did those rated low. The relations between individual attributes and ratings made by the ancillary staff on attitudes toward social problems were very much like the relations between individual attributes and ratings on psychological knowledge. Facility in interpersonal relations was a characteristic of students rated high, although students' attitudes and values were essentially unrelated to this rating.

Although it was the better students (as judged by prior performance) who received high ratings in the GMC, it was the poorer students who were rated as having improved the most. Ratings on improvement were correlated with several scales of the CPI.

COMPARISON OF CORRELATIONAL FLUCTUATIONS AND VARIABILITY OF ATTRIBUTES

One puzzling finding in the study of individual differences in performance in the GMC was the fluctuation in the values of the correlation coefficients between certain attributes and certain staff ratings. Figures 24.1 and 24.2, for example, show the fluctuations in the values of the correlation coefficients between three kinds of individual attributes and ratings on medical knowledge and medical skill. Some of these fluctuations were considerable. For example, the correlation coefficients between previous academic performance and medical skill varied from a high of .70 to a low of −.02; those between previous academic performance and medical knowledge from a high of .80 to a low of .11. The correlations between peer judgments and these ratings fluctuated less —from a high of .50 to a low of .20; but those between personality traits and these ratings ranged from a high of .30 to a low of −.30. The question arose of whether these fluctuations were the result of differences among student groups (i.e., sampling variations) or whether they were attributable to some other cause. Therefore, the correlations between three classes of ratings (medical knowledge and skill, psychological knowledge, and attitudes toward patients' social problems) and individual attributes were further analyzed.

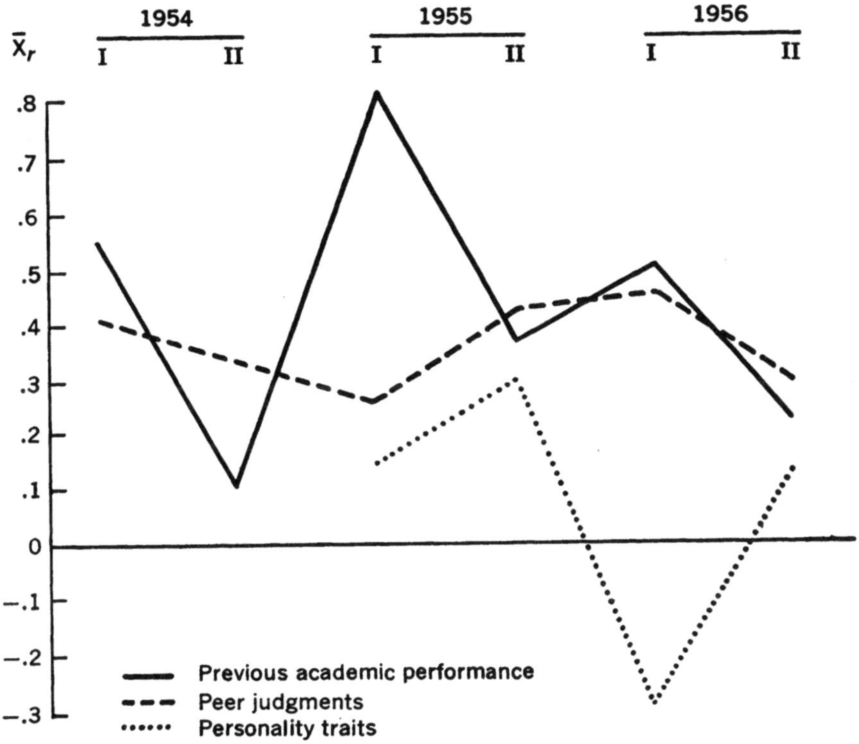

Figure 24.1. Correlations between three individual attributes and staff ratings on medical knowledge (classes of 1954, 1955, and 1956)

The method of analysis was to study the fluctuations in the correlations between these three classes of ratings and three categories of predictor attributes (previous academic performance, peer judgments, and personality traits) to discover whether these fluctuations corresponded to the fluctuations in the degree of variability of the predictor traits. It was assumed that if the correlations between rating and predictor trait fluctuated concomitantly with degree of variability of the predictor trait, then the predictor trait was relevant to the rating; that is, there was a direct or indirect causal link between the predictor trait and the raters' behavior. It is, of course, a statistical truism that when the variability of a trait increases, the correlation between the trait and a second variable increases—provided there is a functional relation between the two variables. However, if the actual results show that the correlation between a predictor trait and a rating does not increase as the variability of the trait increases, it may be assumed that the correlation is an artifact, and that, indeed, the predictor trait and the rating are not functionally related.

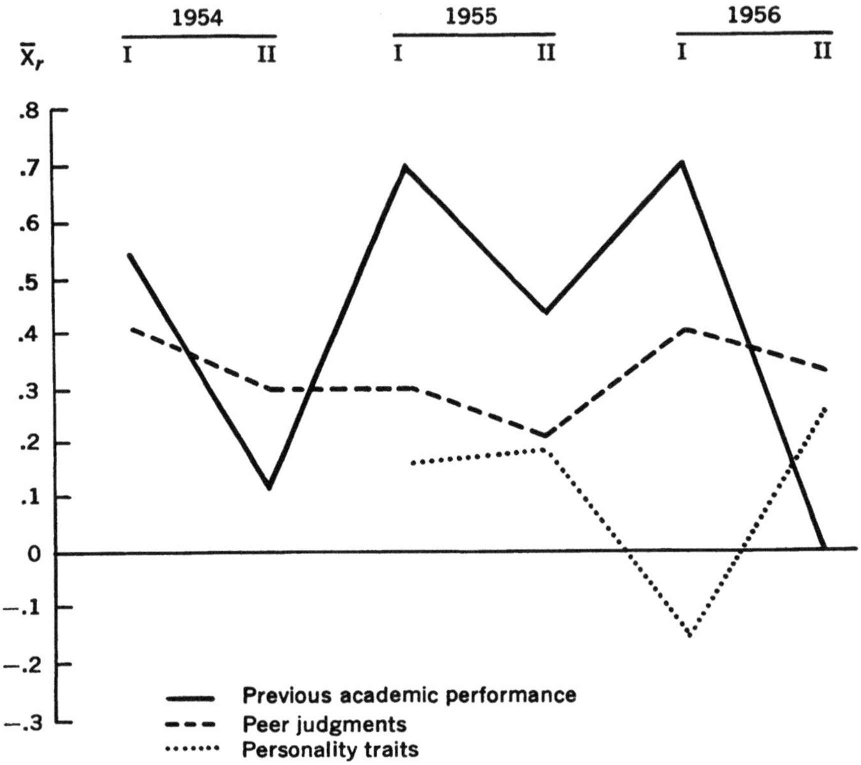

Figure 24.2. Correlations between three individual attributes and staff ratings on medical skill (classes of 1954, 1955, and 1956)

This assumption has a common-sense basis as well as a statistical one. Suppose, for example, that in one group the students are very much like one another in terms of their medical knowledge. (In this case, the variability among the students with respect to previous grade averages would be small.) This homogeneity among the students would make it difficult for the staff to perceive differences among the students, and as a consequence, the correlation between staff ratings on medical knowledge and the students' previous academic performance would be low. Conversely, if the students were very much unlike one another in terms of their medical knowledge, these differences would be readily apparent, and the correlation between previous academic performance and ratings on medical knowledge would be higher—*provided,* however, that such information actually was used by the raters. Thus, the correlation between the trait medical knowledge and the staff rating on medical knowledge would be expected to increase as the students varied more among one another with respect to medical knowledge. One would not, however, expect the correlation with an irrelevant trait, say, height, to increase as the students became more variable with respect to height. Therefore, on common-sense as well as statistical grounds, it should be possible to determine which student traits were relevant or irrelevant to the raters by examining the extent to which the correlation between a given trait and a rating varied concomitantly with the fluctuations in perceivable difference (variability) among students with respect to the given trait.

The following sections compare the fluctuations of the correlation coefficients and the fluctuations in variability of the trait involved in the correlation.

MEDICAL KNOWLEDGE AND SKILL

Figure 24.3 compares the correlations between previous academic performance and ratings on medical knowledge with the degrees of variability of previous academic performance. As can be seen, these two values fluctuated concomitantly; when the variability was high, the correlation was also high, and vice versa. Figure 24.4 presents similar data with ratings on medical skill substituted for ratings on medical knowledge. The values again fluctuated concomitantly. On the assump-

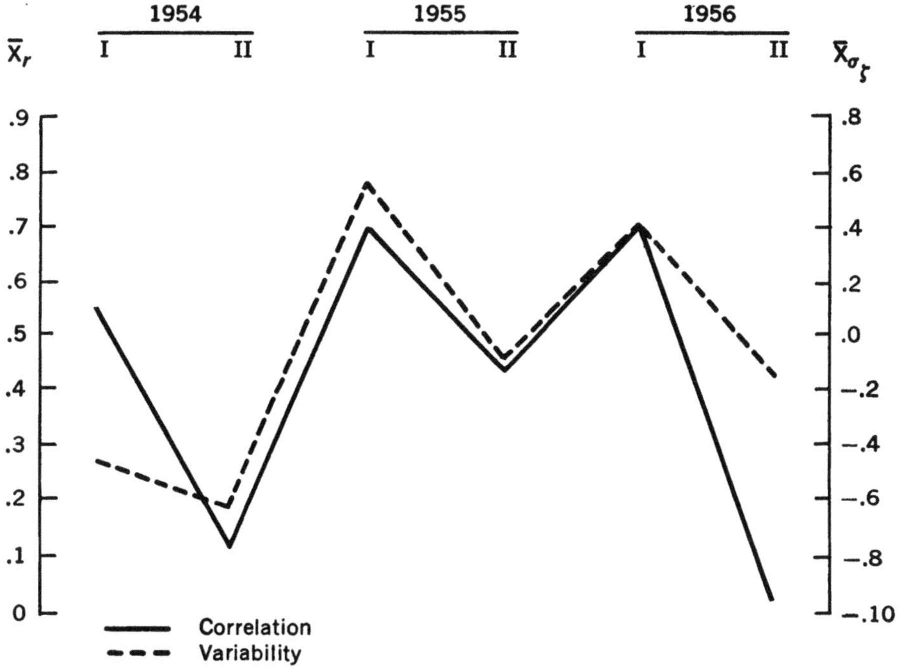

Figure 24.3. Correlations between previous academic performance · and staff ratings on medical knowledge, and variability of previous academic performance (classes of 1954, 1955, and 1956)

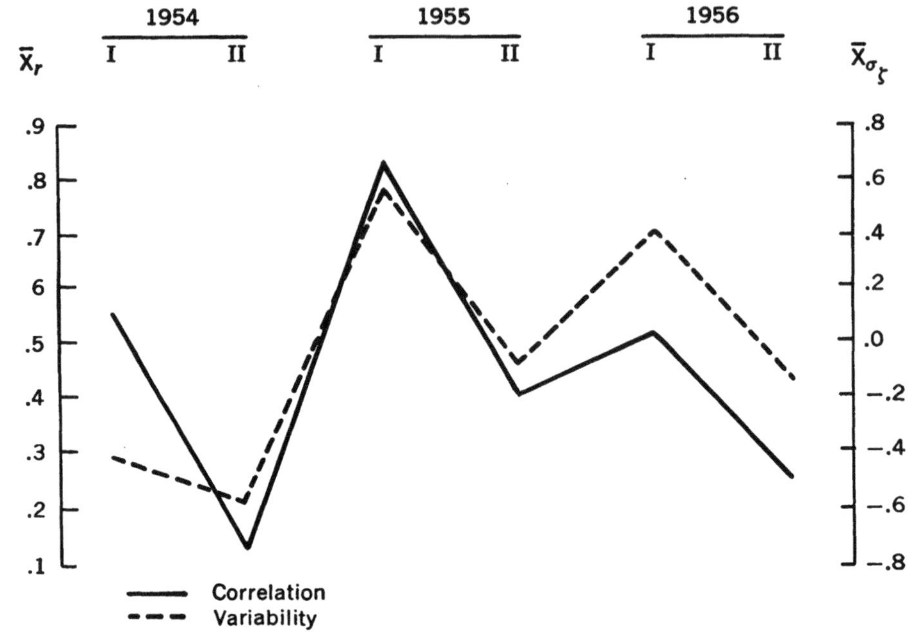

Figure 24.4. Correlations between previous academic performance and staff ratings on medical skill, and variability of previous academic performance (classes of 1954, 1955, and 1956)

tion discussed above, these findings may be interpreted to mean that ratings on medical skill and medical knowledge were functionally related to the students' medical knowledge (as reflected in previous grades); that is, the raters perceived and used this attribute in making their ratings.

Figure 24.5 compares the correlations between peer-judged attributes and ratings on medical knowledge with the degrees of variability of the peer-judged attributes. These two values cannot be said to have fluctuated concomitantly, as did the values discussed immediately above, but the fluctuations show enough similarity to indicate some functional relation between peer-judged attributes and ratings on medical knowledge. Figure 24.6 presents parallel data with ratings on medical skill substituted for ratings on medical knowledge. Here the fluctuations were even more independent of one another than were those shown in Figure 24.5. Since medical knowledge ratings were made by the younger, less experienced physicians, and medical skill ratings were made by the older, more experienced physicians, these findings might be interpreted as indicating that the younger, less experienced physicians, being closer in age and experience to the medical students, somehow utilized cues more nearly identical with the ones

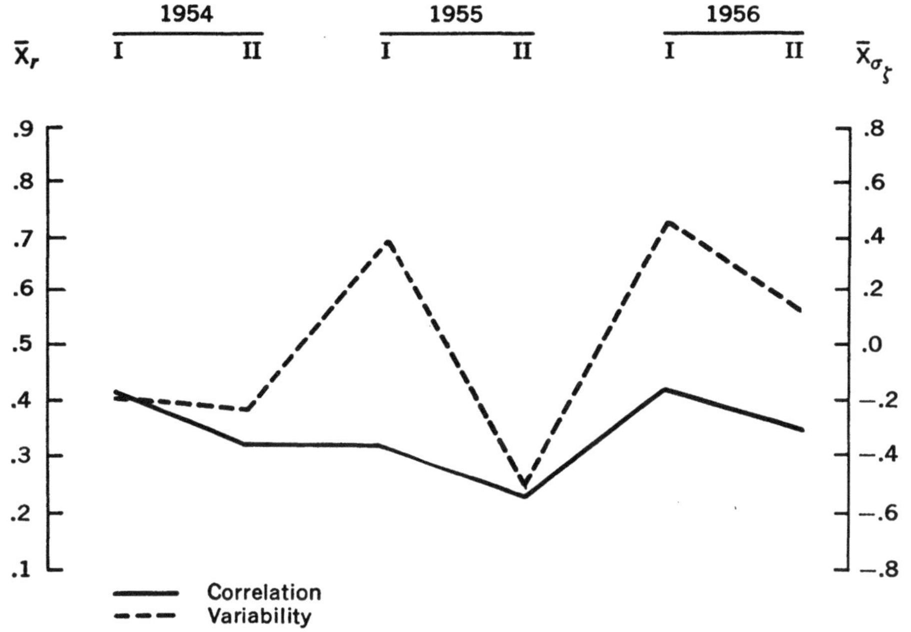

Figure 24.5. Correlations between peer judgments and staff ratings on medical knowledge, and variability of peer judgments (classes of 1954, 1955, and 1956)

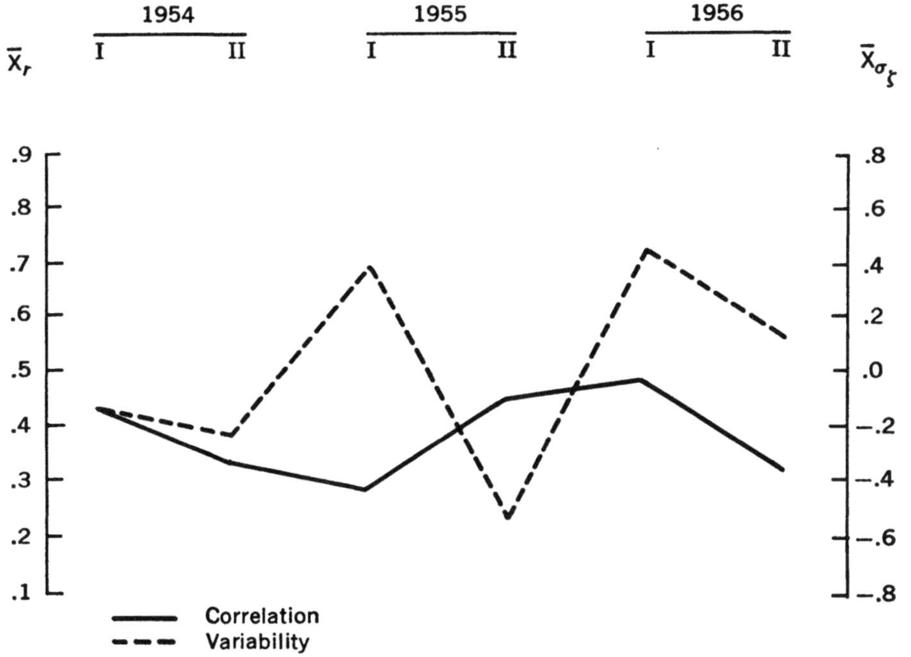

Figure 24.6. Correlations between peer judgments and staff ratings on medical skill, and variability of peer judgments (classes of 1954, 1955, and 1956)

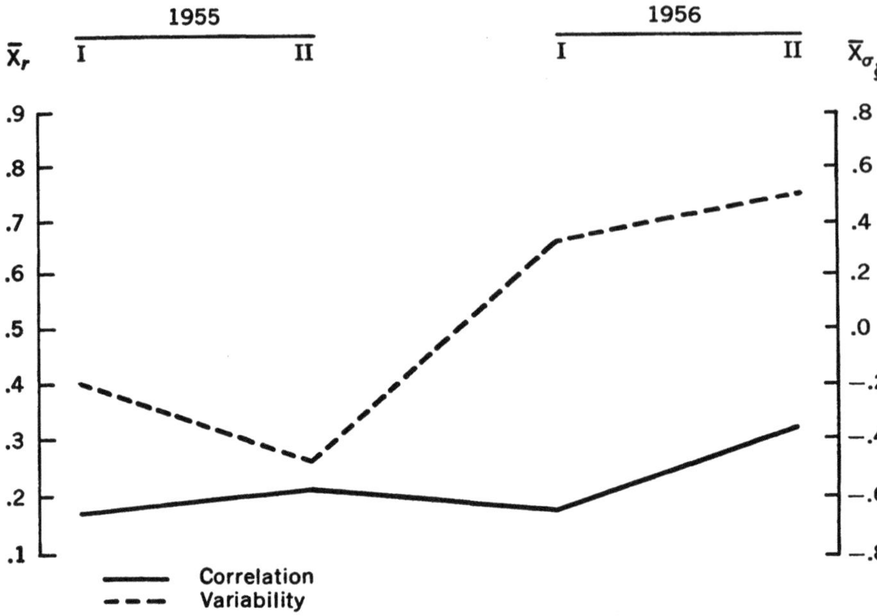

Figure 24.7. Correlations between personality traits and staff ratings on medical knowledge, and variability of personality traits (classes of 1955 and 1956)

used by the students than with those utilized by the older, more experienced physicians. The general conclusion here is that peer-judged attributes were, for the most part, not functionally related to ratings on medical knowledge and medical skill.

Figure 24.7 compares the correlations between ratings on medical knowledge and personality traits with the degrees of variability of the personality traits. It can be seen that the values fluctuated independently of each other; the same was true when ratings on medical skill were substituted for ratings on medical knowledge, as shown in Figure 24.8. The conclusion is that personality traits were not functionally related to ratings on either medical knowledge or medical skill.

PSYCHOLOGICAL KNOWLEDGE

As can be seen in Figure 24.9, correlations between ratings on psychological knowledge and three kinds of individual attributes fluctuated considerably from one student group to another. These fluctuations were studied in the same manner as the fluctuations in the correlations between individual attributes and ratings on medical knowledge and medical skill.

Figure 24.10 compares the correlations between previous academic performance and ratings on psychological knowledge with the degrees

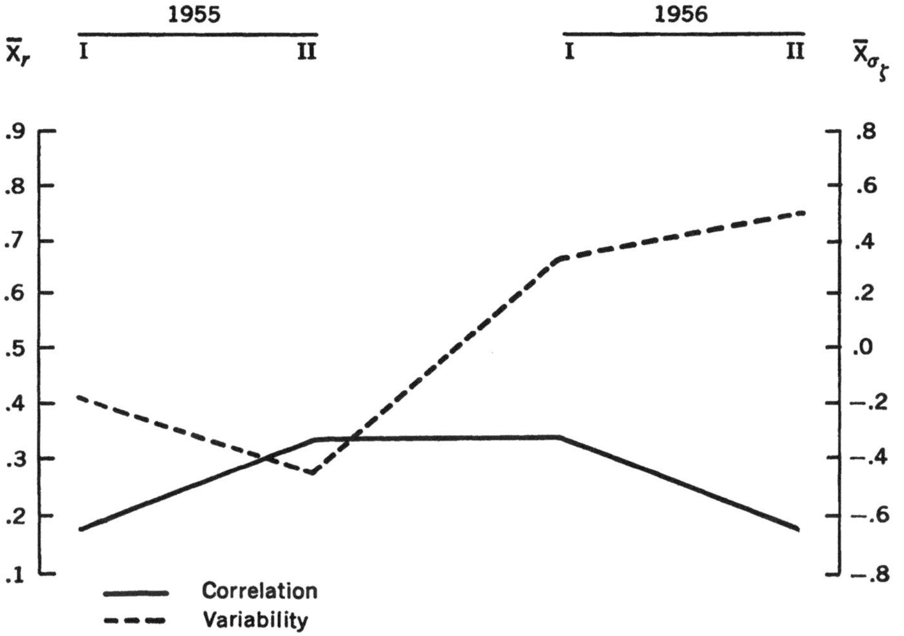

Figure 24.8. Correlations between personality traits and staff ratings on medical skill, and variability of personality traits (classes of 1955 and 1956)

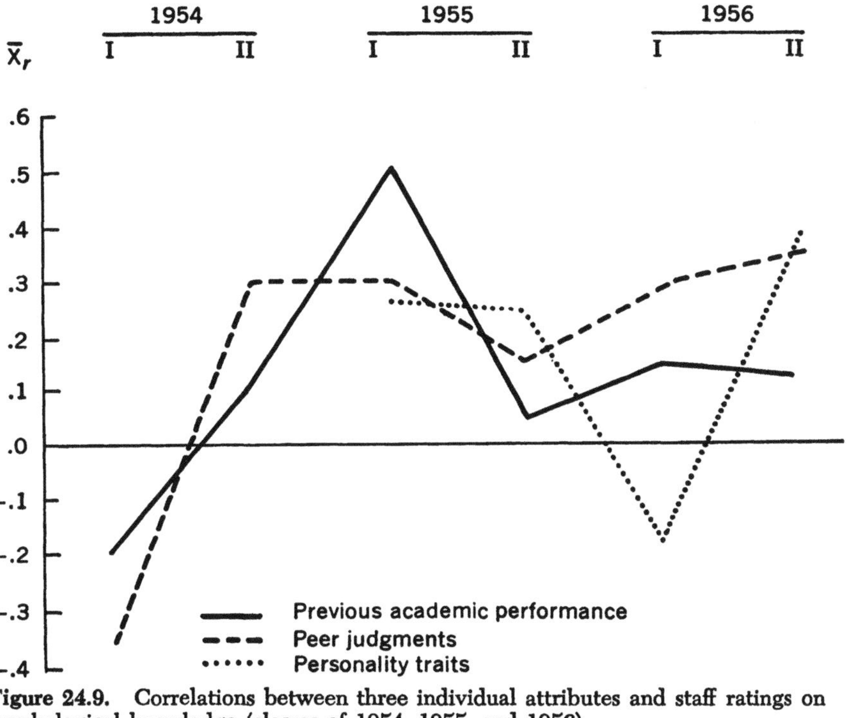

Figure 24.9. Correlations between three individual attributes and staff ratings on psychological knowledge (classes of 1954, 1955, and 1956)

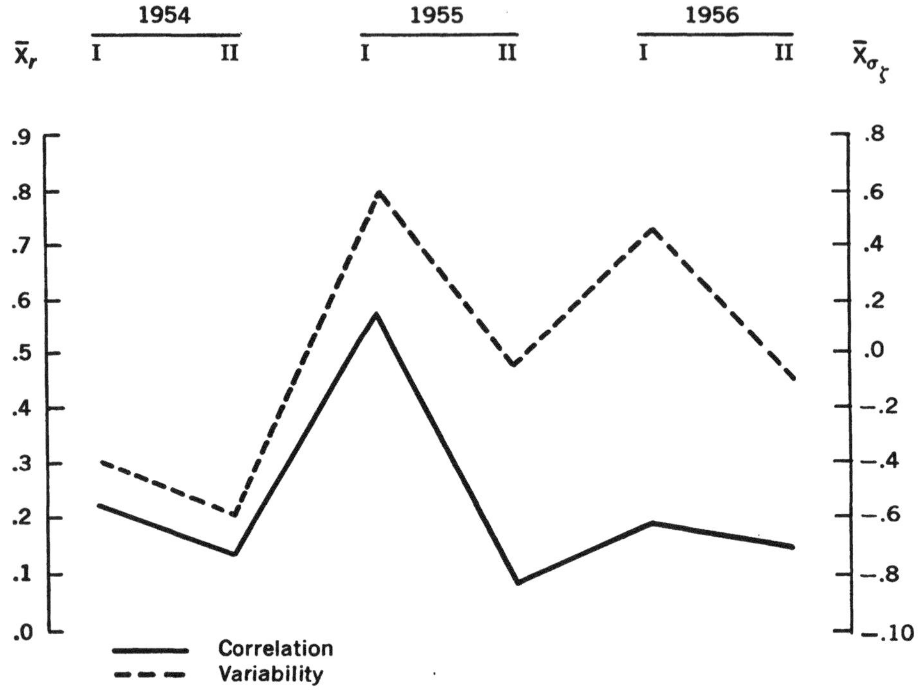

Figure 24.10. Correlations between previous academic performance and staff ratings on psychological knowledge, and variability of previous academic performance (classes of 1954, 1955, and 1956)

of variability of previous academic performance. These values fluctuated concomitantly (though not as markedly so as those shown in Figures 24.3 and 24.4). Thus it may be inferred that ratings on psychological knowledge were functionally related to the students' medical knowledge (as reflected by previous grade averages). However, this functional relation was not so strong as that which existed between ratings on medical knowledge and skill and previous academic performance.

Figure 24.11 compares the correlations between peer-judged attributes and ratings on psychological knowledge with the degrees of variability of peer-judged attributes. These data are rather difficult to interpret. The values tended to fluctuate concomitantly, but not unequivocally so. Possibly the conclusion should be that a functional relation between peer-judged attributes and ratings on psychological knowledge existed, but was rather weak and indirect.

A similar conclusion seems to be indicated by the data shown in Figure 24.12, which compares the degrees of variability of personality traits with the correlations between personality traits and ratings on

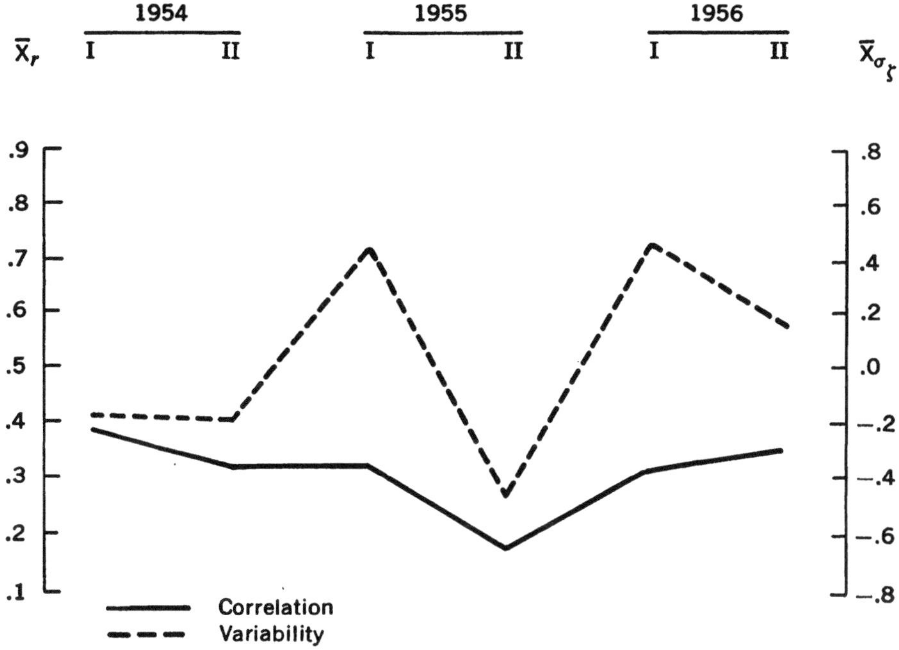

Figure 24.11. Correlations between peer judgments and staff ratings on psychological knowledge, and variability of peer judgments (classes of 1954, 1955, and 1956)

psychological knowledge. Except in the case of the 1956 I group (the group which in other respects provided a definite exception to the results obtained with the other three—see above), the two curves in Figure 24.12 are fairly similar; that is, the values tended to fluctuate concomitantly. Thus, although some functional relation undoubtedly existed between personality traits and ratings on psychological knowledge, that relation was not a strong one.

Attitudes toward patients' social problems

As can be seen in Figure 24.13, the correlations between individual attributes and ratings on attitudes toward patients' social problems (made by the members of the ancillary staff) fluctuated considerably. These fluctuations were compared with the changes in variability of the individual attributes using the procedure described above.

Figure 24.14 compares the degrees of variability of previous academic performance with the correlations between previous academic performance and ratings on attitudes toward patients' social problems. These values fluctuated independently, not concomitantly; hence it may be concluded that no functional relation existed between pre-

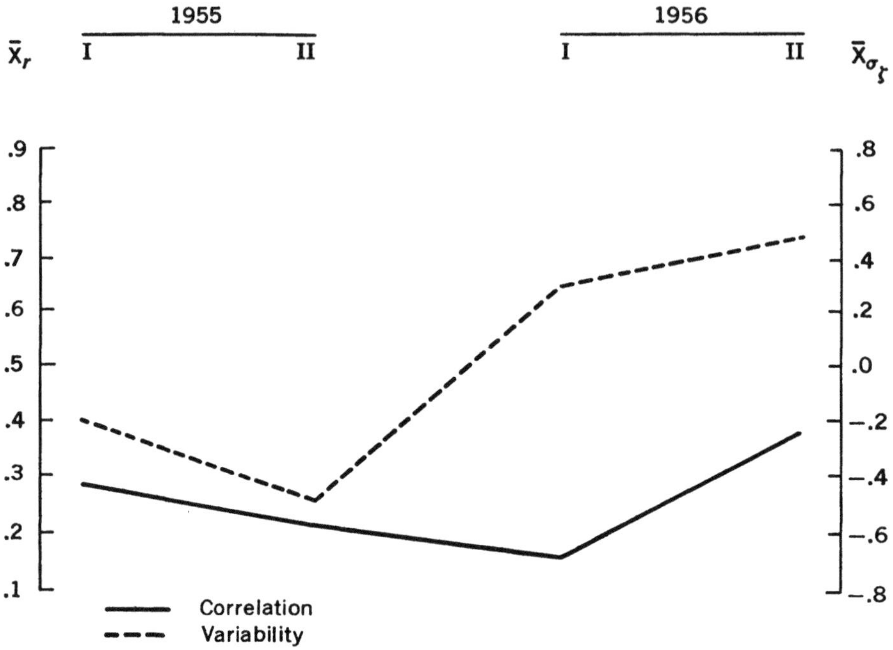

Figure 24.12. Correlations between personality traits and staff ratings on psychological knowledge, and variability of personality traits (classes of 1955 and 1956)

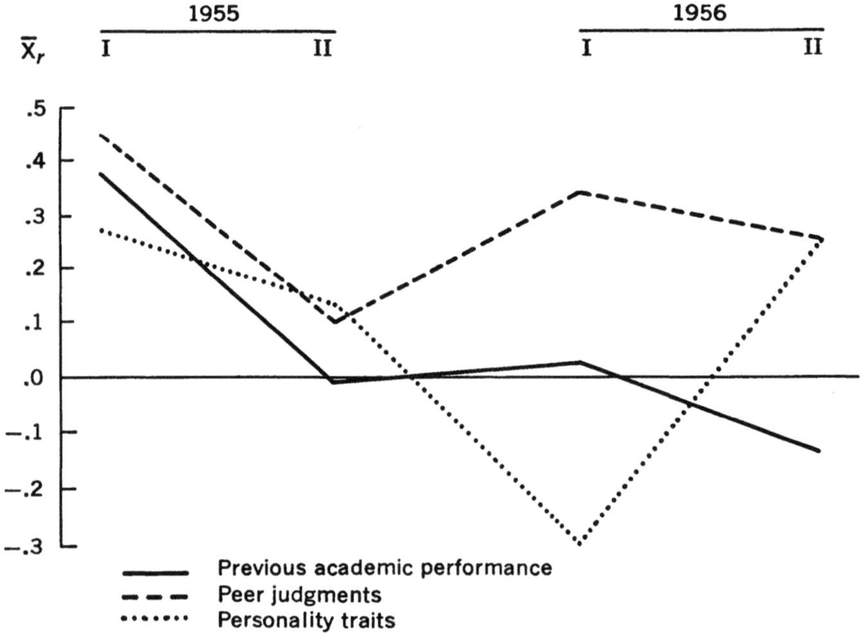

Figure 24.13. Correlations between three individual attributes and staff ratings on attitudes toward patients' social problems (classes of 1955 and 1956)

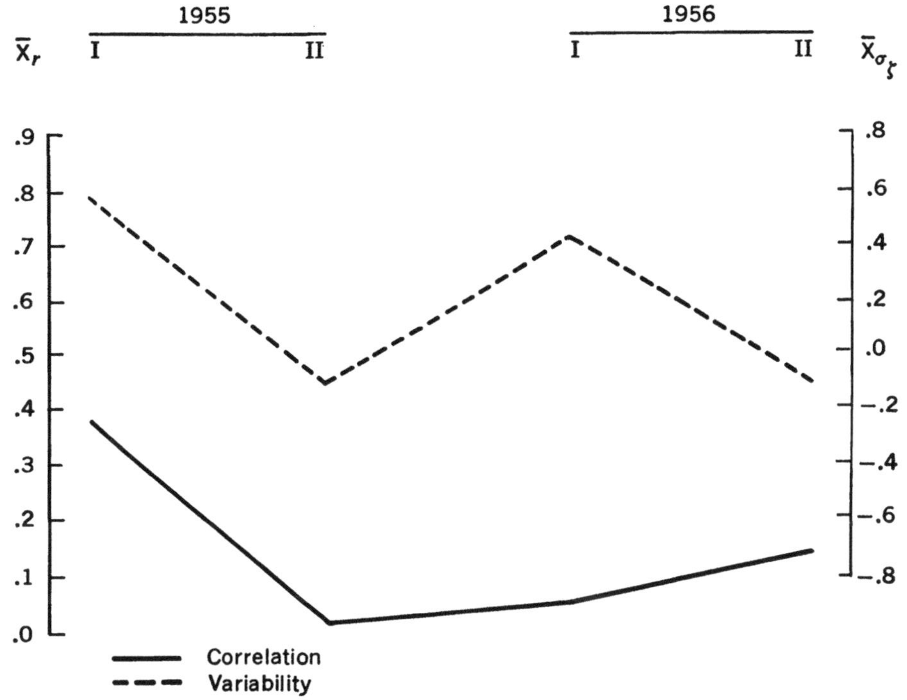

Figure 24.14. Correlations between previous academic performance and staff ratings on attitudes toward patients' social problems, and variability of previous academic performance (classes of 1955 and 1956)

vious academic performance and ratings on attitudes toward patients' social problems.

A different result is indicated by the data shown in Figure 24.15, which compares the degrees of variability of peer-judged attributes with the correlations between peer-judged attributes and ratings on attitudes toward patients' social problems. Here the values fluctuate concomitantly, as do those shown in Figure 24.16, which compares the degrees of variability of personality traits with the correlations between personality traits and ratings on attitudes toward patients' social problems. It may therefore be concluded that functional relations existed between ratings on attitudes toward patients' social problems and both peer-judged attributes and personality traits.

To summarize, this method of analysis—comparison of fluctuations in correlations between traits and ratings with fluctuations in variability of the traits—is based on the hypothesis that if a correlation fluctuates concomitantly with the degree of variability of the trait, a functional relation exists between the trait and the rating. By applying this method to correlations between three kinds of ratings and three classes of individual attributes, the following results were obtained:

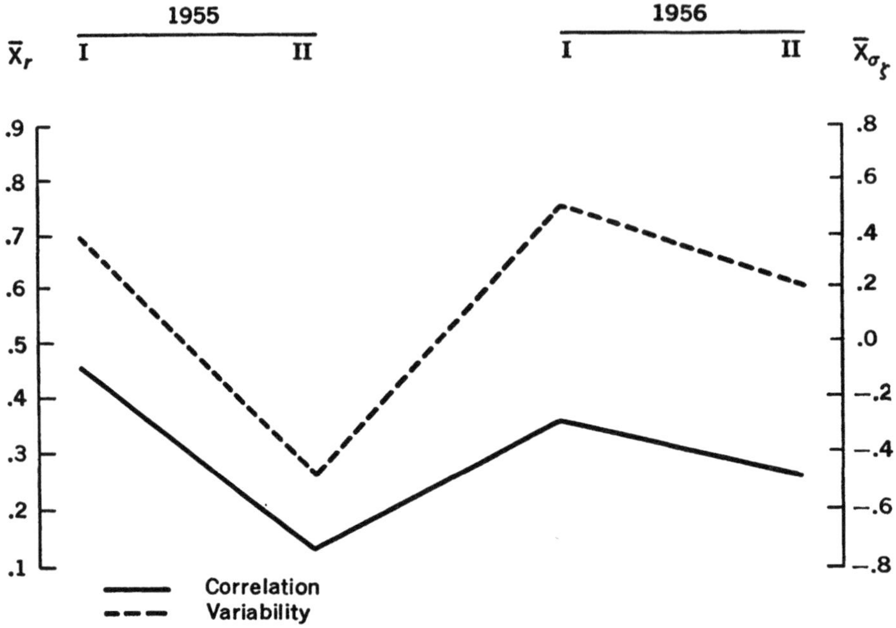

Figure 24.15. Correlations between peer judgments and staff ratings on attitudes toward patients' social problems, and variability of peer judgments (classes of 1955 and 1956)

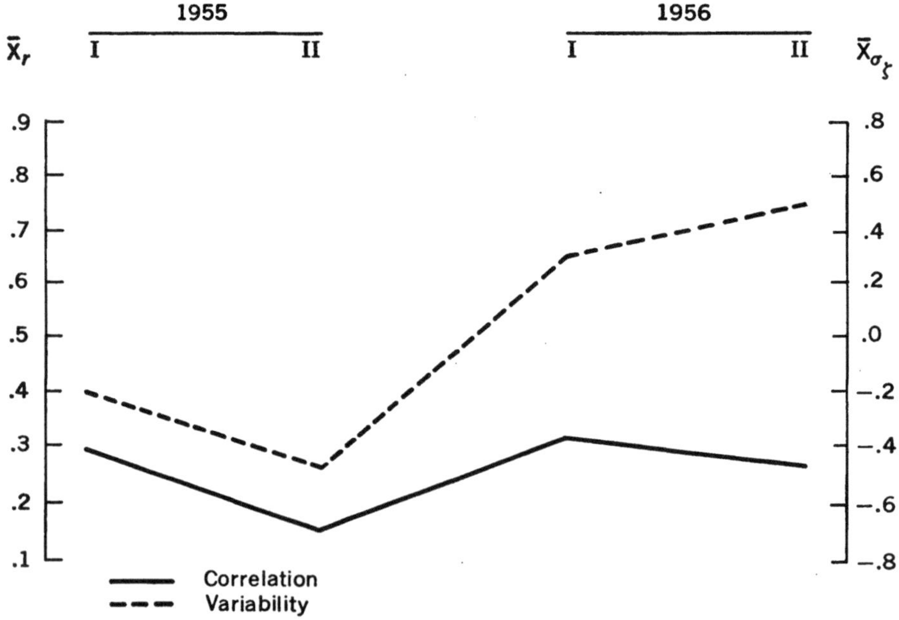

Figure 24.16. Correlations between personality traits and staff ratings on attitudes toward patients' social problems, and variability of personality traits (classes of 1955 and 1956)

1. Ratings on medical knowledge and skill were strongly related to previous academic performance, very weakly related to peer-judged attributes, and unrelated to personality traits.

2. Ratings on psychological knowledge were fairly strongly related to previous academic performance (though not so strongly or directly as were ratings on medical knowledge and skill), and rather weakly related to peer-judged attributes and personality traits.

3. Ratings on attitudes toward patients' social problems were unrelated to previous academic performance, but rather strongly related to peer-judged attributes and personality traits.

Special Problems of the 1956 I GMC Group

One problem encountered in the study of the correlation between individual attributes and ratings made by the GMC staff was particularly perplexing. This was the negative relation between certain personality traits and ratings by *all* raters (see Figures 24.1, 24.2, 24.9, and 24.13) of the students in the 1956 I group. Why should the GMC staff have given high ratings to students who had social poise, who were mature and responsible, and who were interested in achievement, in the 1955 I, 1955 II, and 1956 II groups, but have given high ratings to just the opposite sort of students in the 1956 I group? Some light is thrown on this curious finding by data presented in Figure 24.17, which shows the correlations among the three categories of individual attributes discussed above. It should be noted that the correlation between previous academic performance (in this case, third-year grade average) and peer judgments (in this case, leadership) did not change markedly over the four groups studied. Nor did the correlation between previous academic performance and the personality trait, tolerance, change much over the four groups. The correlation between leadership and tolerance did change markedly, however. In fact, in the 1956 I group the correlation between leadership and tolerance became negative. In other words, those students in the 1956 I group who were highly rated by their peers on leadership were intolerant people. Because of the generally positive correlations among the personality traits in the group of traits of which "tolerance" is a member, it is clear that the student leaders in the 1956 I group—and in that group alone among the groups here studied—were lacking in social poise, maturity, and responsibility. And the leaders in this group, like those in the other groups, also tended to be the students with high grades. The GMC staff, then, was confronted by quite a different situation with this group of students than with the other three. In the other three groups class leaders tended not only to be good students but also "pleasant" people. In the 1956 I group, however, class leaders tended to be those with high grades but not to be "pleasant" people.

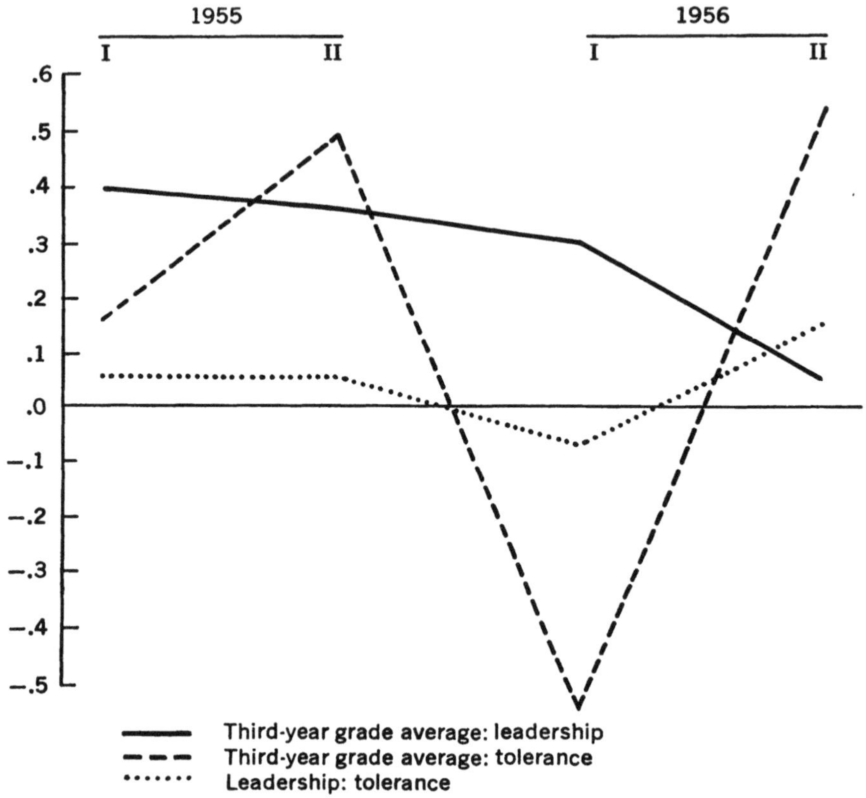

Figure 24.17. Intercorrelations among three individual attributes (classes of 1955 and 1956)

This particular group of students, then, provides a rather interesting opportunity to study the GMC staff as raters; for if staff members were rating students primarily on the basis of personality traits, the correlation between personality traits and ratings would be positive; because of the negative relation between leadership and "pleasant" personality traits, the correlation between leadership and ratings would be negative; and because class leaders tended to have higher grade averages, there would be negative correlations between grade averages and staff ratings. However, quite the contrary result was found. In the 1956 I group the GMC staff ratings were positively correlated with previous academic performance and leadership and negatively correlated with "pleasant" personality traits. Those GMC staff members (social workers and to a certain extent the psychiatrists) who with the other groups utilized personality characteristics when making ratings did not utilize personality characteristics in connection with this particular group, but rated students primarily on the basis of leadership—in spite of the "unpleasant" characteristics of the leaders.

Summary

Fluctuations in the degree of correlation between individual attributes and staff ratings of students are to be expected, and wide fluctuations in correlations occurred in the present study. Although it is customary to attribute such fluctuations to chance (variations due to the use of different samples of students) it seemed likely that a closer examination of the GMC staff's ratings might be useful. Accordingly, certain statistical characteristics of each group of GMC students were studied. It was noted that the extent to which the students differed among one another with respect to previous academic performance varied from group to group. In the first half of each year, students tended to be more unlike one another, whereas in the second half of each year, they tended to be more like one another. On those occasions when the students were unlike one another, the correlation between staff ratings on medical knowledge and skill and previous academic performance was high, and on those occasions when the students were like one another, this correlation was lower. Thus, instead of attributing the fluctuations in correlation between previous academic performance and medical knowledge and skill ratings to chance factors, one may explain these correlations as varying concomitantly with the ease with which discrimination among the students may be made. However, correlations between ratings on medical knowledge and skill and peer judgments, and between ratings on medical knowledge and skill and personality traits did not fluctuate concomitantly with the variability among students. Because these correlations did not vary with the ease of making discriminations among students, it was inferred that previous academic performance was relevant and peer judgments and personality traits irrelevant to the GMC staff's ratings.

The ancillary staff's ratings followed just the opposite pattern. The correlations between peer judgments and ratings on attitudes toward social problems did fluctuate concomitantly with the variability among students, as did the correlation between ancillary staff ratings and personality traits. The correlations between these ratings and previous academic performance, however, did not fluctuate concomitantly with the ease of making discriminations among students' previous academic performance. This finding was taken to mean that previous academic performance was an irrelevant trait, insofar as the ancillary staff were concerned. And, of course, since the ancillary staff were not expected to evaluate students' medical knowledge, this interpretation seems plausible.

The results concerning psychological knowledge ratings seemed to fall somewhere between the results obtained for the two sets of ratings discussed above. Ratings on psychological knowledge seemed to depend in part on all three classes of individual attributes, but not strongly on any one attribute.

A further study of the rating process, involving the intercorrelations among three attributes also indicated that the pediatricians and internists did not include personality characteristics in their evaluations of students, for they rated students in relation to their medical knowledge (as indicated by their previous grades) even on those occasions when the students who were leaders and who had the higher previous grades were relatively unpleasant persons. The results also suggested that the ancillary staff (and to a certain extent the psychiatrists), who ordinarily considered personality characteristics in their evaluation of students, did not always do so. For on the occasions when the class leaders were lacking in social poise and were immature and irresponsible, the ancillary staff rated the leaders high on attitudes toward social problems in spite of their relatively unpleasant personal characteristics.

PERSONALITY TRAITS ASSOCIATED WITH UNEXPECTED PERFORMANCE IN THE GMC

The data presented above showed that, in the main, previous academic performance was positively related to performance in the General Medical Clinic as rated by the internists and pediatricians. However, in each group there were several students whose previous grades were not related in this usual way to their performance in the GMC. The personal attributes of these students were therefore studied more closely to ascertain what attributes were associated with such unexpected performance.

It should be noted that in this study data from several student groups were combined for purposes of analysis, whereas in the previous study of performance each student group was investigated separately. Also, this study made use of a ranking based on the grade assigned to GMC students as an index of over-all performance rather than on the four rating components used above.

Design of the study

The students who participated in the GMC were divided into three groups designated the "plus" group, the "minus" group, and the "R" group. The "plus" group included those students who performed better than previous performance in medical school would lead one to expect. The "minus" group included the students whose conduct in the GMC was noticeably poorer than might have been expected. The "R" group consisted of the remaining GMC students. Differences among the three groups of students with respect to personal attributes were ascertained by noting which attributes distinguished each group of students from the others.

Procedure of the study

The procedure consisted of four steps. The first was to plot the specific index of previous academic performance against over-all performance in the GMC (measured by a ranking based on the GMC clerkship grade). The second step was to identify the three groups of students on the basis of the plotted data. Next, personal attributes were selected which were expected to differentiate "plus" group students, "minus" group students, and "R" group students. Finally, mean scores on attribute measures were computed for each of the three types of students.

Selection of performance indices. The grades assigned at the end of the GMC clerkship represented the staff's evaluation of the students' over-all performance. However, because the grades themselves were too crude an index to use, the students were ranked according to the staff's evaluation of their over-all performance.

The ranks were assigned in the following manner. Prior to the staff meeting in which grades were decided upon, each staff member gave each student a provisional grade. Provisional grades for students were presented during the meeting, and, after some discussion, a final grade for each student was determined. In order to arrive at a rank order, each student was first classified according to final grade. Then distinctions were made among students within the same grade category by referring to the mean *provisional* grade given students by the entire staff.

This procedure was followed for four student groups (1955 I, 1955 II, 1956 I, and 1956 II). The GMC students from the class of 1954 were not used in this study because several measures of personal attributes were not obtained from them.

Several indices of previous academic performance were available: the cumulative grade average, the junior medical clerkship grade, and peer judgment of competence as a physician. Cumulative grade average was chosen because it was based on several grades (hence it was more stable than any single grade), because it represented all of the students' performances in medical school through the third year, and because it would be available in any medical school if replication of this study were to be attempted.

Identification of student types. In order to make distinctions among the three types of students as sharp as possible, only those few students whose performance was markedly better than expected were assigned to the "plus" group, and only those few students whose performance was markedly worse than expected were assigned to the "minus" group. The selection of these students was made from the analysis of scatter diagrams of the relation between cumulative grade average and rank in the group based on GMC grade.[8]

In Figure 24.18 the diagrams of the four student groups are presented. (A rank of 1 on the horizontal axis represents the best GMC student in his group.) Three students in the first group were graded much more highly than would have been predicted from their cumulative grade averages. They were "plus" group students. (They are indicated by x's in the figure.) Two students received very low grades relative to their previous academic performance and were characterized as "minus" group students. (These are indicated by asterisks in the figure.)

In subsequent groups, three, two, and two students, respectively, were classified "plus," making a total of ten students in this group. Similarly, thirteen students were placed in the "minus" group. The remaining GMC students in these two classes numbered forty-seven; a total of seventy students was involved.

Selection of personal attributes. It was decided to use all the individual attributes[9] on which data were available for all four student groups so as to obtain the widest possible coverage.

Analysis of the data. Mean scores on each attribute measure were computed for each of the three categories of students: the "plus," "minus," and "R" groups. Differences between means were inspected and the largest differences were selected. In order to make the differences comparable, all the mean scores were converted to standard scores. Since random sampling techniques were not used in the selection of students, and since the results were not cross validated, no inductive claims can be made for the data. The importance of the analysis lies in the extent to which the results enhance understanding of the nature of the GMC.

RESULTS OF THE STUDY

The individual attributes which distinguished among "plus," "minus," and "R" group students are presented in profile form in Figure 24.19. The "plus" group students had significantly higher peer-judged leadership scores than either the "minus" group or "R" group students. High ratings in several other peer-judged qualities—skill in developing

[8] Although the ranked data and the grade average data do not constitute comparable scales, it was decided to use this method of selecting cases because it made the identification of unexpected performance somewhat simpler.

[9] Except, of course, annual grade averages and grades.

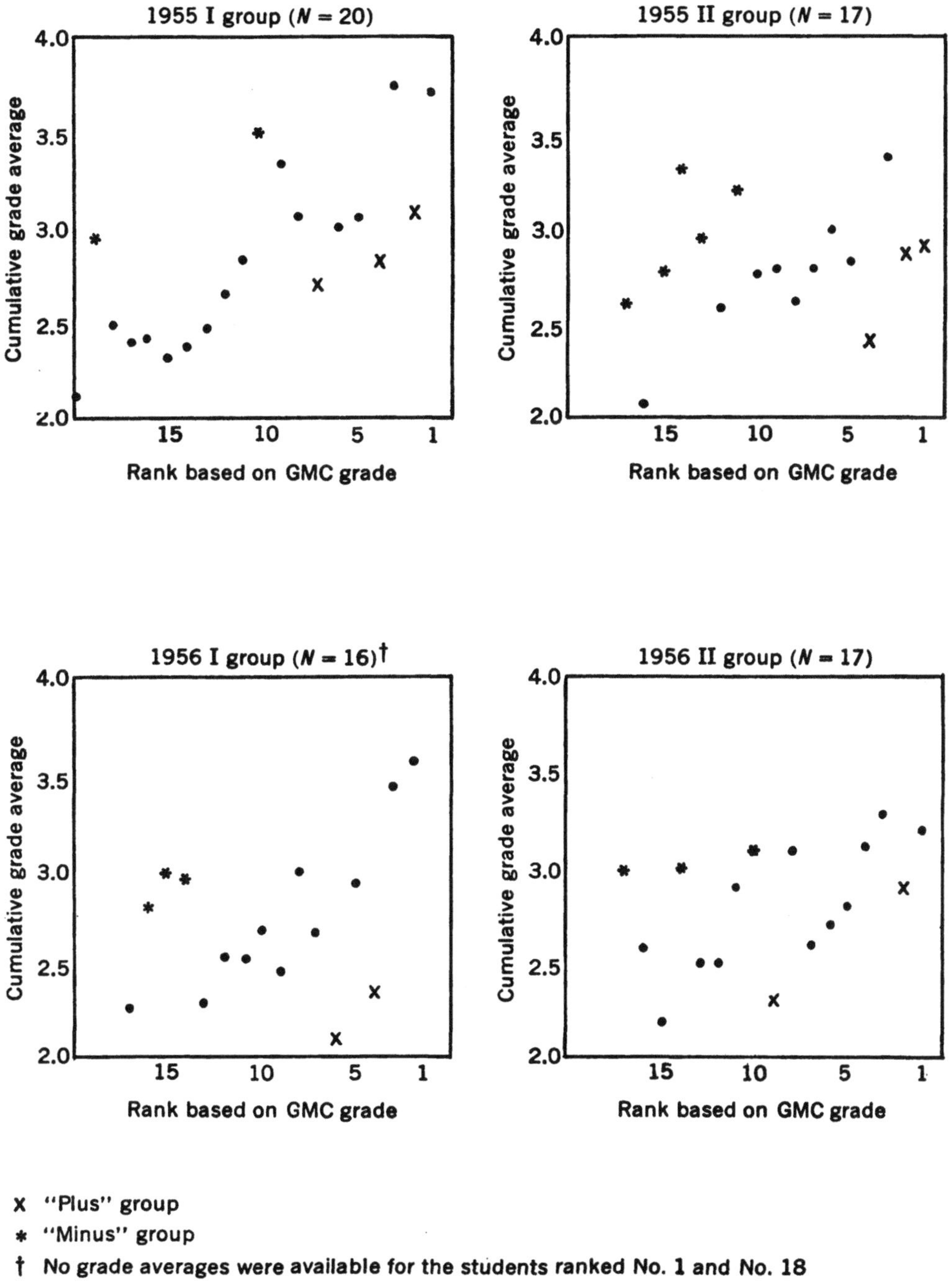

Figure 24.18. Scatter diagrams of the relations between cumulative grade average (prior to senior year) and GMC clerkship grade (classes of 1955 and 1956)

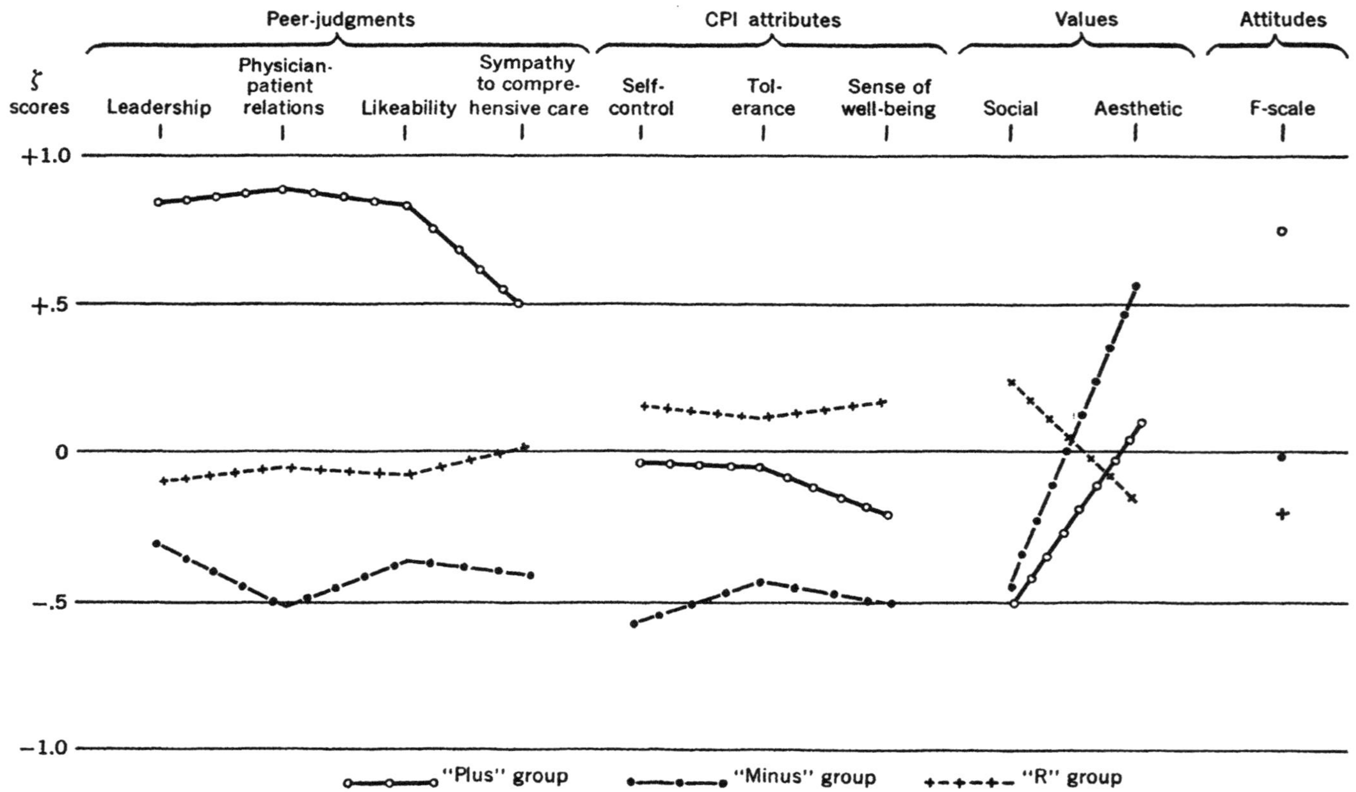

Figure 24.19. Mean standard scores of the "plus," "minus," and "R" groups on selected individual attributes

physician-patient relations, likeability, and sympathy to the comprehensive care concept—also distinguished "plus" group students from students in both other groups. "Minus" students were rated lower on these qualities than "R" students, but the differences were not very great.

"Minus" group students were distinguished from the "R" group in terms of their attitudes, values, and other personality characteristics (as well as their above average academic standing). In Figure 24.19 it can be seen that "minus" group students were relatively authoritarian in their attitudes. That is, they were more intolerant of persons different from themselves, more inflexible in ambiguous situations, and more deferential before authority figures than other GMC students. The relatively low scores of this group on the CPI Tolerance scale tended to confirm this result. Strong aesthetic values and weak social values also distinguished "minus" group students from the others. They were likely to be individualistic and self-sufficient, as well as cold toward other people. "Minus" group students also had less self-control and a weaker sense of well-being (a greater tendency to complain and to entertain strong self-doubts) than other students. Finally, a tendency toward a high degree of general anxiety in these students should be noted.[10]

In general, students who received lower grades from the GMC staff than might have been expected on the basis of their previous performance in medical school were likely to be intolerant, relatively cold toward others, self-doubting, and lacking in self-control.

INTERPRETATION OF THE RESULTS

The attributes which identified "plus" group students could be interpreted separately from those which identified "minus" group students. However, one quality appeared to be characteristic of the "plus" group and not characteristic of the "minus" group. It might be termed "effectiveness in dealing with others." Likeable students and students chosen by their peers as leaders obviously would possess this quality to a relatively high degree; but self-centered, cold, anxious students, lacking in self-control, would be deficient in it.

It was not surprising that this degree of interpersonal effectiveness differentiated unexpected successes from unexpected failures among GMC students. Probably the most striking difference between the academic setting of the early years in medical school and the

[10] Although the mean anxiety score for the "minus" group was higher than that for the "R" group, the difference was not large. However, eleven of the twelve "minus" group students had anxiety scores above the mean score for the "R" group.

clinic setting of the last year is the introduction in the last year of human beings with whom the student must interact to an extensive degree. Lecture notes and memorized facts no longer dominate the student's attention; in their place the live patient appears, whose ailments (which may vary widely from those the student has learned to expect) must be diagnosed and treated. And the patient does not present an artificial, "textbook" diagnostic problem. An ill-considered phrase will arouse his anger or close his mouth during history-taking, or send him away frightened and resentful. In addition, the teacher in the GMC is seldom a lecturer. Instead, he asks many questions of the one other person in the room, the student himself, and not all these questions concern organic medicine. Clearly, a clinic student's effectiveness in dealing with others plays a much more important part in his performance in the GMC than it did in his previous performance in medical school. And, among medical students as a group, effectiveness in dealing with others is not associated to any substantial degree with the quality of previous academic performance. Thus, working with others effectively is an important distinguishing factor among the student types under discussion.

Another very interesting finding was that the "minus" group students had more authoritarian (and less tolerant) attitudes than other GMC students. This result could be interpreted in terms of any one of several components of authoritarianism, but two seem most relevant here. According to theory about authoritarianism, persons with authoritarian attitudes tend to be judgmental toward persons who are perceived to be "weak." For example, psychoneurotic patients and patients from the lower socio-economic class would be thought by authoritarians to be lacking the will power to change their behavior (in the first case) or to raise their socio-economic status (in the second case). There were many of both these types of patients in the GMC, and authoritarian (intolerant) students could be expected to have reacted to these patients in the manner just described. Obviously, such reactions would not allow these students to obtain maximum benefit from their experiences with patients. Intolerant students would not be stimulated to learn more about these patients, but would be repelled by the patients' "weaknesses." In this manner authoritarian attitudes could interfere with the performance of otherwise promising clinical students.

Another characteristic which has been found to be associated with authoritarian attitudes is inflexibility. When it is remembered that clinic functioning presented students with many new situations to master, many frustrations to adjust to, and many complex problems to solve, all of which required flexibility on the students' part, another source of interference with performance of the authoritarian students has obviously been identified. This type of setting could be upsetting to "minus" group students, who, in addition to being relatively authoritarian, tended to lack self-confidence and to be anxious. The many new threats (potential or actual) would probably raise anxiety to a level at which performance would be perceptibly impaired.

The prominence given authoritarian attitudes in this interpretation section is not inconsistent with the importance of the result. And although the relations were not altogether consistent, the F-scale tended to be negatively correlated with the staff ratings in the study reported above. Often these negative correlations were high enough to be regarded as statistically significant.

Chapter 25

The Scheduling Effect

The data presented in the previous chapters showed that a marked difference frequently appeared between the results obtained for the first-half GMC clerkships and those obtained for the second-half GMC clerkships. In general, the first-half clerkships were more successful in attaining the GMC goals than the second-half clerkships.

Description and Explanation

Although this phenomenon, called the scheduling effect, did manifest itself in connection with the traditional objectives which the new program shared with the control program (those objectives most closely associated with organic medicine), it was considerably more pronounced in connection with the special objectives of the General Medical Clinic Program (those particularly associated with the comprehensive care concept). The scheduling effect was apparent, for example, in the test of medical knowledge; for all three years the first-half GMC students performed better than the first-half control students in this test, whereas the control students performed better than the GMC students in all three second-half groups. These differences, however, were small, and most of them could have occurred by chance (see Chapter 16). More striking manifestations of the scheduling effect are shown in Tables 25.1 through 25.3, which present data relevant to the special goals of the GMC.

Table 25.1 indicates the change in students' attitudes toward three aspects of the comprehensive care concept. The pattern seems clear. In the 1956 I group the GMC students' attitudes tended to become more favorable; those of the control group less favorable. In the 1956 II group the attitudes of the GMC students tended to change for the worse, while those of the control students tended to remain unchanged. In other words, the GMC was considerably less successful in attaining

Table 25.1. Change in attitudes toward three aspects of the comprehensive care concept from Pretest to Posttest I (1956 I) and from Posttest I to Posttest II (1956 II)

	1956 I			1956 II		
	Negative change	No change	Positive change	Negative change	No change	Positive change
Attitudes toward behavior disorders						
GMC	3	2	13	9	2	5
Control	8	2	3	6	5	7
Attitudes toward the team concept						
GMC	3	5	10	8	3	5
Control	10	2	1	5	9	4
Attitudes toward the physician-patient relation						
GMC	6	5	7	6	5	5
Control	8	4	1	4	9	5

its special goals with the 1956 II group than it was with the 1956 I group.

Table 25.2 shows the appearance of the scheduling effect in connection with the GMC's effort to increase students' awareness of factors in patients' home lives that might affect their medical problems. The GMC was far more successful in attaining its objectives with the 1955 I and 1956 I groups than with the 1955 II and 1956 II groups. A similar pattern is illustrated in Table 25.3 in connection with the importance attached by students to a number of activities stressed in the GMC.

Examination of the pertinent data suggests that this scheduling effect resulted from a combination of three factors: the students considered learning traditional (organic) medicine more important than learning the techniques of comprehensive care; the GMC students felt that their program presented inadequate opportunities for learning the traditional aspects of medicine; and these attitudes and anxieties were of such a nature that *they tended to intensify as the responsibilities of internship approached.* Apparently this combination of factors interfered with the learning process, particularly during the second half of the senior year, and particularly in those areas specifically associated with the comprehensive care concept.

Evidence supporting the various phases of the foregoing explanation are presented below. These data overlap somewhat; data supporting one phase of the explanation sometimes support another phase also.

Table 25.2. Change in percentage of GMC students responding that a family physician should have various kinds of information as part of his routine information about patients (classes of 1955 and 1956)

	1955 I			1955 II			1956 I			1956 II		
	Pre	Post I	Change	Post I	Post II	Change	Pre	Post I	Change	Post I	Post II	Change
Income	65	80	*15*	77	76	*—1*	50	72	*22*	69	63	*—6*
Nationality, ethnic background	70	90	*20*	59	76	*17*	61	83	*22*	44	44	*0*
Education	60	60	*0*	88	71	*—17*	44	78	*34*	44	50	*6*
Recreational activities	40	70	*30*	53	53	*0*	11	50	*39*	38	38	*0*
Fears, worries, problems	80	95	*15*	71	82	*11*	56	78	*22*	81	69	*—12*

Table 25.3. Change in percentage of GMC students rating certain activities as extremely or very important (class of 1956)

	1956 I			1956 II		
	Pre	Post I	Change	Post I	Post II	Change
Acquiring knowledge of the basic ideas of psychosomatic medicine and psychiatry	17	55	*38*	38	44	*6*
Acquiring skill at applying the basic ideas of psychosomatic medicine and psychiatry to clinical practice	34	66	*32*	25	38	*13*
Having opportunities for psychiatric consultation for your patients	28	50	*22*	32	25	*—7*
Handling the emotional problems of patients	39	66	*27*	50	31	*—19*
Following patients for several months	55	78	*23*	44	31	*—13*
Making home visits	17	17	*0*	19	0	*—19*
Having opportunities to consult with the ancillary services	33	45	*12*	32	19	*—13*
Learning philosophy and point of view of social work	23	33	*10*	19	0	*—19*
Handling the social problems of patients	11	39	*28*	25	19	*—6*
Seeing the families of patients	34	28	*—6*	38	12	*—26*

RATING OF TRADITIONAL MEDICINE ABOVE COMPREHENSIVE CARE

Two kinds of evidence directly indicated that the students considered learning traditional (organic) medicine more important than learning the special techniques of comprehensive care. Another kind of evidence supported this finding indirectly. All students (both GMC and control) were asked to rank nine objectives of the senior program in order of their relative importance. Table 25.4 shows that invariably the objectives relating to traditional medicine were ranked higher than the special goals of the GMC.[1]

Data obtained from interviews with students reinforced the information obtained from the students' rankings. The following comments are typical:

> I feel that, since everything can't be learned in four years of medical school, the organic part comes first.
>
> I'd hate to have any doctor practice on me who was not fully expert in the organic basis because an organic disease can kill you.
>
> People are not going to die as a result of their psychiatric ailments—

[1] Note the perfect rank order correlation between the class of 1955 and the class of 1956 at the end of the senior year (Posttest II), shown in Table 25.4.

Table 25.4. Students' ranking of objectives of senior program in order of importance (1955 II, 1956 I and II)

	Post II 1955	Pretest 1956	Post II 1956
Skill at applying the facts of organic medicine to clinical practice	1	3	1
Knowing how to organize diagnostic and therapeutic regimes	2	1	2
Knowledge of the basic facts of clinical medicine (excluding psychosomatic medicine)	3	2	3
Ability to establish and maintain good physician-patient relations	4	4	4
Knowing the practical application of the principles of comprehensive care in treating patients	5	5	5
Skill at applying the basic ideas of psychosomatic medicine and psychiatry to clinical practice	6	6	6
Knowledge of the basic ideas of psychosomatic medicine and psychiatry	7	9	7
Skill at recognizing and managing social problems in clinical practice	8	8	8
Knowledge and skill at utilizing the ancillary services	9	7	9

at least usually they aren't; but it would be a shame if a person came and trusted his life to you, and you failed to recognize a disease that was a threat to his life.

I agree that this [mental illness] is just as important [as organic disease], that the patient is just as sick, feels just as miserable, as other patients, . . . but if I don't pick up what is troubling him for six months or so, I'm not apt to have altered his life much. On the other hand, if I overlook an organic illness for that long, I may be sued for malpractice—and probably should be.

These remarks also suggest the students' apprehension about the approaching responsibilities of internship, as do others quoted below.

Dissatisfaction with the GMC

Evidence from three sources indicated that the GMC students were dissatisfied with the opportunities their clerkship offered for learning traditional medicine: (1) GMC students judged their clerkship to be less helpful with respect to objectives they considered most important (those connected with traditional medicine) than the control students judged their clerkship; (2) the GMC students judged their gain in proficiency to be least in the areas of traditional medicine, whereas the control students judged their gain in proficiency to be greatest in these

Table 25.5. Students' ranking of the helpfulness of their clerkship with respect to objectives of senior program (class of 1956)

	1956 I		1956 II	
	GMC	Control	GMC	Control
Knowledge of the basic facts of clinical medicine (excluding psychosomatic medicine)	9	3	9	1
Skill at applying the facts of organic medicine to clinical practice	7	2	8	2
Knowledge of the basic ideas of psychosomatic medicine and psychiatry	8	5	1.5	8
Skill at applying the basic ideas of psychosomatic medicine and psychiatry to clinical practice	5	1	1.5	9
Ability to establish and maintain good physician-patient relations	1	4	4	5
Skill at recognizing and managing social problems in clinical practice	3	8	5	7
Knowledge and skill at utilizing the ancillary services	2	9	3	6
Knowing the practical application of the principles of comprehensive care in treating patients	4	7	6	4
Knowing how to organize diagnostic and therapeutic regimes	6	6	7	3

areas;[2] (3) the GMC students indicated that they expected the second-half surgery clerkship to be more helpful with respect to learning traditional medicine than did the control students.

Table 25.5 presents students' judgments of the helpfulness of their respective clerkships in connection with the nine objectives of the senior medical program. There was a strong negative relation between the first-half GMC group and the first-half control group. The GMC clerkship was judged far less helpful in increasing knowledge and skill in the basic aspects of organic medicine, but more helpful in training students to recognize and manage social problems, to utilize ancillary services, etc.; whereas the control clerkship was judged more helpful in the areas of traditional medicine, less helpful in the others. In the second-half groups this negative relation became even stronger—so much so that it can be summarized by saying that those objectives for which the control medical clerkship was judged

[2] It is important to note, however, that objective test data did not support these judgments. The objective measures of changes in (traditional) medical knowledge and skill during the senior year showed that, if any differences existed, it was the GMC students who made the greater gains.

most helpful, the GMC clerkship was judged least helpful, and vice versa. This strengthening of the negative relation in the second half points to intensified dissatisfaction with the special goals of the GMC as students approached the internship period.

Table 25.6 presents the data concerning the students' judgments of their own gains in proficiency in the nine areas. The comparison of Pretest and Posttest I ratings showed little change for the 1956 I GMC students. Skill at using the ancillary services rose from seventh to fourth place, and organizing diagnostic and therapeutic regimes dropped from fifth to eighth place. These changes, however, produced a negative relation between class ratings of objectives' importance and self-ratings of proficiency. On the other hand, these self-ratings changed greatly from

Table 25.6. Students' ranking of their own gain in proficiency with respect to the objectives of the senior program from Pretest to Posttest I and from Posttest I to Posttest II (class of 1956)

	1956 I				1956 II			
	GMC		Control		GMC		Control	
	Pre	Post I	Pre	Post I	Post I	Post II	Post I	Post II
Knowledge of the basic facts of clinical medicine (excluding psychosomatic medicine)	9	9	6	5	4	9	3	3
Skill at applying the facts of organic medicine to clinical practice	6	7	6	3	3	3.5	6	2
Knowledge of the basic ideas of psychosomatic medicine and psychiatry	8	6	4	8	9	8	7	7
Skill at applying the basic ideas of psychosomatic medicine and psychiatry to clinical practice	3	5	3	9	7	7	8	8
Ability to establish and maintain good physician-patient relations	1	1	1	1	1	1	1	1
Skill at recognizing and managing social problems in clinical practice	2	2	2	6	5	5	2	5
Knowledge and skill at utilizing the ancillary services	7	4	9	7	8	6	9	6
Knowing the practical application of the principles of comprehensive care in treating patients	4	3	8	4	2	2	5	4
Knowing how to organize diagnostic and therapeutic regimes	5	8	6	2	6	3.5	4	9

Pretest to Posttest I for the 1956 I control group, and these changes decreased markedly the discrepancy between those goals that the students considered important and those in which they considered themselves proficient. Organizing diagnostic and therapeutic regimes rose from sixth to second place; applying the facts of organic medicine rose from sixth (triple tie score) to third place; and practical application of the principles of comprehensive care rose from eighth to fourth place. At the same time recognizing and managing social problems dropped from second to sixth place; knowledge of the basic ideas of psychosomatic medicine dropped from fourth to eighth place; and skill at applying these facts dropped from third to ninth place. In other words, in the two first-half groups, the control students felt their proficiency had increased most in the areas they considered important, but GMC students did not.

Similar results were found in the 1956 II groups. Again, there was little change in the rankings from Posttest I to Posttest II for the GMC students. The only change of more than three rank order positions was in knowledge of the basic facts of clinical medicine, which dropped from fourth to ninth place. This change was again in the direction of increasing the negative relation between areas the students considered important and areas they considered themselves to be proficient in. On the other hand, several changes occurred in the 1956 II control group ratings. Applying the facts of organic medicine rose from sixth to second place, and recognizing and managing social problems dropped from second to fifth place. Skill at utilizing the ancillary services rose from ninth to sixth place, and organizing diagnostic and therapeutic regimes dropped from fourth to ninth place. The first two of these changes brought students more in line with class ratings of importance, but the second two brought them less in line with these ratings.

A third, somewhat less direct, piece of evidence tending to indicate that the GMC students were dissatisfied with their opportunities for learning traditional medicine was the differences between the expectations of GMC and control students for the helpfulness of their following clerkship (both groups were scheduled for the same clerkship subsequent to GMC or medicine—second-half surgery). Table 25.7 shows the percentages of GMC and control students expecting their second-half surgery clerkship to be extremely or very helpful in attaining the nine objectives of the senior year. It can be seen that a much greater percentage of GMC than control students had high expectations for acquiring more of the basic facts of clinical medicine, acquiring skill at applying the facts of organic medicine to clinical practice, and learning to organize diagnostic and therapeutic regimes—all traditional

Table 25.7. Percentage of students expecting their second-half surgery clerkship to be extremely or very helpful with respect to attaining the objectives of senior program (class of 1956)

	GMC	Control
Knowledge of the basic facts of clinical medicine (excluding psychosomatic medicine)	67	23
Skill at applying the facts of organic medicine to clinical practice	72	30
Knowledge of the basic ideas of psychosomatic medicine and psychiatry	11	16
Skill at applying the basic ideas of psychosomatic medicine and psychiatry to clinical practice	17	16
Ability to establish and maintain good physician-patient relations	28	8
Skill at recognizing and managing social problems in clinical practice	12	8
Knowledge and skill at utilizing the ancillary services	28	8
Knowing the practical application of the principles of comprehensive care in treating patients	33	8
Knowing how to organize diagnostic and therapeutic regimes	67	22

objectives. This finding is pertinent to the hypothesis that the GMC students were dissatisfied with their opportunities for learning traditional medicine. Among the medical students (and among the medical school staff) the surgery and GMC clerkships were generally regarded as representing opposite poles of clinical experience. Thus, if students were particularly critical of the one experience (GMC), it would be reasonable to suppose that they might hold a correspondingly high opinion of an experience (surgery) that they perceived as antithetical.

INTENSIFIED DISSATISFACTION WITH GMC OPPORTUNITIES

Interview data clearly suggested that both dissatisfaction with the opportunities for learning traditional medicine in the GMC and apprehension over the approaching responsibilities of internship and regular practice tended to intensify as the time for actually assuming these responsibilities came closer. Perhaps the most frequent complaint of GMC students was that they "didn't see enough pathology"; another recurring theme (which appeared also in the remarks previously quoted in this chapter) was the fear that a patient would die from some organic disorder overlooked by the physician:

> I feel that I haven't got as much in my senior year as I should have. . . . I feel that because of GMC I haven't seen as much pathology in my senior year as I did in my junior year. . . .
>
> What I'm most interested in is that I don't go out into practice and overlook some pathology that I didn't have the opportunity to see in medical

school because I spent my time down here [in the GMC]. . . . I'm not sure that I've had enough experience with these other diseases [other than psychiatric] to recognize one if it presented itself in my office.

I do feel definitely that when it comes to organic disease—listening to heart murmurs, being able to recognize chest pathology, abdominal disturbances—I probably lack something as compared with my buddies who are over in the other part [in the control clerkship].

I'm going to an internship next year, and the intern has quite a bit of responsibility. The intern has to know how to deal with emergencies as they come up; and it's medical problems he will be faced with more than psychological problems in most of these internships. I will be faced with organic problems and organic emergencies; and I think it is expected of the intern to be acquainted with most of these problems and be able to make some diagnoses and start some treatment, even before the resident gets into the ward.

The interview data were supported by the findings reported in Table 25.8, which shows the percentage of GMC students rating

Table 25.8. Change in percentage of GMC students rating themselves above average with respect to the objectives of senior program (class of 1956)

	1956 I			1956 II		
	Pre	Post I	Change	Post I	Post II	Change
Knowledge of the basic facts of clinical medicine (excluding psychosomatic medicine)	17	45	*28*	37	25	*—12*
Skill in applying the facts of organic medicine to clinical practice	17	62	*45*	37	38	*1*
Knowing how to organize diagnostic and therapeutic regimes	12	40	*28*	37	38	*1*
Knowing the practical application of the principles of comprehensive care in treating patients	12	62	*50*	44	50	*6*
Knowledge of the basic ideas of psychosomatic medicine and psychiatry	11	73	*62*	25	44	*19*
Skill at applying the basic ideas of psychosomatic medicine and psychiatry to clinical practice	23	66	*43*	25	50	*25*
Ability to establish and maintain good physician-patient relations	34	94	*60*	69	69	*0*
Skill at recognizing and managing social problems in clinical practice	17	77	*60*	31	38	*7*
Knowledge and skill at utilizing the ancillary services	12	73	*61*	6	38	*32*

themselves above average in nine areas of medical competence. In every area the increase from Pretest to Posttest I and from Posttest I to Posttest II in the percentage of students who rated themselves above average was greater among 1956 I students than among 1956 II students. (In one area, knowledge of the basic facts of clinical medicine, excluding psychosomatic medicine, fewer 1956 II students rated themselves above average after the GMC experience than had done so before the GMC experience.) This finding is the more striking because almost invariably more 1956 II GMC students rated themselves above average prior to the GMC experience; it is difficult to escape the conclusion that this is another piece of evidence for intensified dissatisfaction with the GMC program among the second-half students.

A final piece of evidence supporting this hypothesis was provided by data on students' reading. Table 25.9 presents the percentages of students reporting various amounts of reading about internal medicine and social phenomena in medicine. In the 1956 I group about the same percentage of GMC and control students reported reading about internal medicine, but in the 1956 II group the percentage of GMC students increased while the percentage of control students decreased markedly. Reports of reading about social phenomena were in striking contrast. In the 1956 I group more GMC than control students reported reading about social phenomena, but in the 1956 II group the percentage of GMC students who reported such reading fell below that of the control students, while the percentage of control students increased.

Another important finding is presented in Table 25.9. A much greater percentage of GMC students than control students reported reading about internal medicine during their second-half surgery clerkship. A smaller proportion of GMC students than control stu-

Table 25.9. Percentage of students reporting some, quite a lot, or very much reading about internal medicine and social phenomena in medicine during various clerkships (class of 1956)

	1956 I		1956 II	
	Social phenomena	Internal medicine	Social phenomena	Internal medicine
GMC	61	67	25	75
Control	31	61	50	39
GMC students in second-half surgery			17	73
Control students in second-half surgery			31	38

dents reported reading about social phenomena during their second-half surgery clerkship.

These results seem to indicate a greater concern on the part of the 1956 II GMC students over their proficiency in internal medicine, and they support the general hypothesis of an intensified dissatisfaction on the part of these students, a dissatisfaction which might well interfere with learning, especially in those non-traditional aspects of comprehensive medical care that were emphasized in the GMC Program.

Implications

It has been shown above that a scheduling effect existed in the results of the GMC Program; the program was definitely less successful in achieving its objectives with the second-half groups than with the first-half groups. This scheduling effect was more markedly apparent in connection with the special goals of the GMC Program (those having to do with the comprehensive care concept) than it was with respect to the more traditional areas of medicine. Analysis of pertinent data supported the following explanation of this scheduling effect: the students considered the traditional objectives of medical training (learning the facts and techniques of organic medicine) more important than the special goals of the GMC Program; they felt that the GMC presented inadequate opportunities for acquiring these traditional facts and techniques as the responsibilities of internship approached—with the apparent result that the GMC Program cannot be said to have attained its objectives during the second half of the senior year.

If the foregoing explanation is accepted, what are its implications for medical education? First of all, it demonstrates the well-known fact that educational efforts risk defeat whenever their objectives are not accepted as important by those who participate in them. Any attempt to convince medical students of the importance of an activity is likely to fail unless the students can readily perceive the importance of that activity in terms of their own goals. Although this research project concerned mainly the attitudes of the students toward a *special* set of objectives, the results may well imply that other, more conventional, objectives may not be reached because of students' attitudes toward them.

A second implication concerns the strategic planning of specific educational experiences for students in relation to the completion of their professional education. Specifically, it places in doubt the assumption that educational innovations *of this sort* will be successful in the senior year of medical school. It was assumed in this program that the "increased maturity" of senior medical students would make the senior year the most effective time to inculcate a broadened concept of medical practice. The results of this research indicate that this assumption is wrong.

The existence of the scheduling effect indicates that the medical students' beliefs about the requirements and responsibilities of the internship year must be considered when planning undergraduate curriculum. Should medical students believe that their major responsibilities as interns will concern matters of life and death, that the psychological and social problems of patients will not be among their major concerns, or among the concerns of their supervisors, then such beliefs must be reckoned with if undergraduate teachers and students are not to work at cross purposes.

Chapter 26

Relations between Individual Attributes and Performance in Medical School

At the time this research project was conceived, the results of many of the studies were expected to have a bearing on the problem of selecting medical students. Some of the findings reported above, the results of the study of students' performance in the GMC and some of the results of the study of changes in knowledge, skill, and attitudes during the senior year are relevant to this problem. However, the data reported in the following pages bear more specifically on the selection process than the material presented elsewhere in this volume.

The study of individual attributes and performance in medical school involved two kinds of analyses. First, correlations were computed between most of the individual attributes measured by the Individual Differences Section and the several annual grade averages; second, correlations were computed between responses to items from the biographical information part of the questionnaires (see Appendix 4) and the annual grade averages. In both analyses annual grade averages were used as measures of students' performance in medical school. Grade averages, despite their technical weaknesses, are the criteria regularly employed in studies of this sort and are likely to continue to be used for this purpose.

Relations between Individual Attributes and Grade Averages

Procedures

A correlational analysis, using the product-moment correlation technique, was carried out in which correlations were computed between a number of individual attributes and various grade averages. The individual attributes were grouped into six sets: conventional selection devices (premedical grade average and the four subtests of the Medical College Admission Test), peer judgments, attitudes (Authoritarian and General Anxiety scales), values, indices of social interaction, and needs. The technical adequacy of the instruments used to measure these individual attributes is discussed in Chapter 15.

Five grade averages were used as measures of performance: first-year, second-year, third-year, fourth-year, and cumulative grade averages. Intercorrelations among these five measures were fairly high, except that those between the fourth-year grade average and the other three tended to be low. Reliabilities of these measures were deemed satisfactory (see Chapter 15).

The subjects were all the students in the classes of 1954, 1955, and 1956. Scores on all tests (except the MCAT and premedical grade average) were obtained when the students were seniors. Hence, the design of this study differed from the usual selection research design in which attributes are measured before entrance into medical school.

Results and interpretation

The correlations between individual attributes and grade averages are presented below in six sections, each dealing with one of the sets of individual attributes listed above.

Conventional selection devices. The correlations between the five grade averages and both the premedical grade average (based on all undergraduate grades) and the four MCAT subtests are presented in Table 26.1. On the basis of this evidence, the premedical grade average appears to be a fairly good predictor of medical school performance. This finding is congruent with those reported by Gottheil and Michael, who, after reviewing the research literature, concluded that this grade average is the best single predictor of performance.[1] (See also below.)

These data (except those for the 1956 class) supported the hypothesis that the MCAT is a better predictor of first- and second-year (preclinical) performance than of third- and fourth-year (clinical) performance. In fact, the chief value of the MCAT appears to be its prediction of first-year grades, although the Knowledge of Premedical Sciences subtest is of some value in predicting second- and third-year grades.

None of the conventional selection devices appears to have been a useful predictor of fourth-year performance. This finding was not particularly surprising, however. First, during the fourth year the students'

[1] See E. Gottheil and C. M. Michael, "Predictor Variables Employed in Research on the Selection of Medical Students," *Journal of Medical Education* 32: 131–147, 1957.

Table 26.1. Correlation coefficients between conventional selection devices and grade averages in medical school (classes of 1954, 1955, and 1956)

		Grade averages				
	Class	First-year	Second-year	Third-year	Fourth-year	Cumulative
Premedical grade average	1954	.33†	.25*	—.02	.02	.14
	1955	.54†	.51†	.38†	.22	.47†
	1956	.35†	.35†	.32*	—.02	.29*
Medical College Admission Test						
Verbal Ability	1954	.22	.09	.09	—.05	.03
	1955	.39†	.21	.30*	.15	.32†
	1956	.09	.19	.18	.08	.18
Quantitative Ability	1954	.25*	—.05	—.09	—.07	—.17
	1955	.42†	.16	.18	.07	.27*
	1956	.07	.16	.00	.12	.08
Knowledge of Modern Society	1954	.14	.20	.21	—.15	.08
	1955	.29*	.12	.16	.04	.19
	1956	.03	.18	.15	.02	.11
Knowledge of Premedical Sciences	1954	.37†	.19	.04	—.08	.02
	1955	.56†	.35†	.30*	.14	.42†
	1956	.18	.25*	.20	.07	.23

* $p < .05$.
† $p < .01$.
Class of 1954, $N=76$; of 1955, $N=70$; of 1956, $N=62$.

activities are markedly different from those they engage in during the earlier years. They are applying their knowledge to actual problems of diagnosis and treatment instead of learning abstract facts and principles. Second, the staff members must base their grading of clinical performance on inferences about students' knowledge and ability instead of on achievement test scores. Third, the MCAT subtests were not designed to predict clinical performance. It would seem desirable to develop other tests for predicting diagnostic ability, skill in treatment, and the other competences of the clinical student.

Peer judgments. The outstanding feature of the correlations between peer judgments and grade averages, shown in Table 26.2, was the general increase in correlation value from first to fourth years (except for the 1954 class). This tendency was particularly noticeable where the leadership attributes were involved. In all three classes, however, judgments reflecting a student's leadership were more closely related to fourth-year performance, whereas aptitude measures and premedical grades were more closely related to first- and second-year performance.

Aside from the fact that the peer judgments were contemporary with the fourth-year grades, at least two interpretations of the correlations between peer judgments and grade averages suggest them-

Table 26.2. Correlation coefficients between peer judgments and grade averages in medical school (classes of 1954, 1955, and 1956)

		Grade averages				
	Class	First-year	Second-year	Third-year	Fourth-year	Cumulative
Leadership (ranking)	1954	.37†	.41†	.31†	.37†	.47†
	1955	.21	.32†	.28*	.56†	.41†
	1956	.27*	.20	.32*	.43†	.42†
Likeability (ranking)	1954	—.03	.04	.20	.04	.10
	1955	—.21	—.06	—.13	.20	—.07
	1956	—.10	—.06	—.13	.25*	.00
Willingness and ability to work independently (ranking)	1954	.32†	.34†	.26*	.21	.34†
	1955	.47†	.52†	.51†	.61†	.63†
	1956	.50†	.54†	.36†	.35†	.57†
Competence as a physician (nomination)	1954	.39†	.47†	.36†	.18	.41†
	1955	.34*	.44†	.47†	.53†	.53†
	1956	.44†	.53†	.56†	.64†	.71†

* $p < .05$.
† $p < .01$.
Class of 1954, $N=77$; of 1955, $N=70$; of 1956, $N=62$.

selves. First, leadership may be more relevant to the tasks of senior medical students than to those of preclinical students. That is, the same qualities that make for leadership, principally initiative, also make students tend to take hold of a case, to assume responsibility for the treatment of patients. This characteristic would probably result in their being favorably judged by the clinical instructors. Second, the staff might be subjectively influenced in their judgments by the leadership qualities of these students and give them better grades as a result.

The strong relation between peer-judged willingness and ability to work independently and grade averages may have resulted partly from the tendency of students to perceive this attribute as closely associated with both medical knowledge and competence as a physician (r = .72 and .53, respectively, in the 1956 class).

The fact that the students were fairly good judges of performance (as reflected in grades) can be seen from the correlations between peer-judged competence as a physician and grade averages. These correlations were spuriously low because of the highly skewed distributions of scores on this peer-nomination measure.

Attitudes. Like the rest of the personality characteristics measured, neither of the two attitudes measured was very highly correlated with performance (see Table 26.3). Authoritarian attitudes showed consistently negative relations with the grade averages, but no correlation value exceeded —.30. However, it is quite reasonable to expect

Table 26.3. Correlation coefficients between attitude scales and grade averages in medical school (classes of 1954, 1955, and 1956)

	Class	*N*	Grade averages: First-year	Second-year	Third-year	Fourth-year	Cumulative
F (Authoritarian) scale	1954	77	—.07	—.21	—.15	—.14	—.25*
	1955	70	—.01	—.06	—.27*	—.15	—.15
	1956	62	—.12	—.20	—.09	—.28*	—.24
General Anxiety scale	1955	62	.12	.17	.15	—.09	.07
	1956	62	.16	.10	.02	—.19	.02

* $p < .05$.

that students whose dispositions tended to be intolerant and inflexible would perform less well in medical school than other students.

The correlations involving the General Anxiety scale were too small to justify any meaningful inferences.

Values. According to Table 26.4, few of the six values measured were related to performance in medical school. In fact, no sizeable correlations were found between value scales and any of the other measures of individual attributes. Because these value scales are interdependent (see Chapter 15), they were not entirely appropriate for use

Table 26.4. Correlation coefficients between Study of Values scales and grade averages in medical school (classes of 1954, 1955, and 1956)

	Class	Grade averages: First-year	Second-year	Third-year	Fourth-year	Cumulative
Theoretical value	1954	—.15	—.01	—.23*	—.02	—.21
	1955	—.20	—.07	—.07	—.08	—.14
	1956	.11	.22	.19	.00	.16
Aesthetic value	1954	.07	.10	—.22	—.10	—.02
	1955	.17	.08	.22	.10	.18
	1956	—.02	.02	—.04	—.05	—.04
Economic value	1954	.14	.13	.09	—.05	.08
	1955	—.07	—.10	—.14	—.21	—.15
	1956	—.19	—.14	—.16	—.06	—.18
Political value	1954	—.06	.11	—.01	.09	.05
	1955	.21	.05	—.01	—.06	.06
	1956	—.06	—.01	—.05	.17	.02
Social value	1954	.00	—.10	.15	.02	.06
	1955	—.01	.07	.13	.12	.10
	1956	.10	.03	.19	.07	.14
Religious value	1954	—.02	—.16	.18	.07	.03
	1955	—.13	—.03	—.13	.09	—.09
	1956	.06	—.04	—.06	—.04	—.01

* $p < .05$.
Class of 1954, $N=78$; of 1955, $N=70$; of 1956, $N=62$.

in correlation studies. Nevertheless, it seems doubtful that these particular values were relevant to any of the variables with which this project was concerned.

Social interaction attributes. The correlations between social interaction attributes (measured by California Personality Inventory scales) and grade averages are presented in Table 26.5. (The CPI was not

Table 26.5. Correlation coefficients between California Psychological Inventory scales and grade averages in medical school (classes of 1955 and 1956)

		Grade averages				
	Class	First-year	Second-year	Third-year	Fourth-year	Cumulative
Achievement via Independence	1955	.14	.18	.23	.29*	.27*
	1956	.14	.17	.13	.15	.20
Intellectual Efficiency	1955	.23	.17	.21	.30*	.30*
	1956	—.05	.07	.00	.07	.05
Tolerance	1955	—.07	.00	.09	.22	.08
	1956	—.01	.01	—.04	.16	.05
Psychological-Mindedness	1955	—.00	.08	.21	.14	.15
	1956	—.08	.07	.01	.08	.04
Responsibility	1955	.14	.10	.23	.30*	.27*
	1956	—.01	.11	—.07	.11	.02
Achievement via Conformance	1955	—.01	.12	.18	.28*	.19
	1956	—.11	.00	.00	.05	—.02
Sense of Well-Being	1955	—.17	—.10	.01	.09	—.04
	1956	—.09	—.08	—.27*	.03	—.12
Self-Control	1955	—.10	.04	.05	.12	.04
	1956	.02	.14	—.10	.09	.03
Good Impression	1955	—.09	.08	.04	.16	.06
	1956	.04	.13	—.07	.11	.08
Socialization	1955	.10	.20	.14	.09	.16
	1956	—.11	—.10	—.04	.03	—.09
Dominance	1955	.11	.08	.15	.14	.15
	1956	—.05	—.06	.08	.02	.01
Sociability	1955	.02	.10	.11	.02	.08
	1956	—.04	—.12	—.03	—.08	—.06
Self-Acceptance	1955	.10	.10	.16	.20	.18
	1956	.00	—.08	.19	.03	.07
Social Presence	1955	.10	.08	.15	.12	.15
	1956	—.05	—.10	—.02	.05	.02
Capacity for Status	1955	.09	.00	.20	.12	.14
	1956	—.22	—.23	—.16	—.06	—.19
Flexibility	1955	—.08	—.19	—.03	—.01	—.07
	1956	—.06	—.13	—.09	—.06	—.07
Communality	1955	—.13	—.14	—.16	—.08	—.15
	1956	—.07	.04	.09	.19	.07
Femininity	1955	—.05	.16	.08	.13	.09
	1956	.17	.10	.00	.00	.07

* $p < .05$.
Class of 1955, $N = 69$; of 1956, $N = 62$.

Table 26.6. Correlation coefficients between Edwards Personal Preference Schedule scales and grade averages in medical school (class of 1956, $N = 62$)

	Grade averages				
	First-year	Second-year	Third-year	Fourth-year	Cumulative
n Achievement	.17	.35†	.21	.24	.32*
n Deference	.02	.24	.04	.15	.14
n Succorance	.06	.05	.10	.07	.11
n Abasement	.05	.08	.00	.08	.04
n Order	.09	.07	—.07	.01	.01
n Aggression	.07	.11	.09	—.04	.06
n Nurturance	.04	.00	.08	—.08	.03
n Endurance	—.09	—.01	—.05	.12	—.01
n Dominance	—.04	.04	—.04	.12	.05
n Intraception	—.01	—.03	—.03	.11	.02
n Autonomy	—.09	—.13	—.17	—.35†	—.27*
n Affiliation	—.16	—.27*	—.05	—.04	—.15
n Exhibition	—.23	—.15	—.02	—.01	—.12
n Heterosexuality	.04	—.15	—.10	—.15	—.11
n Change	—.07	—.13	.02	—.15	—.09
Consistency	.17	.19	.26*	.03	.22

* $p < .05$.
† $p < .01$.

administered to the class of 1954.) None of these relations was very strong; no correlation value exceeded .30. However, the scale intended to measure personal qualities associated with good undergraduate performance, Achievement via Independence, was most closely related to the index of over-all performance in medical school ($r = .27$ and .20 in 1955 and 1956, respectively). In the 1955 class the Intellectual Efficiency and Responsibility scales significantly differentiated the superior students from the less able ones, particularly in fourth-year performance ($r = .30$ for both scales). But in the 1956 class these correlations dropped to nearly zero.[2] The lack of consistency warns against attempting to interpret these findings.

Needs. The last set of correlations to be reported here involves the need scales of the Edwards Personal Preference Schedule (see Table 26.6). It is unfortunate that this instrument was not used with the classes of 1954 and 1955 because the n Achievement and n Autonomy scales appear to have some promise of value as predictors of medical school performance (correlations with cumulative grade average were .32 and —.27, respectively).

The n Achievement scale, which reflects a general concern for doing well and becoming a success, should be of particular interest to educators concerned with medical student selection. One reason is that

[2] It is possible that these results reflect the supposed difference between the class of 1956 and others, see Chapter 10.

the EPPS is so constructed that it is difficult to fake; thus it avoids a common weakness of personality measures used as selection instruments. A second reason is that n Achievement in conjunction with n Affiliation has been shown to be positively related (n Affiliation being negatively related) to graduate performance in clinical psychology.[3] The technique used to measure n Achievement and n Affiliation in the study of students in clinical psychology was different from the EPPS scale. Nevertheless, the similarity of findings was striking, especially when one notes that the pattern of "positive correlation with n Achievement, negative correlation with n Affiliation" holds for second-year grade average to a statistically significant degree ($r = .35$ and $-.27$, respectively, in Table 26.6).

N Autonomy was negatively related to grade averages in the clinical years, but almost unrelated to grade averages in the preclinical years (see Table 26.6). It will be remembered that autonomy needs (as defined by the EPPS) are represented by desires to come and go freely, to say what one thinks, and to feel able to be unconventional if one wishes. Quite possibly students who feel a need for this type of independence do not meet with the approval of clinical instructors, who stress the importance of responsibility to duty and the other kinds of conformity.

Further considerations

It was noted above that, among conventional selection indices, premedical grade average was the best predictor of medical school grades. Analysis has shown that it was also the best single predictor among all the individual attribute tests used in this study. This result matches the conclusion of Gottheil and Michael.[4]

The data discussed above also indicated that the premedical grade average and the MCAT Knowledge of Premedical Sciences subtest were the two best predictors of cumulative grade average. An index of the predictive value of these two measures taken together is a multiple correlation coefficient. The multiple correlation coefficients for the classes of 1955 and 1956 were .55 and .36, respectively. Whitaker, Kelly, and Uhr have reported a multiple r of .61 between the same two predictor measures and a general medical achievement factor, which was closely related to cumulative grade average.[5] Gottheil and Michael

[3] See Byron L. Groesbeck, "Toward Description of Personality in Terms of Configurations of Motives," in J. W. Atkinson (ed.), *Motives in Fantasy, Action, and Society: A Method of Assessment and Study* (Princeton: Van Nostrand, 1958).

[4] *Op. cit.*

[5] See W. L. Whitaker, E. L. Kelly, and L. Uhr, "A Brief Statement Regarding the Michigan Project on the Prediction of Professional Competence in Medicine." Presented at the meeting of the AAMC in Colorado Springs, Colorado, October 1956.

note that several multiple correlation coefficients reported in the literature fall near .60.[6]

More interesting than these statistics, however, was the apparent effect on the teaching staff of the correlation between the MCAT Knowledge of Premedical Sciences subtest and the premedical grade average. When the subtest (a measure of knowledge) and the grade average (a measure of achievement) were highly correlated ($r = .34$ in the 1955 class), it was noted by the research group that the class as a whole was generally well thought of by the faculty. But when the correlation tended to be very low ($r = .07$ in the 1956 class) the research group noted that the staff tended to be rather highly critical of the class as a whole. This effect was probably due to the relation between these variables rather than to the level of knowledge or ability in the class, because the class mean scores on these MCAT tests did not differ in a manner consistent with the latter interpretation. Of course, a sample of two classes is a small number on which to test a hypothesis. Nevertheless, this correlation can be computed from the records in most admissions offices. If the correlation between knowledge and achievement on the one hand and the staff's evaluation of the class on the other is found to hold, it may very well be possible to determine the "teachability" of a class before it enters the classroom. Perhaps such correlations (and their effects) can be altered through the selection process.

A final interesting feature of the correlates of medical school performance was the similarity among the three personality characteristics most closely related to performance throughout the four years. Peer-judged willingness and ability to work independently, the CPI Achievement via Independence scale, and the EPPS n Achievement scale were conceptually[7] related by the common component of independence. This similarity is obvious for the first two measures but less so in the case of need for achievement. However, research on need for achievement has shown that independence training in childhood is related to strength of need for achievement.[8] Other studies have shown the association of qualities involving independence (resistance to group pressures which interfere with good task performance) with need for achievement strength.[9] Hence, it appears that the quality of independ-

[6] *Op. cit.*

[7] Empirically, the three personality measures were not closely related. For the class of 1956 Achievment was correlated .22 and .25 with peer-judged Independence and the CPI Achievement via Independence scale, respectively. But the latter two measures were correlated —.07 and .10 in the 1956 and 1955 classes.

[8] See M. R. Winterbottom, "The Relation of Childhood Training in Independence to Achievement Motivation" (unpublished Ph.D. thesis, University of Michigan, 1953).

[9] See D. C. McClelland, J. W. Atkinson, E. L. Lowell, and R. A. Clark, *The Achievement Motive* (New York: Appleton, 1953).

ence is an important component of success in medical school[10] and that the development of a test of independence in approach to achievement goals (in the medical profession) is a promising project for those interested in the improvement of medical student selection. Also needed is a device for measuring needs (like the Edwards Personal Preference Schedule) in which the items are couched in medical terminology.

Relations between Biographical Data and Grade Averages

Deitrick and Berson have noted the need for more studies of background information as a potential predictor of medical school performance.[11] However, according to Gottheil and Michael, results of investigations of this type "have varied remarkably."[12] None of the conventional items of biographical information has been consistently related to performance. Since the number of these studies is not large, it was decided to carry out such an analysis of data in the attempt to contribute more information.

In addition to conventional background items, the questions found by Barron[13] to predict graduate school performance were used in this study to discover whether similarities existed between attributes predictive of performance in two different kinds of graduate education programs. (The generality of these findings is, of course, restricted by the lack of replication.) Items from the future plans part of the questionnaire were compared with grade averages to find out whether class standing was related to choice of specialty and to type of future professional activity preferred. Again, first-year, second-year, third-year, fourth-year, and cumulative grade averages were used as measures of medical school performance.

Curvilinear as well as linear relations were sought in the analysis of the data obtained from the 1956 class ($N = 63$). (Only incomplete data were available for the other two classes.) The results of the analysis were uniformly negative. Some of the variables found *not* to be related to performance beyond the .05 level of significance were age, marital status, hours of outside work, schooling and occupation of

[10] This statement may need qualification in light of the negative correlation found between n Autonomy and performance. The kind of independence represented by need for Autonomy (independence from group pressures *in general*) may include independence from pressures to do one's work well. If so, need for Autonomy could counteract some of the forces pushing medical students toward better performance and thus result in poorer performance.

[11] See J. E. Deitrick and R. C. Berson, *Medical Schools in the United States at Mid-Century* (New York: McGraw-Hill, 1953).

[12] *Op. cit.*, p. 140.

[13] See F. Barron, *Personal Soundness in University Graduate Students*, University of California Publication in Personality Assessment Research No. 1 (Berkeley: University of California Press, 1954).

parents, incidence of physicians in the family, type of community lived in, religious preference, undergraduate major subject, choice of specialty, and preferred professional activity. Thus, the generally negative results of studies of these variables reported by Gottheil and Michael were replicated in this study; none of the results reported by Barron were found in this study.

It was expected that information pertinent to medical student selection would be obtained by correlating both measures of individual attributes and biographical data with the annual grade averages of the medical students. It was noted that the design of this study was not entirely comparable with that of a selection research project, since some of the data were obtained after the students had been in medical school for three to four years.

Performance in the first two (preclinical) years was best predicted by the subtests of the MCAT and by the premedical grade average. Personality characteristics indicative of independent striving toward achievement were also somewhat related to earlier performance in medical school.

The MCAT scores were related to performance indices for the last two (clinical) years to only a small extent. And the premedical grade average showed only a weak relation to the fourth-year grade average. However, personality characteristics indicative of independent striving toward achievement continued to show a fair amount of correlation with grades. In addition, peer-judged leadership and likeability were quite closely associated with grades for the last two years of medical school. Students with strong autonomy needs tended to be graded down in their senior year.

Over-all performance in medical school (cumulative grade average) was best predicted by premedical grade average and the Knowledge of Premedical Sciences subtest of the MCAT. The biographical information items had no value as predictors of performance.

APPENDICES

Appendix I

Sound-Film Interview Test

Verbatim Account of the Interview

Doctor: Can you tell me just why you came to the hospital?
Patient: Well, yes, I had been in the hospital in Espanola, New Mexico, and this doctor sent me to Dr. ——.
Doctor: What kind of trouble have you been having in the past year or so?
Patient: Oh, pain in my lower left side.
Doctor: Do you have trouble with your bowels?
Patient: Well, not too much, no.
Doctor: Do you ever have diarrhea or constipation?
Patient: Well, not unless I'm taking medicine for pain or a lot of aspirin or things like that.
Doctor: This pain that you've had—has been the main thing that's bothered you?
Patient: Yes.
Doctor: Have you had other illnesses in the past?
Patient: Well, I was operated on a little over a year ago for gall bladder trouble, and I had had two operations before that.
Doctor: Have you ever had any other operations in regard to this pain in your side?
Patient: Two.
Doctor: Two other ones. Have you been taking some medicine recently?
Patient: Well, I took sick the 23rd of February, and they give a lot of IV's and penicillin, streptomycin, sulfa, aureomycin.
Doctor: Was that this pain in your left side?
Patient: Yes.
Doctor: Have you always been overweight?
Patient: Yes. Well, I have been since I was nineteen.
Doctor: Have you been on diets?
Patient: Yes, I've started taking thyroid, took a basal metabolism test, and that's been a little over a year ago.
Doctor: Do you like to eat?
Patient: Well, pretty well. Since my gall bladder's out, not too well; seems I can't hardly stand greasy things.
Doctor: Do you follow a diet pretty closely to try to lose weight?

Patient: Well, I was on this diet and then I took sick, and they took me off of it and put me on strained baby food, and I haven't been back on this diet.

Doctor: When you get this trouble in your left side, do you ever get sick to your stomach?

Patient: Oh, yes, that's the way it starts, is vomiting.

Doctor: Where were you born?

Patient: In Fort Morgan, Colorado.

Doctor: How far did you go in school?

Patient: The first semester of my senior year.

Doctor: What kind of things did you like to do when you were in school?

Patient: Oh, home economics, I liked sewing and cooking.

Doctor: Do you enjoy running a house?

Patient: Yes.

Doctor: What kinds of jobs have you had?

Patient: None, other than just homemaker.

Doctor: How long have you been married?

Patient: It was twenty years the 28th of December.

Doctor: Do you have some children?

Patient: Yes.

Doctor: And how old are they?

Patient: I have a boy that was nineteen the 19th of March, and one that was seventeen the 6th of March, and a daughter that was thirteen the 27th of January.

Doctor: And your children are at home now?

Patient: No, I have a boy that's studying for the ministry at Las Cruces, New Mexico, and the other two are in school.

Doctor: What does your husband do?

Patient: He's a steamfitter for Blank Company at Plainsville, New Mexico.

Doctor: What kind of job did your father have?

Patient: He was a farmer.

Doctor: Did you have a lot of brothers and sisters?

Patient: There was ten of us in the family.

Doctor: When you were a young girl did your family seem to have enough money to get along on?

Patient: Well, we got along, we always worked, we worked on the farm, worked.

Doctor: Did you have a pretty happy childhood?

Patient: Yes.

Doctor: Or did you have to work awfully hard?

Patient: We had to work but Mother and Dad helped; we all worked together and was happy.

Doctor: Do you and your husband have a lot of friends?

Patient: Yes.

Doctor: What kind of things do the two of you like to do when you get a little time off?

Patient: Well, we're so busy in our church work. He's Sunday School superintendent, and I teach Sunday School class, and that keeps us pretty well busy.

Doctor: How often have your menstrual periods been?

Patient: Well, they never have been regular, I never have known.

Doctor: Have they changed at all during the past year?

Patient: Well, ah, they've been more regular in the past, well, in a little more than a year.
Doctor: How do you think this trouble you're having now is going to affect your future health?
Patient: Well, I hope it's better. They seem to think that it will after they take out this part of the intestine, it will help.
Doctor: Are you pretty anxious to have this operation?
Patient: No, I just had one in August. I know it has to be done, but I'm not anxious for it.
Doctor: You don't enjoy surgery.
Patient: No, I don't.
Doctor: Are you afraid of it?
Patient: No, I'm not specially afraid, I just, you kind of remember your suffering in six months.
Doctor: How many children are at home with you?
Patient: Two.
Doctor: Who's taking care of them?
Patient: Oh, a neighbor and then my husband went back yesterday. And he's coming back Sunday and then they have their spring vacation, next week, and then they'll be here with my parents.

Additional Information about Patient

PRESENT ILLNESS

The patient was admitted in March 1953, complaining of pain in the left lower quadrant of her abdomen, intermittently, since August 1951. At that time she suddenly developed left lower quadrant pain, vomiting, and fever, for which she had an abdominal operation in New Mexico. She is said to have had peritonitis, due to a ruptured viscus. There was no prior history of abdominal pain, nausea, vomiting, or disordered bowel function. Since this operation, she has had recurrent episodes of left lower quadrant pain, associated with nausea and vomiting often, and with diarrhea occasionally. Because of this recurrent illness, she was referred to this hospital.

During the past two years, she developed acute cholecystitis, for which a cholecystectomy was performed. Gall bladder disease was not associated with the illness described above.

PAST HISTORY

In 1939 she had an unknown type surgical procedure involving one Fallopian tube; in 1949, pneumonia. *System Review*: The system review is essentially non-contributory. She has had occasional occipital headaches; irregular menses since the menarche, and obesity, for which thyroid extract has been intermittently administered.

PHYSICAL EXAMINATION

T 37 (orally); P 80; R 18; B P 120/70. The patient did not appear ill on admission. The thyroid gland was not palpable. The heart and lungs revealed no remarkable signs. The abdomen was obese with well-healed, right upper quadrant and lower midline scars. The liver was palpated one finger breadth below the right costal margin; there was slight tenderness with slight rebound but little spasm in the left lower quadrant. No masses were palpated. The pelvic and rectal examinations revealed only slight tenderness referred to the left lower quadrant.

LABORATORY

Hgb. 13.8 gms; RBC 4.16; WBC 7,400 with normal differential. The urine was normal. STS negative.

Test of Knowledge and Skill

In all the multiple choice questions, please write on the answer sheet the number of the *one* answer which you think is most nearly correct.

1. At the time of operation in New Mexico in 1951, the most likely ruptured viscus was:
   1. Vermiform appendix
   2. Meckel's diverticulum
   3. Peptic ulcer of the duodenum
   4. Diverticulum of the sigmoid colon
   5. Ileum, involved by regional enteritis
2. If this patient remained in the hospital for a prolonged period of time, considering her background, the following group might logically help in providing care for her children:
   1. Department of Public Welfare
   2. Her church organization
   3. Visiting Nurse Association
   4. Children's and Family Service of the Community Chest
   5. Social Service Department of the Public School System
3. The episodes of left lower quadrant pain, nausea, vomiting, and diarrhea occurring since 1951 are probably due to:
   1. Peritoneal adhesions
   2. Regional enteritis
   3. Sigmoid diverticulitis
   4. Pelvic inflammatory disease
   5. Duodenal ulcer
4. With good comprehensive medical care by the family physician, directed toward the obesity problem in this patient, what are the chances of reducing this patient to a normal weight and keeping her there:
   1. 0%
   2. 10%
   3. 50%
   4. 70%
   5. 90%
5. Assuming that this patient's obesity is related to overeating, the best treatment is a *low calorie diet* and:
   1. Dexedrine sulfate and thyroid extract
   2. Thyroid extract
   3. Dexedrine sulfate

4. Psychotherapy
5. A ten block walk every day

6. In the management of this case, which statement is applicable:
   1. This patient's obesity should respond satisfactorily to dietary restriction and drug therapy
   2. This patient has few emotional problems and psychotherapy is not indicated
   3. A weight reduction diet is contraindicated because of the intestinal pathology
   4. This patient's gastrointestinal symptoms would be accentuated if emotional conflicts are explored, therefore psychotherapy is not indicated
   5. Psychotherapy should be considered a necessary adjunct in the management of this patient's obesity
7. Chronic cholecystitis with cholelithiasis is effectively treated by:
   1. Low fat diet
   2. Low calorie diet
   3. Orally administered bile salts
   4. Tincture of belladonna
   5. None of the above
8. In patients with gastrointestinal disorders, it can generally be stated that:
   1. Intestinal secretions are predominantly under the control of local humoral factors and, therefore, are little influenced by emotions
   2. Emotional problems seen in patients with intestinal disorders occur chiefly as the result of the patient's having the disease
   3. Peptic ulcer and ulcerative colitis are the only gastrointestinal disorders in which emotional stress is thought to play a significant role
   4. The symptoms of all gastrointestinal disorders are influenced by emotional stress
   5. Emotional reactions influence the gastrointestinal motility and secretions, but not the pain threshold
9. Which of the following diseases is *not* associated with obesity:
   1. Hyperinsulinism
   2. Tumor producing destruction of the hypothalamus
   3. Basophilic adenoma of the pituitary gland
   4. Hypogonadism
   5. Infarct of the pituitary
10. During this and previous film interviews, the physician doing the interviewing demonstrated the following:
    1. His warmth automatically makes the patient want to talk about his or her emotional problems
    2. His direct questions bring forth the maximum amount of information
    3. His direct questions often prevent the patient from expressing his emotions freely
    4. He appears concerned about the development of an adequate relation with each patient

5. He frequently tries to probe too deeply into the patient's emotional problems

11. Which of the following would be of no value in the differential diagnosis of acute abdominal pain:
    1. Examination of the gums
    2. Examination of the under side of the tongue
    3. Eosinophil count
    4. Examination of the teeth
    5. Spinal fluid pressure
12. In general, when an adequate physician-patient relation is established, one would anticipate that:
    1. The patient would not question the doctor's decisions
    2. The patient would repress his emotional conflicts
    3. The patient would idealize the physician
    4. The patient would develop some degree of dependence upon the physician
    5. All the above
13. Assume that you were the family physician for this patient in a city of 500,000 population; which of the following (one or more) would you ask to consult with you regarding this case:
    1. Visiting nurse
    2. Social worker
    3. Physical therapist
    4. Dietician
    5. Internist or internal medical subspecialist
    6. Surgeon or surgical subspecialist
    7. Psychiatrist
    8. Other specialist (dermatologist, radiologist, otolaryngologist, gynecologist, etc.)
    9. No need for consultation in this case

Estimation of Age

14. What is the age of this patient?
    Estimate the patient's age and write *one* number in the space provided on the answer sheet.

Estimation of Intelligence

15. Estimate this patient's IQ on the scale below and write the number on the answer sheet that corresponds to the scale point selected.

IQ	80	85	90	95	100 (average)	105	110	115	120
	1	*2*	*3*	*4*	*5*	*6*	*7*	*8*	*9*

Estimation of Vocabulary Level

The Wechsler-Bellevue Form 1 vocabulary test was administered to each patient. The student's task was as follows:

16. Estimate the first word in the list which this patient could not explain.
17. Estimate the first three words missed in a row by this patient.

Estimation of Personality Characteristics

This patient was asked: "How much are you concerned with what the doctor thinks of you as a person?"

18. The patient described himself as being:
19. The patient "really" is:

1. Extremely concerned
2. Very concerned
3. More than most people
4. About the same as most people
5. Less than most people
6. Unconcerned
7. Don't care at all

This patient was asked: "Do you feel that you are . . . ."

20. The patient described himself as being:
21. The patient "really" is:

1. Extremely critical of yourself
2. Overly critical of yourself
3. More critical of yourself than most people
4. Just as critical as most people
5. Less critical than most people
6. Not very critical of yourself
7. Never critical of yourself

This patient was asked: "How do you feel about your health and your past illnesses? Have you had . . . ."

22. The patient described himself as being:
23. The patient "really" is:

1. More trouble than anyone you know
2. Far more than most people
3. More than most people
4. About as much as most people
5. Less than most people
6. Far less than most people
7. Less than anyone you know

This patient was asked: "How has your illness affected your spirits? Has it made you . . . ."

24. The patient described himself as being:
25. The patient "really" is:

1. Extremely depressed and sad
2. Very depressed and sad
3. More depressed and sad than most people would be
4. About as depressed and sad as most people would be
5. Less than most people would be
6. Far less depressed and sad than most people would be
7. Hasn't affected you at all

This patient was asked: "When you have had dealings with people, how have you found them to be? Was there . . . ."

26. The patient described himself as being:

27. The patient "really" is:

1. No one you could really trust
2. A few you could trust
3. Some you could trust
4. You could trust about half the people
5. More than half you could trust
6. Almost all could be trusted
7. No one you couldn't trust

This patient was asked: "Some people are depressed, worry too much, have a lack of confidence, and are unable to concentrate. Would you say that you are usually . . . ."

28. The patient described himself as being:

29. The patient "really" is:

1. Not at all like this
2. Very little like this
3. Some of it fits; most of it doesn't
4. Some of it fits; some of it doesn't
5. Most of it fits you
6. Fits you well
7. Fits you perfectly

This patient was asked: "How active a person have you been? Have you been engaged in . . . ."

30. The patient described himself as being:

31. The patient "really" is:

1. Very many different activities
2. Many activities
3. Quite a few
4. Some
5. Not many
6. A few
7. Very few different activities

This patient was asked: "Do you have your best times when you are . . . ."

32. The patient described himself as being:

33. The patient "really" is:

1. With a large number of strangers
2. With a large number of people, many of them strangers
3. With a large number of friends and strangers
4. With some friends and some strangers
5. With a small group of friends
6. With a few close friends
7. Alone

34. To what extent does this patient's case provide good teaching material for senior medical students?
    1. Provides excellent teaching material
    2. Provides very good teaching material
    3. Provides good teaching material
    4. Provides fair teaching material
    5. Provides poor teaching material
    6. Provides very poor teaching material
    7. Provides terrible teaching material

Differential Memory Test

This is a test of your ability to remember the content of the film interview. In each of the questions below, select the answer that most closely corresponds to the response that the patient gave.

35. Does she ever get sick to her stomach?
    1. Sometimes
    2. Seldom
    3. Yes, vomiting
    4. Constantly
    5. None of the above
36. Did she come from a large family?
    1. Nine children
    2. Two brothers and four sisters
    3. Five sisters and three brothers
    4. Nine brothers and sisters
    5. Four children
37. Did she have to work hard when she was young?
    1. Not especially
    2. Yes, very hard
    3. About the same as most people
    4. They all worked together
    5. Sometimes
38. What does her husband do?
    1. Engineer for Blank Company at Plainsville
    2. Steamfitter
    3. School superintendent
    4. Minister
    5. None of the above
39. How many of her children are at home with her?
    1. The oldest one
    2. The youngest one
    3. The two oldest
    4. The youngest and the oldest
    5. The two youngest
40. When was she married?
    1. Before 1930
    2. 1930–35

3. 1935–40
4. After 1940
5. Film does not give exact information

41. When was her last operation?
    1. Last fall
    2. Last winter
    3. Last spring
    4. Last summer
    5. Over a year ago
42. Which medicine has she *not* received lately?
    1. Thyroid
    2. Penicillin
    3. Streptomycin
    4. Sulfa
    5. Aureomycin

Appendix 2

Medical Attitudes Test

This is a study of what medical students and people in the medical field think about a number of social and medical questions. The best answer to each statement below is *your personal opinion.* We have tried to cover many different points of view. You will find yourself strongly in favor of some and disagree strongly with others. For some statements your opinion will not be as clear cut. Whichever way you feel about any of the statements you can be certain that a good many people feel the way you do. *Be sure to answer every item.* After all, no knowledge, but only your opinion is involved. Think quickly; your immediate reaction to the statement is probably the best one.

Read each statement carefully. Below it are five possible answers numbered 1, 2, 3, 4, and 5, to correspond with your answer sheet. Choose the answer you think best represents the way you feel.

1. How important do you think it is for the doctor to know the effect of the patient's illness on his family in order to provide adequate treatment?
   1. Not important at all
   2. Pretty unimportant
   3. Not so important
   4. Pretty important
   5. Very important

2. The greatest service a physician can provide is in following long term health and adjustment of patients and families rather than in concentrating only on the treatment of immediate illness complaints of his patients.
   1. Strongly disagree
   2. Disagree
   3. Undecided
   4. Agree
   5. Strongly agree

3. In medical practice today there are sufficient specialists so that a physician in general practice should not assume long term responsibility for his patients.
   1. Completely disagree
   2. Disagree
   3. Undecided
   4. Agree for the most part
   5. Completely agree

4. The medical school should train students for specialties rather than general practice.
   1. Disagree completely
   2. Disagree
   3. Undecided
   4. Agree
   5. Agree completely

5. Do you think that as a physician you would prefer to have for your patients all members of a family rather than patients as individuals?
   1. Definitely not
   2. No
   3. Undecided
   4. Yes
   5. Definitely yes

6. The most important function of the physician is to immediately relieve the suffering of the patient.
   1. Strongly disagree
   2. Disagree
   3. Undecided
   4. Agree
   5. Strongly agree

7. In a general practice there is no reason to stress good health and promote disease prevention since the average patient only wants to pay for the alleviation of his disease.
   1. For practically no cases at all
   2. For very few cases
   3. For some cases
   4. For most cases
   5. For practically all cases

8. How practical do you think it is for a doctor in clinical practice to take time to follow up provocative clues other than the presenting symptoms?
   1. It is always impractical
   2. It is usually impractical

3. Undecided
4. It is usually practical
5. It is always practical

9. Do you think medical training in the clinical years should concentrate most of the student's time on evaluation and treatment of specific disease processes?
   1. Definitely not
   2. No
   3. Undecided
   4. Yes
   5. Definitely yes

10. A specialist such as an otologist, gynecologist, psychiatrist, etc., generally would be less effective on a routine home call than a general practitioner.
    1. Strongly disagree
    2. Disagree
    3. Undecided
    4. Agree
    5. Strongly agree

11. Do you think that in a medical setting, the doctor should have all personnel involved in the treatment of patients participate in case discussions regardless of their profession?
    1. Almost never
    2. Not very often
    3. Quite often
    4. Usually
    5. Almost always

12. To what extent do you think a medical doctor in a clinical team should consult with the team members, such as social worker, psychologist, etc., before making basic decisions in the management of the patient, such as discharge, referrals, or pronounced changes in therapy?
    1. In none of his cases
    2. In some of his cases
    3. In about half of his cases
    4. In most of his cases
    5. In nearly all of his cases

13. How important do you think it is to have nonmedical specialists included on a treatment team in a medical setting?
    1. Not important at all
    2. Pretty unimportant
    3. Not so important
    4. Pretty important
    5. Very important

14. The medical doctor in a clinical team consisting of psychologist, social worker, nurse, therapists, and technicians should take a decidedly directive rather than coordinating position if treatment is to be effective.
    1. Strongly disagree
    2. Disagree
    3. Undecided
    4. Agree
    5. Strongly agree

15. How important do you think it is for a physician to actively participate in organized state public health programs?
    1. Not important at all
    2. Pretty unimportant
    3. Not so important
    4. Pretty important
    5. Very important

16. A medical doctor is free to decide whether or not he wants to accept the opinion of a consultant.
    1. Almost never
    2. Seldom
    3. Undecided
    4. Quite often
    5. Almost always

17. In general clinical practice a medical social worker is unnecessary provided an experienced nurse is available.
    1. Disagree completely
    2. Disagree
    3. Undecided
    4. Agree for the most part
    5. Agree completely

18. A medical doctor should accept the opinion of a consultant without reservation.
    1. Never
    2. Seldom
    3. Undecided
    4. Most of the time
    5. Always

19. After a physician has explained the medical diagnosis and prognosis of a patient to his relatives he refers the family to the social worker for further discussion of their reactions to the patient's diagnosis and illness. How good a practice do you think this is?
    1. A very poor practice

2. A somewhat poor practice
3. Undecided
4. A fairly good practice
5. A very good practice

20. A patient's ability to pay for medical services should not influence treatment given by the doctor.
    1. Strongly disagree
    2. Disagree
    3. Undecided
    4. Agree
    5. Strongly agree

21. Adequate treatment cannot be done unless personal relations with patients are kept to a minimum.
    1. Disagree completely
    2. Disagree
    3. Undecided
    4. Agree for the most part
    5. Agree completely

22. A doctor generally should refuse to care for patients that definitely indicate unfavorable response to treatment.
    1. Completely disagree
    2. Disagree
    3. Undecided
    4. Agree for the most part
    5. Completely agree

23. How often do you think that to do an adequate job as a doctor, your personal life should be subordinated to the demands of caring for patients?
    1. Not very often
    2. Quite often
    3. About half the time
    4. Almost always
    5. Always

24. In general practice a doctor should refuse to treat patients with disease processes because he is not interested in them. To what extent do you agree?
    1. Strongly disagree
    2. Disagree
    3. Undecided
    4. Agree
    5. Strongly agree

25. Do you think a doctor should feel free to refuse the care of patients who he thinks will be uncooperative?
    1. He almost never should refuse
    2. He usually should not refuse
    3. Undecided
    4. He occasionally should refuse
    5. He almost always should refuse

26. Generally the more illnesses a doctor sees the less concerned he will be with the suffering of patients.
    1. Completely disagree
    2. Disagree
    3. Undecided
    4. Agree for most part
    5. Completely agree

27. How much should a doctor try to find out about the personal problems of his patients in addition to problems related to their illnesses?
    1. Hardly anything at all
    2. Very little
    3. Not so much
    4. Very much
    5. As much as possible

28. How much do you think patients can contribute to the treatment process during their illness?
    1. Practically nothing
    2. Very little
    3. Only a limited amount
    4. Quite a lot
    5. A very large amount

29. Do you think that in a regular office practice a busy doctor can provide time to talk with each individual patient about problems other than his immediate complaints?
    1. Almost never
    2. Not very often
    3. Undecided
    4. Usually
    5. Almost always

30. Most people who are interested in psychiatry have emotional problems of their own.
    1. Disagree completely
    2. Disagree somewhat
    3. Undecided
    4. Agree somewhat
    5. Agree completely

31. The great majority of so-called mental disorders can be traced directly to an hereditary tendency of some sort.
   1. Disagree completely
   2. Disagree somewhat
   3. Undecided
   4. Agree somewhat
   5. Agree completely

32. Psychiatric treatment is a luxury rather than a real necessity to most patients who ask for it.
   1. Disagree completely
   2. Disagree somewhat
   3. Undecided
   4. Agree somewhat
   5. Agree completely

33. An emotional upset should be as acceptable an excuse for missing a final examination as would a severe cold.
   1. Disagree completely
   2. Disagree somewhat
   3. Undecided
   4. Agree somewhat
   5. Agree completely

34. A sound practitioner reserves his time for really ill persons rather than neurotic ones.
   1. Disagree completely
   2. Disagree somewhat
   3. Undecided
   4. Agree somewhat
   5. Agree completely

35. The exclusive use of simple reassurance and placebos (e.g., sugar pills and other palliative techniques) in the treatment of neurotics is justified in view of the lack of evidence concerning the effectiveness of more complicated therapy.
   1. Disagree completely
   2. Disagree somewhat
   3. Undecided
   4. Agree somewhat
   5. Agree completely

36. It is useful for society to divide people into categories of "sane" or "insane."
   1. Disagree completely
   2. Disagree somewhat
   3. Undecided

4. Agree somewhat
5. Agree completely

37. Patients ill with emotional disorders number more than the total of civilian patients in our hospitals for all the medical and surgical illnesses put together.
    1. Disagree completely
    2. Disagree somewhat
    3. Undecided
    4. Agree somewhat
    5. Agree completely

38. Behavior patterns can be altered at most any life period—in childhood, adolescence, and adulthood.
    1. Disagree completely
    2. Disagree somewhat
    3. Undecided
    4. Agree somewhat
    5. Agree completely

39. Psychiatric knowledge is essential to the treatment of more than half of the patients a physician sees in his practice.
    1. Disagree completely
    2. Disagree somewhat
    3. Undecided
    4. Agree somewhat
    5. Agree completely

40. Intellectually gifted children are likely to be weak and retarded physically and emotionally unstable.
    1. Disagree completely
    2. Disagree somewhat
    3. Undecided
    4. Agree somewhat
    5. Agree completely

41. Health supervision as compared with curative medicine is uninteresting and unprofitable to the physician.
    1. Definitely not
    2. No
    3. Undecided
    4. Yes
    5. Definitely yes

42. Hygiene, often defined as the science of health, is as much a science as internal medicine and pediatrics.
    1. Disagree completely

2. Disagree
3. Undecided
4. Agree
5. Agree completely

43. Specific knowledge necessary for prevention of disease is so limited at this stage of development that the time of a practicing physician is much better spent in curative medicine.
    1. Completely disagree
    2. Disagree
    3. Undecided
    4. Agree for the most part
    5. Completely agree

44. For a well-rounded medical education, work in pediatrics and surgery is decidedly more important than work in preventive medicine.
    1. Strongly disagree
    2. Disagree
    3. Undecided
    4. Agree
    5. Strongly agree

45. Preventive medicine necessitates a degree of understanding of patient's attitude toward health and disease that is unusual in the current practice of medicine.
    1. Completely disagree
    2. Disagree
    3. Undecided
    4. Agree for the most part
    5. Completely agree

46. In present day practice the demand for treatment of disease is so great that hardly any time can be spared to concern oneself with prevention of illness.
    1. Completely disagree
    2. Disagree
    3. Undecided
    4. Agree for the most part
    5. Completely agree

47. How important do you think it is for a physician to participate in programs of accident prevention?
    1. Not important at all
    2. Pretty unimportant
    3. Not so important
    4. Pretty important
    5. Very important

48. Since prevention of disease is directly related to the properties of disease itself, there is no special reason to teach the preventive aspects in separate courses.
    1. Disagree completely
    2. Disagree
    3. Undecided
    4. Agree
    5. Agree completely

49. There is little value in stressing principles of disease prevention as personal habits of most adult patients are so firmly established that the possibility of effecting more lasting change is rather unlikely.
    1. Disagree completely
    2. Disagree
    3. Undecided
    4. Agree
    5. Agree completely

50. Prevention of disease as a medical activity is primarily the responsibility of health departments rather than the responsibility of bedside physicians.
    1. Disagree completely
    2. Disagree
    3. Undecided
    4. Agree for the most part
    5. Agree completely

Appendix 3

Staff Description Checklists[1]

Put a check mark in front of each adjective on the following page which you consider to be descriptive of (1) the typical surgery staff man, (2) the typical internist or pediatrician, and (3) the typical psychiatrist. Do not worry about contradictions, duplications, and so forth.

1. – adaptable
2. – adventurous
3. – aggressive
4. – alert
5. – aloof
6. – anxious
7. – appreciative
8. – argumentative
9. – arrogant
10. – assertive
11. – autocratic
12. – bossy
13. – calm
14. – capable
15. – changeable
16. – cheerful
17. – clear-thinking
18. – clever
19. – cold
20. – complicated
21. – conscientious
22. – conservative
23. – considerate
24. – conventional
25. – cool
26. – cooperative
27. – curious
28. – defensive
29. – deliberate
30. – dependable
31. – determined
32. – dominant
33. – easy going
34. – efficient
35. – egotistical
36. – emotional
37. – energetic
38. – enterprising
39. – enthusiastic
40. – fair-minded
41. – forceful
42. – foresighted
43. – forgetful
44. – frank
45. – friendly
46. – gentle
47. – good-natured
48. – hasty
49. – helpful
50. – humorous
51. – hurried
52. – idealistic
53. – impatient
54. – impulsive
55. – individualistic
56. – informal
57. – ingenious
58. – insightful
59. – intelligent
60. – irritable
61. – kind
62. – leisurely
63. – logical
64. – mannerly
65. – masculine
66. – methodical
67. – mild
68. – moderate
69. – natural
70. – obliging
71. – opinionated
72. – opportunistic
73. – organized
74. – patient
75. – persistent
76. – planful
77. – pleasant
78. – polished
79. – practical
80. – praising
81. – precise
82. – preoccupied
83. – progressive
84. – rational
85. – realistic
86. – reflective
87. – relaxed
88. – reserved
89. – resourceful
90. – responsible
91. – restless
92. – rigid
93. – sarcastic
94. – self-confident
95. – sensitive
96. – sharp-witted
97. – sincere
98. – soft-hearted
99. – stable
100. – strong
101. – stubborn
102. – sympathetic
103. – tactful
104. – temperamental
105. – tense
106. – thorough
107. – tolerant
108. – unassuming
109. – unconventional
110. – understanding
111. – unemotional
112. – unrealistic
113. – versatile
114. – warm
115. – wise
116. – witty
117. – worrying

[1] Taken from the Gough Adjective Check-List. See H. G. Gough, *Reference Handbook for the Gough Adjective Check-List* (Berkeley: University of California Institute of Personality Assessment and Research, 1955). In actual practice these were administered as three separate tests. However, since the same adjectives were used for all these checklists, they are combined here.

Appendix 4

Questionnaire Used in Connection with Dependent Variables Measures

1. Do you look upon your contact with patients while in medical school
   1. Primarily as an opportunity to learn medicine
   2. Primarily as an opportunity to help patients
   3. As presenting equal opportunities to learn medicine and to help patients
2. How much satisfaction did you derive from the physician-patient relationships you have had in the past six months?
   1. A great deal
   2. A moderate amount
   3. Very little
   4. None at all
3. With respect to responsibility for the *diagnosis* of patients, would you say that during the past six months you have had
   1. Too little responsibility
   2. Enough responsibility
   3. Too much responsibility
4. How about responsibility for *treating* patients—would you say that during the past six months you have had
   1. Too little responsibility
   2. Enough responsibility
   3. Too much responsibility

Although you are not yet a doctor officially, many people probably think of you as one. We'd like to find out how you feel about yourself in this respect. For each of the following write

1. If you have thought of yourself *primarily as a doctor* rather than as a student
2. If you have thought of yourself *primarily as a student* rather than as a doctor

5. In the most recent dealings you have had with *patients* how have you tended to think of yourself?
6. What about when you have talked with your *classmates* in recent weeks—how have you tended to think of yourself then?
7. And when you have had contacts with your *instructors* in recent weeks—how have you tended to think of yourself?
8. Finally, when you had contacts with *nurses* in clinics or on the wards in the past month or so, how have you tended to think of yourself?

In your opinion, how have these different people thought about you in this respect? For the following write:

1. If you have been thought of *primarily as a doctor* rather than as a student
2. If you have been thought of *primarily as a student* rather than as a doctor

9. In your recent dealings with *patients*, how have they thought of you, by and large?
10. When you talked with your *classmates* in recent weeks, how, in your opinion, did they think of you?
11. And in your recent contacts with your *instructors*, how have they thought of you?
12. Finally, when you came in contact with *nurses* in clinics or on the wards in the past month or so, how did they seem to think of you?
13. To what extent do you worry that patients with whom you are dealing will lose respect for you if they learn that you are a student?
    1. A great deal
    2. Quite a bit
    3. Not very much
    4. Not at all
14. By and large, have patients generally been discussed with you as individual persons or as specific disease entities?
    1. As individual persons
    2. As specific disease entities
15. If you, as a fourth-year student, make a mistake in the *diagnosis* of a patient under your care, do you feel that this is
    1. Primarily your own responsibility
    2. Primarily the responsibility of the hospital staff
16. If you make a mistake in the *treatment* of a patient under your care, do you feel that this is
    1. Primarily your own responsibility
    2. Primarily the responsibility of the hospital staff

Everyone recognizes that it is difficult to generalize about "the faculty." But in your own experience, how much *interest*—on the average—did the members of the following groups at Colorado take in their students during the past six months? Select one of the following for each:

1. A great deal

2. A moderate amount
3. Little
17. House staff
18. Full-time clinical faculty
19. Practitioners who teach part time

Do you believe that a family physician should have information about the following characteristics of a patient:

1. As part of a doctor's *routine* information, or
2. As part of a doctor's information *only where specifically indicated*

Write either 1 or 2 on the answer sheet for each of the following:

20. Income
21. Diet
22. Physical environment—home and neighborhood
23. Occupation
24. Social standing in the community
25. Relationships with friends, relatives, associates
26. Religion
27. Nationality or ethnic group
28. Education
29. Political affiliation
30. Aspirations and goals in life
31. Fears, worries, problems
32. Recreational activities
33. Marital status

Below is a list of problems and situations which many medical students meet in their dealings with patients. How confident do you feel about your ability to deal with each of these problems *at the present time?* Select one of the following for each:

1. Completely confident
2. Fairly confident
3. Not really confident
4. Completely lacking in confidence

34. When a patient has an emotional outburst of crying, swearing, or something like that.
35. Preventing a patient from becoming embarrassed during a pelvic examination.
36. Talking with the family of a patient who has just died.
37. Having to tell a patient that the tests performed on him do not reveal the cause of his problems.
38. Deciding what to tell a patient who has a serious and irremediable illness.
39. Knowing what to do in an emergency.
40. Being able to do a venipuncture without any difficulty.
41. Having a doctor as one of your patients.
42. Being able to make a diagnosis in a difficult case.
43. Deciding on appropriate medication and dosage.

44. In your judgment, who should take *primary responsibility* for seeing to it that an investigation is made of social and environmental factors which may be affecting the health of a given patient?
   1. Patient's doctor
   2. Medical social worker
   3. Nurse
   4. Other. Who?
45. Who should *actually carry out* the investigation of social and environmental factors that may be affecting the health of a patient?
   1. Patient's doctor
   2. Medical social worker
   3. Nurse
   4. Other. Who?

Below is a list of problems which practicing physicians sometimes meet. To what extent have you thought about each of these problems?
   1. Have thought quite a lot
   2. Have thought a little
   3. Have thought not at all

Answer for each of the following:
46. The uncertainties of diagnosis and therapy that one meets in practice.
47. The possibility of becoming too attached to a patient.
48. The possibility of reacting negatively to a patient.
49. The difficulty of maintaining the proper degree of detachment from patients.
50. The problem of ordering valuable diagnostic tests which are painful or unpleasant.
51. The problem of ordering valuable diagnostic tests which are painful, unpleasant, or expensive.
52. The problem of employing necessary therapy which may have serious adverse side-effects on the patient.
53. The difficulties of providing high quality medical care and still make a decent living in practice.

Below is a list of problems which practicing physicians sometimes meet. Do you feel that you now can solve these problems?
   1. Almost sure I can solve this
   2. Believe I can solve this
   3. Almost sure I cannot solve this

Answer for each of the following:
54. The uncertainties of diagnosis and therapy that one meets in practice.
55. The possibility of becoming too attached to a patient.
56. The possibility of reacting negatively to a patient.
57. The difficulty of maintaining the proper degree of detachment from patients.
58. The problem of ordering valuable diagnostic tests which are painful or unpleasant.

59. The problem of employing valuable therapeutic measures which are painful, unpleasant, or expensive.
60. The problem of employing necessary therapy which may have serious adverse side-effects on the patient.
61. The difficulties of providing high quality medical care and still make a decent living in practice.

Because of the scope of the field of medicine, it is likely that students select areas of major interest. We would like to ascertain *your own* interests as a fourth-year medical student.

How important is it to you to be able to devote attention to the following topics in your senior year? Select one of the following alternatives for each of the questions below.

1. Not important at all
2. Of minimal importance
3. Less than average importance
4. Of average importance
5. More than average importance
6. Very important
7. Extremely important

62. To acquire more of the basic facts of clinical medicine (excluding psychosomatic medicine).
63. To acquire skill at applying the facts of organic medicine to the practice of clinical medicine.
64. To acquire knowledge of the basic ideas of psychosomatic medicine and psychiatry.
65. To acquire skill at applying the basic ideas of psychosomatic medicine and psychiatry to the practice of clinical medicine.
66. To improve your ability to establish and maintain good physician-patient relationships.
67. To acquire skill at recognizing and managing social problems in the practice of clinical medicine.
68. To acquire knowledge and skill at utilizing the ancillary services (social service and public health nurse).
69. To learn the practical application of the principles of comprehensive care in treating patients.
70. To learn to organize diagnostic and therapeutic regimes.

On the basis of your experience, *how helpful* do you think the clerkship you have just completed (GMC, surgery, or med-ob-gyn-peds) was with respect to the topics below? Select one of the alternatives below for each of the questions that follow.

1. Was extremely helpful
2. Was very helpful
3. Was moderately helpful
4. Was somewhat helpful
5. Was only slightly helpful

6. Was not at all helpful
7. Was a hindrance

71. In acquiring more of the basic facts of clinical medicine (excluding psychosomatic medicine).
72. In acquiring skill in applying the facts of organic medicine to the practice of clinical medicine.
73. In acquiring knowledge of the basic ideas of psychosomatic medicine and psychiatry.
74. In acquiring skill in applying the basic ideas of psychosomatic medicine and psychiatry to the practice of clinical medicine.
75. In improving your ability to establish and maintain good physician-patient relationships.
76. In acquiring skill in recognizing and managing social problems in the practice of clinical medicine.
77. In acquiring knowledge and skill in utilizing the ancillary services (social service and public health nurse).
78. In learning the practical application of the principles of comprehensive care in treating patients.
79. In learning to organize diagnostic and therapeutic regimes.

With respect to the clerkship you have just completed (GMC, surgery, or med-ob-gyn-peds), how *proficient* was the staff in each of the areas below? Select one of the alternatives below for each of the questions that follow.

1. Staff was extremely poor
2. Staff was very poor
3. Staff was poor
4. Staff was average
5. Staff was good
6. Staff was very good
7. Staff was extremely good

80. In knowledge of the basic facts of clinical medicine (excluding psychosomatic medicine).
81. In skill at applying the facts of organic medicine to the practice of clinical medicine.
82. In knowledge of the basic ideas of psychosomatic medicine and psychiatry.
83. In skill at applying the basic ideas of psychosomatic medicine and psychiatry to the practice of clinical medicine.
84. In ability to establish and maintain good physician-patient relationships.
85. In skill at recognizing and managing social problems in the practice of clinical medicine.
86. In knowledge and skill at utilizing the ancillary services (social service and public health nurse).
87. In the practical application of the principles of comprehensive care in treating patients.
88. In knowing how to organize diagnostic and therapeutic regimes.

Below is a list of activities or circumstances that could help or hinder a student in his senior year. In order to obtain what *you* want from your senior year, *how important* would it be to you to have the following conditions present or to engage in the following activities?

Select one of the alternatives below for each of the questions that follow.

1. Not important at all
2. Of minimal importance
3. Of less than average importance
4. Of average importance
5. Of more than average importance
6. Very important
7. Extremely important

89. To follow patients for several months.
90. To make home visits.
91. To have responsibility for diagnosis of patients.
92. To have responsibility for treatment of patients.
93. To engage in activities yourself rather than observe the staff.
94. To have opportunities to explain to patients their prognosis, limitations, etc.
95. To have the staff give direct instruction in physician-patient relationships.
96. To have opportunities for psychiatric consultation for your patients.
97. To have opportunities to give psychotherapy.
98. To have opportunities for consultation with the medical specialties.
99. To have opportunities to get to know the staff personally.
100. To have opportunities to consult with the ancillary services (social worker, public health nurse).
101. To use ancillary services in patient care.
102. To learn the skills that the social worker has and when to utilize them.
103. To learn the philosophy and point of view of social work.
104. To have staff supervision time readily available.
105. To have a high quality of staff supervision.
106. To have specific staff suggestions for the interpretation of symptoms and treatment.
107. To learn the amount and dosage schedule for specific therapies.
108. To learn the principles of therapy.
109. To develop physical examination skills.
110. To develop skill in history taking.
111. To do laboratory procedures.
112. To attend conferences.
113. To handle the emotional problems of patients.
114. To handle the social problems of patients.
115. To handle the medical problems of patients.
116. To make rounds.
117. To work with diagnostic problems.
118. To observe a doctor in private practice.
119. To see the families of patients.

120. To see a wide variety of illnesses.
121. To see unusual pathological conditions.
122. To attend didactic lectures.
123. To have patients with a definite pathology.
124. To take complete social histories.
125. To have little delay in waiting to be checked.
126. To have little or no paper work to do.
127. To have little or no "scut" work to do.
128. To have very few "crocks."
129. To have very few broken appointments.
130. To have little delay in getting laboratory reports.
131. To have laboratory reports of unquestionable reliability.
132. To have charts readily accessible.
133. To have nursing help readily available.
134. To have few or no interruptions during student-staff "checking."
135. To have few or no hospital policies which restrict patient care or lead to inefficiency.
136. To have an avenue available for the expression of student criticism.
137. To have the responsibilities and duties of students clearly defined.
138. To "scrub" on operations.
139. To follow the latest medical advances in books and journals.
140. To present cases in some conference or seminar.
141. To handle routine medical problems.
142. To spend a lot of time exploring social and emotional factors when taking a history.
143. To spend more than an hour-and-a-half working up a patient.
144. To advise patients on their personal problems.
145. To work at some interesting research problem.
146. To learn how to function as a member of a clinic team.

Below is a line representing the distance between the average medical student in each class and the house officer. Where would you place yourself with respect to your *present proficiency?*

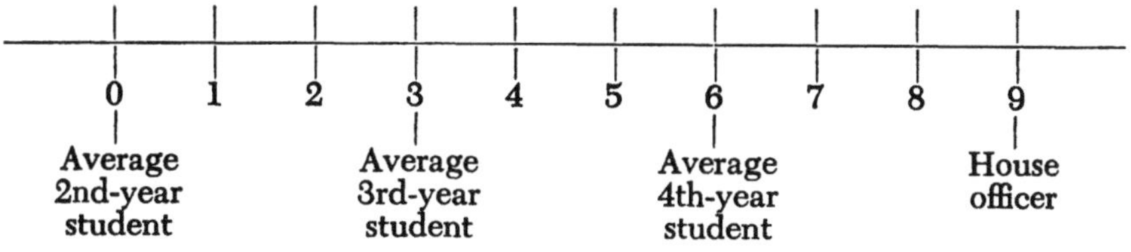

147. In knowledge of the basic facts of clinical medicine (excluding psychosomatic medicine).
148. In skill at applying the facts of organic medicine to the practice of clinical medicine.
149. In knowledge of the basic ideas of psychosomatic medicine and psychiatry.
150. In skill at applying the basic ideas of psychosomatic medicine and psychiatry to the practice of clinical medicine.

151. In ability to establish and maintain good physician-patient relationships.
152. In skill at recognizing and managing social problems in the practice of clinical medicine.
153. In knowledge and skill at utilizing the ancillary services (social service and public health nurse).
154. In the practical application of the principles of comprehensive care in treating patients.
155. In knowing how to organize diagnostic and therapeutic regimes.

During your *previous* clerkship (GMC, surgery, or med-ob-gyn-peds) how much did the staff actively contribute to your proficiency in each of the areas below; i.e., excluding the effects of your own efforts or other factors, how helpful was the staff? Select one of the alternatives below for each of the questions that follow.

1. Staff was extremely helpful
2. Staff was very helpful
3. Staff was moderately helpful
4. Staff was somewhat helpful
5. Staff was only slightly helpful
6. Staff was not at all helpful
7. Staff was a hindrance

156. In acquiring more of the basic facts of clinical medicine (excluding psychosomatic medicine).
157. In acquiring skill at applying the facts of organic medicine to the practice of clinical medicine.
158. In acquiring knowledge of the basic ideas of psychosomatic medicine and psychiatry.
159. In acquiring skill at applying the basic ideas of psychosomatic medicine and psychiatry to the practice of clinical medicine.
160. In improving your ability to establish and maintain good physician-patient relationships.
161. In acquiring skill at recognizing and managing social problems in the practice of clinical medicine.
162. In acquiring knowledge and skill at utilizing the ancillary services (social service and public health nurse).
163. In learning the practical application of the principles of comprehensive care in treating patients.
164. In learning to organize diagnostic and therapeutic regimes.

During your previous clerkship (GMC, surgery, or med-ob-gyn-peds) how helpful was the patient material as aids to achieving proficiency in each of the areas below? That is to say, considering the types of patients, their number and variety, how much did the patient material contribute to your achieving proficiency? Select one of the alternatives below for each of the questions that follow.

1. Patient material was extremely helpful

2. Patient material was very helpful
3. Patient material was moderately helpful
4. Patient material was somewhat helpful
5. Patient material was only slightly helpful
6. Patient material was not at all helpful
7. Patient material was a hindrance

165. In acquiring more of the basic facts of clinical medicine (excluding psychosomatic medicine).
166. In acquiring skill at applying the facts of organic medicine to the practice of clinical medicine.
167. In acquiring knowledge of the basic ideas of psychosomatic medicine and psychiatry.
168. In acquiring skill at applying the basic ideas of psychosomatic medicine and psychiatry to the practice of clinical medicine.
169. In improving your ability to establish and maintain good physician-patient relationships.
170. In acquiring skill at recognizing and managing social problems in the practice of clinical medicine.
171. In acquiring knowledge and skill at utilizing the ancillary services (social service and public health nurse).
172. In learning the practical application of the principles of comprehensive care in treating patients.
173. In learning to organize diagnostic and therapeutic regimes.

174. During your previous clerkship (GMC, surgery, or med-ob-gyn-peds), what sort of attitude did you feel the staff had toward Social Service?
   1. A very negative attitude
   2. A slightly negative attitude
   3. A neutral attitude
   4. A slightly positive attitude
   5. A very positive attitude

175. During your previous clerkship (GMC, surgery, or med-ob-gyn-peds), what sort of attitude did you feel the staff had toward psychosomatic medicine and psychiatry?
   1. A very favorable attitude
   2. A slightly favorable attitude
   3. A neutral attitude
   4. A slightly unfavorable attitude
   5. A very unfavorable attitude

176. From your own experience or from what you have observed with other students do you think that personality conflicts or personality affinities with staff members played an important role in students' experiences during your previous clerkship (GMC, surgery, or med-ob-gyn-peds)?
   1. Personality factors were an insignificant aspect of student experience

2. Personality factors were present but were not of great importance
3. Personality factors were a significant aspect of student experience
4. Personality factors were a very important aspect of student experience
5. Personality factors played a predominant role in student experience

177. In your personal experience how useful has it been to take a thorough personal and social history?
1. It has rarely been of use in the treatment and management of patients for me
2. It has occasionally been of use in the treatment and management of patients for me
3. It has frequently been of use in the treatment and management of patients for me
4. It has almost always been of use in the treatment and management of patients for me

178. During your previous clerkship (GMC, surgery, or med-ob-gyn-peds), how much independence did you have and how much do you think you should have had?
How much independence *did* you have? Select one of the alternatives below.

No independence at all	Very little independence	A moderate amount	Very much independence	Complete independence
/	/	/	/	/
1.	2.	3.	4.	5.

How much independence *should you have had?*

Much less independence	Somewhat less independence	The same amount of independence	Somewhat more independence	Much more independence
/	/	/	/	/
1.	2.	3.	4.	5.

Below is a list of activities that senior students could engage in or circumstances that could be present. To what extent did you engage in each of these activities or to what extent was each of these conditions present *for you during your previous clerkship* (GMC, surgery, or med-ob-gyn-peds)? Select one of the alternatives below for each of the activities or circumstances that follow.

1. Never present
2. Seldom present
3. Occasionally present
4. Sometimes present, sometimes not
5. Frequently present
6. Very frequently present
7. Always present

179. Following patients for several months.
180. Making home visits.
181. Having responsibility for diagnosis of patients.
182. Having responsibility for treatment of patients.
183. Engaging in activities yourself rather than observing the staff.
184. Having opportunities to explain to patients their prognosis, limitations, etc.
185. Having the staff give direct instruction in physician-patient relationships.
186. Having opportunities for psychiatric consultation for your patients.
187. Having opportunities to give psychotherapy.
188. Having opportunities for consultation with the medical specialties.
189. Having opportunities to get to know the staff personally.
190. Having opportunities to consult with the ancillary services (social worker, public health nurse).
191. Using ancillary services in patient care.
192. Learning the skills that the social worker has and when to utilize them.
193. Learning the philosophy and point of view of social work.
194. Having staff supervision time readily available.
195. Having a high quality of staff supervision.
196. Having specific staff suggestions for the interpretation of symptoms and treatment.
197. Learning the amount and dosage schedule for specific therapies.
198. Learning the principles of therapy.
199. Developing physical examination skills.
200. Developing skill in history taking.
201. Doing laboratory procedures.
202. Attending conferences.
203. Handling the emotional problems of patients.
204. Handling the social problems of patients.
205. Handling the medical problems of patients.
206. Making rounds.
207. Working with diagnostic problems.
208. Observing a doctor in private practice.
209. Seeing the families of patients.
210. Seeing a wide variety of illnesses.
211. Seeing unusual pathological conditions.
212. Attending didactic lectures.
213. Having patients with a definite pathology.
214. Taking complete social histories.
215. Having little delay in waiting to be checked.
216. Having little or no paper work to do.
217. Having little or no "scut" work to do.
218. Having very few "crocks."
219. Having very few broken appointments.
220. Having little delay in getting laboratory reports.

221. Having laboratory reports of unquestionable reliability.
222. Having charts readily accessible.
223. Having nursing help readily available.
224. Having few or no interruptions during student-staff "checking."
225. Having few or no hospital policies which restrict patient care or lead to inefficiency.
226. Having an avenue available for the expression of student criticism.
227. Having the responsibilities and duties of students clearly defined.
228. "Scrubbing" on operations.
229. Following the latest medical advances in books and journals.
230. Presenting cases in some conference or seminar.
231. Handling routine medical problems.
232. Spending a lot of time exploring social and emotional factors when taking a history.
233. Spending more than an hour-and-a-half working up a patient.
234. Advising patients on their personal problems.
235. Working at some interesting research problem.
236. Learning how to function as a member of a clinic team.

237. Choose one of the alternatives below to describe your experience with psychotherapy during your previous clerkship (GMC, surgery, or med-ob-gyn-peds). Please read all the alternatives before choosing.
    1. I did not engage in psychotherapy and would have liked to.
    2. I did not engage in psychotherapy and would not have liked to.
    3. I did engage in psychotherapy and liked it.
    4. I did engage in psychotherapy and did not particularly like it.

During your previous clerkship (GMC, surgery, or med-ob-gyn-peds) how much reading did you do in each of the areas below? Select one of the alternatives below for each of the areas that follow.

1. No reading at all
2. Very little reading
3. Some reading
4. Quite a lot of reading
5. Very much reading

238. How much reading did you do in the area of surgery?
239. How much reading did you do in the area of internal medicine?
240. How much reading did you do in the area of pediatrics?
241. How much reading did you do in the area of obstetrics and gynecology?
242. How much reading did you do in the area of psychosomatic medicine and psychiatry?
243. How much reading did you do in the area of social phenomena in medicine?

Below is listed a number of third and fourth year clerkships. *How helpful* were these clerkships to you in gaining proficiency in each of the areas below? For each of the questions that follow select the clerkship that was *most helpful to you* and the clerkship that was *least* helpful to you.

1. 3rd-year pediatrics
2. 3rd-year medicine
3. 3rd-year ob-gyn
4. 3rd-year surgery
5. 4th-year pediatrics
6. 4th-year medicine
7. 4th-year ob-gyn
8. 4th-year surgery
9. 4th-year GMC

244. Most helpful clerkship in acquiring more of the basic facts of clinical medicine (excluding psychosomatic medicine).
245. Least helpful clerkship in acquiring more of the basic facts of clinical medicine (excluding psychosomatic medicine).
246. Most helpful clerkship in acquiring skill in applying the facts of organic medicine to the practice of clinical medicine.
247. Least helpful clerkship in acquiring skill in applying the facts of organic medicine to the practice of clinical medicine.
248. Most helpful clerkship in acquiring knowledge of the basic ideas of psychosomatic medicine and psychiatry.
249. Least helpful clerkship in acquiring knowledge of the basic ideas of psychosomatic medicine and psychiatry.
250. Most helpful clerkship in acquiring skill in applying the basic ideas of psychosomatic medicine and psychiatry to the practice of clinical medicine.
251. Least helpful clerkship in acquiring skill in applying the basic ideas of psychosomatic medicine and psychiatry to the practice of clinical medicine.
252. Most helpful clerkship in improving your ability to establish and maintain good physician-patient relationships.
253. Least helpful clerkship in improving your ability to establish and maintain good physician-patient relationships.
254. Most helpful clerkship in acquiring skill in recognizing and managing social problems in the practice of clinical medicine.
255. Least helpful clerkship in acquiring skill in recognizing and managing social problems in the practice of clinical medicine.
256. Most helpful clerkship in acquiring knowledge and skill in utilizing the ancillary services (social service and public health nurse).
257. Least helpful clerkship in acquiring knowledge and skill in utilizing the ancillary services (social service and public health nurse).
258. Most helpful clerkship in learning the practical application of the principles of comprehensive care in treating patients.
259. Least helpful clerkship in learning the practical application of the principles of comprehensive care in treating patients.
260. Most helpful clerkship in learning to organize diagnostic and therapeutic regimes.

261. Least helpful clerkship in learning to organize diagnostic and therapeutic regimes.

This section deals with your professional plans and ambitions for the future. Even though you may not be certain of your plans, please answer the questions on the basis of your present feelings.

262. How much have you thought about the kind of career you would like to have in medicine?
1. A great deal
2. A fair amount
3. Only a little
4. Not at all

263. (a) What kind of internship have you applied for? Write the number of your first choice *and second choice.*
1. Rotating
2. Straight medical
3. Straight surgical
4. Straight pathology
5. Mixed medical and surgical
6. Obstetrics and gynecology
7. Straight pediatrics
8. Other. What?

(b) In what kind of hospital do you hope to intern?
1. Public hospital in a small town not affiliated with a university
2. Public hospital in a large city not affiliated with a university
3. Public hospital in a small town closely affiliated with a university
4. Public hospital in a large city closely affiliated with a university
5. University hospital
6. Private hospital in a small town
7. Private hospital in a large city
8. Army, Navy, Air Force, or public health service hospital
9. Other. What?

264. (a) Do you intend to take a residency in some specialty?
1. Yes
2. No
3. Uncertain

(b) How certain do you feel about this intention?
1. Very certain
2. Fairly certain
3. Not at all certain

(c) Why do you intend—or not intend—to take a residency?

(d) (For students who intend or hope to take a residency)

In what specialty do you intend to take your residency? Even though you may not have decided definitely yet, please select your first *two choices* in the order of your preference. Write the number of your first choice and second choice.
1. Medicine

2. Surgery
3. Obstetrics and gynecology
4. Pediatrics
5. Pathology
6. Psychiatry
7. Ophthalmology
8. Ear, nose, and throat
9. Urology
10. Neurosurgery
11. Plastic surgery
12. Orthopedics
13. General practice
14. Other. What?

(e) (For students who intend or hope to take a residency)
How certain are you of your first choice?
1. Very certain
2. Fairly certain
3. Not at all certain

265. What fields of medicine do you feel *least* inclined to enter? Please select *three* choices.
1. Medicine
2. Surgery
3. Obstetrics and gynecology
4. Pediatrics
5. Pathology
6. Psychiatry
7. Ophthalmology
8. Ear, nose, and throat
9. Urology
10. Neurosurgery
11. Plastic surgery
12. Orthopedics
13. General practice
14. Other. What?

266. When you have finished your formal medical training (including work beyond your MD):
(a) To what type of professional activity in the list below would you *prefer* to give *most* of your working time? Select a first choice and a *second choice.*
1. General practice
2. Specialty practice
3. Teaching some medical specialty
4. Doing research
5. Other. What?

(b) How certain are you about your choices in question (a) above?
1. Very certain
2. Fairly certain

3. Not at all certain

(c) Apart from what you would like, to what type of professional activity in the list below do you expect to give *most* of your working time? Select a first choice *and a second choice.*

1. General practice
2. Specialty practice
3. Teaching some medical specialty
4. Doing research
5. Other. What?

(d) If you could arrange it, in which *one* of the following situations would you carry out the professional activity which you have indicated you prefer most?

1. Own professional office with hospital affiliation
2. Own professional office without hospital affiliation
3. Large private clinic or hospital
4. Small group clinic
5. Medical school
6. Government or military service
7. Industrial firm
8. Research foundation or institute
9. Other. What?

267. When did you decide on the career which you have indicated in the previous question?

1. Senior year in medical school
2. Junior year in medical school
3. Sophomore year in medical school
4. Freshman year in medical school
5. Before entering medical school

268. Describe the professional situation you would most *like* to be in ten years from now.

269. List the fraternal organizations to which you have belonged (or now belong), the year you joined, and the number of years you have been (were) a member.

Appendix 5

Measures of Individual Attributes

Numerous measures of individual attributes were employed in the effort to gain insight into and understanding of the senior medical students' experiences. These measures are listed on the following pages.

In addition, a tabular presentation is made of the relationships studied between the measures of individual attributes and the measures of psychological change, students' performance in the GMC, and students' response to the GMC clerkship. An "x" indicates a relationship involving an individual attribute which was measured only once. The other symbols refer to the times at which the individual attributes were measured.

Pr = Pretest scores
PI = Posttest I scores
PII = Posttest II scores
1st = First half-year (change period)
2nd = Second half-year (change period)

List of measures of individual attributes used in the studies of correlates of psychological change, students' performance in the GMC, and students' response to the GMC clerkship*

	Correlates of change (change periods, by half-year)						Students' performance in the GMC (six student groups)						Students' response to the GMC clerkship: Biographical items and preferred professional activity			
	1954	1955		1956			1954		1955		1956		1955		1956	
Measures of individual attributes	I	I	II	I	II	Over-all	I	II	I	II	I	II	I	II	I	II
Aptitude for medical education																
Medical College Admission Test																
Verbal Ability	x	x	x	x	x	x	x	x	x	x	x	x	x	x	x	x
Quantitative Ability	x	x	x	x	x	x	x	x	x	x	x	x	x	x	x	x
General Ability	x						x	x								
Knowledge of Modern Society	x	x	x	x	x	x	x	x	x	x	x	x	x	x	x	x
Knowledge of Premedical Sciences	x	x	x	x	x	x	x	x	x	x	x	x	x	x	x	x
Previous academic performance																
Premedical grade average		x	x	x	x	x	x	x	x	x	x	x	x	x	x	x
Number of courses (or credit hours) in psychology		x	x	x	x	x			x	x	x	x				
Number of courses (or credit hours) in sociology																
Number of courses in philosophy				x	x	x					x	x				
First-year grade average	x			x	x	x	x	x	x	x	x	x				
Second-year grade average	x	x	x	x	x	x	x	x	x	x	x	x	x	x	x	x
Third-year grade average	x	x	x	x	x	x	x	x	x	x	x	x	x	x	x	x
Fourth-year grade average																
Eight-quarter cumulative grade average	x	x	x	x	x	x			x	x	x	x	x	x	x	x
Over-all cumulative grade average																
Psychiatry course grade		x	x													
Psychopathology course grade		x	x	x	x	x			x	x	x	x				
Psychosomatics course grade		x	x						x	x						
Functional psychoses course grade																
Public health course grade		x	x	x	x	x			x	x	x	x				
Junior medical clerkship grade		x	x	x	x	x			x	x	x	x				
Junior pediatrics clerkship grade		x	x						x	x						
Junior obstetrics-gynecology clerkship grade		x	x						x	x						
Junior surgical clerkship grade		x	x	x	x	x			x	x	x	x				
Junior comprehensive examination scores	x						x	x								

* See page 615 for key.

Measures of individual attributes	Correlates of change (change periods, by half-year) 1954 I	1955 I	1955 II	1956 I	1956 II	1956 Over-all	Students' performance in the GMC (six student groups) 1954 I	1954 II	1955 I	1955 II	1956 I	1956 II	Students' response to the GMC clerkship: Biographical items and preferred professional activity 1955 I	1955 II	1956 I	1956 II
Personality characteristics																
A. Peer judgments																
Leadership (peer ranking)	Pr	Pr		Pr	Pr	Pr	Pr	Pr	Pr		Pr	PI	Pr	Pr	Pr	PI
Leadership (peer nomination)	Pr		PI		Pr	Pr	Pr	Pr		PI		Pr				
Likeability (peer ranking)	Pr	Pr		Pr	Pr	Pr	Pr	Pr	Pr		Pr	PI	Pr	Pr	Pr	PI
Likeability (peer nomination)	Pr		PI		Pr	Pr	Pr	Pr		PI		Pr				
Cooperativeness (peer ranking)	Pr	Pr					Pr	Pr	Pr							
Cooperativeness (peer nomination)	Pr		PI				Pr	Pr		PI						
Competence as a physician (peer nomination)	Pr	Pr	PI	Pr	Pr	Pr	Pr	Pr	Pr	PI	Pr	Pr	Pr	PI	Pr	Pr
Skill in developing good relations with patients (peer ranking)		Pr	PI	Pr	Pr	Pr			Pr	PI	Pr	PI	Pr	PI	Pr	PI
Willingness and ability to work independently (peer ranking)		Pr	PI	Pr	Pr	Pr			Pr	PI	Pr	PI	Pr	PI	Pr	PI
Sympathy to the notion of comprehensive medical care (peer ranking)		Pr	PI	Pr	Pr	Pr			Pr	PI	Pr	PI	Pr	PI	Pr	PI
Responsibility and maturity (peer ranking)				Pr	Pr	Pr					Pr	PI			Pr	PI
Amount of medical knowledge (peer ranking)				Pr	Pr	Pr					Pr	PI				
Future excellence as a physician (peer ranking)																
B. Self-ratings																
Q4 (for those who work) How many hours per week do you work?		x	x													
Q25 (1) Amount of reward for scholastic success as an adolescent		x	x	x	x	x				x	x	x				
(2) Amount of reward for showing initiative as an adolescent				x	x	x				x	x	x				
(3) Amount of reward for ability to get along with others as an adolescent				x	x	x				x	x	x				
(4) Amount of reward for showing responsibility as an adolescent				x	x	x				x	x	x				
(5) Amount of reward for being influential (among friends) as an adolescent				x	x	x				x	x	x				

Measures of individual attributes	Correlates of change (change periods, by half-year)						Students' performance in the GMC (six student groups)						Students' response to the GMC clerkship Biographical items and preferred professional activity			
	1954	1955		1956			1954		1955		1956		1955		1956	
	I	I	II	I	II	Over-all	I	II	I	II	I	II	I	II	I	II
Q32 (a) Amount of interest in research		x	x													
(b) Amount of interest in considering the patient's social circumstances															Pr	Pr
(c) Amount of interest in working with social service or public health nurse		x	x													
(d) Amount of interest in consideration of the welfare of the patient's family		x	x	x	x	x					x	x			Pr	Pr
(e) Amount of interest in minor surgery		x	x	x	x	x					x	x				
(f) Amount of interest in major surgery		x	x	x	x	x					x	x				
(g) Amount of interest in taking an administrative position in a hospital				x	x	x					x	x				
Q33 How early in life did you feel confident in your ability to develop satisfying relationships with others?		x	x	x	x	x					x	x				
A5 In comparison with other people that you know who are of approximately the same age as yourself, how would you rate yourself in terms of the importance you attach to intellectual and professional accomplishments?					PI	Pr						PI			Pr	PI
A9 When you fantasy or day-dream, how frequently do they concern intellectual or professional accomplishments?					PI	Pr						PI				
A14 When you are in a situation in which you are competing with someone who is also present, to what extent is your efficiency interfered with by the fear that you are not doing or will not do well?					PI	Pr					Pr	PI			Pr	PI
A17 To what extent is the adequacy of your social adjustment a source of worry to you?					PI	Pr						PI				
A41 To what extent do you find yourself worrying about whether or not your fellow students accept you as a friend?					PI	PI						PI			PI	PI
A42 How often do you experience some anxiety when a patient presents an ambiguous problem in diagnosis?					PI	PI						PI			PI	PI

Measures of individual attributes	Correlates of change (change periods, by half-year)						Students' performance in the GMC (six student groups)						Students' response to the GMC clerkship: Biographical items and preferred professional activity			
	1954	1955		1956			1954		1955		1956		1955		1956	
	I	I	II	I	II	Over-all	I	II	I	II	I	II	I	II	I	II
A43 When you think of the responsibilities you will have for your patients when you are practicing medicine, to what extent do you experience fear or anxiety?					PI	PI						PI			PI	PI
A44 To what extent do you find yourself worrying about the adequacy of your knowledge of differential diagnosis?					PI	PI						PI			PI	PI
C. Attitudes																
California F scale	Pr	Pr	PI	Pr	PI	Pr	Pr	Pr	Pr	PI	Pr	PI	Pr	Pr	Pr	PI
Liberal Attitude scale	x	x	x	x	x	x	x	x	x	x	x	x				
General Anxiety scale		x	x	Pr	PI	Pr			x	x	Pr	PI			Pr	PI
Self-Acceptance scale		x	x	x	x	x			x	x	x	x				
Self-Criticality scale		x	x	x	x	x			x	x	x	x				
D. Values																
Study of Values																
Theoretical	x	x	x		x	x	x	x	x	x	x	x	x	x	x	x
Aesthetic	x	x	x		x	x	x	x	x	x	x	x	x	x	x	x
Economic	x	x	x		x	x	x	x	x	x	x	x	x	x	x	x
Political	x	x	x		x	x	x	x	x	x	x	x				
Social	x	x	x		x	x	x	x	x	x	x	x	x	x	x	x
Religious	x	x	x		x	x	x	x	x	x	x	x				
E. Social interaction variables																
California Psychological Inventory																
Good Impression		x	x	x	x	x			x	x	x	x				
Self-Control		x	x	x	x	x			x	x	x	x	x	x	x	x
Sense of Well-Being		x	x	x	x	x			x	x	x	x	x	x	x	x
Socialization		x	x	x	x	x			x	x	x	x				
Responsibility		x	x	x	x	x			x	x	x	x	x	x	x	x
Achievement via Conformance		x	x	x	x	x			x	x	x	x	x	x	x	x
Dominance		x	x	x	x	x			x	x	x	x	x	x	x	x
Sociability		x	x	x	x	x			x	x	x	x	x	x	x	x
Self-Acceptance		x	x	x	x	x			x	x	x	x				
Social Presence		x	x	x	x	x			x	x	x	x				
Capacity for Status		x	x	x	x	x			x	x	x	x				

Measures of individual attributes	Correlates of change (change periods, by half-year)						Students' performance in the GMC (six student groups)						Students' response to the GMC clerkship Biographical items and preferred professional activity			
	1954	1955		1956			1954		1955		1956		1955		1956	
	I	I	II	I	II	Over-all	I	II	I	II	I	II	I	II	I	II
Tolerance		x	x	x	x	x			x	x	x	x	x	x	x	x
Intellectual Efficiency		x	x	x	x	x			x	x	x	x	x	x	x	x
Psychological-Mindedness		x	x	x	x	x			x	x	x	x	x	x	x	x
Achievement via Independence		x	x	x	x	x			x	x	x	x	x	x	x	x
Flexibility		x	x	x	x	x			x	x	x	x	x	x	x	x
Femininity		x	x	x	x	x			x	x	x	x				
Communality				x	x	x			x	x	x	x				
F. Needs																
Edwards Personal Preference Schedule																
n(eed) Affiliation					x	x					x	x			x	x
n(eed) Nurturance					x	x					x	x			x	x
n(eed) Succorance					x	x					x	x			x	x
n(eed) Endurance					x	x					x	x			x	x
n(eed) Order					x	x					x	x			x	x
n(eed) Deference					x	x					x	x			x	x
n(eed) Abasement					x	x					x	x			x	x
n(eed) Dominance					x	x					x	x			x	x
n(eed) Aggression					x	x					x	x			x	x
n(eed) Achievement					x	x					x	x			x	x
n(eed) Exhibition					x	x					x	x			x	x
n(eed) Autonomy					x	x					x	x			x	x
n(eed) Intraception					x	x					x	x			x	x
n(eed) Change					x	x					x	x			x	x
n(eed) Heterosexuality					x	x					x	x			x	x
Biographical Items and Preferred Professional Activity																
Age													x	x	x	x
Marital status													x	x	x	x
Number of relatives holding MD													x	x	x	x
Preferred professional activity (after formal training) (also employed as an index of student response, see Appendix 6)													x	x	x	x
Measures of students' knowledge, skill, and attitudes (including questionnaire items)																
Sound-Film Interview																
Medical knowledge															Pr	PI
Medical knowledge (change)															1st	2nd

	Correlates of change (change periods, by half-year)						Students' performance in the GMC (six student groups)						Students' response to the GMC clerkship Biographical items and preferred professional activity			
	1954	1955		1956			1954		1955		1956		1955		1956	
Measures of individual attributes	I	I	II	I	II	Over-all	I	II	I	II	I	II	I	II	I	II
Medical skill															Pr	PI
Medical skill (change)															1st	2nd
Psychological knowledge															Pr	PI
Psychological knowledge (change)															1st	2nd
Psychological skill															Pr	PI
Psychological skill (change)															1st	2nd
Sociological knowledge and skill															Pr	PI
Sociological knowledge and skill (change)															1st	2nd
Accuracy of estimates of age															Pr	PI
Accuracy of estimates of age (change)															1st	2nd
Variability in estimates of age															Pr	PI
Variability in estimates of age (change)															1st	2nd
Accuracy of estimates of intelligence															Pr	PI
Accuracy of estimates of intelligence (change)															1st	2nd
Variability in estimates of intelligence															Pr	PI
Variability in estimates of intelligence (change)															1st	2nd
Mean variability in estimates of personality traits (measured by self-ratings)															Pr	PI
Mean variability in estimates of personality traits (measured by self-ratings) (change)															1st	2nd
Mean variability in estimates of personality traits (measured by tests)															Pr	PI
Mean variability in estimates of personality traits (measured by tests) (change)															1st	2nd
Differential memory score															Pr	PI
Differential memory score (change)															1st	2nd
Medical team: choice of visiting nurse as consultant															Pr	PI
Medical team: choice of visiting nurse as consultant (change)															1st	2nd
Medical team: choice of social worker as consultant															Pr	PI
Medical team: choice of social worker as consultant (change)															1st	2nd
Medical team: choice of psychiatrist as consultant															Pr	PI
Medical team: choice of psychiatrist as consultant (change)															1st	2nd

Measures of individual attributes	Correlates of change (change periods, by half-year)						Students' performance in the GMC (six student groups)						Students' response to the GMC clerkship Biographical items and preferred professional activity			
	1954	1955		1956			1954		1955		1956		1955		1956	
	I	I	II	I	II	Over-all	I	II	I	II	I	II	I	II	I	II
Medical Attitudes test																
Attitudes toward comprehensive care															Pr	PI
Attitudes toward comprehensive care (change)															1st	2nd
Attitudes toward team concept															Pr	PI
Attitudes toward team concept (change)															1st	2nd
Attitudes toward doctor-patient relation															Pr	PI
Attitudes toward doctor-patient relation (change)															1st	2nd
Attitudes toward behavior disorders															Pr	PI
Attitudes toward behavior disorders (change)															1st	2nd
Attitudes toward health supervision															Pr	PI
Attitudes toward health supervision (change)															1st	2nd
Total score on five scales															Pr	PI
Total score on five scales (change)															1st	2nd
F (Authoritarian) scale													Pr	PI	Pr	PI
F (Authoritarian) scale (change)													1st	2nd	1st	2nd
Questionnaire items																
How helpful was GMC in increasing your proficiency in																
Acquiring facts of clinical medicine															PI	PII
Acquiring skill in applying facts of organic medicine															PI	PII
Learning how to make diagnoses and treat patients													PI	PII		
Acquiring knowledge of psychosomatic medicine and psychiatry															PI	PII
Acquiring skill in applying facts of psychosomatic medicine and psychiatry															PI	PII
Improving physician-patient relation ability															PI	PII
Learning to maintain good relation with patients													PI	PII		
Acquiring skill in managing social problems															PI	PII
Acquiring knowledge and skills in utilizing ancillary services															PI	PII
Learning practical applications of principles of comprehensive care															PI	PII
Seeing patients' problems in their total setting													PI	PII		
Learning to organize diagnoses and therapeutic regimes															PI	PII
How important is it to devote your attention to the following topics in your senior year? (pretest–posttest change)																
Acquiring facts of clinical medicine															1st	2nd
Acquiring skill in applying facts of organic medicine															1st	2nd

Measures of individual attributes	Correlates of change (change periods, by half-year)						Students' performance in the GMC (six student groups)						Students' response to the GMC clerkship Biographical items and preferred professional activity			
	1954	1955		1956			1954		1955		1956		1955		1956	
	I	I	II	I	II	Over-all	I	II	I	II	I	II	I	II	I	II
Acquiring knowledge of psychosomatic medicine and psychiatry															1st	2nd
Acquiring skill in applying facts of psychosomatic medicine and psychiatry															1st	2nd
Improving physician-patient relation ability															1st	2nd
Acquiring skill in managing social problems															1st	2nd
Acquiring knowledge and skill in utilizing ancillary services															1st	2nd
Learning practical applications of principles of comprehensive care															1st	2nd
Learning to organize diagnoses and therapeutic regimes															1st	2nd
How important is it to you to engage in the following activities in your senior year? (pretest–posttest change)																
To follow patients for several months															1st	2nd
To make home visits															1st	2nd
To have responsibility for diagnoses															1st	2nd
To have responsibility for treatment															1st	2nd
To have opportunities for psychiatric consultations															1st	2nd
To have opportunities to give psychotherapy															1st	2nd
To have opportunity to consult ancillary services															1st	2nd
To learn skills and usefulness of social worker															1st	2nd
To handle emotional problems of the patient															1st	2nd
To handle social problems of the patient															1st	2nd
To see the families of the patients															1st	2nd
To spend a lot of time exploring social and emotional factors when taking a history															1st	2nd
To learn how to function as a member of the clinic team															1st	2nd
GMC Staff Ratings (*adjusted*)																
Medical knowledge													x	x	x	x
Medical skill													x	x	x	x
Psychological knowledge													x	x	x	x
Attitude toward patients' social problems													x	x	x	x
Change toward ideal student															x	x

Appendix 6

Students' Response to the GMC Program

Distribution of scores on indices of students' response to the GMC (classes of 1955 and 1956)

Number of students				
1955 I	1955 II	1956 I	1956 II	Indices of response
				Index of extensive patient contact
				Number of patients seen
0	1	0	0	30 or fewer
3	1	0	0	31–35
4	1	3	1	36–40
4	5	7	0	41–45
4	3	4	4	46–50
3	3	4	4	51–55
2	3	0	6	56–60
0	0	0	2	61 or more
				Indices of intensive patient contact (continuity of care)
				Mean number of visits per patient
6	2	2	1	2.1–2.5
7	10	7	3	2.6–3.0
4	4	4	8	3.1–3.5
3	1	4	3	3.6–4.0
0	0	1	2	4.1+
				To what extent was this condition present during the GMC clerkship: following patients for several months?
		0	1	1. Never present
		0	0	2.
		1	1	3.
		0	1	4.
		3	4	5.
		10	4	6.
		4	6	7. Always present

Number of students				
1955 I	1955 II	1956 I	1956 II	Indices of response
				How valuable was the opportunity to follow patients continuously in the GMC clerkship?
5	10			1. Very valuable
12	6			2.
3	1			3. Not particularly valuable
0	0			4. Don't know
				Index of presentation of patients
				By and large, have patients generally been discussed with you as individual persons or as specific disease entities?
14	13	15	10	1. Individual persons
6	4	3	7	2. Specific disease entities
				Indices of student responsibility for patients
				With respect to responsibility for the diagnosis and treatment of patients, would you say that during the past six months you have had:
1	2	1	3	2. Too little responsibility
5	5	2	4	3.
14	10	14	10	4.
0	0	1	0	5.
0	0	0	0	6. Too much responsibility
				To what extent was this condition present for you, during the GMC clerkship: having responsibility for diagnosis of patients?
		0	1	1. Never present
		0	1	2.
		0	1	3.
		6	0	4.
		4	9	5.
		5	3	6.
		3	2	7. Always present
				To what extent was this condition present during the GMC clerkship: having responsibility for treatment of patients?
		0	1	1. Never present
		0	0	2.
		0	1	3.
		5	1	4.
		4	7	5.
		7	5	6.
		2	2	7. Always present

Number of students				
1955 I	1955 II	1956 I	1956 II	Indices of response
				If you, as a fourth-year student, make a mistake in the diagnosis or treatment of a patient under your care, do you feel that this is:
14	11	16	13	2. Primarily your own responsibility
5	4	0	4	3. Sometimes your own responsibility and sometimes the responsibility of the hospital staff
1	2	2	0	4. Primarily the responsibility of the hospital staff
				How helpful was the GMC clerkship in making a student feel more like a doctor?
5	12			1. Extremely helpful
10	4			2.
4	1			3. Not at all helpful
1	0			4. No opinion
				In the most recent dealings you have had with patients, how have you tended to think of yourself?
14	14	15	14	1. Primarily as a doctor
6	3	3	3	2. Primarily as a student
				Finally, when you have had contacts with nurses in clinics or on the wards in the past month or so, how have you tended to think of yourself?
9	11	13	11	1. Primarily as a doctor
11	6	5	6	2. Primarily as a student
				And when you have had contacts with your instructors in recent weeks, how have you tended to think of yourself?
2	5	7	2	1. Primarily as a doctor
18	12	11	15	2. Primarily as a student
				What about when you have talked with your classmates in recent weeks—how have you tended to think of yourself then?
1	8	8	4	1. Primarily as a doctor
19	9	10	13	2. Primarily as a student
				Number of broken appointments:
5	1	1	0	3– 5
6	5	4	2	6– 8
5	3	4	3	9–11
3	4	3	7	12–14
1	2	4	4	15–17
0	2	2	1	18+

Number of students				
1955 I	1955 II	1956 I	1956 II	Indices of response
				Indices of the physician-patient relation
				How much satisfaction did you derive from the physician-patient relations you have had in the past six months?
13	13	15	9	1. A great deal
7	3	3	6	2.
0	1	0	2	3.
0	0	0	0	4. None at all
				To what extent was this condition present during the GMC clerkship: having the staff give direct instruction in physician-patient relations?
		0	2	1. Never present
		8	3	2.
		4	2	3.
		4	4	4.
		0	2	5.
		1	1	6.
		1	3	7. Always present
				How helpful was the GMC clerkship with respect to learning how to maintain good relations with patients?
12	11			1. Extremely helpful
7	6			2.
1	0			3. Not at all helpful
0	0			4. No opinion
				Number of broken appointments per number of patients seen:
3	0	1	0	.10 or less
6	4	2	2	.11–.15
2	1	2	2	.16–.20
3	6	1	5	.21–.25
4	2	8	6	.26–.30
1	2	0	2	.31–.35
0	2	3	0	.36–.40
1	0	1	0	.41+
				Indices of response to families of patients (Family Care Program)
				Total number of contacts with families:
8	5	3	6	0– 5
8	5	10	6	6–15
4	4	4	5	16–25
0	1	1	0	26–35
0	2	0	0	36+
				Number of home contacts with families:
17	13	16	14	0– 2
3	1	2	1	3– 5
0	1	0	1	6– 8
0	1	0	0	9–11
0	1	0	1	12+

Number of students				
1955 I	1955 II	1956 I	1956 II	Indices of response
				Number of GMC contacts with families:
8	6	4	8	0– 5
6	2	6	3	6–10
6	5	7	6	11–15
0	2	1	0	16–20
0	2	0	0	21+
				Number of ward contacts with families:
17	13	14	13	0– 2
2	1	2	4	3– 5
1	1	0	0	6– 8
0	2	2	0	9+
				Number of hours of GMC time spent with families:
9	6	4	9	0– 5
5	2	6	3	6–10
4	5	7	3	11–15
1	2	0	1	16–20
1	2	0	1	21+
				To what extent was this condition present during the GMC clerkship: making home visits?
		5	4	1. Never present
		4	3	2.
		6	2	3.
		2	2	4.
		0	4	5.
		1	0	6.
		0	2	7. Always present
				How helpful was the GMC clerkship in getting experience outside the hospital?
10	7			1. Extremely helpful
7	7			2.
2	2			3. Not at all helpful
1	1			4. No opinion
				Indices of response to the teaching staff as consultants
				Number of times student conferred with psychiatrist (estimated by psychiatrist)
		5	3	0– 2
		1	4	3– 5
		5	3	6– 8
		2	3	9–11
		5	2	12–14
		0	2	15+

Number of students				
1955 I	1955 II	1956 I	1956 II	Indices of response
				Number of times student conferred with social workers and public health nurse (estimated by social workers and public health nurse)
		0	1	0– 5
		0	7	6–10
		5	1	11–15
		5	6	16–20
		4	1	21–25
		4	1	26+
				To what extent was this condition present during the GMC clerkship: learning how to function as a member of a clinic team?
		0	0	1. Never present
		1	1	2.
		0	2	3.
		4	4	4.
		6	3	5.
		3	4	6.
		4	3	7. Always present
				How helpful was the GMC clerkship in learning how to function as a member of a clinic team?
7	7			1. Extremely helpful
8	10			2.
4	0			3. Not at all helpful
1	0			4. No opinion
				Change in attitude. Helpfulness of GMC with respect to learning how to function as a member of a clinic team:
0	1			—3 more helpful than expected
1	0			—2
3	3			—1
10	9			0
5	4			1
0	0			2
1	0			3 less helpful than expected
				Initial attitude toward GMC. On the basis of your experience and from what you have heard, how helpful do you think the GMC clerkship will be
				In acquiring more of the basic facts of clinical medicine (excluding psychosomatic medicine):
		1	7	1. Will be extremely helpful
		9	5	2.
		7	4	3.
		1	1	4.
		0	0	5.
		0	0	6.
		0	0	7. Will be a hindrance

Number of students				
1955 I	1955 II	1956 I	1956 II	Indices of response
				In acquiring skill at applying the facts of organic medicine to the practice of clinical medicine
		2	7	1. Will be extremely helpful
		11	6	2.
		2	3	3.
		0	1	4.
		3	0	5.
		0	0	6.
		0	0	7. Will be a hindrance
				In learning to organize diagnostic and therapeutic regimes
		6	9	1. Will be extremely helpful
		8	7	2.
		1	1	3.
		2	0	4.
		0	0	5.
		0	0	6.
		1	0	7. Will be a hindrance
				In learning how to make diagnoses and how to treat patients
0	0			1. Will be extremely helpful
11	3			2.
6	8			3. Will be not at all helpful
3	6			4. No opinion
				In acquiring knowledge of the basic ideas of psychosomatic medicine and psychiatry
		1	1	1. Will be extremely helpful
		3	6	2.
		7	4	3.
		5	3	4.
		2	2	5.
		0	1	6.
		0	0	7. Will be a hindrance
				In acquiring skill at applying the basic ideas of psychosomatic medicine and psychiatry to the practice of clinical medicine
		1	3	1. Will be extremely helpful
		7	5	2.
		4	2	3.
		6	3	4.
		0	3	5.
		0	1	6.
		0	0	7. Will be a hindrance

Number of students				
1955 I	1955 II	1956 I	1956 II	Indices of response
				In improving your ability to establish and maintain good physician-patient relations
		7	9	1. Will be extremely helpful
		6	4	2.
		4	2	3.
		0	2	4.
		0	0	5.
		1	0	6.
		0	0	7. Will be a hindrance
				In learning to maintain good relations with patients
17	9			1. Will be extremely helpful
3	6			2.
0	1			3. Will be not at all helpful
0	1			4. No opinion
				In acquiring skill at recognizing and managing social problems in the practice of clinical medicine
		1	2	1. Will be extremely helpful
		8	7	2.
		4	3	3.
		2	3	4.
		2	1	5.
		1	1	6.
		0	0	7. Will be a hindrance
				In acquiring knowledge and skill at utilizing the ancillary services (social service and public health nurse)
		2	2	1. Will be extremely helpful
		10	5	2.
		3	3	3.
		2	6	4.
		1	1	5.
		0	0	6.
		0	0	7. Will be a hindrance
				In learning the practical application of the principles of comprehensive care in treating patients
		6	5	1. Will be extremely helpful
		7	8	2.
		4	2	3.
		1	2	4.
		0	0	5.
		0	0	6.
		0	0	7. Will be a hindrance
				In seeing the patients' problems in their total setting
14	8			1. Will be extremely helpful
5	7			2.
0	1			3. Will be not at all helpful
1	1			4. No opinion

Number of students: 1955 I	1955 II	1956 I	1956 II	Indices of response
				Change in attitude toward the GMC (The rating a student makes on a questionnaire variable before entering the GMC is subtracted from his rating on the same variable after leaving the GMC)
				Helpfulness in acquiring more of the basic facts of clinical medicine (excluding psychosomatic medicine)
		0	0	—3 & —4 more helpful than expected
		0	1	—2
		3	0	—1
		8	2	0
		6	2	+1
		0	6	+2
		0	5	+3 & 4
		1	1	+5 & 6 less helpful than expected
				Helpfulness in acquiring skill at applying the facts of organic medicine to the practice of clinical medicine
		2	0	—3 & —4 more helpful than expected
		1	1	—2
		4	1	—1
		4	2	0
		6	4	+1
		0	3	+2
		0	5	+3 & 4
		1	1	+5 & 6 less helpful than expected
				Helpfulness in learning to organize diagnostic and therapeutic regimes
		2	0	—3 & —4 more helpful than expected
		1	0	—2
		2	2	—1
		4	2	0
		6	2	+1
		2	4	+2
		0	6	+3 & 4
		1	1	+5 & 6 less helpful than expected
				Helpfulness in learning how to make diagnoses and how to treat patients
0	1			—3 & —4 more helpful than expected
0	0			—2
4	4			—1
5	6			0
2	5			+1
6	1			+2
3	0			+3 & 4 less helpful than expected

Number of students				
1955 I	1955 II	1956 I	1956 II	Indices of response
				Helpfulness in acquiring knowledge of the basic ideas of psychosomatic medicine and psychiatry
		3	2	—3 & —4 more helpful than expected
		4	2	—2
		3	2	—1
		4	8	0
		3	1	+1
		0	1	+2
		0	1	+3 & 4
		1	0	+5 & 6 less helpful than expected
				Helpfulness in acquiring skill at applying the basic ideas of psychosomatic medicine and psychiatry to the practice of clinical medicine
		1	3	—3 & —4 more helpful than expected
		5	1	—2
		5	3	—1
		3	5	0
		2	3	+1
		1	0	+2
		0	2	+3 & 4
		1	0	+5 & 6 less helpful than expected
				Helpfulness in improving your ability to establish and maintain good physician-patient relations
		1	0	—3 & —4 more helpful than expected
		2	1	—2
		3	0	—1
		9	9	0
		2	4	+1
		0	1	+2
		0	0	+3 & 4
		1	2	+5 & 6 less helpful than expected
				Helpfulness in learning to maintain good relations with patients
0	0			—3 & —4 more helpful than expected
0	2			—2
0	4			—1
14	8			0
6	3			+1
0	0			+2
0	0			+3 & 4 less helpful than expected

Number of students				
1955 I	1955 II	1956 I	1956 II	Indices of response
				Helpfulness in acquiring skill at recognizing and managing social problems in the practice of clinical medicine
		5	1	—3 & —4 more helpful than expected
		2	2	—2
		3	5	—1
		6	2	0
		0	4	+1
		1	1	+2
		0	0	+3 & 4
		1	2	+5 & 6 less helpful than expected
				Helpfulness in acquiring knowledge and skill at utilizing the ancillary services (social service and public health nurse)
		1	1	—3 & —4 more helpful than expected
		2	3	—2
		6	2	—1
		8	6	0
		0	3	+1
		0	1	+2
		0	1	+3 & 4
		1	0	+5 & 6 less helpful than expected
				Helpfulness in learning the practical application of the principles of comprehensive care in treating patients
		1	1	—3 & —4 more helpful than expected
		1	1	—2
		4	2	—1
		6	3	0
		4	3	+1
		0	3	+2
		1	2	+3 & 4
		1	2	+5 & 6 less helpful than expected
				Helpfulness in seeing the patients' problems in their total setting
0	1			—3 & —4 more helpful than expected
1	0			—2
0	4			—1
9	6			0
10	5			+1
0	1			+2
0	0			+3 & 4 less helpful than expected
				Preferred professional activity (after formal training)
13	10	9	7	1. General practice
1	2	3	5	2. Surgery
3	2	3	3	3. Obstetrics–gynecology
0	0	0	1	4. Pediatrics
0	1	1	0	5. Psychiatry
0	0	1	0	6. Ophthalmology
1	0	0	0	7. Orthopedics
1	0	1	0	8. Neurosurgery and neurology
1	2	0	0	9. Medicine

INDEX

Index

Adjective Check-List: use of, 287; Self-Acceptance scale, 288; Self-Criticality scale, 288
Allport-Vernon-Lindzey Study of Values, 291–292
Ancillary staff ratings, 136–137
Attitudes: summary of GMC effect on, 133–134, 141; findings related to individual attributes, 143–144; toward patients' social problems, 514–520. *See also* Medical attitudes; Psychological attitudes; Sociological attitudes
Attitudes (individual differences measures): relevance of, 288–289; technical characteristics of, 289–290; statistical description of, 290–291
Attitudes toward behavior disorders, 410, 440–441
Attitudes toward health supervision, 342, 344–345, 367–369
Attitudes toward patients' social problems, 535–539

Biographical data: questionnaire, 304; and grade averages, 572–573

California F scale: *see* F (Authoritarian) scale
California Psychological Inventory: methodology, 294–299; relevance of, 296; statistical description of, 296–299
Chronology of the project, 112–113
Clerkship experience analysis: medical knowledge, 321–322, 337; psychological knowledge, 376–377; psychological skill, 400–402; psychological attitudes, 433–435; sociological knowledge and skill, 451–453; sociological attitudes, 467
Cognitive dimensions: computation of (Teaching Conference Record), 239–245; (Post-Conference Interview), 250–255; correlations between, 260–264; Teaching Conference Record correlations, 260–262; Post-Conference Interview correlations, 262–264; relations between learning and, 264–274; hypothesis 1 studies, 265–274; hypothesis 2 studies, 274
——— definitions: differentiation, 216–217; unity, 217–219; maximum centrality, 219–220; sum of dependences, 220; maximum determinance, 221; segmentation, 221–223; homogeneity, 223–224; relations ratio, 224
——— procedures: organic diagnosis, 241–242; psycho-social diagnosis, 242; total diagnosis including therapy, 242–243, 245; total diagnosis, 244; organic and psycho-social diagnosis, 244
Cognitive structure and learning, 257–259
Comprehensive care: rationale, 3–4; definition of, 4; problems of teaching, 17–20; psychologist's general comments on, 148–152; implications of, 157–158; attitudes toward, 342–343, 364–367; vs. traditional medicine (scheduling effect), 553–554
Comprehensive care conferences: goals, 80–82; importance of, 83–84; changes in, 89
Control group: distribution of time, 12–14; formation of, 103; attitudes of, 123–124; adequacy of, 154
Criterion problem: emergence of, 482–485; preliminary attempts to solve, 485–487; study of GMC staff raters,

487–491; independent observations, 490–491; solutions to, 491–494; summary, 494–497
Curriculum: changes in, 87–88; importance of sequence, 103–105; sequence, 104

Diaries: procedure, 276; analysis of, 361–362, 456–457, 472–474; excerpts from, 362, 456–457, 472–474
Differential Memory test: description of, 177–178; reliability of, 178; validity of, 178; analysis of, 412–417
Dependent Variables Section: organization of, 108–110; function of, 130–131; contribution of, 146
—— findings: medical knowledge, 313–316; medical skill, 330–333; medical attitudes, 342–353; psychological knowledge, 370–373; psychological skill, 390–398; psychological attitudes, 410–431; sociological knowledge and skill, 448–449; sociological attitudes, 459–466
—— methodology: Sound-Film Interview, 130–131; Medical Attitudes test, 131; Self-Description Checklist, 131; questionnaire, 131
—— test development: Sound-Film Interview, 166–204; Medical Attitudes test, 205–206; Staff Description Checklist, 207; questionnaire, 208; summary, 208–209

Edwards Personal Preference Schedule: methodology, 299–304; relevance of, 301; technical characteristics of, 301; statistical description of, 301–304
Estimation of age test: description, 192–193; reliability, 193–194; analysis of, 393, 417–418
Estimation of intelligence test: description of, 194; reliability, 194–195; analysis of, 393, 418
Estimation of personality characteristics test: description of, 199–202; analysis of, 396–398, 419–446
Estimation of vocabulary level test: description of, 195–196; reliability, 196; analysis of, 394–396, 418–419
Experimental design: description of, 103–106; problems caused by, 123
Experimental variables, 105–107

Family and Home Care Program: excerpts from student summaries, 54–58, 75–78; selection of families for, 61; operation of, 61–62; patients, 62–66; families' suitability to, 66–71; patients' reactions to, 71–72; student experiences, 72–75; importance of, 75–79; changes in, 90–91
—— patients: ages and family structures, 62–63; economic status and ethnic background, 63; medical characteristics, 63–66; reactions, 71–72
F (Authoritarian) scale (California F scale), 287

General Anxiety scale, 288
General Medical Clinic: initiated, 3; goals, 4–5, 114–115, 118–119, 156; policies, 5–6; methods, 6–7, 158; curriculum, 8–10, 87–88; student time distribution, 10–12; staff, 15–17, 20–23, 88–89; patients, 36–48, 54–59; students' patient load, 49–51; Family and Home Care Program, 60–79, 90–91; comprehensive care conferences, 80–84, 89; seminars, 82, psychosomatic conferences, 82; preceptorial program, 82–83, 89–90; obstetrical program, 85; well-baby program, 85–86; changes in, 87–91; problems, 92–97; effects of, 133–137; reasons for effects, 137–141; implications of, 153–161; suggestions for improvement of, 159–160; present functioning, 160–161; student dissatisfaction with, 554–561
—— group: formation of, 103; special problems, 539–541
—— patients: social characteristics of, 36–43; medical characteristics of, 44–48; importance of, 54–59
—— problems: communication, 92–93; with medical school, 93–94; with hospital, 94–97
Gough Adjective Check-List, 207
Grade averages: individual attributes study results, 563–572; and biographical data, 572–573

Independent Variables Section: organization of, 107–108; function of, 131–132; contribution of, 146–147; criticism of, 154–155; theory, 210–213; hypotheses, 213–214
—— findings: medical knowledge, 316–326; medical skill, 333–339; medical attitudes, 347–364; psychological knowledge, 373–385; psychological skill, 398–404; psychological attitudes, 431–440; sociological knowledge and skill, 449–457; sociological attitudes, 466–474

——— methodology: Teaching Conference Record, 214–215; Post-Conference Interview, 215–216; cognitive dimensions definitions, 216–224
———procedure: Teaching Conference Record, 225–247; Post-Conference Interview, 247–255; cognitive structure and learning, 257–259; diaries, 276; summary, 276–277
Individual attributes: function of, 132
——— and student performance: staff ratings, 497–524; summary, 524–526
——— and grade averages: procedures, 563–564; results, 564–570, discussion, 570–572
——— findings: correlation with GMC performance, 136–137; medical knowledge, 141–142, 326–328; medical skill, 141–142, 339–340; medical attitudes, 364–369; psychological knowledge, 142–143, 385–388; psychological skill, 142–143, 404–408; psychological attitudes, 143–144, 440–446; sociological knowledge and skill, 457–458; sociological attitudes, 474–475
Individual differences methodology: organization, 110–111; contribution of, 147; aptitude for medical education, 278–281; previous academic performance, 281–284; peer-judged attributes, 284–287; Liberal Attitude scale, 287; ACL Self-Criticality scale, 288; General Anxiety scale, 288; ACL Self-Acceptance scale, 288; values measures, 291–294; Allport-Vernon-Lindzey Study of Values, 291–294; social interaction variables, 294–299; California Psychological Inventory, 294–299; needs measures, 299–304; Edwards Personal Preference Schedule, 299–304; background information, 304; self-ratings, 304–306
Interpersonal perception measures: description, 179–180; components, 180–189; Random Comparison Method, 189–202; reliability and validity, 202–203; analysis, 407–408

Liberal Attitude scale, 287–288

Measures: Sound-Film Interview, 166–204; Medical Attitudes test, 205–206; Staff Description Checklist, 207; questionnaire, 208, (background information) 304, (self-ratings) 304–306; Teaching Conference Record, 214–215, 225–247; Post-Conference Interview, 247–255; diaries, 276; Medical College Admission Test, 278–281; previous academic performance, 281–284; peer-judged attributes, 284–287; Liberal Attitude scale, 287; F (Authoritarian) scale, 287; General Anxiety scale, 288; Adjective Check-List Self-Acceptance scale, 288; Adjective Check-List Self-Criticality scale, 288; Allport-Vernon-Lindzey Study of Values, 291–292; California Psychological Inventory, 294–299; Edwards Personal Preference Schedule, 299–304
Medical attitudes: as GMC objective, 116; findings summary, 341; toward health supervision, 342, 344–345, 367–369; toward comprehensive care, 342–343, 364–367; dependent variables findings, 342–353; questionnaire responses, 345–347; students' conceptions of specialists, 347–353; student interviews, 352–353, 360–361; independent variables findings, 353–364; teaching conferences, 353–354; student activities, 354–355; general clerkship experience, 354–358; special GMC techniques, 358–360; staff's student evaluation, 360; diaries, 361–362; staff interviews, 363–364; individual attributes findings, 364–369
Medical Attitudes test: function of, 131; validity of, 205–206; description of, 205–206
Medical College Admission Test: methodology, 278–281; relevance, 279; technical characteristics, 279–280; statistical description, 280–281
Medical knowledge: as objective of GMC, 115; GMC effect on, 133, 137–140; individual attributes findings, 141–142, 326–328; Sound-Film Interview test of, 168–171; findings summary, 312–313; objective tests findings, 313–315; dependent variables findings, 313–316; questionnaire findings, 315–316; independent variables findings, 316–326; teaching conferences, 317–319; student activities, 319–321; general clerkship experience, 321–322; special GMC techniques, 322–323; staff's student evaluation, 323; student interviews, 323–324; staff interviews, 324–326; adjusted GMC staff ratings study, 500–532

Medical skill: as GMC objective, 116; summary of GMC effect on, 133, 137–140; individual attributes findings, 141–142, 339–340; Sound-Film Interview test of, 171–173; findings summary, 329–330; dependent variables findings, 330–333; independent variables findings, 333–339; teaching conferences, 335; student activities, 335–337; general clerkship experience, 337; special GMC educational techniques, 337–338; staff's student evaluation, 338; student and staff interviews, 338–339; adjusted GMC staff ratings, 505–532
Minnesota Multiphasic Personality Inventory, 199–200

Obstetrical program, 85–86

Patients: students' load, 49–51; missed appointments, 51–54
——— characteristics: social, 24–26, 36–43; demographic, 26–36; medical, 44–48
Peer-judged attributes: methodology, 284–287; relevance, 285; technical characteristics, 285; statistical description, 286–287
Physician-patient relations, 392–398, 410–412, 441–442
Post-Conference Interview: description of, 215–216; procedure, 247–255; method of analysis, 249–250; cognitive dimensions computation, 250–255; sampling, 257; cognitive dimensions correlations, 262–264
Preceptorial program: description of, 82–83; changes in, 89–90
Previous academic performance: methodology, 281–282; relevance, 282–283; technical characteristics, 283; statistical description, 283–284
Psychological attitudes: as GMC objective, 117; findings summary, 409; dependent variables findings, 410–431; behavior disorders, 410; physician-patient relations, 410–412; differential memory, 412–417; toward patients, 417–423; questionnaire responses, 423–426; student interviews, 426–431, 436–437; independent variables findings, 431–440; teaching conferences, 432–433; general clerkship experience, 433–435; special GMC techniques, 435–436; staff interviews, 437–440; individual attributes findings, 440–446; toward behavior disorders, 440–441; physician-patient relations, 441–442; perception of patients' individual differences, 442–446
Psychological knowledge: as GMC objective, 116; GMC effect on, 133, 140; individual attributes findings, 142–143, 385–388; Sound-Film Interview, 173–174; findings summary, 370; dependent variables findings, 370–373; independent variables findings, 373–385; teaching conference, 373–375; student activities, 374–376; general clerkship experience, 376–377; special GMC techniques, 377; staff's student evaluation, 377; student interviews, 377–379; staff interviews, 379–385; students' skill in applying, 391–392; adjusted staff ratings study, 510–514; correlational fluctuations compared with attributes variability, 532–535
Psychological skill: as GMC objective, 117; GMC effect on, 133, 140; individual attributes findings, 142–143, 404–408; Sound-Film Interview, 174–176; findings summary, 389–390; dependent variables findings, 390–398; at applying psychological knowledge, 391–392; in developing physician-patient relations, 392–398; independent variables findings, 398–404; teaching conference, 399–400; student activities, 400; general clerkship experience, 400; special GMC techniques, 402–403; staff's student evaluation, 403; student interviews, 403–404; objective test measurement, 404–407; interpersonal perception tasks, 407–408
Psychosomatic conferences, 82

Questionnaire: function of, 131; description of, 208; background information, 304; self-ratings, 304–306

Random Comparison Method, 187–192
Ratings of students: *see* Criterion problem
Research project: goals, 102–103, 113–114; organization of, 107–112, 129–130; chronology, 112–113; limitations, 119–128; contributions of sections, 146–147; medical educator's viewpoint, 153–155
Research project limitations: facilities, 119; manipulation of environment, 119–120; liaison with GMC staff,

120–121; staff time, 121; student time, 121; staff attitudes, 121–122, 124–125; student attitudes, 121–122, 124; experimental design, 123; summary, 125–128

Scheduling effect: findings summary, 134–136; description of, 550–553; rating traditional vs. comprehensive medicine, 553–554; implications of, 561–562
Seminars: description of, 82; importance of, 85
Sociological attitudes: as GMC objective, 117–118; findings summary, 459; dependent variables findings, 459–466; independent variables findings, 466–474; teaching conferences, 466–467; general clerkship experience, 467; special GMC techniques, 467–469; student interviews, 469–472; diaries, 472–474; individual attributes findings, 474–475
Sociological knowledge and skill: as GMC objective, 117–118; GMC effect on, 133, 140; Sound-Film Interview, 176–177; findings summary, 447–448; dependent variables findings, 448–449; independent variables findings, 449–457; teaching conference, 450–451; student activities, 451; general clerkship experience, 451–453; special GMC techniques, 453–454; student interviews, 454–456; diaries, 456–457; individual attributes findings, 457–458
Sound-Film Interview: function of, 130–131; description of, 166–167; conducting filmed interview, 167
——— Interpersonal Perception tests: estimation of age, 192–195; estimation of intelligence, 194–195; estimation of vocabulary level, 195–198; use of MMPI with, 199–200; estimation of personality characteristics, 199–202; reliability and validity, 202–203; value of, 203–204
——— multiple-choice tests: medical knowledge, 168–171; medical skill, 171–173; psychological knowledge, 173–174; psychological skill, 174–176; sociological knowledge and skill, 176–177; differential memory, 177–178; suggestions for improvement, 178–179
Special GMC techniques: medical knowledge, 322–323; medical skill, 337–338; medical attitudes, 358–360; psychological knowledge, 377; psychological skill, 402–403; psychological attitudes, 435–436; sociological knowledge and skill, 453–454; sociological attitudes, 467–469
Staff: composition, 15–16; selection criteria for, 17; training requirements for, 20–21; recruiting and maintaining, 21–23; effectiveness of, 23; changes in, 88–89; attitudes, 121–122, 124–125; as raters of student performance, 487–491
——— interviews: excerpts from, 139–140, 324–325, 363, 379–385, 437–439; analysis of, 324–326, 338–339, 363–364, 379–385, 437–440
——— (adjusted) ratings: medical knowledge, 500–505; student performance, 500–524; medical skill, 505–510; psychological knowledge, 510–514; attitudes toward patients' social problems, 514–520; general improvement, 520–524
——— ratings: summary of findings, 136–137; preliminary study original student performance, 497–500; student performance–individual attributes, 497–526
Staff Description Checklist, 207
Student activities analyses: 319–321, 335–337, 451
Student interview analyses: medical knowledge, 323–324; medical skill, 338–339; medical attitudes, 352–353, 360–361; psychological knowledge, 377–379; psychological skill, 403–404; psychological attitudes, 426–431, 436–437; sociological knowledge and skill, 454–456; sociological attitudes, 469–472
Student interview excerpts, 378–379, 430–431, 436–437, 455, 470–472
Students: Family and Home Care Program experiences, 72–75; attitudes toward, 121–122, 124, 138–140, 141; influence of scheduling effect on, 135; effect of internship on, 135–136; staff evaluations of, 323, 338, 360, 377, 403; conceptions of specialists, 347–352; activities, 354–355, 374–376, 400; general clerkship experience, 354–358
——— GMC performance: ratings of, 480–481; analysis procedures, 481; criterion problem, 481–497; relations between individual attributes and staff ratings, 497–526; personality traits associated with, 542–549

Teaching Conference Record: description of, 214–215; sample conference, 225–231; procedure, 225–247; computation of cognitive dimensions, 239–245; interview sampling, 255–257; accuracy of, 259; cognitive dimensions correlations, 260–262
—— analysis: method, 232–245; problems, 245–247; medical knowledge, 317–319; medical skill, 335; medical attitudes, 353–354; psychological knowledge, 373–375; psychological skill, 399–400; psychological attitudes, 432–433; sociological knowledge and skill, 450–451; sociological attitudes, 466–467
Test administration, 105
Test development, 166–209

Values: use of Allport-Vernon-Lindzey Study of Values, 291–292; relevance of, 292; technical characteristics, 292; statistical description of, 292–294
Variability compared with correlational fluctuations: medical knowledge and skill, 529–532; psychological knowledge, 532–535; attitudes toward patients' social problems, 535–539; summary, 541–542

Well-baby program: description of, 85; importance of, 86

Bei Fragen zur Produktsicherheit wenden Sie sich bitte an:
If you have any questions regarding product safety,
please contact:

Walter de Gruyter GmbH
Genthiner Straße 13
10785 Berlin
productsafety@degruyterbrill.com